CLINICAL COMPANION

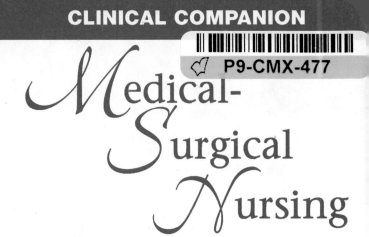

Medical-Surgical Nursing

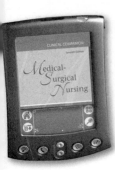

Seventh Edition

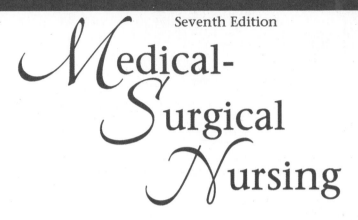

Medical-Surgical Nursing

Prepared by

Patricia Graber O'Brien, APRN-BC, MA, MSN

Instructor, College of Nursing
University of New Mexico;
Clinical Research Coordinator
Lovelace Scientific Resources
Albuquerque, New Mexico

Shannon Ruff Dirksen, RN, PhD
Patricia Graber O'Brien, APRN-BC, MA, MSN
Sharon L. Lewis, RN, PhD, FAAN
Margaret McLean Heitkemper, RN, PhD, FAAN
Linda Bucher, RN, DNSc

with 32 illustrations

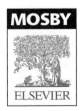

MOSBY

ELSEVIER

MOSBY
ELSEVIER

11830 Westline Industrial Drive
St. Louis, Missouri 63146

Clinical Companion to Medical-Surgical Nursing, ed. 7   ISBN: 978-0-323-03689-4

Notice

Knowledge and best practice in this field are constantly changing. As new research and
experience broaden our knowledge, changes in practice, treatment and drug therapy
may become necessary or appropriate. Readers are advised to check the most current
information provided (i) on procedures featured or (ii) by the manufacturer of each
product to be administered, to verify the recommended dose or formula, the method
and duration of administration, and contraindications. It is the responsibility of the
practitioner, relying on their own experience and knowledge of the patient, to make
diagnoses, to determine dosages and the best treatment for each individual patient, and to
take all appropriate safety precautions. To the fullest extent of the law, neither the
Publisher nor the Authors assumes any liability for any injury and/or damage to persons
or property arising out or related to any use of the material contained in this book.

The Publisher

Previous editions copyrighted 2004, 2000, 1996

ISBN: 978-0-323-03689-4

Acquisitions Editor: Kristin Geen
Senior Developmental Editor: Lauren Lake
Publishing Services Manager: Jeff Patterson
Project Manager: Mary G. Stueck
Design Direction: Mark Oberkrom
Cover Designer: Paula Ruckenbrod
Text Designer: Paula Ruckenbrod

Printed in the United States of America

Last digit is the print number: 9   8   7   6   5   4   3

Working together to grow
libraries in developing countries

www.elsevier.com | www.bookaid.org | www.sabre.org

ELSEVIER   BOOK AID International   Sabre Foundation

PREFACE

The *Clinical Companion* for Lewis, Heitkemper, Dirksen, O'Brien, and Bucher's *Medical-Surgical Nursing: Assessment and Management of Clinical Problems,* seventh edition, has been updated as a condensed reference of essential information on over 200 medical-surgical diseases, disorders, and clinically related topics. The seventh edition of this pocket-sized book provides nurses and nursing students quick access to current, concise, and important information when caring for patients.

Additional disorders, tables, and figures have been added to this edition. Patient and family teaching content has been expanded. The *Clinical Companion* can be used separately as a reference or in conjunction with *Medical-Surgical Nursing: Assessment and Management of Clinical Problems,* seventh edition.

The book is divided into three sections. Part One contains commonly encountered medical-surgical diseases and disorders arranged alphabetically and organized in an easy-to-use format. The disorders are extensively cross-referenced to *Medical-Surgical Nursing,* seventh edition, for the reader who desires additional information. Part Two contains brief explanations of common medical-surgical treatments and procedures (e.g., pacemakers, oxygen therapy) in which the role of the nurse is emphasized. Part Three contains reference material related to information frequently used in nursing clinical practice (e.g., heart and breath sounds, medication administration, and blood and urine laboratory values). This section also contains a list of commonly-used abbreviations and key phrases translated into Spanish. An extensive index is provided for easy location of information, and content updates and weblinks may be found at http://evolve.elsevier.com/Lewis/medsurg.

The authors hope the *Clinical Companion* will become an invaluable reference and resource in helping nurses meet the challenges of caring for patients and their families during states of altered health and well-being.

Patricia Graber O'Brien
Shannon Ruff Dirksen
Sharon L. Lewis
Margaret McLean Heitkemper
Linda Bucher

CONTENTS

Part Two
Treatments and Procedures

Part Three
Reference Appendix

PART ONE

Disorders

Description

Acute abdominal pain is a symptom of many different types of tissue injury and can arise from damage to abdominal or pelvic organs and blood vessels. The most common causes of acute abdominal pain are listed in Table 1. Some causes (e.g., hemorrhage, obstruction) are life threatening because of large fluid losses, but other problems require only conservative medical treatment.

Clinical Manifestations

Pain is the most common presenting symptom of an acute abdominal problem. Patients may also complain of nausea, vomiting, diarrhea, constipation, flatulence, fatigue, fever, and an increase in abdominal girth.

Diagnostic Studies

- Diagnosis begins with a complete history and physical examination. Physical examination should include both a rectal and pelvic examination in addition to the abdomen.
- Complete blood count (CBC), urinalysis, abdominal x-ray, and an electrocardiogram (ECG) are done initially, along with an ultrasound or computed tomography (CT) scan.
- Pregnancy tests should be performed on women of childbearing age who have acute abdominal pain to rule out ectopic pregnancy.

Collaborative Care

The goals of management are to identify and treat the cause and monitor and treat complications, especially shock. A differential diagnosis needs to be made because many causes of abdominal pain do not require surgery.

- Appropriate pain management that does not result in altered consciousness (e.g., ketorolac [Toradol]) can decrease diffuse pain and abdominal rigidity and help localize the pain.
- In addition to being a therapeutic measure, surgery can be diagnostic. An *exploratory laparotomy,* in which an opening is made through the abdominal wall into the peritoneal cavity, can be done to determine the cause of acute abdominal pain. Operative exploration is justified when "look and see" is better than "wait and see."

Table 1	Common Causes of Abdominal Pain

- Appendicitis
- Bowel obstruction
- Cholecystitis
- Diverticulitis
- Gastroenteritis
- Pancreatitis
- Pelvic inflammatory disease
- Perforated gastric or duodenal ulcer
- Peritonitis
- Ruptured abdominal aneurysm
- Ruptured ectopic pregnancy

- If the cause of acute pain can be surgically removed (e.g., inflamed appendix) or surgically repaired (e.g., ruptured abdominal aneurysm), then surgery is considered definitive therapy.

Nursing Management

Goals

The patient will have resolution of inflammation, relief of abdominal pain, freedom from complications (especially hypovolemic shock), and normal nutritional status.

Nursing Diagnoses

- Acute pain
- Risk for deficient fluid volume
- Imbalanced nutrition: less than body requirements
- Anxiety

Nursing Interventions

General care for the patient involves monitoring and managing fluid and electrolyte balance, vital signs, pain, and anxiety. If the patient has an exploratory laparotomy or other surgery, the nurse provides preoperative and postoperative care.

- Preoperative emergency preparation of the patient with acute abdominal pain may include a CBC count, typing and crossmatching of blood, and clotting studies. Catheterization, preparation of abdominal skin, and insertion of a nasogastric (NG) tube may be done in the emergency department (ED) or operating room (OR).

The increased use of laparoscopic procedures has reduced the risk of postoperative complications related to wound care and altered gastrointestinal (GI) motility. These procedures generally result in shorter hospital stays. A general nursing care plan for the postoperative patient is presented in Chapter 20, Lewis and others, *Medical-Surgical Nursing,* edition 7, pp. 383 to 386.

- An NG tube with low suction may be used to empty the stomach of secretions and gas. If the upper GI tract has been

entered, drainage from the NG tube may be dark brown
to dark red for the first 12 hours. Later it should be light
yellowish brown or greenish. Continuing dark red or bright
red blood can indicate hemorrhage, and "coffee ground"
granules in the drainage are due to the presence of blood
acted on by acidic gastric secretions.

- The NG tube is checked frequently for patency, because it
  may become obstructed with mucus, sediment, or old blood.
  An order is usually written to irrigate the tube with 20 to
  30 ml of normal saline solution if needed. Repositioning the
  tube may facilitate drainage. Mouth care and nasal care are
  essential.
- Parenteral fluids are administered to provide the patient
  with fluids and electrolytes until bowel sounds return.
  Occasionally, ice chips may be ordered because they prevent
  dry mouth. The diet may be supplemented with multivitamins and iron.
- Nausea and vomiting are not uncommon after abdominal
  surgery; these problems are often self-limiting. Observation
  is important in determining the cause. Antiemetics such as
  prochlorperazine (Compazine), promethazine (Phenergan),
  ondansetron (Zofran), or trimethobenzamide (Tigan) may
  be ordered (see Nausea and Vomiting, p. 426).
- Abdominal distention and gas pains are also common after
  surgery; these are due to swallowed air and impaired peristalsis resulting from immobility, manipulation of abdominal contents during surgery, and side effects of anesthesia.
  Early ambulation helps restore peristalsis and eliminate
  flatus and gas pain. For severe gas pain, a medication (e.g.,
  metoclopramide [Reglan]) may be given to stimulate peristalsis. The health care provider should be informed of
  abdominal distention and rigidity. Gradually, as intestinal
  activity increases, distention and gas pains decrease.

▼ **Patient and Family Teaching**
Preparation for discharge begins soon after surgery. Instructions
to the patient and family should include any modifications in activity, care of the incision, diet, and drug therapy.

- Clear liquids are given initially after surgery, and if tolerated, the patient progresses to a regular diet.
- Normal activities should be resumed gradually with planned
  rest periods.
- The patient should be aware of possible complications after
  surgery and should notify the physician immediately if
  vomiting, pain, weight loss, incisional drainage, or changes
  in bowel function occur.

ACUTE CORONARY SYNDROME

Description

Acute coronary syndrome (ACS) is a term used to reflect the relationships among the pathophysiology, diagnosis, prognosis, and interventions of the serious manifestations of coronary artery disease (CAD). These manifestations include unstable angina (UA), non–ST-segment-elevation myocardial infarction (NSTEMI), and ST-segment-elevation myocardial infarction (STEMI).

Pathophysiology

ACS occurs when a stable coronary artery atherosclerotic plaque ruptures, exposing the intima to blood and stimulating platelet aggregation and local vasoconstriction with thrombus formation. If this unstable lesion is *partially* occluded by a thrombus, it manifests as UA or a NSTEMI. If the lesion is *totally* occluded by a thrombus, it manifests as a STEMI. It is not well understood what causes a coronary plaque to suddenly become unstable, but systemic inflammation is thought to play a role.

Unstable Angina. UA occurs as a result of the ischemia associated with thrombus formation and vasoconstriction. The chest pain is new in onset, occurs at rest, or has a worsening pattern. The patient with chronic stable angina may develop UA, or UA may be the first clinical manifestation of CAD.

Myocardial Infarction. A myocardial infarction (MI) occurs as a result of sustained ischemia, causing irreversible myocardial cell death (necrosis). Thrombus formation is responsible for 80% to 90% of all acute MIs. When a thrombus develops, perfusion to the myocardium distal to the occlusion is blocked, resulting in an infarction. Contractile function of the heart stops in the necrotic areas. The degree of altered function depends on the area of the heart involved and the size of the infarction. Most MIs involve some portion of the left ventricle.

Cardiac cells can withstand ischemic conditions for approximately 20 minutes before cellular death (necrosis) begins. If ischemia persists, it takes approximately 4 to 6 hours for the entire thickness of the heart muscle to become necrosed.

- Infarctions are described by the area of occurrence as anterior, inferior, lateral, or posterior wall infarctions. Common combinations of areas are the anterolateral or anteroseptal MI. An inferior MI is also called a diaphragmatic MI.
- The degree of preestablished collateral circulation also determines the infarction's severity. In an individual with a

history of CAD, adequate collateral channels may have been established that provide the area surrounding the infarction site with blood supply and oxygen (O_2). **A**

The body's response to cell death is the inflammatory process. Within 24 hours, leukocytes infiltrate the area. Enzymes are released from the dead cardiac cells and are important diagnostic indicators of MI. Proteolytic enzymes from neutrophils and macrophages remove all necrotic tissue by the second or third day.

- The necrotic zone is identifiable by electrocardiogram (ECG) changes and by nuclear scanning after the onset of symptoms.
- At 10 to 14 days after an MI, the beginning scar tissue is still weak. The myocardium is considered to be especially vulnerable to increased stress because of the unstable state of the healing heart wall.
- By 6 weeks after MI, scar tissue has replaced necrotic tissue. At this time, the injured area is said to be healed. The scarred area is often less compliant than the surrounding fibers. This condition may be manifested by uncoordinated wall motion, ventricular dysfunction, or pump failure.

Clinical Manifestations

Unstable Angina. UA is unpredictable, occurs with increasing frequency, and is easily provoked by minimal or no exertion. Women have prodromal symptoms such as fatigue, shortness of breath, indigestion, and anxiety that are early manifestations of CAD. Because these symptoms are not recognized as manifestations of CAD, many women present with UA before CAD has been diagnosed.

Myocardial Infarction. Severe, immobilizing, and persistent chest pain not relieved by rest or nitrate administration is the hallmark of an MI.

- Persistent and unlike any other pain, it is usually described as a heaviness, pressure, burning, crushing, tightness, or constriction.
- Common locations are epigastric, substernal, or retrosternal. The pain may radiate to the neck, jaw, and arms or to the back. It may occur while the patient is active or at rest, asleep or awake, and commonly occurs in the early morning hours.
- The pain usually lasts for 20 minutes or more and is more severe than usual anginal pain. When epigastric pain is present, the patient may take antacids without relief.
- Some patients may not have pain but may have "discomfort," weakness, fatigue, or shortness of breath. Women may experience atypical discomfort, shortness of breath, or fatigue.

Additional manifestations may include nausea and vomiting, diaphoresis, and constriction of peripheral blood vessels. On physical examination, the patient's skin is ashen, clammy, and cool (cold sweat). Fever occurs within the first 24 hours (up to 100.4° F [38° C]) and may continue for 1 week. Blood pressure (BP) and pulse rate are also elevated initially. BP then drops, with decreased urine output, lung crackles, hepatic engorgement, and peripheral edema. Jugular veins may be distended with obvious pulsations.

Complications
Dysrhythmias are the most common complication after an MI and are the most common cause of death in patients in the prehospital period. Dysrhythmias are caused by any condition that affects the myocardial cell's sensitivity to nerve impulses, such as ischemia, electrolyte imbalances, and sympathetic nervous system stimulation. The intrinsic rhythm of the heartbeat is disrupted, causing either a very fast heart rate (HR) (tachycardia), a very slow HR (bradycardia), or an irregular HR. Life-threatening dysrhythmias occur most often with anterior wall infarction, pump failure, and shock. Complete heart block is seen in massive infarction (see Dysrhythmias, p. 199).
- Ventricular fibrillation, a common cause of sudden death, is a lethal dysrhythmia that most often occurs within the first 4 hours after the onset of pain. Premature ventricular contractions (PVCs) may precede ventricular tachycardia and fibrillation. Ventricular dysrhythmias need immediate treatment.

Heart failure (HF) occurs when the pumping power of the heart has diminished. Depending on the severity and extent of the injury, HF occurs initially with subtle signs such as slight dyspnea, restlessness, agitation, or slight tachycardia.
- Pulmonary congestion, crackles in the lungs, the presence of an S_3 or S_4 heart sound, or jugular vein distention from right-sided heart failure may be found.

Cardiogenic shock occurs when inadequate oxygen and nutrients are supplied to the tissues because of severe left ventricular failure.
- Cardiogenic shock requires aggressive management, including control of dysrhythmias, intraaortic balloon pump therapy, and support of contractility with vasoactive drugs.

Diagnostic Studies
In addition to the patient's history of pain, risk factors, and health history, the primary diagnostic studies used to determine whether a person has UA or an MI, and the type of MI, include an ECG and serum cardiac markers.

- Changes in the QRS complex, ST segment, and T wave caused by ischemia and infarction can help differentiate among UA, STEMI, and NSTEMI.
- Patients with STEMI tend to have a more extensive MI that is associated with prolonged and complete coronary occlusion and the development of a pathologic Q wave on the ECG.
- Patients with UA or NSTEMI usually have transient thrombosis or incomplete coronary occlusion and usually do not develop pathologic Q waves.
- Because an MI evolves over time, the ECG can reveal the time sequence of ischemia, injury, infarction, and resolution of the infarction.
- When the ECG is normal or nondiagnostic at the time the patient presents with chest pain, the ECG may change to reflect an infarction within a few hours.

Certain proteins, called *serum cardiac markers,* are released into the blood in large quantities from necrotic heart muscle after an MI.

- The MB band of creatine kinase (CK-MB) and troponin are two important specific markers that can indicate the presence and extent of cardiac damage.

Other diagnostic measures can include coronary angiography, exercise stress testing, and echocardiograms.

Collaborative Care

It is extremely important that a patient with ACS is rapidly diagnosed and treated to preserve cardiac muscle. Initial management of the patient with chest pain most often occurs in the emergency department (ED).

- After an intravenous (IV) route is established, sublingual nitroglycerin and a chewable aspirin are given, O_2 is usually administered by nasal cannula at a rate of 2 to 4 L/min, and morphine sulfate is given IV if pain is unrelieved by nitroglycerin.
- The patient will receive ongoing care in a critical care unit where continuous ECG monitoring is available and dysrhythmias can be detected and treated.
- Vital signs, including pulse oximetry, are taken frequently during the first few hours after admission and monitored closely thereafter. Bed rest and limitation of activity are initially used, with a gradual increase in activity.
- For patients with UA or NSTEMI with negative cardiac markers and ongoing angina, a combination of aspirin, heparin, and a glycoprotein IIb/IIIa inhibitor (e.g., abcix-

imab [ReoPro], eptifibatide [Integrilin], tirofiban [Aggra-stat]) is recommended. *Percutaneous coronary intervention* (PCI) is considered once the patient is stabilized and angina is controlled.

- For patients with STEMI or NSTEMI with positive cardiac markers, reperfusion therapy is indicated.

Reperfusion therapy can include emergent percutaneous coronary intervention (PCI) or fibrinolytic (thrombolytic) therapy. The goal in treatment of acute MI is to salvage as much myocardial muscle as possible.

- Emergent PCI is recommended as the first line of treatment for patients with confirmed MI when specialized cardiac centers are available. The patient undergoes cardiac catheterization to evaluate the blockage, and stents may be placed (see Angina, Chronic Stable, p. 44).

Fibrinolytic therapy can be performed in facilities that do not have an interventional cardiac catheterization lab. Treatment of MI with fibrinolytic therapy is aimed at stopping the infarction process by dissolving the thrombus in the coronary artery and reperfusing the myocardium. Commonly used thrombolytics are tissue plasminogen activator (tPA), streptokinase, and reteplase (Retavase). To be of the most benefit, thrombolytics must be given as soon as possible, ideally within the first hour of onset of symptoms and preferably within the first 6 hours after the onset of pain. Contraindications and complications with thrombolytic therapy are described in Lewis and others, *Medical-Surgical Nursing,* edition 7, pp. 807 to 808.

Drug therapy includes IV nitroglycerin (Tridil), aspirin, β-adrenergic blockers, and systemic anticoagulation with either low-molecular-weight heparin given subcutaneously or IV unfractionated heparin as initial drug treatments of choice. ACE inhibitors are added for select patients following MI, and calcium channel blockers may be used if the patient is already taking adequate doses of β-adrenergic blockers or does not tolerate β-adrenergic blockers. Morphine sulfate is used for chest pain unrelieved by nitroglycerin. It also decreases cardiac workload and reduces anxiety and fear. Antidysrhythmic drugs are used to treat life-threatening dysrhythmias.

Coronary artery bypass graft surgery (CABG) consists of the construction of new vessels between the aorta or other major arteries and the myocardium distal to the obstructed coronary artery (or arteries). It requires a sternotomy (opening of the chest cavity) and the use of cardiopulmonary bypass (CPB). It is a palliative treatment for CAD and not a cure. Newer techniques include minimally invasive direct coronary artery bypass and

transmyocardial laser revascularization. These surgical procedures and related nursing care are further discussed in Lewis and
others, *Medical-Surgical Nursing,* edition 7, pp. 808 to 810.

Nursing Management
Goals
The patient with an MI will experience relief of pain, preservation
of myocardium, immediate and appropriate treatment, effective
coping with illness-associated anxiety, participation in a rehabilitation plan, and reduction of risk factors.

See NCP 34-1 for the patient with acute coronary syndrome,
Lewis and others, *Medical-Surgical Nursing,* edition 7, pp. 811 to
812.

Nursing Diagnoses
- Acute pain
- Ineffective tissue perfusion
- Anxiety
- Activity intolerance
- Ineffective therapeutic regimen management

Nursing Interventions
Priorities for nursing interventions in the initial phase include pain
assessment and relief, physiologic monitoring, promotion of rest
and comfort, alleviation of stress and anxiety, and understanding
of the patient's emotional and behavioral reactions. Proper management of these priorities decreases the O_2 needs of a compromised
myocardium. In addition, the nurse needs to institute measures to
avoid the hazards of immobility while encouraging rest.

- Nitroglycerin and morphine should be given as needed to
  eliminate or reduce chest pain. Once pain is relieved, the
  nurse may have to deal with denial in a patient who inter-
  prets the absence of pain as an absence of cardiac disease.
- The nurse should be trained in ECG interpretation so that
  dysrhythmias causing further deterioration of the cardiovascular status can be identified and treated.
- In addition to frequent vital signs, intake and output should
  be evaluated at least once per shift, and physical assessment
  should be carried out to detect deviations from the patient's
  baseline parameters; included are the assessment of lung
  and heart sounds and inspection for evidence of early heart
  failure (e.g., dyspnea, tachycardia, pulmonary congestions,
  distended neck veins).
- Assessment of the patient's oxygenation status is helpful,
  especially if the patient is receiving O_2. The nares also
  should be checked for irritation or dryness (see Oxygen
  Therapy, p. 734).

- It is important to plan nursing and therapeutic actions to ensure adequate rest periods free from interruption.
- Anxiety is present in all patients in various degrees. The nurse's role is to identify the source of anxiety and assist the patient in reducing it. If the patient is afraid of being alone, a family member should be allowed to sit quietly by the bedside or to check in frequently with the patient. If a source of anxiety is fear of the unknown, the nurse should explore these concerns with the patient and help with appropriate reality testing.

▼ **Patient and Family Teaching**

Teaching begins with the ED nurse and progresses through the staff nurse to the community health nurse. Cardiac rehabilitation is the restoration of a person to an optimal state of function in six areas: physiologic, psychologic, mental, spiritual, economic, and vocational. The purpose of teaching is to give the patient and family the tools they need for successful rehabilitation (Table 2).

- Anticipatory guidance involves preparing the patient and family for what to expect in the course of recovery and

Table 2	Patient and Family Teaching Guide: Myocardial Infarction

The nurse needs to teach the following to the patient and the family:
- Anatomy and physiology of the heart and vessels
- Cause and effect of atherosclerosis
- Definition of terms (e.g., CAD, angina, MI, sudden cardiac death, HF)
- Signs and symptoms of angina and MI and reasons they occur*
- Healing after infarction
- Identification and modification of risk factors (Table 34-3, Lewis and others, *Medical-Surgical Nursing*, edition 7, p. 792.
- Rationale for tests and treatments, including ECG, blood tests, and angiography, and monitoring rest, diet, and medications*
- Appropriate expectations about recovery and rehabilitation (anticipatory guidance)
- Resumption of work, physical activity, and sexual activity
- Measures to take to promote recovery and health
- Importance of the gradual, progressive resumption of activity*

CAD, Coronary artery disease; *ECG*, electrocardiogram; *HF*, heart failure; *MI*, myocardial infarction.
* Identified by patients as most important to learn before discharge.

rehabilitation. By learning what to expect during treatment and recovery, the patient gains a sense of control over his or her life.

A

- The patient should be taught the parameters within which to exercise and how to check pulse rate. The patient should be told the maximum HR that should be present at any point. If the HR exceeds this level or does not return to the rate of the resting pulse within a few minutes, the patient should stop. The patient should be instructed to stop exercising if pain or dyspnea occurs. Basic guidelines for cardiac conditioning are presented in Table 34-20, Lewis and others, *Medical-Surgical Nursing,* edition 7, p. 816.
- Because of the short hospitalization, it is critical to give the patient specific guidelines for activity and exercise so that overexertion does not occur. It is helpful to stress that when the patient "listens to what the body is saying," uncomplicated recovery should proceed.
- It is important to include sexual counseling for cardiac patients and their partners. Reading material on resumption of sexual activity may be presented to the patient to facilitate discussion. The nurse should return to clarify and explain as necessary.

ACUTE RESPIRATORY DISTRESS SYNDROME

Description

Acute respiratory distress syndrome (ARDS) is a sudden and progressive form of acute respiratory failure in which the alveolar-capillary membrane becomes damaged and more permeable to intravascular fluid. The alveoli fill with fluid, resulting in severe dyspnea, hypoxemia refractory to supplemental oxygen (O_2), reduced lung compliance, and diffuse pulmonary infiltrates.

The incidence of ARDS in the United States is estimated at more than 150,000 cases annually. Despite supportive therapy, mortality from ARDS is approximately 50%. Patients who have both gram-negative septic shock and ARDS have a mortality rate of 70% to 90%.

- Table 3 lists conditions that predispose patients to the development of ARDS. The most common cause is sepsis. Patients with multiple risk factors are three or four times more likely to develop ARDS.
- Direct lung injury may cause ARDS, or ARDS may develop as a consequence of the systemic inflammatory response

Table 3	Conditions Predisposing to Acute Respiratory Distress Syndrome

Direct Lung Injury	Indirect Lung Injury
Common causes	**Common causes**
Aspiration of gastric contents or other substances	Sepsis (especially gram-negative infection)
Viral/bacterial pneumonia	Severe massive trauma
Less common causes	**Less common causes**
Chest trauma	Acute pancreatitis
Embolism: fat, air, amniotic fluid, thrombus	Anaphylaxis
Inhalation of toxic substances	Cardiopulmonary bypass
Near-drowning	Disseminated intravascular coagulation
O_2 toxicity	Multiple blood transfusions
Radiation pneumonitis	Opioid drug overdose (e.g., heroin)
	Nonpulmonary systemic diseases
	Severe head injury
	Shock states

syndrome (SIRS). ARDS may also develop as a result of multiple organ dysfunction syndrome (MODS) (see Systemic Inflammatory Response Syndrome and Multiple Organ Dysfunction Syndrome, p. 617).

Pathophysiology

An exact cause for damage to the alveolar-capillary membrane is not known. However, many changes are thought to be due to stimulation of the inflammatory and immune systems, which causes an attraction of neutrophils to the pulmonary interstitium. The neutrophils cause a release of biochemical, humoral, and cellular mediators that produce changes in the lung, including increased pulmonary capillary membrane permeability, destruction of elastin and collagen, formation of pulmonary microemboli, and pulmonary artery vasoconstriction. Pathophysiologic changes in ARDS are divided into three phases: injury or exudative, reparative or proliferative, and fibrotic.

The *injury* or *exudative phase* occurs approximately 1 to 7 days (usually 24 to 48 hours) after the initial direct lung injury or host insult. The primary changes of this phase are interstitial and alveolar edema (noncardiogenic pulmonary edema) and atelectasis.

- Neutrophils adhere to the pulmonary microcirculation, causing damage to the vascular endothelium and increased capillary permeability.

- Alveolar cells that produce surfactant are damaged by the changes caused by ARDS. This damage, in addition to further fluid and protein accumulation, results in surfactant dysfunction. The widespread atelectasis that occurs further decreases lung compliance, compromises gas exchange, and contributes to hypoxemia.
- Hyaline begins to line the alveolar membrane. Hyaline membranes contribute to fibrosis and atelectasis, leading to a decrease in gas exchange capability and lung compliance.
- Severe ventilation-perfusion (V/Q) mismatch and shunting of pulmonary capillary blood result in hypoxemia unresponsive to increasing concentrations of O_2 (*refractory hypoxemia*).

The *reparative* or *proliferative phase* begins 1 to 2 weeks after the initial lung injury. During this phase there is an influx of granulocytes, monocytes, and lymphocytes and fibroblast proliferation. The injured lung has an immense regenerative capacity after acute injury.

- Increased pulmonary vascular resistance and pulmonary hypertension may occur in this stage because fibroblasts and inflammatory cells destroy the pulmonary vasculature.
- Lung compliance continues to decrease, and hypoxemia worsens because of fibrotic changes.
- If this phase persists, widespread fibrosis results. If this phase is arrested, the lesions resolve.

The *fibrotic phase* occurs approximately 2 to 3 weeks after the initial lung injury. This phase is also called the chronic or late phase of ARDS. By this time the lung is completely remodeled by sparsely placed collagenous and fibrous tissues. Diffuse scarring and fibrosis result in decreased lung compliance and decreased surface area for gas exchange. Pulmonary hypertension results from fibrosis.

Progression of ARDS varies among patients. Some persons survive the acute phase of lung injury; pulmonary edema resolves, and complete recovery occurs in a few days. Others go on to the fibrotic (late or chronic) phase requiring long-term mechanical ventilation, with a poor chance of survival.

Clinical Manifestations

At the time of initial injury and for several hours to 1 to 2 days afterward, the patient may not exhibit respiratory symptoms.

- Initial presentation of ARDS is often insidious. The patient may exhibit dyspnea, cough, and restlessness. Chest auscultation may be normal or reveal fine, scattered crackles.

Arterial blood gases (ABGs) demonstrate mild hypoxemia and respiratory alkalosis. Chest x-ray may be normal or exhibit evidence of minimal scattered interstitial infiltrates. Edema may not manifest until there is a 30% increase in lung fluid content.

- As ARDS progresses, symptoms worsen because of increased fluid accumulation in the lungs and decreased lung compliance. Tachycardia, tachypnea, diaphoresis, changes in sensorium with decreased mentation, cyanosis, and pallor may be present. Chest auscultation usually reveals scattered to diffuse crackles and rhonchi.

- Refractory hypoxemia, despite increased fraction of inspired oxygen concentration (FIO_2) by mask, cannula, or endotracheal tube, is a hallmark of ARDS. Hypercapnia signifies that hypoventilation is occurring.

- As ARDS progresses, profound respiratory distress occurs, requiring endotracheal intubation and positive pressure ventilation (PPV). The chest x-ray reveals *whiteout* or *white lung* because consolidation and coalescing infiltrates pervade the lungs, leaving few recognizable air spaces.

- Pleural effusions may be present. Severe hypoxemia, hypercapnia, and metabolic acidosis, with symptoms of target organ or tissue hypoxemia, may ensue if prompt therapy is not instituted.

Complications may develop as a result of ARDS itself or its treatment. The major cause of death in ARDS is MODS, often accompanied by sepsis. The vital organs most commonly involved are the kidneys, liver, and heart. The organ systems most often involved are the central nervous system (CNS) and hematologic and gastrointestinal systems.

Diagnostic Studies

There are no precise criteria that define ARDS. ARDS is considered to be present if the patient presents with refractory hypoxemia, a chest x-ray with new bilateral interstitial or alveolar infiltrates, a pulmonary artery wedge pressure ≤18 mm Hg and no evidence of heart failure, and a predisposing condition consistent for ARDS within 48 hours of clinical manifestations.

Nursing and Collaborative Management
Goals

During therapy, the patient with ARDS will have a partial pressure of oxygen in arterial blood (PaO_2) of at least 60 mm Hg and adequate lung volume to maintain normal pH. A patient recovering from ARDS will experience a PaO_2 within limits of normal for age or baseline values on room air (FIO_2 of 21%), oxygen saturation in arterial blood (SaO_2) >90%, a patent airway, and clear lungs on auscultation.

The collaborative care for acute respiratory failure is applicable to ARDS (see NCP 68-1, Lewis and others, *Medical-Surgical Nursing,* edition 7, pp. 1807 to 1809). Patients with ARDS are commonly cared for in critical care units.

Nursing Diagnoses
- Impaired gas exchange
- Ineffective airway clearance
- Ineffective breathing pattern
- Risk for fluid volume excess
- Anxiety
- Imbalanced nutrition: less than body requirements

Respiratory Therapy

O_2 Administration. The goal of O_2 therapy is to correct hypoxemia (see Oxygen Therapy, p. 734). Masks with high-flow systems that deliver higher O_2 concentrations are initially utilized to maximize O_2 delivery. The general standard for O_2 administration is to give the lowest concentration that results in a PaO_2 of 60 mm Hg or greater. When FIO_2 exceeds 60% for more than 48 hours, the risk for O_2 toxicity increases. Patients with ARDS often need intubation with mechanical ventilation (see NCP 66-1, Lewis and others, *Medical-Surgical Nursing,* edition 7, pp. 1754 to 1756, and Artificial Airways: Endotracheal Tubes, p. 693) because the PaO_2 cannot otherwise be maintained at acceptable levels.

Mechanical Ventilation. Endotracheal intubation and mechanical ventilation provide additional respiratory support. In patients with ARDS, positive expiratory-end pressure (PEEP) is often used. When PEEP is applied, the lung is kept partially expanded, which prevents alveoli from totally collapsing. If hypoxemic failure persists in spite of high levels of PEEP, alternative modes and therapies may be used. These include pressure support ventilation, pressure release ventilation, pressure control ventilation, inverse ratio ventilation, high-frequency ventilation, and permissive hypercapnia (low tidal volumes that allow partial pressure of carbon dioxide in arterial blood [$PaCO_2$] to increase slowly, maintaining normal pH and low airway pressures).

Extracorporeal membrane oxygenation (ECMO) and extracorporeal carbon dioxide (CO_2) removal pass blood across a gas-exchanging membrane outside the body and then return oxygenated blood back to the body.

Positioning. Some patients with ARDS demonstrate a marked improvement in PaO_2 when turned from the supine to the prone position (e.g., PaO_2 70 mm Hg supine, PaO_2 90 mm Hg prone) with no change in inspired O_2 concentration. The response may be sufficient to allow a reduction in inspired O_2 concentration or PEEP. When this positioning is used, there must be a plan in place for immediate positioning for cardiopulmonary resuscitation (CPR) in the event of a cardiac arrest.

Another positioning strategy that can be considered for patients with ARDS is lateral rotation therapy. The purpose of this therapy is to provide continuous, slow, side-to-side turning of the patient by rotating the actual bed frame. The lateral movement of the bed is maintained for 18 of every 24 hours to stimulate postural drainage and help to mobilize pulmonary secretions. In addition, the bed may also contain a vibrator pack that can provide chest physiotherapy to further assist with secretion mobilization and removal.

Medical Supportive Therapy

Maintenance of Cardiac Output and Tissue Perfusion. Patients on PPV and PEEP frequently experience decreased cardiac output. Continuous hemodynamic monitoring is essential to detect these changes and titrate therapy. An arterial catheter is inserted for continuous monitoring of blood pressure (BP) and to withdraw blood for ABGs. A pulmonary artery catheter is inserted to allow monitoring of pulmonary artery pressures, pulmonary artery wedge pressures (which indicate fluid status of the left side of the heart), and cardiac output. Use of inotropic drugs, such as dobutamine (Dobutrex) or dopamine (Intropin), may be necessary.

Maintenance of Nutrition and Fluid Balance. Maintenance of nutrition and fluid balance is challenging in the patient with ARDS. Parenteral or enteral feedings are started to meet the high energy requirements of these patients. Leaky pulmonary capillaries cause increased fluid in the lungs, resulting in pulmonary edema. At the same time, the patient may be volume depleted and therefore prone to hypotension and decreased cardiac output from mechanical ventilation and PEEP. Controversy exists as to the benefits of fluid replacement with crystalloids versus colloids. To limit pulmonary edema, the pulmonary artery wedge pressure is kept as low as possible without impairing cardiac output. The patient is usually placed on mild fluid restriction, and diuretics are used as necessary.

▼ Patient and Family Teaching

Fear of suffocation or death is not uncommon in patients with ARDS.

- Providing reassurance, spending time with the patient, and ensuring that help can be received immediately (e.g., call light is readily available) may help to decrease patient anxiety level. Anxiety may also be reduced through instruction and use of progressive relaxation, guided imagery, and music therapy.

- It is helpful to explain to the patient any possible sensations that may be encountered with each new experience (e.g., suctioning, drawing ABGs) so that coping strategies can be purposefully selected.

ADDISON'S DISEASE

Description

Addison's disease is a primary adrenocortical insufficiency in which all three classes of adrenal steroids (glucocorticoids, mineralocorticoids, and androgens) are reduced because of hypofunction of the adrenal cortex. In secondary adrenocortical insufficiency, which is caused by a lack of pituitary adrenocorticotropic hormone (ACTH) secretion, corticosteroids and androgens are deficient but mineralocorticoids rarely are. The most common cause of Addison's disease is an autoimmune disorder; adrenal tissue is destroyed by antibodies against the patient's own adrenal cortex. Often, other endocrine conditions are present and Addison's disease is considered a component of *polyendocrine deficiency syndrome*. Other causes include infarction, fungal infections (e.g., histoplasmosis), acquired immunodeficiency syndrome (AIDS), and metastatic cancer. Iatrogenic Addison's disease may be due to adrenal hemorrhage (often related to anticoagulant therapy), antineoplastic chemotherapy, ketoconazole (Nizoral) therapy for AIDS, or bilateral adrenalectomy.

Clinical Manifestations

Manifestations have a very slow (insidious) onset and include progressive weakness, fatigue, weight loss, and anorexia. Skin hyperpigmentation, a striking feature, is seen primarily in sun-exposed areas of the body, at pressure points, over joints, and in creases, especially palmar creases.

- Other frequent manifestations are orthostatic hypotension, hyponatremia, hyperkalemia, nausea and vomiting, and diarrhea.

Patients with adrenocortical insufficiency are at risk for acute adrenal insufficiency *(addisonian crisis),* a life-threatening emergency caused by insufficient adrenocortical hormones or a sudden, sharp decrease in these hormones.

- The most dangerous feature is hypotension, which may cause shock, especially during stress. Circulatory collapse from this cause is often unresponsive to the usual treatment (vasopressors and fluid replacement) and requires corticosteroid administration.
- Addisonian crisis may be triggered by stress (e.g., from infection, surgery, trauma, or psychologic distress), sudden cessation of corticosteroid hormone replacement therapy (often done by a patient who lacks knowledge regarding replacement therapy), adrenal surgery, or sudden pituitary gland destruction.

Diagnostic Studies

- In Addison's disease, plasma cortisol levels are subnormal or fail to rise over basal levels with an ACTH stimulation test.
- A positive response to ACTH stimulation indicates a functioning adrenal gland and points to pituitary disease rather than adrenal disease.
- Free cortisol levels in the urine are decreased.
- Serum electrolytes show hyperkalemia, hypochloremia, and hyponatremia.
- Computed tomography (CT) and magnetic resonance imaging (MRI) are used to localize tumors or identify adrenal changes.

Collaborative Care

Treatment is focused on management of the underlying cause when possible. The mainstay of treatment is replacement therapy with corticosteroids (e.g., hydrocortisone) with glucocorticoid and mineralocorticoid activity. Mineralocorticoid replacement with fludrocortisone acetate (Florinef) is administered daily with increased salt in the diet.

- When any illness or stress occurs, whether mild or acute, the corticosteroid dosage must be increased to prevent adrenal crisis. The patient usually is instructed to take 2 to 3 times the usual dose.

If vomiting or diarrhea occurs, as may happen with influenza, the health care provider must be notified immediately because electrolyte replacement may be necessary. In addition, these symptoms may be early indicators of crisis.

Management of addisonian crisis requires immediate aggressive management. Treatment must be directed toward shock management and high-dose hydrocortisone replacement. Large volumes of 0.9% saline solution and 5% dextrose are administered to reverse hypotension and electrolyte imbalances until blood pressure returns to normal.

Nursing Management

When the patient with Addison's disease is hospitalized, whether for diagnosis, an acute crisis, or some other health problem, frequent nursing assessment is necessary.

- Vital signs and signs of fluid volume deficit and electrolyte imbalance should be assessed every 30 minutes to 4 hours for the first 24 hours, depending on the patient's instability.
- Nursing interventions include daily weights, corticosteroid administration, protection against exposure to infection (reverse isolation), and assistance with daily hygiene.
- The patient should be protected from noise, light, and environmental temperature extremes. The patient cannot cope with these stresses because corticosteroids cannot be produced.
- If hospitalization was due to an adrenal crisis, patients usually respond by the second day and can start oral corticosteroid replacement.
- Because discharge frequently occurs before the usual maintenance dose of corticosteroids is reached, the patient should be instructed on the importance of keeping scheduled follow-up appointments.

▼ **Patient and Family Teaching**

Because of the serious nature of the disease and the need for lifelong replacement therapy, a well-organized and carefully presented teaching plan is important (Table 4).

- Patients must be taught the signs and symptoms of corticosteroid deficiency and excess and to report to their clinicians so that the dose can be adjusted to each patient's need.
- It is critical that the patient wear an identification bracelet (Medic-Alert) and carry a wallet card stating the patient has Addison's disease so that appropriate therapy can be initiated in case of an unexpected trauma, accident, or crisis.
- Patients should carry an emergency kit with them at all times. The kit should consist of 100 mg of intramuscular (IM) hydrocortisone (Solu-Medrol), syringes, and instructions for use.
- The patient and significant others should be instructed in how to give an IM injection if replacement therapy cannot be taken orally. The patient should verbalize instructions, practice IM injections with saline, and have written instructions as to when to alter the dose.

Table 4	Patient and Family Teaching Guide: Addison's Disease

The following should be included in a teaching plan for the patient and family:
1. Names, dosages, and actions of drugs
2. Symptoms of overdosage and underdosage
3. Conditions requiring increased medication (e.g., trauma, infection, surgery, emotional crisis)
4. Course of action to take relative to changes in medication
   - Increase in dose of corticosteroid
   - Administration of large dose of intramuscular corticosteroid, including demonstration and return demonstration
   - Consultation with health care provider
5. Prevention of infection and need for prompt and vigorous treatment of existing infections
6. Need for lifelong replacement therapy
7. Need for lifelong medical supervision
8. Need for medical identification device

ALZHEIMER'S DISEASE

Description
Alzheimer's disease (AD) is a chronic, progressive, degenerative disease of the brain. It is the most common form of dementia, accounting for approximately 60% to 80% of all cases of dementia. Dementia is a syndrome characterized by dysfunction or loss of memory, orientation, attention, language, judgment, and reasoning, and changes in behavior. Approximately 4.5 million people in the United States have AD. Most patients live 8 to 10 years after being diagnosed, although some patients live for 20 years.

Pathophysiology
The exact etiology of AD is unknown. Although age is the most important risk factor for developing AD (affecting 50% of those over age 85 years), AD is not a normal part of aging. When AD develops in someone younger than 60 years, it is referred to as *early-onset AD*. AD that becomes evident in individuals after the age of 60 years is called *late-onset AD*.

Characteristic findings of AD include the abnormal presence of amyloid plaques and neurofibrillary tangles in the brain, loss of connections among cells, and cell death.

- Amyloid plaques consist of clusters of insoluble deposits of a protein called β-amyloid, other proteins, remnants of neurons, non-nerve cells such as microglia, and other cells. In AD the plaques develop first in brain areas used for memory and cognitive function, and eventually the cerebral cortex areas responsible for language and reasoning are affected.

- Neurofibrillary tangles are abnormal collections of twisted protein threads inside nerve cells. The main component of these structures is a protein called *tau*. Normally tau proteins maintain cellular structure by holding intracellular microtubules together. In AD the tau protein is altered, and as a result, the microtubules twist together in a helical fashion, ultimately forming neurofibrillary tangles.

- The third feature of AD, the gradual loss of connections among neurons, causes damage and death of neurons. This causes the brain shrinkage (atrophy) seen in AD.

Etiologic factors that are being studied include genetic factors, the role of inflammation in the development of AD, links between cardiovascular disease and AD, and lifestyle factors such as dietary patterns, leisure activities, and educational attainment.

Clinical Manifestations

Pathologic changes often precede clinical manifestations of dementia by 5 to 20 years. (Early warning signs of AD are listed in Table 5.)

- An initial sign is subtle deterioration in memory. Inevitably this progresses to more profound memory loss that interferes with the patient's ability to function. Recent events and new information cannot be recalled. Personal hygiene deteriorates as does the ability to maintain attention.

- Behavioral manifestations (e.g., agitation) and psychotic manifestations (e.g., delusion, illusions) may occur as a result of changes in the brain and are neither intentional nor controllable by the patient with AD.

- Later in the disease, long-term memories cannot be recalled, and patients lose the ability to recognize family members. Eventually the ability to communicate and perform activities of daily living (ADLs) is lost.

- In the late or final stages, the patient is unresponsive and incontinent and requires total care.

Diagnostic Studies

The diagnosis of AD is a diagnosis of exclusion. When all other possible conditions that can cause mental impairment have been ruled out and manifestations of dementia persist, the diagnosis of AD can be made.

Table 5	Patient and Family Teaching Guide: Early Warning Signs of Alzheimer's Disease

1. *Memory loss that affects job skills.* Frequent forgetfulness or unexplainable confusion at home or in the workplace may signal that something is wrong. This type of memory loss goes beyond forgetting an assignment, colleague's name, deadline, or phone number.
2. *Difficulty performing familiar tasks.* It is not abnormal for most people to become distracted and to forget something (e.g., leave something on the stove too long). People with Alzheimer's disease (AD) may cook a meal but then forget not only to serve it but also that they made it.
3. *Problems with language.* Most people have trouble with finding the "right" word from time to time. A person with AD may forget simple words or substitute inappropriate words, making their speech difficult to understand.
4. *Disorientation to time and place.* Although most individuals occasionally forget the day of the week or what they need from the store, people with AD can become lost on their own street, not knowing where they are, how they got there, or how to get back home.
5. *Poor or decreased judgment.* Many individuals from time to time may choose not to dress appropriately for the weather (e.g., not bringing a coat or sweater on a cold evening). A person with AD may dress inappropriately in more noticeable ways, such as wearing a bathrobe to the store or a sweater on a hot day.
6. *Problems with abstract thinking.* For the person with AD this goes beyond challenges such as balancing a checkbook. The person with AD may have difficulty recognizing numbers or doing even basic calculations.
7. *Misplacing things.* For many individuals temporarily misplacing keys, purses, or wallets is a normal albeit frustrating event. The person with AD may put items in inappropriate places (e.g., eating utensils in clothing drawers) but have no memory of how they got there.
8. *Changes in mood or behavior.* Most individuals experience mood changes. The person with AD tends to exhibit more rapid mood swings for no apparent reason.
9. *Changes in personality.* As most individuals age they may demonstrate some change in personality (e.g., become less tolerant). The person with AD can change dramatically, either suddenly or over a period of time. For example, someone who is generally easygoing may become angry, suspicious, or fearful.
10. *Loss of initiative.* The person with AD may become and remain uninterested and uninvolved in many or all of his or her usual pursuits.

Adapted from Alzheimer's Association: *Ten warning signs of Alzheimer's disease.*

- A computed tomography (CT) scan or magnetic resonance imaging (MRI) may show brain atrophy and enlarged ventricles in the later stages of the disease, although this finding occurs in other diseases and in persons without cognitive impairment.
- Newer techniques, including single photon emission computed tomography (SPECT), magnetic resonance spectroscopy (MRS), and positron emission tomography (PET), allow for detection of changes early in the disease, as well as monitoring treatment response.
- Laboratory tests may be used to examine genetic markers and to rule out other causes of cognitive impairment (e.g., thyroid disease, anemias, renal disease).
- Neuropsychologic testing can help document the degree of cognitive dysfunction in early stages.
- Definitive diagnosis of AD can be made only at autopsy when the presence of neurofibrillary tangles and neuritic plaques is observed.

Collaborative Care

Management of AD is aimed at improving or controlling the decline in cognition and undesirable symptoms that the patient may exhibit. Table 60-8, Lewis and others, *Medical-Surgical Nursing,* edition 7, p. 1569 details drug therapy for AD.

- Cholinesterase inhibitors that are used in the treatment of mild and moderate dementia include donepezil (Aricept), rivastigmine (Exelon), and galantamine (Razadyne). These drugs have been shown to either improve or stabilize cognitive decline in some people with AD. However, these drugs do not reverse disease progression.
- Memantine (Namenda) is used for the treatment of middle to late stages of AD. It appears to protect the brain's nerve cells by blocking the damaging effects of glutamate, which is released in large amounts by cells damaged by AD.
- Drug therapy is often used for the management of behavioral problems. Because of side effects associated with conventional antipsychotic drugs such as haloperidol (Haldol), atypical antipsychotics are also used for behavioral management in AD. Risperidone (Risperdal), olanzapine (Zyprexa), and quetiapine (Seroquel) reduce aggression and improve behavior.
- Treating the depression often associated with AD may improve cognitive ability. Depression is often treated with selective serotonin reuptake inhibitors (SSRIs), including fluoxetine (Prozac), sertraline (Zoloft), fluvoxamine

(Luvox), and citalopram (Celexa). Antiseizure medications (neuroleptics) are also used to manage behavior problems.
- Under study is the role of ginkgo biloba, hormone replacement therapy, nonsteroidal antiinflammatory drugs (NSAIDs), statins, and antioxidants in the prevention and/ or treatment of AD.

Nursing Management
Goals
The patient with AD will maintain functional ability for as long as possible, be maintained in a safe environment with a minimum of injuries, have personal care needs met, and have dignity maintained.

See NCP 60-1 for the patient with AD, Lewis and others, *Medical-Surgical Nursing,* edition 7, pp. 1571 to 1572.
Nursing Diagnoses
- Disturbed thought processes
- Self-care deficit
- Risk for injury
- Grieving
- Wandering
Nursing Interventions
Nursing care is focused on decreasing clinical manifestations, preventing harm, and supporting the patient and caregiver through the disease process.

Although there is no current treatment for reversing AD, there is a need for ongoing monitoring of both the patient and the patient's caregiver. An important nursing responsibility is to work collaboratively with the patient's health care provider to manage symptoms effectively as they change over time.
- The nurse is often responsible for teaching the caregiver to perform essential tasks for the patient. The nurse also should work with the caregiver to assess stressors and to identify coping strategies to reduce the burden of caregiving. To aid in identifying caregiver problems, a nursing care plan for the caregiver of a person with AD is available at *http://evolve.elsevier.com/Lewis/medsurg.*
- Adult day care is one of the options available to the person with AD. Common goals of all day-care programs are to provide respite for the family and a protective environment for the patient.
- As the disease progresses, the demands on the caregivers eventually exceed the resources. The person with AD may need to be placed in a long-term care facility, where special

units to care for persons with AD are becoming increasingly common.

- Patients with AD are subject to acute and other chronic illnesses. Their inability to communicate health symptoms and problems places responsibility for assessment and diagnosis on caregivers and health professionals. Hospitalization of the patient can be a traumatic event for both patient and caregiver and can precipitate a worsening of the disease.

- Support groups for caregivers and family members have been formed throughout the United States and other countries to provide an atmosphere of understanding and to give current information about the disease itself and related topics such as safety, legal, ethical, and financial issues.

- Decisions related to care should be made with the patient, family members, and health care team early in the disease. The nurse has a role in advising the patient and caregiver to initiate health care and advance directives and decisions while the patient still has the capacity to do so.

AMYOTROPHIC LATERAL SCLEROSIS

Amyotrophic lateral sclerosis (ALS) is a rare, progressive neurologic disease characterized by loss of motor neurons. This disease became known as Lou Gehrig's disease when the famous baseball player was stricken with it in the early 1940s. The onset is between the ages of 40 and 70 years, and twice as many men as women are affected. ALS usually leads to death within 2 to 6 years of diagnosis.

- For unknown reasons, motor neurons in the brainstem and spinal cord gradually degenerate in ALS. Consequently, messages originating in the brain never reach the muscles to activate them.

- Typical symptoms are weakness of the upper extremities, dysarthria, and dysphagia. Muscle wasting and fasciculations result from denervation of the muscles and lack of stimulation and use.

- Death usually results from respiratory infection secondary to compromised respiratory function.

- There is no cure for ALS. This illness is devastating because the patient remains cognitively intact while wasting away.

■ Riluzole (Rilutek) slows the progression of ALS. This drug works to decrease the amount of glutamate (an excitatory neurotransmitter) in the brain. In clinical trials, riluzole has been shown to delay the need for tracheostomy and death by a few months.

The challenge of nursing care is to support the patient's cognitive and emotional functions by facilitating communication, reducing risk of aspiration, decreasing pain secondary to muscle weakness, decreasing risk of injury related to falls, providing diversional activities such as reading and human companionship, and helping the patient and family with anticipatory grieving related to loss of motor function and ultimately death.

ANEMIA

Description

Anemia is a deficiency in the number of red blood cells (RBCs), or erythrocytes, the quantity of hemoglobin (Hb), and/or the volume of packed red cells (hematocrit). Anemia can be caused by blood loss, impaired production of erythrocytes, or increased destruction of erythrocytes.

■ Because RBCs transport oxygen (O_2), erythrocyte disorders can lead to tissue hypoxia. This hypoxia accounts for many of the clinical manifestations of anemia.

■ Anemia is not a specific disease; it is a manifestation of a pathologic process.

■ Anemia is identified and classified by laboratory evaluation.

■ Anemia can result from primary hematologic problems or can develop as a secondary consequence of defects in other body systems.

The different types of anemia can be classified according to either morphology (cell characteristics) or etiology.

■ Morphologic classification is based on descriptive, objective laboratory information about erythrocyte size and color.

■ Etiologic classification is related to clinical conditions causing anemia, such as decreased erythrocyte production, blood loss, or increased erythrocyte destruction (Table 6).

■ Although the morphologic system is the most accurate means of classifying anemia, it is easier to discuss patient care by focusing on the etiologic problem. Table 7 relates morphologic classifications to various etiologies.

■ Although the Hb level is decreased in all anemias, other
laboratory findings are characteristic of specific anemias
and are used in diagnosis of anemias (Table 8).

A

Clinical Manifestations

■ Manifestations of anemia are caused by the body's response to
tissue hypoxia. The specific manifestations vary depending on

Table 6	Etiologic Classification of Anemia

Decreased Erythrocyte Production
Decreased hemoglobin synthesis
■ Iron deficiency
■ Thalassemias (decreased globin synthesis)
■ Sideroblastic anemia (decreased porphyrin)
Defective DNA synthesis
■ Cobalamin (vitamin B_{12}) deficiency
■ Folic acid deficiency
Decreased number of erythrocyte precursors
■ Aplastic anemia
■ Anemia of leukemia and myelodysplasia
■ Chronic diseases or disorders
Chemotherapy

Blood Loss
Acute
■ Trauma
■ Blood vessel rupture
Chronic
■ Gastritis
■ Menstrual flow
■ Hemorrhoids

Increased Erythrocyte Destruction*
Intrinsic
■ Abnormal hemoglobin (Hb S—sickle cell anemia)
■ Enzyme deficiency (G6PD)
■ Membrane abnormalities (paroxysmal nocturnal
hemoglobinuria, hereditary spherocytosis)
Extrinsic
■ Physical trauma (prosthetic heart valves, extracorporeal
circulation)
■ Antibodies (isoimmune and autoimmune)
■ Infectious agents and toxins (malaria)

DNA, Deoxyribonucleic acid; *G6PD,* glucose-6-phosphate dehydrogenase;
Hb S, hemoglobin S.
* Hemolytic anemias.

Table 7	Relationship of Morphologic Classification and Etiologies of Anemia

Morphology	Etiology
Normocytic, normochromic (normal size and color)	Acute blood loss, hemolysis, chronic renal disease, chronic disease, cancers, sideroblastic anemia, refractory anemia, diseases of endocrine dysfunction, aplastic anemia, sickle cell disease, pregnancy
Macrocytic, normochromic (large size, normal color)	Cobalamin (vitamin B_{12}) deficiency, folic acid deficiency, liver disease (including effects of alcohol abuse), postsplenectomy
Microcytic, hypochromic (small size, pale color)	Iron deficiency anemia, thalassemia, lead poisoning

the severity of anemia and the presence of coexisting disease. Hb levels may determine the severity of anemia.

- Mild states of anemia (Hb 10 to 14 g/dl [100 to 140 g/L]) may exist without causing symptoms. If symptoms develop, they are usually caused by an underlying disease or a compensatory response to heavy exercise. These symptoms include palpitations, dyspnea, and diaphoresis.
- In cases of moderate anemia (Hb 6 to 10 g/dl [60 to 100 g/L]), cardiopulmonary symptoms (e.g., increased heart rate) may be present with rest as well as activity.
- Patients with severe anemia (Hb < 6 g/dl [<60 g/L]) display many clinical manifestations involving multiple body systems (Table 9).

Nursing Management
Goals
The patient with anemia will assume normal activities of daily living (ADLs), maintain adequate nutrition, and develop no complications related to anemia. See NCP 31-1 for the patient with anemia, Lewis and others, *Medical-Surgical Nursing*, ed. 7, pp. 688 to 689.
Nursing Diagnoses/Collaborative Problems
- Activity intolerance
- Imbalanced nutrition: less than body requirements
- Ineffective therapeutic regimen management
- Potential complication: hypoxemia

Table 8   Laboratory Study Findings in Anemias

	Iron Deficiency	Thalassemia Major	Cobalamin (Vitamin B₁₂) Deficiency	Folic Acid Deficiency	Aplastic Anemia	Sickle Cell Anemia
Hb/Hct	↓	↓	↓	↓	↓	↓
MCV	↓	↓	↑	↑	N	N
MCH	↓	↓	N or slight ↑	N or slight ↑	N	N
MCHC	↓	↓	N	N	N	N
Reticulocytes	N or ↓	↑	↓ to N	↓	↓	↑
Serum iron	↓	↑	N	N	± N	N to ↑
TIBC	↑	↑	N	N	± N	N to ↑
Transferrin	N or ↓	↓	Slight ↑	Slight ↑	N	N
Ferritin	↓	N or ↑	↑	↑	N	N
Bilirubin	N to ↓	↑	N to ↑	N	N	↑
Platelets	—	—	↓	N	↓	↑
Other findings	—	—	Cobalamin, positive Schilling test, achlorhydria	↓ Folate	↓ WBC	—

Hb, Hemoglobin; *Hct*, hematocrit; *MCH*, mean corpuscular hemoglobin; *MCHC*, mean corpuscular hemoglobin concentration; *MCV*, mean corpuscular volume; *N*, normal; *TIBC*, total iron-binding capacity; *WBC*, white blood cell.

A

Table 9 Clinical Manifestations of Anemia

Body System	Mild (Hb 10-14 g/dl [100-140 g/L])	Moderate (Hb 6-10 g/dl [60-100 g/L])	Severe (Hb < 6 g/dl [<60 g/L])
			Severity of Anemia
Integument	None	None	Pallor, jaundice,* pruritus*
Eyes	None	None	Icteric conjunctiva and sclera,* retinal hemorrhage, blurred vision
Mouth	None	None	Glossitis, smooth tongue, sore mouth
Cardiovascular	Palpitations	Increased palpitations	Tachycardia, increased pulse pressure, systolic murmurs, intermittent claudication, angina, HF, MI
Pulmonary	Exertional dyspnea	Dyspnea	Tachypnea, orthopnea, dyspnea at rest
Neurologic	None	None	Headache, vertigo, irritability, depression, impaired thought processes
Gastrointestinal	None	None	Anorexia, hepatomegaly, splenomegaly, difficulty swallowing
Musculoskeletal	None	None	Bone pain
General	None	Fatigue	Sensitivity to cold, weight loss, lethargy

Hb, Hemoglobin; *HF*, heart failure; *MI*, myocardial infarction.
* Caused by hemolysis.

Nursing Interventions
The numerous causes of anemia necessitate different nursing interventions specific to patient needs. General components of care for all patients with anemia may include:

- Correction of the etiology of the anemia as the ultimate goal of therapy
- Dietary and lifestyle changes that may reverse some anemias and return patients to their former state of health
- Acute interventions such as blood transfusions, drug therapy (e.g., erythropoietin, vitamin replacements), and O_2 therapy
- Ongoing assessment of the patient's knowledge regarding adequate nutritional intake and compliance to drug therapies should be included in the plan of care

Specific types of anemia are listed under separate headings.

ANEMIA, APLASTIC

Description
Aplastic anemia is a disease in which the patient has peripheral blood pancytopenia (decrease of all blood types: red blood cells [RBCs], white blood cells [WBCs], and platelets) and hypocellular bone marrow. Signs and symptoms can range from a chronic condition managed with erythropoietin or blood transfusions to a critical condition with hemorrhage and sepsis.

Pathophysiology
There are various etiologic classifications for aplastic anemia, but they can be divided into two major groups: congenital (idiopathic) or acquired.

- Congenital aplastic anemia is caused by chromosomal alterations.
- Acquired aplastic anemia is a result of exposure to ionizing radiation, chemical agents (e.g., benzene, insecticides, arsenic, alcohol), viral and bacterial infections (e.g., hepatitis, parvovirus, miliary tuberculosis), and prescribed medications (e.g., alkylating agents, antiseizure medications, antimetabolites, antimicrobials, gold). Approximately 70% of the acquired aplastic anemias are idiopathic.

Clinical Manifestations
Aplastic anemia may develop abruptly over days or insidiously over weeks and months. It can vary from mild to severe. Clinically

the patient may have symptoms caused by suppression of any or all bone marrow elements.

- General manifestations of anemia such as fatigue and dyspnea, as well as cardiovascular and cerebral signs, may be seen (Table 9).
- The patient with neutropenia (low neutrophil count) is susceptible to infection and may be febrile.
- Thrombocytopenia is manifested by a predisposition to bleeding (e.g., petechiae, ecchymoses, epistaxis).

Diagnostic Studies

Diagnosis is confirmed by laboratory studies.

- All marrow elements are affected: hemoglobin (Hb), WBC, and platelet values are often decreased (see Table 8).
- Reticulocyte count is low, and bleeding time is prolonged.
- Serum iron and total iron-binding capacity (TIBC) are elevated as initial signs of erythroid suppression.
- Bone marrow examination may be done for any anemic state, but findings are especially important in aplastic anemia because the marrow is hypocellular with increased yellow marrow (fat content).

Nursing and Collaborative Management

Management of aplastic anemia is based on identifying and removing the causative agent (when possible) and providing supportive care until pancytopenia reverses.

Nursing interventions appropriate for the patient with pancytopenia from aplastic anemia are presented in the nursing care plans for patients with anemia, thrombocytopenia, and neutropenia (see NCPs 31-1, pp. 688 to 689, 31-2, p. 706, and 31-3, p. 716, Lewis and others, *Medical-Surgical Nursing,* edition 7). Nursing actions are directed at preventing complications from infection and hemorrhage.

- Prognosis of untreated aplastic anemia is poor (approximately 75% fatal). However, advances in medical management, including hematopoietic stem cell transplant (HSCT) and immunosuppressive therapy with antithymocyte globulin (ATG) and cyclosporine or high-dose cyclophosphamide (Cytoxan), have improved outcomes significantly. ATG is a horse serum containing polyclonal antibodies against human T cells. Rationale for this therapy is that aplastic anemia is an immune-mediated disease.
- Treatment of choice for adults less than 45 years old who do not respond to immunosuppressive therapy and who have

a human leukocyte antigen (HLA)–matched donor is HSCT. **A**
Best results occur in a younger patient who has not had
previous blood transfusions. Prior transfusions increase the
risk of graft rejection.
- For the older adult or the patient without an HLA-matched
donor, the treatment of choice is immunosuppression with
ATG or cyclosporine or high-dose cyclophosphamide.
Response to this therapy may only be partial, but usually
transfusions can be avoided.

ANEMIA, COBALAMIN (VITAMIN B$_{12}$) DEFICIENCY

Description
Anemia resulting from a cobalamin (vitamin B$_{12}$) deficiency is a
type of megaloblastic anemia caused by impaired DNA synthesis.
When DNA synthesis is impaired, defective red blood cell (RBC)
maturation results in large, abnormal RBCs. Normally a protein
known as *intrinsic factor* (IF) is secreted by parietal cells of the
gastric mucosa. IF is required for cobalamin (extrinsic factor)
absorption in the distal ileum. Therefore if IF is not secreted,
cobalamin cannot be absorbed.
- In *pernicious anemia,* the most common cause of cobalamin deficiency, the gastric mucosa does not secrete IF.
- Other causes of cobalamin deficiency include gastrointestinal (GI) surgery and diseases that impair secretion of IF,
nutritional deficiency, chronic alcoholism, and hereditary
enzymatic defects of cobalamin utilization.

Pathophysiology
Cobalamin deficiency can occur in patients who have had GI
surgery, such as gastrectomy; patients who have had a small bowel
resection involving the ileum; and patients with Crohn's disease,
ileitis, diverticuli of the small intestine, and/or chronic atrophic
gastritis. In these cases, cobalamin deficiency results from the loss
of IF-secreting gastric mucosal surface or impaired absorption of
cobalamin in the distal ileum. Because an acid environment in the
stomach is required for the secretion of IF, cobalamin deficiency is
also found in long-term users of H$_2$-histamine receptor blockers.
Pernicious anemia is caused by an absence of IF, either from
gastric mucosal atrophy or autoimmune destruction of parietal

cells. Destruction of the parietal cells prevents both IF and hydrochloric acid secretion. Pernicious anemia has an insidious onset
that generally begins in middle age or later (usually after age 40
years). It occurs frequently in persons of northern European
ancestry (particularly Scandinavians) and African Americans. In
African Americans, the disease tends to begin early (with a high
frequency in women) and is often severe.

Clinical Manifestations

Manifestations of anemia related to cobalamin deficiency usually
develop over months and are related to tissue hypoxia (see Table
9, p. 32).

- GI manifestations include a sore tongue, anorexia, nausea,
  vomiting, and abdominal pain.
- Neuromuscular manifestations include weakness, paresthesias of feet and hands, reduced vibratory and position
  senses, ataxia, muscle weakness, and impaired thought processes ranging from confusion to dementia.

Diagnostic Studies

Laboratory data reflective of cobalamin deficiency anemia are
presented in Table 8, p. 31.

- Erythrocytes appear large (macrocytic) and have abnormal
  shapes. This structure contributes to erythrocyte destruction because the cell membrane is fragile.
- Serum cobalamin levels are reduced.
- A Schilling test can be used to assess parietal cell function
  and is diagnostic of pernicious anemia if orally administered radioactive cobalamin is absorbed following the parenteral administration of IF.

Collaborative Care

Regardless of how much cobalamin is ingested, the patient is not
able to absorb it if IF is lacking or if there is impaired ileum
absorption, so dietary management is not used for cobalamin
replacement.

- The anemia can be reversed with supplemental cobalamin.
  Parenteral (cyanocobalamin or hydroxocobalamin) or intranasal (Nascobal) administration of cobalamin is the treatment of choice. A typical treatment schedule consists of
  1000 mg cobalamin IM daily for 2 weeks, then weekly until
  hematocrit is normal, and then monthly for life. High-dose
  oral cobalamin and sublingual cobalamin are also available. Regular supplemental cobalamin will reverse the
  anemia, but long-standing neuromuscular complications
  may not be reversible.

Nursing Management

- Patients who have a positive family history of pernicious anemia should be evaluated for symptoms. Although disease development cannot be prevented, early detection and treatment can lead to reversal of symptoms.
- Nursing interventions for the patient with anemia are appropriate for the patient with cobalamin deficiency (see Anemia, p. 28). In addition to these measures, the patient should be protected from burns and trauma because of diminished sensation to heat and pain as a result of neurologic impairment.
- Ongoing care is primarily related to ensuring good patient compliance with treatment. There must be careful follow-up evaluation to assess for neurologic difficulties that were not fully corrected by cobalamin replacement therapy. Because the potential for stomach cancer is increased in pernicious anemia, the patient should have frequent and careful evaluation for this problem.

ANEMIA, FOLIC ACID DEFICIENCY

Folic acid is required for DNA synthesis leading to red blood cell (RBC) (erythrocyte) formation and maturation. A deficiency of folic acid results in a megaloblastic anemia with large, immature RBCs. Common causes of folic acid deficiency are (1) poor nutrition, especially a lack of leafy green vegetables, liver, citrus fruits, yeast, dried beans, nuts, and grains; (2) malabsorption syndromes, particularly small bowel disorders; (3) drugs that impede absorption and use of folic acid (e.g., methotrexate), antiseizure medications (e.g., phenobarbital, phenytoin [Dilantin]), and others (e.g., trimethoprim, sulfasalazine); (4) alcohol abuse and anorexia; and (5) hemodialysis treatments, since folic acid is lost during dialysis.

Clinical Manifestations

Clinical manifestations of folic acid deficiency are similar to those of cobalamin deficiency. The disease develops insidiously, and the patient's symptoms may be attributed to other coexisting problems, such as cirrhosis or esophageal varices.

- Gastrointestinal (GI) disturbances include dyspepsia and a smooth, beefy red tongue.
- Absence of neurologic problems is an important diagnostic finding; this lack of neurologic involvement differentiates folic acid deficiency from cobalamin deficiency.

- Diagnostic findings for folic acid deficiency are presented in Table 8, p. 31. A normal serum cobalamin level and a gastric analysis positive for hydrochloric acid help differentiate folic acid deficiency from cobalamin deficiency.

Folic acid deficiency is treated by replacement therapy with the usual dose of 1 mg/day by mouth. In malabsorption states, up to 5 mg/day may be required. Duration of treatment depends on the reason for the deficiency. The patient should be encouraged to eat foods containing large amounts of folic acid.

Nursing interventions for the patient with anemia are appropriate for the patient with folic acid deficiency (see Anemia, p. 28).

ANEMIA, IRON DEFICIENCY

Description
Iron deficiency anemia, one of the most common chronic hematologic disorders, is found in 30% of the world's population. In the United States, iron deficiency anemia is most common in the very young, those on poor diets, and women in their reproductive years.

Pathophysiology
Iron deficiency may develop from inadequate dietary intake, malabsorption, blood loss, or hemolysis. Iron is obtained from dietary intake, but only 5% to 10% of all ingested iron is absorbed in the duodenum. This amount of dietary iron is adequate to meet needs of men and older women, but it may be inadequate for those individuals who have higher iron needs (e.g., menstruating or pregnant women).

Iron absorption occurs in the duodenum, and absorption can be altered after surgical procedures that involve removal of or bypass of the duodenum. Malabsorption syndromes may also involve disease of the duodenum, affecting iron absorption.

Blood loss is a major cause of iron deficiency in adults. Major sources of chronic blood loss are from the gastrointestinal (GI) and genitourinary (GU) systems.

- GI bleeding is often not apparent and therefore may exist for a considerable time before the problem is identified. Loss of 50 to 75 ml of blood from the upper GI tract is required to cause stools to appear black (melena). This color results from iron in the red blood cells (RBCs).

- Common causes of GI blood loss are peptic ulcer, esophagitis, diverticuli, hemorrhoids, and neoplasia. GU blood loss
occurs primarily from menstrual bleeding. The average
monthly menstrual blood loss is about 45 ml, which causes
a loss of about 22 mg of iron.
- In addition to the anemia of chronic kidney disease, dialysis
treatment may induce iron deficiency anemia because of the
blood lost in the dialysis equipment and frequent blood
sampling.
- Pregnancy contributes to iron deficiency because of iron
diversion to the fetus for erythropoiesis, blood loss at delivery, and lactation.

Clinical Manifestations
In the early course of iron deficiency anemia, the patient may be
free of symptoms. As the disease becomes chronic, any of the
general manifestations of anemia may develop (see Table 9, p. 32).
In addition, specific clinical symptoms related to iron deficiency
anemia may occur.
- Pallor is the most common finding, and glossitis (inflammation of tongue) is the second most common; another
finding is cheilitis (inflammation of lips).
- In addition, the patient may report headache, paresthesias,
and a burning sensation of the tongue, all of which are
caused by lack of iron in the tissues.

Diagnostic Studies
Laboratory abnormalities characteristic of iron deficiency anemia
are presented in Table 8, p. 31. Other diagnostic studies are done
to determine the cause of iron deficiency. For example, endoscopy
and colonoscopy may be used to detect GI bleeding.

Collaborative Care
The main goal in iron deficiency anemia is to treat the underlying
cause of reduced intake (e.g., malnutrition, alcoholism) or absorption of iron. Efforts are directed toward replacing iron, which may
be done through increasing iron intake.
- The patient should be taught which foods are good sources
of iron. If nutrition is adequate, increasing iron intake by
dietary means may not be practical. Consequently, oral or
occasionally parenteral iron supplements are used.
- Drug therapy with iron supplements requires special considerations related to administration and side effects (see
Drug Therapy, Iron Deficiency Anemia, Lewis and others,
Medical-Surgical Nursing, edition 7, pp. 690 to 691).

- If iron deficiency is from acute blood loss, transfusion of packed RBCs may be required.

Nursing Management
It is important to recognize groups of individuals who are at increased risk for development of iron deficiency anemia, including premenopausal and pregnant women, persons from low socio-economic backgrounds, older adults, and individuals experiencing blood loss. Dietary teaching, with an emphasis on foods high in iron, is important for these groups. Supplemental iron is especially important for pregnant women.

Appropriate nursing measures are presented in NCP 31-1, Lewis and others, *Medical-Surgical Nursing,* edition 7, pp. 688 to 689.

▼ **Patient and Family Teaching**
- It is important to discuss with the patient the need for diagnostic studies to identify the cause. The hemoglobin (Hb) level and RBC count are reassessed to evaluate the response to therapy.
- Compliance with dietary and drug therapy needs to be emphasized. To replenish the body's iron stores, the patient should take iron therapy for 2 to 3 months after the Hb level returns to normal.

ANEURYSM

Description
An aneurysm is an outpouching or dilation of the arterial wall and is a common problem involving the aorta. Aneurysms of peripheral and cerebral arteries also can occur but are far less common. Aortic aneurysms may involve the aortic arch, thoracic aorta, and/or abdominal aorta, but most aneurysms are found in the abdominal aorta below the level of the renal arteries. The dilated aortic wall becomes lined with thrombi that can embolize, leading to acute ischemic symptoms to distal (downstream) branches. The growth rate of an aneurysm is unpredictable, but the larger the aneurysm, the greater the risk of rupture.

Pathophysiology
Although the cause is unknown, several theories of pathogenesis exist. The most common etiology of descending and abdominal aneurysms is atherosclerosis. Atherosclerotic plaques deposited beneath the intima (the innermost layer of the artery) are thought to cause degenerative changes in the media (middle layer of arte-

rial wall), leading to loss of elasticity, weakening, and eventual
dilation of the aorta.

- A strong genetic component may exist in the development
  of abdominal aortic aneurysms (AAAs).
- Less common causes of aneurysms include blunt or penetrating trauma and inflammatory or infectious aortitis.
- Aneurysms are generally divided into two basic classifications: true and false.
- A *true aneurysm* is one in which the wall of the artery
  forms the aneurysm, with at least one vessel layer still
  intact. True aneurysms can be further subdivided into fusiform and saccular dilations. A fusiform aneurysm is circumferential and relatively uniform in shape; a saccular
  aneurysm is pouchlike, with a narrow neck connecting the
  bulge to one side of the arterial wall.
- A *false aneurysm,* or *pseudoaneurysm,* is not an aneurysm
  but a disruption of all layers of the arterial wall resulting in
  bleeding that is contained by surrounding structures. False
  aneurysms may result from trauma, from infection, or after
  peripheral artery bypass graft surgery at the site of the
  graft-to-artery anastomosis. They may also result from
  arterial leakage after removal of cannulae, such as upper or
  lower extremity arterial catheters and intraaortic balloon
  pump devices.

Clinical Manifestations

Thoracic aorta aneurysms are usually asymptomatic. When manifestations are present, they are varied, with deep, diffuse chest
pain the most common symptom.

Aneurysms in the ascending aorta and aortic arch can produce
angina from disruption of blood flow to the coronary arteries and
hoarseness as a result of pressure on the recurrent laryngeal nerve.
Pressure on the esophagus can cause dysphagia. If the aneurysm
presses on the superior vena cava, it can cause distended neck
veins and head and arm edema.

AAAs also are often asymptomatic and may be detected on
routine physical examination or coincidentally when the patient is
being examined for an unrelated problem (e.g., abdominal x-ray).
On examination a pulsatile mass in the periumbilical area slightly
to the left of midline may be detected. Bruits may be audible with
a stethoscope placed over the aneurysm.

- Symptoms of an AAA may mimic pain associated with any
  abdominal or back disorder. Symptoms may result from
  compression of nearby anatomic structures (e.g., back pain
  caused by lumbar nerve compression).

- Occasionally aneurysms spontaneously embolize plaque and thrombi. This can cause "blue toe syndrome," in which patchy mottling of the feet and toes occurs in the presence of peripheral pulses.

Complications

The most serious complication is rupture.

- If rupture occurs posteriorly into the retroperitoneal space, bleeding may be tamponaded by surrounding structures, preventing exsanguination. In this case the patient has severe back pain and may have back and/or flank ecchymosis *(Grey Turner's sign)*.
- If rupture occurs anteriorly into the abdominal cavity, death from massive hemorrhage is likely. If the patient does reach the hospital, the presence of hypovolemic shock is indicated by tachycardia; hypotension; pale, clammy skin; decreased urine output; altered sensorium; and abdominal tenderness.

Diagnostic Studies

- Chest x-ray demonstrates mediastinal silhouette and abnormal widening of the thoracic aorta.
- Echocardiography may show aortic insufficiency related to ascending aortic dilation.
- Ultrasonography is useful to screen for aneurysms and to serially monitor aneurysm size.
- An electrocardiogram (ECG) is done to rule out a myocardial infarction (MI) because patients with thoracic aneurysms have symptoms suggestive of angina.
- Computed tomography (CT) determines anterior-posterior and cross-sectional diameter of the aneurysm.
- Magnetic resonance imaging (MRI) may also be used to diagnose and assess severity of the aneurysm.

Collaborative Care

The goal of management is to prevent rupture of the aneurysm; therefore early detection and prompt treatment are imperative. Once an aneurysm is suspected, studies are performed to determine its exact size and location. Generally, if coexisting problems are stable, surgical repair is the treatment of choice.

- Before surgery, the patient is hydrated and any abnormalities in electrolytes, coagulation, and hematocrit are corrected.
- If the aneurysm has ruptured, immediate surgical intervention is required. Even with prompt care, the mortality rate after rupture is high (33% to 94%) and increases with

the patient's age. Illustrations of surgical techniques are presented in Fig. 38-4 in Lewis and others, *Medical-Surgical Nursing,* edition 7, p. 896.

- An alternative to conventional surgical repair of an AAA is the minimally invasive endovascular grafting technique. This technique involves placement of a sutureless aortic graft into the abdominal aorta through the femoral artery.

Nursing Management
Goals
The patient undergoing aortic surgery will have normal tissue perfusion, intact motor and sensory function, and no complications related to surgical repair, such as infection or thrombosis.

Nursing Diagnoses
- Ineffective tissue perfusion
- Risk for infection

Nursing Interventions
- The patient should be encouraged to reduce cardiovascular risk factors, including blood pressure (BP) control, smoking cessation, increasing physical activity, and maintaining normal body weight and serum lipid levels. These measures are also done to ensure continued graft patency after surgical repair.
- The nursing role during the preoperative period includes patient and family teaching, providing support for the patient and family, and careful assessment of all body systems.
- In the postoperative period adequate respiratory function, fluid and electrolyte balance, and pain control need to be maintained. The nurse must monitor graft patency and renal perfusion. The nurse can also assist in preventing dysrhythmias, infections, and neurologic complications. A nursing care plan for the patient with an aneurysm repair is available at *http://evolve.elsevier.com/Lewis/medsurg.*

▼ **Patient and Family Teaching**
The patient may be apprehensive about returning home after major surgery involving the aorta.

- Encourage the patient to express any concerns, and reassure the patient that normal activities can be gradually resumed.
- Fatigue, poor appetite, and irregular bowel habits are to be expected.
- Heavy lifting is to be avoided for at least 4 to 6 weeks after traditional surgery.
- Observation of incisions for signs and symptoms of infection is encouraged. Any redness, increased pain, fever >100° F (>37.8° C), or drainage from incisions should be reported to the physician.

- The patient should be taught to observe for changes in extremity color or warmth and how to palpate peripheral pulses and to assess changes in their quality.
- The patient who has received a synthetic graft should be aware that prophylactic antibiotics may be required before future invasive procedures.
- Sexual dysfunction in male patients is not uncommon after aortic surgery. This may occur because the internal hypogastric artery is disrupted, leading to altered blood flow to the penis.
- Patients who do not undergo surgical repair should be urged to receive regular routine physical examinations and reminded that any symptom, no matter how minor, must be investigated if it persists.

ANGINA, CHRONIC STABLE

Description
Angina, or chest pain, is the clinical manifestation of reversible myocardial ischemia that occurs when the demand for myocardial oxygen exceeds the ability of the coronary arteries to supply the heart with oxygen. The primary cause of myocardial ischemia is insufficient blood flow to the myocardium through coronary arteries narrowed by atherosclerosis (see Coronary Artery Disease, p. 150). Chronic stable angina and acute coronary syndrome are clinical manifestations of coronary artery disease (CAD).

Chronic Stable Angina
Chronic stable angina refers to chest pain that occurs intermittently over a long period with the same pattern of onset, duration, and intensity of symptoms. The pain usually lasts for only a few minutes (3 to 5 minutes) and commonly subsides when the precipitating factor is relieved. Pain at rest is unusual.

- An electrocardiogram (ECG) usually reveals ST-segment depression, indicating ischemia.
- Chronic stable angina can be controlled with medications on an outpatient basis. Because stable angina is often predictable, medications can be timed to provide peak effects during the time of day when angina is likely to occur.

Variants of chronic stable angina include:

- *Silent ischemia,* in which ischemia occurs in the absence of any subjective symptoms

- *Nocturnal ischemia,* which occurs only at night but not necessarily when the person is lying down or sleeping
- *Angina decubitus,* which is chest pain that occurs only when the person is lying down and is usually relieved by standing or sitting

Pathophysiology

On the cellular level, the myocardium becomes cyanotic within the first 10 seconds of coronary occlusion, and ECG changes appear. With total occlusion of the coronary arteries, contractility ceases after several minutes, depriving myocardial cells of oxygen and glucose for aerobic metabolism. Myocardial nerve fibers are irritated by the lactic acid formed by anerobic metabolism and transmit a pain message to cardiac nerves and upper thoracic posterior roots (the reason for referred cardiac pain to the left shoulder and arm).

- Under ischemic conditions, cardiac cells are viable for about 20 minutes. With restoration of blood flow, aerobic metabolism resumes and contractility is restored. Cellular repair begins.
- Ischemia with pain (angina) or without pain has the same prognosis. Diabetes mellitus is associated with an increased prevalence of silent ischemia.

Clinical Manifestations

Chronic stable angina may occur when precipitating factors alter the balance of myocardial oxygen demand and oxygen supply (e.g., physical exertion, temperature extremes, strong emotions, heavy meals, smoking, sexual activity, use of stimulants); it is described by patients in a variety of ways. Table 10 provides a memory device to assess the characteristics of angina.

- On direct questioning, some patients may deny feeling pain but will refer to a vague sensation, pressure, or ache in chest. It is an unpleasant feeling, often described as a constrictive, squeezing, heavy, choking, or suffocating sensation.
- Many persons complain of severe indigestion or burning. Although discomfort is usually felt substernally, the sensation may occur in the neck or radiate to various locations, including the jaw, shoulders, and down the arms.
- Often people will complain of pain between the shoulder blades and dismiss it as not being related to the heart.
- Relief of chronic stable angina pectoris is usually obtained with rest or relief of the precipitating factor.

Table 10	PQRST Assessment of Angina

The following can be used as a memory device to assist in obtaining information from the patient who has chest pain.

	Factor	Questions to Ask Patient
P	Precipitating events	What events or activities precipitated the pain (e.g., argument, exercise, resting)?
Q	Quality of pain	What does the pain feel like (e.g., pressure, dull, aching, tight, squeezing)?
R	Radiation of pain	Where is the pain located? Does the pain radiate to other areas (e.g., back, arms, jaw, teeth, shoulder, elbow)?
S	Severity of pain	On a scale of 0 to 10 with 10 being the most severe pain you could imagine, how would you rate the pain?
T	Timing	When did the pain begin? Has the pain changed since this time? Have you had pain like this before?

Diagnostic Studies

Diagnostic studies used to evaluate angina are the same as those used to diagnose CAD (see Coronary Artery Disease, p. 150). For patients with known CAD and chronic stable angina, two studies are commonly used to evaluate coronary artery perfusion.

- Treadmill exercise testing is important because ST-segment and T-wave changes that occur during exercise are an indirect assessment of coronary perfusion. Severely abnormal ECGs during exercise testing indicate a significant disease process and may indicate the need for coronary angiography.
- Cardiac catheterization and coronary angiography can identify a coronary lesion that may be amenable to an intervention that can be done at the time of the catheterization.

Collaborative Care

The treatment of chronic stable angina is aimed at decreasing oxygen demand and/or increasing oxygen supply. Continued

emphasis on reduction of CAD risk factors is a priority. In addition
to antiplatelet and cholesterol-lowering drug therapy, the most
common therapeutic intervention for chronic stable angina is the
use of nitrate therapy to enhance coronary blood flow. Emergency
care of the patient with chest pain is presented in Table 34-13,
Lewis and others, *Medical-Surgical Nursing*, edition 7, p. 806.
Treatment of chronic stable angina may also include percutaneous coronary intervention with balloon angioplasty and stent
placement.

Drug Therapy

- Antiplatelet aggregation therapy is the first line of drug therapy
  in the treatment of chronic stable angina. Aspirin is the drug
  of choice to reduce the progression of angina to myocardial
  infarction (MI).
- Short-acting nitrates are first-line therapy for the treatment of
  angina. Nitrates produce their principal effects by dilating
  peripheral blood vessels, coronary arteries, and collateral
  vessels. Sublingual nitroglycerin will usually relieve pain in
  approximately 3 minutes and has a duration of approximately
  30 to 60 minutes. If symptoms are unchanged or worse after 5
  minutes, the patient should activate the emergency medication
  services system. Nitroglycerin sublingually can be used prophylactically before undertaking an activity that the patient
  knows may precipitate an anginal attack.
- Long-acting nitrates can be used to reduce the incidence of
  anginal attacks. Longer-acting nitrates are available in oral
  preparations, ointments, and transdermal controlled-release
  patches.
- β-Adrenergic blocking agents, such as propranolol (Inderal)
  and metoprolol (Lopressor), are preferred drugs for management of chronic stable angina. These drugs decrease myocardial contractility, heart rate, systemic vascular resistance
  (SVR), and blood pressure (BP), all of which reduce myocardial O$_2$ demand.
- Calcium blocking agents, such as nifedipine (Procardia),
  verapamil (Calan), diltiazem (Cardizem), and nicardipine
  (Cardene), are used if β-adrenergic blocking agents are contraindicated, poorly tolerated, or do not control symptoms. The
  primary effects of calcium channel blockers are systemic vasodilation with decreased SVR, decreased myocardial contractility, and coronary vasodilation.

Percutaneous Coronary Intervention (PCI)

If a coronary lesion is amenable to an intervention during cardiac
catheterization, coronary revascularization with an elective percutaneous coronary intervention (PCI) may be done.

- A *balloon angioplasty* is performed in a catheterization laboratory. A catheter equipped with a balloon tip is inserted into the narrowed coronary artery. When the lesion is located, the catheter is passed through and just past the lesion, the balloon is inflated, and the atherosclerotic plaque is compressed, resulting in vessel dilation.
- *Intracoronary stents* are often inserted in conjunction with balloon angioplasty. Stents are used to treat abrupt or threatened abrupt closure and restenosis after balloon angioplasty. Stents are expandable, meshlike structures designed to maintain vessel patency by compressing arterial walls and resisting vasoconstriction. Because stents are thrombogenic, patients are usually treated with antiplatelet agents, such as aspirin.
- The most serious complication of PCI is dissection of the newly dilated artery. If the damage is extensive, the coronary artery could rupture, causing cardiac tamponade, ischemia and infarction, and possibly death.
- Primary complications from stent placement are hemorrhage and vascular injury. Additional complications are acute MI, stent embolization, coronary spasm, and emergent coronary artery bypass graft (CABG) surgery. The possibility of dysrhythmias is always present.

Nursing Management
Goals
The patient with chronic stable angina will experience pain relief, have reduced anxiety, have adequate knowledge of the problem and prescribed treatment, and modify or alter risk factors.
Nursing Diagnoses
- Acute pain
- Anxiety
- Ineffective tissue perfusion (cardiac)
- Activity intolerance
Nursing Interventions
- If a nurse is present during an anginal attack, the following measures should be instituted: (1) administration of O_2, (2) determination of vital signs, (3) 12-lead ECG, (4) prompt pain relief with a nitrate followed by an opioid analgesic if needed, (5) auscultation of heart sounds, and (6) comfortable positioning of the patient.

▼ **Patient and Family Teaching**
The patient with a history of chronic stable angina should be reassured that a long, productive life is possible.

- Teaching tools, such as pamphlets, films at the bedside, a heart model, and especially written information, are important components of patient and family education.
- The patient should be assisted in identifying factors that precipitate angina and given instruction on how to avoid or control these factors.
- The patient needs to be assisted in identifying personal risk factors for CAD. Once these risk factors are known, various methods of decreasing them should be discussed.
- Teaching the patient and family about diets that are low in sodium and saturated fat may be appropriate. Maintaining ideal body weight is important in controlling angina, because weight above this level increases myocardial workload.
- Adhering to a regular, individualized exercise program that conditions the myocardium rather than overstressing it is important. Most patients can be advised to walk briskly on a flat surface 30 minutes per day at least 4 or 5 days per week.
- The patient and family should be taught the proper use of nitroglycerin and other medications.
- Counseling should be provided to assess psychologic adjustment of the patient and family to the diagnosis of CAD and resulting angina. Many patients feel a threat to their identity and self-esteem.

ANGINA, PRINZMETAL'S

Description

Prinzmetal's angina *(variant angina)* is a rare form of angina that is frequently seen in patients with a history of migraine headaches and Raynaud's phenomenon. It often occurs at rest, usually in response to spasm of a major coronary artery. The spasm may occur in the absence of coronary artery disease, as well as with documented disease.

- Factors that may precipitate coronary artery spasm include increased myocardial O_2 demand and increased levels of a variety of vasoactive substances, such as histamine, angiotensin, epinephrine, norepinephrine, and prostaglandins.
- When spasm occurs, the patient experiences angina and transient ST-segment elevation. The pain may occur during rapid eye movement (REM) sleep when myocardial O_2 consumption increases. It may be relieved by moderate exercise, or it may disappear spontaneously.

- Cyclic, short bursts of pain at a usual time each day may also occur with this type of angina.
- Coronary angiography is the only way to confirm the diagnosis of Prinzmetal's angina.
- Treatment includes the use of calcium channel blockers and/or nitrates.

ANGINA, UNSTABLE

See Acute Coronary Syndrome.

ANKYLOSING SPONDYLITIS

Description

Ankylosing spondylitis (AS) is a chronic inflammatory disease that primarily affects the axial skeleton, including the sacroiliac joints, intervertebral disk spaces, and costovertebral articulations. Approximately 90% of whites and 50% of African Americans with AS are positive for the HLA-B27 antigen. The highest incidence of AS is in persons 25 to 34 years of age. Men are five times more likely to develop AS than women.

Pathophysiology

The cause of AS is unknown. Genetic predisposition appears to play an important role in disease pathogenesis, but the precise mechanisms are unknown. Aseptic synovial inflammation in joints and adjacent tissue causes the formation of granulation tissue and the development of dense fibrous scars that lead to fusion of articular tissues. Extraarticular inflammation can affect the eyes, lungs, heart, kidneys, and peripheral nervous system.

Clinical Manifestations

Symptoms of inflammatory spine pain are usually the first indications of AS. These include lower back pain, stiffness, and limitation of motion that are worse during the night and in the morning but improve with mild activity. General symptoms such as fever, fatigue, anorexia, and weight loss are rarely present.

Iritis is the most common nonskeletal symptom. It can appear as an initial presentation of the disease years before arthritic symptoms develop.

Severe postural abnormalities and deformity can lead to significant disability. Aortic insufficiency and pulmonary fibrosis are frequent complications. Cauda equina syndrome can also result, contributing to lower extremity weakness and bladder dysfunction.

A

Diagnostic Studies

- Pelvic x-rays demonstrate sacroiliac changes ranging from subtle erosion to completely fused joints in which joint spaces have been obliterated.
- Laboratory testing is not specific, but an elevated erythrocyte sedimentation rate (ESR) and mild anemia may be seen.
- HLA-B27 testing is often done and can be used to exclude AS if negative.

Collaborative Care

Prevention of AS is not possible; however, families with diagnosed HLA-B27–positive rheumatic diseases should be alert to signs of lower back pain and arthritis symptoms so that early therapy can be initiated.

Care of the patient is aimed at maintaining maximal skeletal mobility while decreasing pain and inflammation. Heat applications, nonsteroidal antiinflammatory drugs (NSAIDs) and salicylates, and disease-modifying antirheumatic drugs (DMARDs), such as sulfasalazine (Azulfidine) or methotrexate, can help in the relief of symptoms. Etanercept (Enbrel), a type of biologic therapy, inhibits the action of tumor necrosis factor (TNF) and has been shown to reduce disease activity and improve patient functioning.

Postural control with stretching exercises of the back, neck, and chest is important to minimize spinal deformity. Surgery may be indicated for severe deformity and mobility impairment. Spinal osteotomy and total joint replacement are the most commonly performed procedures.

Nursing Management

Nursing responsibilities include education about the nature of the disease and principles of therapy. A home management program consists of local moist heat, regular exercise, and knowledgeable use of medications.

- Excessive physical exertion during periods of active inflammation should be discouraged.
- Proper positioning at rest is essential. The mattress should be firm, and the patient should sleep on the back with a flat pillow, avoiding positions that encourage flexion deformity.
- Postural training emphasizes avoiding spinal flexion (e.g., leaning over a desk), heavy lifting, and prolonged walking,

standing, or sitting. Sports that facilitate natural stretching, such as swimming and racquet games, should be encouraged.
- Family counseling and vocational rehabilitation are important.

ANORECTAL ABSCESS

Anorectal abscesses are collections of perianal pus resulting from obstruction of the anal glands, leading to infection and abscess formation.
- Common causative organisms are *Escherichia coli,* staphylococci, and streptococci. Manifestations include local pain and swelling, foul-smelling drainage, tenderness, and elevated temperature. Sepsis can occur as a complication. Diagnosis is by rectal examination.
- Surgical therapy consists of abscess drainage. If packing is used, it should be impregnated with petroleum jelly and the area should be allowed to heal by granulation. The packing is changed every day, and moist, hot compresses are applied to the area. Care must be taken to avoid soiling the dressing during urination or defecation. A low-fiber diet is given. The patient may leave the hospital with the area open.
- Discharge teaching should include wound care, importance of sitz baths, thorough cleaning after bowel movements, and follow-up visits to a health care provider.

AORTIC DISSECTION

Description
Aortic dissection is the result of a tear in the intimal (innermost) lining of the arterial wall that allows blood to enter between the intima and media, thus creating a false lumen of blood flow. This process is usually acute and life threatening.
- As the heart contracts, each systolic pulsation causes increased pressure, which further increases dissection. As it extends proximally or distally, it may occlude major branches of the aorta, cutting off blood supply to the brain, abdominal organs, spinal cord, and extremities.

- The exact cause is uncertain. Most people with dissection problems are older or have chronic hypertension. Persons with Marfan syndrome (a connective tissue disease) have a high incidence of dissection. Pregnancy promotes vascular stress because of increased blood volume. Areas prone to dissection are the ascending aorta, aortic arch, and, most commonly, the descending thoracic aorta beyond the origin of the left subclavian artery.

Clinical Manifestations and Complications

The patient with aortic dissection usually has sudden, severe pain in the back, chest, or abdomen. The pain is described as "tearing" or "ripping" and may mimic that of a myocardial infarction. As the dissection progresses, pain may be located both above and below the diaphragm.

- If the arch of the aorta is involved, the patient may exhibit neurologic deficiencies, including altered level of consciousness, dizziness, and weakened or absent carotid and temporal pulses.
- An ascending aortic dissection usually produces some disruption of coronary blood flow and some degree of aortic valvular insufficiency.
- When either subclavian artery is involved, pulse quality and blood pressure (BP) readings may differ significantly between the left and right arms.
- As dissection progresses down the aorta, the abdominal organs and lower extremities may demonstrate evidence of altered tissue perfusion.
- A severe complication of dissection of the ascending aortic arch is *cardiac tamponade,* which occurs when blood escapes from the dissection into the pericardial sac. Clinical manifestations include hypotension, narrowed pulse pressure, distended neck veins, muffled heart sounds, and pulsus paradoxus.
- Because the aorta is weakened by medial dissection, it may rupture. Hemorrhage may occur into the mediastinal, pleural, or abdominal cavities.
- Dissection can lead to occlusion of the arterial supply to many vital organs, including the spinal cord, kidneys, and abdominal structures. Ischemia of the spinal cord produces symptoms varying from weakness to paralysis in lower extremities and decreased pain sensation. Renal ischemia can lead to renal failure. Signs of abdominal ischemia include abdominal pain, decreased bowel sounds, and altered bowel elimination.

Diagnostic Studies
- Chest x-ray indicates widening of the mediastinal silhouette and pleural effusion.
- Computed tomography (CT) scan or magnetic resonance imaging (MRI) is the emergency diagnostic procedure of choice to assess presence and severity of dissection.
- Echocardiogram may indicate left ventricular hypertrophy.
- Angiography may be necessary to assess the extent of dissection after the patient is stabilized.

Collaborative Care
The goal of therapy for aortic dissection without complications is to lower BP and myocardial contractility to decrease the pulsatile forces within the aorta.
- An intravenous (IV) β-adrenergic blocker, such as esmolol (Brevibloc), is typically used to decrease the BP and the force of myocardial contractility. Esmolol is particularly useful since it has a rapid onset and a short half-life.
- Other antihypertensive agents, such as sodium nitroprusside (Nipride), calcium channel blockers, and angiotensin-converting enzyme (ACE) inhibitors, may also be used.
- The patient without complications can be conservatively treated for a period. Supportive treatment is directed toward pain relief, blood transfusion (if required), and management of heart failure (if indicated).
- If dissection involves the ascending aorta, imminent surgery is indicated. Surgery is also indicated when drug therapy is ineffective or when complications of aortic dissection (e.g., heart failure, leaking dissection, occlusion of artery) are present. Surgery is delayed for as long as possible to allow time for edema in the area of dissection to resolve and to permit clotting of blood in the false lumen.
- Surgery for aortic dissection involves resection of the aortic segment containing the intimal tear and replacement with synthetic graft material.

Nursing Management
Interventions related to an aortic dissection include keeping the patient in bed in semi-Fowler's position and maintaining a quiet environment. These measures assist in keeping systolic BP at the lowest possible level to maintain vital organ perfusion. Opioids and tranquilizers should be administered as ordered. Pain and anxiety must be managed because they increase BP.
- Continuous IV administration of antihypertensive agents requires close nursing supervision. Continuous cardiac and

intraarterial pressure monitoring is required. The nurse
should observe for changes in the quality of peripheral
pulses and for signs of increasing pain, restlessness, and
anxiety. If blood vessels branching off the aortic arch are
involved, decreased cerebral blood flow may alter sensorium and level of consciousness.

Postoperative care after surgery to correct the dissection
is similar to that after aortic aneurysm repair (see a nursing care
plan for the patient having surgical repair of the aorta, available
at *http://evolve.elsevier.com/Lewis/medsurg*).

▼ **Patient and Family Teaching**

■ The therapeutic regimen at discharge includes antihypertensive
drugs. The patient needs to understand that these drugs must
be taken to control BP. β-Adrenergic blockers (e.g., metoprolol
[Toprol-XL]) can be taken orally to continue to decrease myocardial contractility.

■ It is important that the patient understand the drug regimen and
potential side effects and to seek immediate help if pain returns
or other symptoms progress.

APPENDICITIS

Description
Appendicitis is an inflammation of the appendix, a narrow blind
tube that extends from the inferior part of the cecum. Appendicitis
occurs in 7% to 12% of the general population, most commonly
in young adults.

Pathophysiology
The most common causes of appendicitis are obstruction of the
lumen by a fecalith (accumulated feces), foreign bodies, a tumor
of the cecum or appendix, or intramural thickening resulting from
hypergrowth of lymphoid tissue. Obstruction results in distention,
venous engorgement, and the accumulation of mucus and bacteria,
which can lead to gangrene and perforation.

Clinical Manifestations and Complications
Appendicitis typically begins with periumbilical pain, followed by
anorexia, nausea, and vomiting. The pain is persistent and continuous, eventually shifting to the right lower quadrant and localizing
at McBurney's point (located halfway between the umbilicus and
right iliac crest).

- Further assessment reveals localized and rebound tenderness with muscle guarding. The patient usually prefers to lie still, often with right leg flexed. Low-grade fever may be present, and coughing aggravates the pain. Rovsing's sign may be elicited by palpation of the left lower quadrant, causing pain to be felt in the right lower quadrant.

Complications of acute appendicitis are perforation, peritonitis, and abscesses.

Diagnostic Studies
- Because diagnosis can be difficult, the standard for diagnosis is an ultrasound or a computed tomography (CT) scan.
- White blood cell (WBC) count may be elevated but is not diagnostic.
- Urinalysis may be done to rule out genitourinary conditions that mimic manifestations of appendicitis.
- A new technique to diagnose appendictitis, NeutroSpec imaging, uses a technetium-labeled anti–CD 15 monoclonal antibody that selectively binds to neutrophils at the infection site. An infection can be detected using a gamma camera, resulting in a diagnosis in less than 1 hour.

Collaborative Care
If diagnosis and treatment are delayed, the appendix can rupture, and the resulting peritonitis can be fatal. Treatment is immediate surgical removal *(appendectomy)* if the inflammation is localized. If the appendix has ruptured and there is evidence of peritonitis or an abscess, conservative treatment, consisting of antibiotic therapy and parenteral fluids, may be used to prevent sepsis and dehydration for 6 to 8 hours before an appendectomy is performed.

Nursing Management
The patient with abdominal pain is encouraged to see a physician and to avoid self-treatment, particularly the use of laxatives and enemas. Increased peristalsis from these procedures may cause perforation.

- Until a health care provider sees the patient, nothing should be taken by mouth (NPO) to ensure the stomach will be empty if surgery is needed.
- An ice bag may be applied to the right lower quadrant to decrease the flow of blood to the area and impede the inflammatory process. Heat is never used because it may cause the appendix to rupture.

Surgery is performed, generally laparoscopically, as soon as a diagnosis is made. Postoperative nursing management is similar to postoperative care of a patient after laparotomy (see Abdominal

Pain, Acute, p. 3). In addition, the patient should be observed for
evidence of peritonitis. Ambulation begins the day of surgery or
the first postoperative day. Diet is advanced as tolerated.

- The patient is usually discharged on the first or second
  postoperative day, and normal activities are resumed 2 to 3
  weeks after surgery.

ASTHMA

Description
Asthma is a chronic inflammatory disease that causes an increase
in airway hyperresponsiveness that leads to recurrent episodes of
wheezing, breathlessness, chest tightness, and cough, particularly
at night and in the early morning. These episodes are associated
with widespread but variable airflow obstruction that is usually
reversible, either spontaneously or with treatment. The clinical
course of asthma is unpredictable, ranging from paroxysms of
dyspnea and wheezing to unremitting symptoms.

- Asthma affects an estimated 20 million people in the United
  States. Mortality and morbidity rates from asthma appear
  to have plateaued and/or decreased, yet there are more than
  4000 deaths per year from asthma. The death rate is 42%
  higher in females than in males and three times higher in
  African Americans than in whites.

Pathophysiology
The primary pathophysiologic process in asthma is chronic inflammation that leads to airway hyperresponsiveness (hyperreactivity)
and acute airflow limitation. Although the exact mechanisms that
cause asthma are unknown, triggers are involved and exposure
to allergens or irritants initiates the inflammatory cascade
(Table 11).

Table 11	Triggers of Acute Asthma Attacks
Allergen inhalation	Drugs
Air pollutants	Occupational exposure
Viral upper respiratory infection	Food additives
Sinusitis	Hormones/menses
Exercise and cold, dry air	Gastroesophageal reflux
Stress	disease (GERD)

- As the inflammatory process begins, mast cells in the bronchial wall degranulate and release multiple inflammatory mediators. Common mediators are leukotrienes, histamine, cytokines, prostaglandins, and nitric oxide.
- The resulting inflammatory process results in vascular congestion; edema formation; production of thick, tenacious mucus; bronchial muscle spasm; thickening of airway walls; and increased bronchial hyperresponsiveness.
- This process can occur within 30 to 60 minutes after exposure to a trigger or irritant and is sometimes referred to as the *early-phase response* in asthma.

Symptoms can recur 4 to 10 hours after the initial attack because of eosinophil and lymphocyte activation and further release of more inflammatory mediators.

- This delayed response is called the *late-phase response* in asthma. It can be more severe than the early-phase response and can persist for 24 hours or more.
- A self-sustaining cycle of inflammation occurs, limiting airflow as a result of airway swelling with or without bronchoconstriction. Corticosteroids are effective in treating this inflammation.

Chronic, untreated inflammation results in structural changes in the bronchial wall known as *remodeling*.

- The bronchial smooth mucles hypertrophy, collagen is deposited in the airway walls, and mucus-secreting cells undergo hyperplasia. There is evidence that remodeling can be prevented by early introduction of inhaled corticosteroids.

During an asthma attack, decreased perfusion and ventilation of the alveoli and increased alveolar gas pressure lead to ventilation-perfusion abnormalities in the lungs.

- The patient will be hypoxemic early on with decreased $PaCO_2$ and increased pH (respiratory alkalosis) as a result of hyperventilation.
- As the airflow limitation worsens with air trapping, the $PaCO_2$ normalizes and then rises to produce respiratory acidosis, which is an ominous sign signifying respiratory failure.

Clinical Manifestations

Asthma attacks may have an abrupt or gradual onset and may last a few minutes to several hours; a person may be asymptomatic with normal pulmonary function between attacks.

- Characteristic manifestations are wheezing, cough, dyspnea, and chest tightness. Expiration may be prolonged with an inspiratory/expiratory (I/E) ratio of 1:3 or 1:4.

- Wheezing is an unreliable sign to gauge the severity of an attack because many patients with minor attacks wheeze loudly, whereas others with severe attacks do not wheeze.
- In some patients with asthma, cough is the only symptom. The cough may be nonproductive because secretions may be so thick, tenacious, and gelatinous that their removal is difficult.
- During an acute attack, the patient usually sits upright or slightly bent forward using accessory muscles of respiration, and the respiratory rate is usually more than 30 breaths per minute.
- Signs of hypoxemia include restlessness, increased anxiety, inappropriate behavior, and increased pulse and blood pressure (BP).
- Percussion reveals hyperresonance of the lungs. Auscultation usually reveals inspiratory or expiratory wheezing.
- Severely diminished breath sounds, or a "silent chest," is an ominous sign, indicating severe obstruction and impending respiratory failure. Diminished or absent breath sounds may also indicate atelectasis or pneumothorax.

Classification of Asthma

Asthma can be classified as mild intermittent, mild persistent, moderate persistent, or severe persistent (Table 12). Patients may progress up or down in asthma level severity over the course of their disease. Good asthma control correlates with minimal symptoms, ability to sleep through the night, and ability to participate in sports, exercise, and strenuous activity.

Complications

Severe acute asthma can result in complications such as rib fractures, pneumothorax, pneumomediastinum, atelectasis, pneumonia, and status asthmaticus.

Status asthmaticus is a severe, life-threatening complication of asthma that is refractory to usual treatment and places the patient at risk for respiratory failure.

- Causes of status asthmaticus include viral illnesses, ingestion of aspirin or nonsteroidal antiinflammatory drugs (NSAIDs), emotional stress, an increase in allergen exposure, abrupt discontinuation of drug therapy (especially corticosteroids), abuse of aerosol medication, and ingestion of β-adrenergic blockers. The patient usually reports a history of poorly controlled asthma progressing over days or weeks.

Table 12 Classification of Asthma Severity

Classification	Symptoms	Nighttime Symptoms	Pulmonary Function*
Step 1 Mild Intermittent	Symptoms ≤2 times/wk Asymptomatic and with normal PEFR between exacerbations Exacerbations brief (hours to days) Intensity of exacerbations varies	≤2 times/mo	FEV_1/PEFR ≥80% of that predicted PEFR variability <20%
Step 2 Mild Persistent	Symptoms >2 times/wk but <1 time/day Exacerbations may affect activity	>2 times/mo	FEV_1/PEFR ≥80% of predicted PEFR variability 20%-30%
Step 3 Moderate Persistent	Daily symptoms Daily use of inhaled short-acting β_2-agonist Exacerbations affect activity Exacerbations at least 2 times/wk and may last for days	>1 time/wk	FEV_1/PEFR >60% but <80% of predicted PEFR variability >30%
Step 4 Severe Persistent	Continual symptoms Limited physical activity Frequent exacerbations	Frequent	FEV_1/PEFR ≤60% of predicted PEFR variability >30%

From *Practical guide for the diagnosis and management of asthma, based on expert panel report 2: guidelines for the diagnosis and management of asthma,* Washington, DC, 1997, National Institutes of Health.
* Percent predicted values for forced expiratory volume in 1 second (FEV_1) and percent of personal best for peak expiratory flow rate (PEFR). Patients should be assigned to the most severe step in which any feature occurs. Clinical features for individual patients may overlap across steps. An individual's classification may change over time.

■ Clinical manifestations are similar to those of asthma, but they are more severe and prolonged. Extreme anxiety, fear of suffocation, severely increased work of breathing, and diaphoresis are common.

■ Hypertension, sinus tachycardia, and ventricular dysrhythmias may also occur.

■ Complications from status asthmaticus include pneumothorax, pneumomediastinum, acute cor pulmonale, and respiratory muscle fatigue leading to respiratory arrest.

■ Death from status asthmaticus is usually the result of respiratory arrest or cardiac failure.

Diagnostic Studies

■ Detailed history may help identify asthma triggers.

■ Pulmonary function studies including response to bronchodilator therapy are necessary to diagnose asthma and give an objective measure of airflow obstruction.

■ Sputum specimen, if indicated, can rule out bacterial infection.

■ Elevated serum IgE levels and eosinophil count are suggestive of allergic tendency.

■ Chest x-ray during an attack shows hyperinflation.

■ Arterial blood gases (ABGs) with mild attack show respiratory alkalosis with an arterial O_2 pressure (PaO_2) near normal. Hypercapnia and respiratory acidosis indicate severe disease.

■ Nitric oxide levels are increased in the breath of people with asthma.

■ Serial peak expiratory flow rates (PEFR), pulse oximetry, and ABGs provide information about severity of attack and response to treatment.

■ Allergy testing may indicate the specific allergen causing the attack.

Collaborative Care

■ Education remains the cornerstone of asthma management and should start at the time of asthma diagnosis and be integrated into every step of clinical asthma care.

■ Prevention management includes teaching the patient who has persistent airflow obstruction and frequent attacks of asthma to avoid triggers of acute attacks and to premedicate before exercising.

Drug therapy for asthma depends on the patient's classification of severity of symptoms (see Table 12).

■ The patient with *mild intermittent asthma* should use inhaled β_2-adrenergic agonists, cromolyn (Intal), or nedo-

cromil (Tilade) before exercising or when expecting exposure to triggers.

In all patients with *persistent asthma,* inhaled corticosteroids
(ICSs) are the preferred treatment as the daily, long-term control
medication.

- In *mild persistent asthma,* cromolyn, nedocromil, or one
  of the leukotriene receptor blockers (e.g., montelukast
  [Singulair]) is an alternate treatment if the desired effect is
  not reached with low-dose ICS.

- *Moderate persistent asthma* requires daily use of inhaled
  low- or medium-dose ICS that may be combined with a long-
  acting inhaled β_2 agonist (e.g., salmeterol [Serevent]) either
  as a separate medication or in combination (e.g., fluticasone/
  salmeterol [Advair]). Alternatively, in conjunction with the
  ICS, montelukast or theophylline can be used.

- For *severe persistent asthma,* a combination of high-dose
  ICS and inhaled β_2 agonists (e.g., Advair) is used to alleviate symptoms. Some persons require continuous oral corticosteroids, which should be maintained at as low a dosage
  as possible and administered on alternate days (if possible)
  to reduce systemic side effects.

For a list of drugs used in the treatment of asthma and chronic
obstructive pulmonary disease (COPD), see Table 29-7, Lewis and
others, *Medical-Surgical Nursing,* edition 7, pp. 618 to 620.

The choice of treatment of an *acute asthma attack* depends on
the severity of the attack and response to initial therapy.

- Oxygen therapy should be started immediately and monitored with pulse oximetry or ABGs.

- Initial therapy includes an inhaled β_2-adrenergic agonist
  administered by metered-dose inhaler (MDI) or nebulizer
  every 20 minutes for 1 hour; the anticholinergic medication
  ipratropium (Atrovent) is nebulized with the β_2-agonist if
  the exacerbation is severe.

- Corticosteroids are indicated if the initial response to the
  β_2-agonist is insufficient, and therapy is continued until the
  patient is breathing comfortably, wheezing has disappeared,
  and pulmonary function study results are near baseline values.

Management of the patient with *status asthmaticus* includes
most of the therapeutic measures for acute asthma.

- The frequency and dose of inhaled bronchodilators may be
  increased, and intravenous (IV) corticosteroids are
  administered.

- Supplemental oxygen, IV fluids, and an arterial catheter are
  initiated. If there is no response to treatment, intubation and
  mechanical ventilation may be indicated.

Nursing Management

Goals

The patient with asthma will maintain >80% of personal best PEFR or FEV_1 and will have minimal symptoms during the day and night, acceptable activity levels (including exercise and other physical activity), no recurrent exacerbations of asthma or decreased incidence of asthma attacks, and adequate knowledge to participate in and carry out management.

See NCP 29-1 for the patient with asthma, Lewis and others, *Medical-Surgical Nursing,* edition 7, pp. 625 to 626.

Nursing Diagnoses

- Ineffective airway clearance
- Anxiety
- Deficient knowledge

Nursing Interventions

During an acute attack of asthma, it is important to monitor the patient's respiratory and cardiovascular systems. This includes auscultating lung sounds; taking pulse rate, respiratory rate, and BP; and monitoring ABGs, pulse oximetry, and PEFR. The patient's work of breathing (i.e., use of accessory muscles, degree of fatigue) and response to therapy should also be evaluated. Findings that warrant urgent medical intervention to avoid respiratory failure include:

- Heart rate >120 beats/min, pulsus paradoxus, respiratory rate >30 breaths/min, wheezes heard on auscultation that turn silent, speaking only in words (not sentences), oxygen saturation <90%, PaO_2 <60 mm Hg, $PaCO_2$ >45 mm Hg, PEFR < 100 L/min, and agitation.
- Nursing interventions include administering oxygen (O_2), bronchodilators, and medications (as ordered) and ongoing patient monitoring (especially lung auscultation).
- An important nursing goal during an acute attack is to decrease the patient's sense of panic. A calm, quiet, reassuring attitude may help the patient relax. The patient should be positioned comfortably (usually sitting) to maximize chest expansion. Staying with the patient and being available to the patient provide additional comfort. Encouraging slow breathing through pursed lips can be helpful.

▼ Patient and Family Teaching

The nursing role in preventing asthma attacks or decreasing their severity focuses on teaching the patient and family (Table 13).

- The patient should be taught to avoid known personal triggers for asthma (e.g., cigarette smoke, pet dander) and irritants (e.g., cold air, aspirin, foods, cats). If cold air cannot be avoided, dressing properly with a scarf or mask helps

Table 13	Patient and Family Teaching Guide: Asthma

Teaching Topic
- What Is Asthma?
- What Is Good Asthma Control?
- Hindrances to Asthma Treatment and Control
- Environmental/Trigger Control
- Medications
- Correct Use of Metered-Dose Inhaler, Dry Powder Inhaler, Spacer, and Nebulizer
- Breathing Techniques
- Correct Use of Peak Flowmeter
- Asthma Action Plan

reduce the risk of an asthma attack. Aspirin and NSAIDs should be avoided if they are known to precipitate an attack. Many over-the-counter (OTC) drugs contain aspirin, and the patient should be instructed to read labels carefully.

- β-Adrenergic blocking agents (e.g., propranolol [Inderal]) should not be used because they inhibit bronchodilation.
- Because the patient with asthma takes several different medications with different routes and frequencies, the drug regimen can be confusing and complex. The patient must learn about the numerous medications and develop self-management strategies. Some patients may benefit from keeping a diary to record medication use, presence of wheezing or coughing, PEFR, drug side effects, and activity level. This information will be valuable in helping the health care provider adjust the medication.

A written asthma management plan should be developed together with the patient and family (see Table 29-13, Lewis and others, *Medical-Surgical Nursing,* edition 7, p. 627). Most plans are based on the patient's asthma symptoms and peak flow monitoring. The plan should require peak flow monitoring at least daily and should describe what the patient and family need to do when symptoms become worse. Family members need to know where the patient's inhalers, oral medication, and emergency phone numbers are located. Family members can also be instructed on how to decrease patient anxiety if an asthma attack occurs.

- The patient should be taught to maintain a fluid intake of 2 to 3 L/day, good nutrition, and adequate rest. Physical exercise (e.g., swimming, walking, stationary cycling) within the patient's limit of tolerance can be performed with the use of preexercise bronchodilators.

- Counseling may be indicated to help the patient and family resolve personal, family, social, and occupational problems that have resulted from asthma.

BELL'S PALSY

Description
Bell's palsy (peripheral facial paralysis, acute benign cranial polyneuritis) is a disorder characterized by a disruption of motor branches of the facial nerve (CN VII) on one side of the face in the absence of any other disease, such as a stroke.

- The exact etiology is not known, but current theories suggest that reactivated herpes simplex virus (HSV) may be involved in some cases.
- Onset of Bell's palsy is often accompanied by an outbreak of herpes vesicles in or around the ear.
- Bell's palsy is considered benign with full recovery after 6 months in about 85% of patients, especially if treatment is instituted immediately.

Clinical Manifestations
Paralysis of the motor branches of the facial nerve typically results in a flaccidity of the affected side of the face, with drooping of the mouth accompanied by drooling. Inability to close the eyelid, with an upward movement of the eyeball when closure is attempted, is also evident.

- A widened palpebral fissure (opening between the eyelids), flattening of the nasolabial fold, unilateral loss of taste, and inability to smile, frown, or whistle are also common.
- Fever, tinnitus, and a hearing deficit may occur.
- Decreased muscle movement may alter chewing ability, and some patients may experience a loss of tearing or excessive tearing.
- Pain may be present behind the ear on the affected side, especially before the onset of paralysis.

Complications can include psychologic withdrawal because of changes in appearance, malnutrition and dehydration, mucous membrane trauma, corneal abrasions, and facial spasms and contractures.

Diagnosis of Bell's palsy is one of exclusion. Diagnosis and prognosis are indicated by observation of the typical pattern of onset and the testing of percutaneous nerve excitability by electromyogram (EMG).

Collaborative Care
Methods of treatment include moist heat, gentle massage, and electrical stimulation of the nerve. Stimulation may maintain muscle tone and prevent atrophy. Care is primarily focused on relief of symptoms and prevention of complications.

- Corticosteroids, especially prednisone, are started immediately, and best results are obtained if corticosteroids are initiated before paralysis is complete. When the patient improves to the point that corticosteroids are no longer necessary, they should be tapered off over 2 weeks. Usually corticosteroid treatment decreases edema and pain, but mild analgesics can be used if necessary.
- Because HSV is implicated in many cases of Bell's palsy, treatment with acyclovir (Zovirax) alone or in conjunction with prednisone is used. Valacyclovir (Valtrex) and famciclovir (Famvir) have also been used.

Nursing Management
Goals
The patient with Bell's palsy will be pain free or have pain controlled, maintain adequate nutritional status, maintain appropriate oral hygiene, not experience injury to the eye, return to normal or previous perception of body image, and be optimistic about disease outcome.
Nursing Diagnoses
- Acute pain
- Imbalanced nutrition: less than body requirements
- Risk for injury (corneal abrasion)
- Disturbed body image
Nursing Interventions
- Mild analgesics can relieve pain. Hot wet packs can reduce discomfort of herpetic lesions, aid circulation, and relieve pain.
- The face should be protected from cold and drafts because trigeminal hyperesthesia (extreme sensitivity to pain or touch) may accompany the syndrome.
- Maintenance of good nutrition is important. The patient should be taught to chew on the unaffected side of the mouth to avoid trapping food and to improve taste. Thorough oral hygiene must be carried out after each meal to prevent development of

parotitis, caries, and periodontal disease from accumulated residual food.

- Dark glasses may be worn for protective and cosmetic reasons. Artificial tears (methylcellulose) should be instilled frequently during the day to prevent corneal drying. Ointment and an impermeable eye shield can be used at night to retain moisture. In some patients taping the lids closed at night may be necessary to provide protection.

- A facial sling may be helpful to support affected muscles, improve lip alignment, and facilitate eating. Vigorous massage can break down tissues, but gentle upward massage has psychologic benefits. When function begins to return, active facial exercises are performed several times per day.

- Change in physical appearance can be devastating; the patient needs to be reassured that a stroke did not occur and that chances for a full recovery are good. The patient's need for privacy should be respected, especially during meals. Enlisting support from family and friends is important.

BENIGN PROSTATIC HYPERPLASIA

Description

Benign prostatic hyperplasia (BPH) is an enlargement of the prostate gland resulting from an increase in the number of epithelial cells and stromal tissue. It is the most common urologic problem of the adult male.

- BPH occurs in about 50% of men older than 50 years and 90% of men older than 80 years. Approximately 25% of men require treatment by age 80 years.
- Prostatic hyperplasia does not predispose a patient to the development of prostate cancer.

Pathophysiology

Although the cause is not completely understood, it is thought that BPH results from endocrine changes associated with aging.

- Excessive accumulation of dihydroxytestosterone (the principal intraprostatic androgen), estrogen stimulation, and local growth hormone action are proposed causes.
- The enlargement of the gland gradually compresses the urethra, causing partial or complete obstruction.
- The location of the enlargement rather than the size of the prostate is most significant in the development of obstructive symptoms.

Clinical Manifestations

The patient seeks assistance for relief of symptoms that have worsened as urethral obstruction has gradually increased. Symptoms fall into one of two groups: obstructive symptoms and irritative symptoms.

- Obstructive symptoms of BPH develop as a result of urinary retention and include a decrease in the caliber and force of the urinary stream, difficulty in initiating voiding, and dribbling at the end of urination.
- Irritative symptoms, including urinary frequency, urgency, dysuria, bladder pain, nocturia, and incontinence, are related to inflammation and infection.

The majority of complications result from urinary obstruction and urinary retention.

- Acute urinary retention is common and is an indication for surgical intervention in about 25% to 30% of patients.
- Urinary tract infection is also a common complication because of incomplete bladder emptying and residual urine that provides a favorable environment for bacterial growth.
- Calculi may develop in the bladder because of alkalination of the residual urine.
- Hydronephrosis and pyelonephritis caused by back pressure of urine in an obstructed system may lead to renal failure.

Diagnostic Studies

- Physical examination including digital rectal examination (DRE) for prostate size, symmetry, and consistency
- Urinalysis with culture to identify infection or inflammation
- Postvoid residual urine volume to assess degree of urine flow obstruction
- Prostate-specific antigen (PSA) measured to rule out prostate cancer
- Urodynamic flow studies and transrectal ultrasound scan of prostate
- Cystourethroscopy to evaluate bladder neck obstruction for surgical candidates

Collaborative Care

The initial conservative treatment for BPH is referred to as "watchful waiting." If the patient begins to have signs or symptoms that are bothersome or indicate a complication, further treatment is indicated. There are numerous treatment options for BPH.

Drug Therapy. Drugs are often used to treat BPH with variable results.

- 5-α-Reductase inhibitors reduce the size of the prostate gland. Finasteride (Proscar) blocks the enzyme needed to convert testosterone to dihydroxytestosterone, the principal intraprostatic androgen. This results in a regression of hyperplastic tissue. Dutasteride (Duagen) has the same effect as finasteride and may also be used.

- α₁-Adrenergic receptor blockers cause smooth muscle relaxation in prostate tissue, which ultimately facilitates urinary flow through the urethra. α₁-Adrenergic receptor blockers, such as alfuzosin (Uroxatral), doxazosin (Cardura), terazosin (Hytrin), and tamsulosin (Flomax), are currently being used.

Herbal Therapy. Plant extracts have been used in the management of BPH. Saw palmetto *(Serenoa repens),* specifically, has been shown to improve urinary symptoms and urinary flow measures.

Invasive Therapy. Invasive therapy is indicated when there is a decrease in urine flow sufficient to cause discomfort, persistent residual urine, acute urinary retention because of obstruction with no reversible precipitating cause, or hydronephrosis. Advantages and disadvantages of the various nonsurgical invasive treatment options are compared in Table 55-3, Lewis and others, *Medical-Surgical Nursing,* edition 7, p. 1418.

- Invasive treatment of symptomatic BPH primarily involves resection or ablation of the prostate. The selection of a surgical approach depends on size and position of the prostatic enlargement as well as surgical risk.

Transurethral resection of the prostate (TURP) is a surgical procedure involving removal of prostate tissue using a resectoscope inserted through the urethra. TURP has long been considered the "gold standard" surgical treatment of obstructing BPH. A large three-way indwelling catheter with a 30-ml balloon containing sterile water is usually inserted into the bladder after the procedure to provide hemostasis and facilitate urinary drainage. The bladder is irrigated, either continuously or intermittently, for at least 24 hours to prevent obstruction from mucous threads and blood clots.

Transurethral incision of the prostate (TUIP) is performed with the patient under local anesthesia and is indicated for men with moderate to severe symptoms and small prostates who are poor surgical candidates.

Minimally Invasive Therapy. Minimally invasive therapies generally do not require hospitalization or catheterization and have lower risk of complications.

Transurethral microwave thermotherapy (TUMT) is an outpatient procedure that involves the delivery of microwaves directly to the prostate through a transurethral probe. The temperature of the prostate tissue is raised to about 113° F (45° C) causing necrosis, thus relieving the obstruction.

Transurethral needle ablation (TUNA) is another outpatient procedure that increases the temperature of prostate tissue, thus causing localized necrosis. TUNA differs from TUMT in that only prostate tissue in direct contact with the needle is affected, allowing greater precision in removal of the target tissue.

Laser procedures to treat BPH are used in a variety of approaches. The laser beam is delivered transurethrally through a fiber instrument and is used for cutting, coagulation, and vaporization of prostatic tissue.

Nursing Management

Because the nurse is most directly involved with the care of patients having prostatic surgery, the focus of nursing management is on preoperative and postoperative care.

Goals

Overall preoperative goals for the patient having prostatic surgery are to have restoration of urinary drainage, treatment of any urinary tract infection, and understanding of the upcoming surgery. Overall postoperative goals are that the patient will have no complications, complete bladder emptying, restoration of urinary control, and satisfying sexual expression.

See NCP 55-1 for the patient undergoing prostate surgery, Lewis and others, *Medical-Surgical Nursing,* edition 7, p. 1420.

Nursing Diagnoses

Preoperative
- Acute pain
- Fear
- Risk for infection

Postoperative
- Acute pain
- Urge urinary incontinence
- Risk for infection
- Ineffective therapeutic regimen management

Nursing Interventions

The cause of BPH is largely attributed to the aging process. The focus of health promotion is on early detection and treatment. The American Cancer Society recommends a yearly medical history and digital rectal examination (DRE) for men over 50 years old for early detection of prostate problems. When symptoms of prostatic hyperplasia become evident, further diagnostic screening may be necessary.

- Some men find that ingestion of alcohol and caffeine tends to increase prostatic symptoms because of the diuretic effect that increases bladder distention. Compounds found in common cough and cold remedies, such as pseudoephed-

rine (in Sudafed) and phenylephrine (in Allerest or Cori-
cidin preparations), often worsen BPH symptoms.

- Patients with obstructive symptoms should be advised to
  urinate every 2 to 3 hours or when they first feel the urge
  to minimize urinary stasis and acute urinary retention.

Preoperative Care. Urinary drainage must be restored before
surgery; a urethral catheter such as a coudé (curved-tip) catheter
may be needed.

- Any infection of the urinary tract must be treated before
  surgery. Restoring drainage and encouraging a high fluid
  intake (2 to 3 L/day) are helpful.
- The patient is usually concerned about the impact of
  impending surgery on sexual function. The nurse should
  provide an opportunity for the patient and his partner to
  express their concerns.

Postoperative Care. The plan of care should be adjusted to the
type of surgery, reasons for surgery, and patient response to
surgery. Main complications after surgery are infection, urinary
incontinence, hemorrhage, and bladder spasms.

- After prostatectomy, the bladder may be continuously irrigated with sterile normal saline solution to remove clotted
  blood from the bladder and ensure drainage of urine. Some
  form of irrigation (continuous or intermittent) may be used
  for 24 hours or until no clots are noted draining from the
  bladder.
- Blood clots are normal for the first 24 to 36 hours. However,
  large amounts of bright red blood in the urine can indicate
  hemorrhage.
- The rate of infusion of continuous bladder irrigation (CBI)
  fluid should be at a rate to keep the urine drainage light pink
  without clots.
- The catheter should be connected to a closed drainage
  system and not disconnected unless it is being removed,
  changed, or irrigated. Secretions that accumulate around
  the meatus can be cleansed daily with soap and water.
- Bladder spasms occur as a result of irritation of the bladder
  mucosa from insertion of a resectoscope, presence of a
  catheter, or clots leading to obstruction of the catheter. The
  patient should be instructed not to attempt to urinate around
  the catheter because this increases the likelihood of spasm.
  If bladder spasms develop, the catheter should be checked
  for clots. If present, the clots should be removed by irrigation so urine can flow freely. Belladonna and opium suppositories, along with relaxation techniques, are used to
  relieve pain and decrease spasm.

- Sphincter tone may be poor immediately after catheter removal, resulting in urinary incontinence or dribbling. Sphincter tone can be strengthened by having the patient practice Kegel exercises (pelvic floor muscle technique). Continence can improve for up to 12 months. If continence has not been achieved by that time, the patient may be referred to a continence clinic; a variety of methods, including biofeedback, have been used to achieve positive results. The patient can also use a penile clamp, condom catheter, or incontinent briefs to avoid embarrassment from dribbling.
- The patient should be observed for signs of postoperative infection. If an external wound is present, the area should be observed for redness, heat, swelling, and purulent drainage. Rectal procedures, such as rectal temperatures and enemas (except insertion of well-lubricated belladonna and opium suppositories), should be avoided.
- Activities that increase abdominal pressure, such as sitting or walking for prolonged periods and straining to have a bowel movement, should be avoided.
- Dietary intervention and stool softeners are important to prevent the patient from straining while having bowel movements. Straining increases intraabdominal pressure, which can lead to bleeding at the operative site. A diet high in fiber facilitates the passage of stool.

▼ Patient and Family Teaching

Discharge planning and home care issues are important aspects of postprostatectomy care.

- Instructions include (1) caring for an indwelling catheter, if one is in place; (2) managing urinary incontinence; (3) maintaining oral fluids between 2 and 3 L/day; (4) observing for signs and symptoms of urinary tract and wound infection; (5) preventing constipation; (6) avoiding heavy lifting (>10 lb [>4.5 kg]); and (7) refraining from driving or sexual intercourse as directed by the physician.
- Many men experience retrograde ejaculation after prostatectomy because of trauma to the internal sphincter. Semen is discharged into the bladder at orgasm and may produce cloudy urine when the patient urinates after orgasm. The nurse should discuss these changes with the patient and his partner and allow them to ask questions and express their concerns.
- Sexual counseling and treatment options may be necessary if erectile dysfunction becomes a chronic or permanent problem.
- The bladder may take up to 2 months to return to its normal capacity. The patient should be instructed to drink at least

2 L of fluid per day and to urinate every 2 to 3 hours to flush the urinary tract. Bladder irritants such as caffeine products, citrus juices, and alcohol should be avoided or limited to small amounts.

- The patient must be advised that he should continue to have yearly DREs if he has had any procedure other than complete removal of the prostate. Hyperplasia or cancer can occur in the remaining prostatic tissue.

BLADDER CANCER

Description
The most frequent malignant tumor of the urinary tract is transitional cell carcinoma of the bladder, which accounts for nearly 1 in every 20 cancers diagnosed in the United States. Cancer of the bladder is most common between the ages of 60 and 70 years and is at least three times as common in men as in women.

Risk factors for bladder cancer include cigarette smoking, exposure to dyes used in the rubber and cable industries, and long-term use of phenacetin-containing analgesics. Individuals with chronic, recurrent renal calculi and chronic lower urinary tract infections also have an increased risk of squamous cell bladder cancer. Women treated with radiation for cervical cancer and patients receiving cyclophosphamide (Cytoxan) also have an increased risk; the reason is unknown.

Clinical Manifestations
- Gross, painless hematuria (chronic or intermittent) is the most common clinical finding. Bladder irritability with dysuria, frequency, and urgency may also occur.
- When cancer is suspected, urine specimens for cytology can be obtained to determine the presence of neoplastic or atypical cells.

Diagnostic Studies
Bladder cancer can be detected by intravenous pyelogram (IVP), ultrasound, computed tomography (CT), or magnetic resonance imaging (MRI). Bladder cancer is confirmed by cystoscopy and biopsy.

Clinical staging is determined by the depth of invasion of the bladder wall and surrounding tissue. Bladder tumors are staged using the Jewett-Strong-Marshall system. This system broadly classifies bladder cancer as superficial, invasive, or metastatic disease.

- Pathologic grading systems are also used to classify the malignant potential of tumor cells, indicating a scale ranging from well differentiated to anaplastic.
- Low-stage, low-grade, superficial bladder cancers are most common, most responsive to treatment, and more easily cured.

Nursing and Collaborative Management

Surgical therapy may involve a variety of procedures including the following:

- *Transurethral resection with fulguration* (electrocautery) is used for diagnosis and treatment of superficial lesions with a low recurrence rate. This procedure is also used to control bleeding in patients who are poor operative risks or who have advanced tumors.
- *Laser photocoagulation* can be repeated a number of times for superficial bladder cancer and recurrence. Advantages of this procedure include bloodless destruction of lesions, minimal risk of perforation, and the lack of a need for a urinary catheter.
- *Open loop resection* (snaring of polyp-type lesions) *with fulguration* is used to control bleeding for large superficial tumors and multiple lesions. Treatment of large lesions entails a segmental resection of the bladder.

Postoperative management of the patient who has had one of these surgical procedures includes instructions to drink large amounts of fluid each day for the first week after the procedure, avoid alcoholic beverages, use opioid analgesics and stool softeners if necessary, and take sitz baths to promote muscle relaxation and reduce urinary retention.

- The nurse should also help the patient and family cope with fears about cancer, surgery, and sexuality and should emphasize the importance of regular follow-up care. Frequent routine cystoscopies are required.

When the tumor is invasive or involves the trigone (area where ureters insert into the bladder) and the patient is free from metastases beyond the pelvic area, a partial or radical cystectomy with urinary diversion is the treatment of choice.

- A *partial cystectomy* includes resection of that portion of the bladder wall containing the tumor, along with a margin of normal tissue.
- A *radical cystectomy* involves removal of the bladder, prostate, and seminal vesicles in men and the bladder, uterus, cervix, urethra, and ovaries in women.

Radiation therapy is used with cystectomy or as the primary therapy when the cancer is inoperable or when surgery is refused. Increasingly, radiation therapy is being combined with systemic chemotherapy.

- Cisplatin (Platinol), vinblastine (Velban), doxorubicin (Adriamycin), and methotrexate (Folex) are chemotherapeutic agents that may be used systemically before surgery, before radiation, or for distant metastases.

Chemotherapy with local instillation of chemotherapeutic or immune-stimulating agents can be delivered into the bladder through a urethral catheter, usually at weekly intervals for 6 to 12 weeks.

- These intravesical agents are instilled directly into the patient's bladder and retained for about 2 hours; position of the patient may be changed every 15 minutes for maximum contact in all areas of the bladder.
- Bacille Calmette-Guérin (BCG), a weakened strain of *Mycobacterium bovis,* is the treatment of choice for carcinoma in situ. When BCG is ineffective, α-interferon, thiotepa (Thioplex) and/or valrubicin (Valstar) may be used.
- Most patients have irritative voiding symptoms and hemorrhagic cystitis following intravesical therapy.

It is important for the nurse to encourage the patient to increase daily fluid intake and to quit smoking, assess the patient for secondary urinary infection, and stress the need for routine urology follow-up care. The patient may have fears or concerns about sexual activity or bladder function that will also need to be addressed.

BONE CANCER

Description

Primary malignant bone neoplasms are rare in adults. Metastatic bone cancer in which the cancer has spread from another site is a more common problem. Primary bone cancer is called *sarcoma.* The more common types of primary bone cancer are osteogenic sarcoma, chondrosarcoma, Ewing's sarcoma, and chordoma (Table 14).

Osteogenic Sarcoma (Osteosarcoma)

Osteogenic sarcoma is a primary neoplasm of bone that is extremely aggressive and rapidly metastasizes to distant sites. It

Table 14	Types of Primary Bone Cancer
Type	**Description**
Osteogenic sarcoma	Most common type of bone cancer; occurs mostly in young males between ages 10-25 yr; most often in bones of arms, legs, or pelvis
Chondrosarcoma	Occurs in cartilage cells most commonly in the arms, legs, and pelvic bones of adults ages 50-70 yr; can also arise from benign bone tumors; wide surgical resection most effective treatment
Ewing's sarcoma	Develops in medullary cavity of long bones, especially the femur, humerus, pelvis, and tibia; usually occurs in children and teenagers; use of surgery, chemotherapy, and radiation has increased 5-yr survival rate to 60%
Chordoma	Rare tumor that occurs in base of skull and vertebral bones of adults ages 50-70 yr; involvement of spinal cord and nerves limits use of surgery and radiation; may recur 10 or more yr after treatment

usually occurs in the metaphyseal region of long bones of the extremities, particularly in regions of the distal femur, proximal tibia, and proximal humerus, as well as the pelvis.

Clinical manifestations are usually associated with a past history of minor injury and gradual onset of pain and swelling, especially around the knee. The injury does not cause the neoplasm but rather serves to bring the preexisting condition to medical attention. Joint motion can be restricted if the tumor is close to a joint structure.

Diagnosis is confirmed from biopsy tissue specimens, elevation of serum alkaline phosphatase and calcium levels, and findings on x-ray, computed tomography (CT) or positron emission tomography (PET) scans, and magnetic resonance imaging (MRI). Metastasis is present in 10% to 20% of individuals on diagnosis, with the lung being the most frequent site.

Major advances are being made in treatment. Preoperative chemotherapy is used to decrease tumor size. As a result, limb-salvage surgical procedures are being used more frequently. Amputation (see p. 691) may be necessary. Adjunct chemotherapy after surgery has increased the survival rate.

Metastatic Bone Cancer

The most common type of malignant bone tumor occurs as a result of metastasis from a primary tumor. Common sites for the primary tumor include the breast, prostate, gastrointestinal tract, lung, kidney, ovary, and thyroid. Metastatic bone lesions are commonly found in the vertebrae, pelvis, femur, humerus, or ribs and may occur at any time following diagnosis and treatment of the primary tumor.

Metastasis to the bone should be suspected in any patient who has local bone pain and a past history of cancer. Treatment may be palliative and consists of radiation and pain management.

Nursing Management

Goals

The patient with bone cancer will have satisfactory pain relief; maintain preferred activities as long as possible; demonstrate acceptance of body image changes resulting from chemotherapy, radiation, and surgery; be free from injury; and verbalize a realistic idea of disease progression and prognosis.

Nursing Diagnoses

- Acute pain
- Impaired physical mobility
- Disturbed body image
- Grieving
- Risk for injury
- Impaired home maintenance

Nursing Interventions

Nursing care of the patient with a malignant bone neoplasm does not differ significantly from care given to the patient with a malignant disease of any other body system. However, special attention is required to reduce complications associated with prolonged bed rest and to prevent pathologic fractures. The patient is often reluctant to participate in therapeutic activities because of weakness and fear of pain. Regular rest periods should be provided between activities. Careful handling of the affected extremity is important to prevent pathologic fractures.

The nurse must be able to assist the patient and family in accepting the guarded prognosis associated with bone cancer. Inability to accomplish age-specific developmental tasks can increase the frustrations with this condition. Special attention is necessary for problems of pain and dysfunction, chemotherapy, and specific surgery, such as spinal cord decompression or amputation.

BRAIN TUMORS

Description

Tumors of the brain may be primary, arising from tissues within the brain, or secondary, resulting from a metastasis from a malignant neoplasm elsewhere in the body. Secondary brain tumors are the most common type. Brain tumors are generally classified according to the tissue from which they arise.

- The most common primary brain tumors originate in astrocytes. These tumors are called *gliomas,* including astrocytoma and glioblastoma multiforme. Glioblastoma multiforme is the most common primary brain tumor, followed by meningioma and astrocytoma.
- More than half of brain tumors are malignant; they infiltrate the brain parenchyma and are not amenable to complete surgical removal. Other tumors may be histologically benign but are located such that complete removal is not possible.
- Unless treated, all brain tumors eventually cause death from increasing tumor volume leading to increased intracranial pressure (ICP). (For a comparison of the major brain tumors, see Table 57-12, Lewis and others, *Medical-Surgical Nursing,* edition 7, p. 1488.)

Clinical Manifestations

The appearance of manifestations depends on the location, size, and rate of tumor growth. A wide range of clinical manifestations are associated with brain tumors.

- Headache is a common problem. Tumor-related headaches tend to be worse at night and may awaken the patient. The headaches are usually dull and constant but occasionally throbbing.
- Seizures are common in gliomas and brain metastases. Brain tumors can cause nausea and vomiting from increased ICP.
- Cognitive dysfunction, including memory problems and mood or personality changes, is common in patients with brain metastases. As the tumor expands, it may produce signs of increased ICP, cerebral edema, or obstruction of the cerebrospinal fluid (CSF) pathways.
- Manifestations may clearly indicate the location of the tumor by an alteration in the function controlled by the affected area (see Table 57-13, Lewis and others, *Medical-Surgical Nursing,* edition 7, p. 1489).

If the tumor mass obstructs the ventricles or occludes the outlet, ventricular enlargement (hydrocephalus) can occur. Surgical treatment is needed to relieve pressure and involves placement of a ventriculoatrial or a ventriculoperitoneal shunt. Shunt malfunction is evidenced by signs of increased ICP, such as headache, blurred vision, vomiting without nausea, decreasing level of consciousness (LOC), or restlessness. These signs, as well as those of an infected shunt, such as high fever, persistent headache, and stiff neck, warrant investigation.

Diagnostic Studies

- Magnetic resonance imaging (MRI) and positron emission tomography (PET) scans allow for detection of very small tumors.
- Cerebral angiography determines blood flow and localization of tumor.
- Computed tomography (CT) and brain scanning assist in tumor location.
- Other useful diagnostic studies include single photon emission computed tomography (SPECT) and electroencephalogram.

Collaborative Care

Treatment goals are aimed at identifying the tumor type and location, removing or decreasing tumor mass, and preventing or managing increased ICP.

Surgical removal is the preferred treatment for brain tumors (see the section on cranial surgery in Lewis and others, *Medical-Surgical Nursing,* Chapter 57, edition 7, pp. 1491 to 1493). Surgical outcome depends on the type, size, and location of the tumor. Meningiomas and oligodendrogliomas can usually be completely removed, whereas more invasive gliomas and medulloblastomas can be only partially removed. Even if complete surgical removal of the tumor is not possible, surgery can reduce tumor mass, which decreases ICP and provides relief of symptoms with an extension of survival time. Tumors located in deep central areas of the dominant hemisphere, posterior corpus callosum, or upper brain-stem cause extensive neurologic damage and are considered inoperable.

Radiation therapy is commonly used as a follow-up measure after surgery. Radiation seeds can also be implanted into the brain. Cerebral edema and rapidly increasing ICP may be a complication of radiation therapy, but they can be managed with high doses of corticosteroids (dexamethasone [Decadron], prednisone).

Normally the blood-brain barrier prohibits the entry of most drugs into brain parenchyma. However, the most malignant brain tumors cause a breakdown of the blood-brain barrier in the tumor area, allowing chemotherapeutic agents to be used. Nitrosoureas such as carmustine (BCNU) and lomustine (CCNU) are commonly used; methotrexate and procarbazine (Matulane) are also used. Temozolomide (Temodar) is the first oral chemotherapy being used to cross the blood-brain barrier. Chemotherapy-laden biodegradable wafers implanted during surgery can deliver chemotherapy directly to the tumor site. Intrathecal administration also allows direct delivery of chemotherapeutic drugs to the central nervous system.

Many techniques to control and treat brain tumors are under investigation, including local hyperthermia and biologic therapy.

- Although progress in treatment has increased the length and quality of survival of patients with gliomas, outcomes remain poor.

Nursing Management
Goals
The patient with a brain tumor will maintain normal ICP, maximize neurologic functioning, achieve control of pain and discomfort, and be aware of the long-term implications with respect to prognosis and cognitive and physical functioning.

Nursing Diagnoses/Collaborative Problems
- Ineffective tissue perfusion
- Acute pain (headache)
- Self-care deficits
- Anxiety
- Potential complication: seizures
- Potential complication: increased ICP

Nursing Interventions
Behavioral changes associated with a frontal lobe lesion, such as loss of emotional control, confusion, memory loss, and depression, are often not perceived by the patient but can be very disturbing and frightening to the family. Assisting the family in understanding what is happening is an important role for the nurse.

- The confused patient with behavioral instability can be a challenge. Close supervision of activity, use of side rails, judicious use of restraints, padding of rails, and a calm, reassuring approach are all essential care techniques.
- Minimization of environmental stimuli, creation of a routine, and use of reality orientation can be incorporated into the care plan for the confused patient.
- Seizures often occur with brain tumors, and seizure precautions should be instituted for the protection of the patient (see Seizure Disorders, p. 556).
- Motor and sensory dysfunctions are problems that interfere with the activities of daily living. Alterations in mobility

must be managed, and the patient needs to be encouraged to provide as much self-care as physically possible. Self-image often depends on the patient's ability to participate in care within the limitations of the physical deficits.

- Motor (expressive) or sensory (receptive) dysphasia may occur. Disturbances in communication can be frustrating for the patient and may interfere with the nurse's ability to meet patient needs. Attempts should be made to establish a communication system that can be used by both the patient and staff.

- Nutritional intake may be decreased because of the patient's inability to eat, loss of appetite, or loss of desire to eat. Assessing the nutritional status of the patient and ensuring adequate nutritional intake are important aspects of care. The patient may need encouragement to eat or, in some cases, may have to be fed orally by gastrostomy or nasogastric tube or by parenteral nutrition (PN) (see Tube Feeding, p. 751, and Parenteral Nutrition, p. 743).

The patient with a brain tumor who undergoes cranial surgery requires complex nursing care (see the section on cranial surgery, Lewis and others, *Medical-Surgical Nursing,* edition 7, pp. 1491 to 1493).

BREAST CANCER

Description

Breast cancer is the most common malignancy in women in the United States except for skin cancer and is second only to lung cancer as the leading cause of death from cancer in women. More than 211,000 new cases of breast cancer are diagnosed in women in the United States each year. Although the vast majority of breast problems occur in women, men can have breast problems. About 1700 new cases of breast cancer are diagnosed in men annually.

Pathophysiology

Although the etiology is not completely understood, a number of factors are thought to be related to the development of breast cancer. Risk factors appear to be cumulative and interacting, and the overall risk for breast cancer may be greatly increased in women with a positive family history and the presence of additional risk factors. Table 15 identifies some major risk factors for breast cancer.

Table 15	Risk Factors for Breast Cancer

Increased Risk	Comments
Female	Women account for 99% of breast cancer cases.
Age 50 yr or over	Majority of breast cancers are found in postmenopausal women. After age 60 yr, incidence greatly increases.
Family history	Breast cancer in a first-degree relative, particularly when premenopausal or bilateral, increases risk. Gene mutations (BRCA-1 or BRCA-2) play a role in 5%-10% of breast cancer cases.
Personal history of cancer of breast, colon, endometrium, or ovary	Personal cancer history significantly increases risk of breast cancer, cancer in other breast, and recurrence.
Early menarche (<12 yr); late menopause (>55 yr)	Long menstrual history increases risk of breast cancer.
First full-term pregnancy after age 30 yr; nulliparity	Prolonged exposure to unopposed estrogen increases risk for breast cancer.
Benign breast disease with atypical epithelial hyperplasia, lobular carcinoma in situ	Atypical changes found on breast biopsy increase the risk of breast cancer.
Weight gain and obesity after menopause; high dietary fat intake	Fat cells store estrogen.
Exposure to ionizing radiation	Radiation damages DNA (e.g., prior treatment for Hodgkin's lymphoma).
Combined hormone replacement (estrogen and progesterone)	Estrogen exposure and unknown hormonal regulation and tumor promotion increase risk.

Table 16	Types of Breast Cancer	
Type	**Frequency of Occurrence**	
Infiltrating ductal carcinoma	63%-68%	
▪ Colloid (mucinous)		
▪ Inflammatory		
▪ Paget's disease		
▪ Medullary		
▪ Papillary		
▪ Tubular		
Infiltrating lobular carcinoma	10%-15%	
Noninvasive	4%-6%	
▪ Ductal carcinoma in situ		

B

The various types of breast cancer identified in Table 16 are based on histologic characteristics and tumor growth pattern. The natural history of breast cancer varies considerably from patient to patient. Cancer growth can range from slow to rapid.

- Factors that affect cancer prognosis are tumor size, axillary node involvement (the more nodes involved, the worse the prognosis), tumor differentiation (morphology of malignant cells), *HER-2/neu* status (a genetic marker), and estrogen and progesterone receptor status.

Clinical Manifestations

Breast cancer is usually first detected as a single lump or as a mammographic breast abnormality. It occurs most often in the upper outer quadrant of the breast because most of the glandular tissue is there.

- If palpable, breast cancer is characteristically hard, irregularly shaped, poorly delineated, nonmobile, and nontender. Malignant lesions are characteristically painless and nontender.
- A small percentage of breast cancers cause nipple discharge. The discharge is usually unilateral and may be clear or bloody. Nipple retraction may occur.
- Plugging of the dermal lymphatics can cause skin thickening and exaggeration of the usual skin markings, giving skin the appearance of an orange peel (peau d'orange).
- In large cancers, infiltration, induration, and dimpling (pulling in) of the overlying skin may occur.

. Recurrence may be local or regional (skin or soft tissue near mastectomy site, axillary lymph nodes) or distant (most commonly bone, lung, brain, and liver).

Diagnostic Studies
Screening
- Physical examination of breast and lymphatics
- Mammography and ultrasound
- Breast magnetic resonance imaging (MRI)
- Biopsy
  - Stereotactic core biopsy
  - Fine needle aspiration

After Diagnosis
- *Axillary node dissection* is often performed. Axillary lymph node involvement is one of the most important prognostic factors in breast cancer. The more nodes involved, the greater the risk of recurrence.
- *Lymphatic mapping and sentinel lymph node dissection (SLND)* help the surgeon identify the lymph node or nodes that drain first from the tumor site *(sentinel node)*. Assessment of this node can be used to determine the extent of tumor spread to axillary lymph nodes.
- Tumor size is a valuable prognostic variable: the larger the tumor, the poorer the prognosis. In addition, poorly differentiated tumors appear morphologically disorganized and are more aggressive.
- Estrogen and progesterone receptor status is useful to determine treatment decisions and prognosis. Receptor-positive tumors commonly (1) show histologic evidence of being well differentiated, (2) have a lower chance for recurrence, and (3) are frequently responsive to hormonal therapy. Receptor-negative tumors (1) are often poorly differentiated histologically, (2) frequently recur, and (3) are usually unresponsive to hormonal therapy.
- DNA content (ploidy status) correlates with tumor aggressiveness. Diploid tumors have been shown to have a significantly lower risk of recurrence than aneuploid tumors.

Collaborative Care
All of the prognostic factors are considered in treatment decisions, and tumor size (T), nodal involvement (N), and presence of metastasis (M), are used to stage breast cancer with the TNM system (see TNM Classification System, p. 796).
Surgical Therapy. Breast conservation surgery (lumpectomy) with radiation therapy and modified radical mastectomy with or

without reconstruction are currently the most common options for resectable breast cancer. The overall survival with lumpectomy and radiation is about the same as that with modified radical mastectomy.

Breast conservation surgery (lumpectomy) involves removal of **B** the entire tumor along with a margin of normal tissue. An axillary lymph node dissection (ALND) is usually done along with a lumpectomy. If there is evidence of systemic disease, chemotherapy may be given before radiation therapy.

- An ALND involves the removal of 12 to 20 nodes and is usually performed if the sentinel lymph node or nodes contain malignant cells. A sentinal lymph node dissection (SLND) has replaced ALND for patients who do not have malignant cells identified in the sentinel nodes.
- One of the main advantages of breast conservation surgery and radiation is that it preserves the breast, including the nipple. The goal of combined surgery and radiation is to maximize the benefits of both cancer treatment and cosmetic outcome while minimizing the risks.

Modified radical mastectomy includes removal of the breast and axillary lymph nodes but preserves the pectoralis major muscle. This surgery is selected over breast conservation therapy if the tumor is too large to excise with good margins and attain a reasonable cosmetic result. Some patients may select this procedure over lumpectomy when presented with the choice of either procedure. See Table 52-7, Lewis and others, *Medical-Surgical Nursing,* edition 7, p. 1353 for treatment options, side effects, complications, and patient issues related to common surgical procedures to treat breast cancer.

After surgery, the woman must be monitored for the rest of her life at regular intervals. Most women have professional examinations every 6 months for the first 2 years, and then annually thereafter.

- In addition, the woman must continue to practice monthly breast self-examinations (BSEs) on both breasts or on the remaining breast and mastectomy site. The woman should also have yearly mammography of the remaining breast or breast tissue.
- The most common sites of cancer recurrence are at the surgical site and in the opposite breast.

Adjuvant Therapy. The decision to recommend adjuvant (additional) therapy after surgery depends on the number of involved nodes, menstrual status, age, cell type, size and extent of the cancer, presence or absence of estrogen receptors, and other preexisting health problems that can complicate treatment.

Adjuvant therapies include radiation therapy and systemic therapies such as chemotherapy, hormonal manipulation, and biologic and targeted therapy.

Radiation Therapy. The three situations in which radiation therapy may be used for breast cancer are (1) as primary treatment to prevent local breast recurrences after breast conservation surgery, (2) as adjuvant treatment following mastectomy to prevent local and nodal recurrences, and (3) as palliative treatment for pain caused by local recurrence and metastases. Lumpectomy is almost always followed by radiation.

Chemotherapy. Cytotoxic drugs are used to destroy cancer cells. Breast cancer is one of the solid tumors that is the most responsive to chemotherapy. In some patients chemotherapy is given preoperatively to decrease the size of the primary tumor. The incidence and severity of the side effects that accompany chemotherapy are influenced by the specific drug combinations, drug schedule, and dose of the drugs (see Chemotherapy, p. 712).

Hormonal Therapy. Estrogen can promote growth of breast cancer cells if cells are estrogen-receptor positive. Hormonal therapy removes or blocks the source of estrogen, thus promoting tumor regression, and may be used as an adjuvant to primary treatment or in patients with recurrent or metastatic cancer. Hormone receptor assays can identify women who are likely to respond to hormone therapy, and drugs have been developed that can inactivate the hormone-secreting glands as effectively as surgery or radiation. Women who are postmenopausal are more likely to have hormone-dependent tumors, with significantly greater chances of tumor regression. Tamoxifen (Nolvadex) has been the agent of choice in postmenopausal, estrogen-receptor positive women with all stages of breast cancer for the past 30 years. (See Table 17 for hormonal therapy for breast cancer.)

Biologic Therapy. Trastuzumab (Herceptin) is an antibody that targets HER-2/neu, an antigen that often appears on the surface of breast cancer cells. After the antibody attaches to the antigen, it is taken into the cells and eventually kills them. It can be used alone or in combination with other chemotherapy to treat patients with breast cancer whose tumors overexpress the HER-2 gene.

Nursing Management
Goals
The patient with breast cancer will actively participate in the decision-making process related to treatment options, fully comply with the therapeutic plan, manage side effects of adjuvant therapy, and be satisfied with support provided by significant others and health care providers.

Table 17	Drug Therapy: Hormonal Therapy for Breast Cancer

Mechanism of Action	Examples
Blocks estrogen receptors	tamoxifen (Nolvadex) toremifene (Fareston)
Destroys estrogen receptors	fulvestrant (Faslodex)
Prevents production of estrogen by inhibiting aromatase	anastrozole (Arimidex) letrozole (Femara) exemestane (Aromasin) aminoglutethimide (Cytadren)

See NCP 52-1 for the patient after a mastectomy or lumpectomy, Lewis and others, *Medical-Surgical Nursing,* edition 7, pp. 1357 to 1358.

Nursing Diagnoses/Collaborative Problems

After a diagnosis of breast cancer and before a treatment plan has been selected, the following diagnoses apply:

- Decisional conflict
- Fear
- Disturbed body image

If the patient undergoes a lumpectomy or modified radical mastectomy, nursing diagnoses may include:

- Acute pain
- Anxiety
- Disturbed body image
- Ineffective therapeutic regimen management
- Impaired physical mobility
- Risk for injury

Nursing Interventions

The time between the diagnosis of breast cancer and the selection of a treatment plan is a difficult period for the woman and her family. Although the primary care provider discusses treatment options, the woman often relies on the nurse to clarify and expand on these options.

- Appropriate nursing interventions during this period include exploring the woman's usual decision-making patterns, helping the woman accurately evaluate the advantages and disadvantages of the options, providing information relevant to the decision, and supporting the patient once a decision is made.
- Regardless of the surgery planned, the patient needs to be provided with sufficient information to ensure informed

consent. Teaching in the preoperative phase includes instruction in turning and deep breathing, a review of postoperative exercises, and an explanation of the recovery period from the time of surgery until discharge.

The woman who has breast conservation surgery usually has an uneventful postoperative course with only a moderate amount of pain. The woman who has had a modified radical mastectomy needs nursing interventions specific to this surgery.

- Restoring arm function on the affected side after mastectomy and axillary lymph node dissection is an important goal.
- The woman should be placed in semi-Fowler's position with the arm on the affected side elevated on a pillow. Flexing and extending the fingers should begin in the recovery room, with progressive increases in activity.
- Postoperative arm and shoulder exercises are instituted gradually at the surgeon's direction.
- Postoperative discomfort can be minimized by administering analgesics about 30 minutes before initiating exercises. When showering is appropriate, warm water running over the involved shoulder often has a soothing effect and reduces joint stiffness.

Whenever possible, the same nurse should work with the woman so that progress can be monitored.

Lymphedema (accumulation of lymph in soft tissue) can occur as a result of excision or radiation of the lymph nodes. The patient may experience heaviness, pain, impaired motor function in the arm, and numbness and paresthesia of the fingers. The patient must understand that she is at risk of developing lymphedema for the rest of her life. Measures to prevent or reduce lymphedema must be taught including:

- The affected arm should never be dependent, even while the person is sleeping.
- Blood pressure (BP) readings, venipunctures, and injections should not be done on the affected arm.
- The woman must be instructed to protect the arm on the operative side from even minor trauma such as a pinprick or sunburn.
- If trauma to the arm occurs, the area should be washed thoroughly with soap and water, and a topical antibiotic ointment and bandage should be applied.
- Frequent and sustained elevation of the arm, regular use of a custom-fitted pressure sleeve, and treatment with an inflatable sleeve (pneumomassage) may also be helpful.

Throughout interactions the nurse must keep in mind the extensive psychologic impact of the disease. All aspects of care must include sensitivity to the woman's efforts to cope with a life-threatening disease. The nurse can help meet the woman's psychologic needs by doing the following:

- Assisting her to develop a positive but realistic attitude
- Helping identify sources of support and strength to her, such as her partner, family, and spiritual practices
- Encouraging her to verbalize anger and fears about her diagnosis
- Promoting open communication of thoughts and feelings between the patient and her family
- Providing accurate and complete answers to questions about the disease, treatment options, and reproductive or lactation issues (if appropriate)
- Offering information about community resources, such as Reach to Recovery, Y-ME, CanSurmount, Encore, and local support organizations and groups

▼ **Patient and Family Teaching**
- The nurse should emphasize the importance of an annual mammography and breast self-awareness. Future symptoms that should be reported to the clinician include new back pain, weakness, constipation, shortness of breath, and confusion.
- The nurse should stress the importance of wearing a well-fitting prosthesis designed for women who have had a mastectomy.
- A preoperative sexual assessment provides baseline data that the nurse can use to plan postoperative interventions. Often, the husband, sexual partner, or family members may need assistance in dealing with their emotional reactions to the diagnosis and surgery so that they can act as effective means of support for the patient.
- Depression may occur with the continued stress of a cancer diagnosis. Special nursing interventions are necessary for both psychologic support and self-care teaching if a recurrence is found.

Breast reconstruction is discussed in Chapter 52, Lewis and others, *Medical-Surgical Nursing,* edition 7.

BURNS

Description
Burns are tissue injuries resulting from exposure to or direct contact with heat, chemicals, electrical current, or radiation. An

estimated 1.1 million North Americans seek medical care each year for burns.

Pathophysiology

The extent of burn injury is influenced by energy intensity, duration of exposure, and type of tissue injured. Immediately after the injury occurs, there is an increase in blood flow to the area surrounding the wound. This is followed by the release of various vasoactive substances from burned tissue, which results in increased capillary permeability. Fluid then shifts from the intravascular compartment to the interstitial space, producing edema and hypovolemia. After several days, diuresis from fluid mobilization occurs and healing begins.

Types of Burn Injury

Various types of burns may be seen alone or in combination with other burns.

- Thermal injury is the most common type of burn and can be caused by flame, flash, scald, or contact with hot objects.
- Chemical burns are the result of tissue injury and destruction from necrotizing substances such as acids and alkali substances. Chemicals can cause respiratory, skin, eye, and systemic injury for up to 72 hours after the exposure.
- Smoke and inhalation injury results from the inhalation of hot air or noxious chemicals that can cause damage to the respiratory tract. These injuries include carbon monoxide poisoning, thermal burn above the glottis, or chemical burn below the glottis.
- Electrical burns result from coagulation necrosis caused by intense heat from an electric current.

Classification of Burn Injury

The treatment of burns is related to injury severity. A variety of methods exist for determining burn severity.

1. The *depth of burn* is described according to the depth of skin destruction (epidermis, dermis, or subcutaneous tissue) (Table 18).
   - Partial-thickness burn.
     1. Superficial (first degree) with erythema, pain, mild swelling, no vesicles or blisters.
     2. Deep (second degree) with fluid-filled vesicles, severe pain, mild to moderate edema.
   - Full-thickness burn (third and fourth degree) with dry, waxy, leathery, or hard skin; pain insensitivity; possible bone, muscle, and tendon involvement.

Table 18 Classification of Burn Injury Depth

Classification	Clinical Appearance	Cause	Structure
Partial-Thickness Skin Destruction			
■ Superficial (first-degree)	Erythema, blanching on pressure, pain and mild swelling, no vesicles or blisters (although after 24 hr skin may blister and peel)	Superficial sunburn Quick heat flash	Only superficial devitalization with hyperemia is present. Tactile and pain sensation intact.
■ Deep (second-degree)	Fluid-filled vesicles that are red, shiny, wet (if vesicles have ruptured); severe pain caused by nerve injury; mild to moderate edema	Flame Flash Scald Contact burns Chemical tar	Epidermis and dermis involved to varying depth. Some skin elements, from which epithelial regeneration can occur, remain viable.
Full-Thickness Skin Destruction			
■ Third- and fourth-degree	Dry, waxy white, leathery, or hard skin; visibly thrombosed vessels; insensitivity to pain and pressure because of nerve destruction; possible involvement of muscles, tendons, and bones	Flame Scald Chemical Tar Electric current	All skin elements and nerve endings destroyed. Coagulation necrosis present. Surgical intervention for wound closure.

B

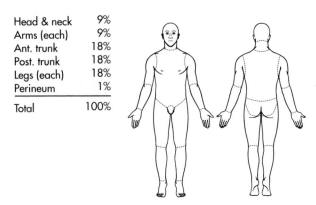

Head & neck	9%
Arms (each)	9%
Ant. trunk	18%
Post. trunk	18%
Legs (each)	18%
Perineum	1%
Total	100%

Fig. 1. Rule of nines chart.

2. The extent of burn is calculated as the percent of total body surface area (TBSA) that has been burned. Two common methods for determining the extent of a burn include:
   - Lund-Browder chart, which takes into account the patient's age and relative body area.
   - Rule of nines chart, which is easy to remember and adequate for initial assessment (Fig. 1).
3. Burn location has a direct relationship to the severity of the injury. For example, face and neck burns may inhibit respiratory function; hands, feet, joint, and eye burns may limit self-care and functioning.
4. Patient risk factors include older age, which contributes to slower healing and longer rehabilitation, and preexisting disorders such as cardiovascular, pulmonary, or renal disease that reduce the patient's ability to recover from the tremendous demands of burn injury.

The American Burn Association (ABA) has established referral criteria that recommend which burn injuries should be treated in a burn unit (see Table 19).

Clinical Manifestations

- *Emergent phase:* Characterized by possible shock from pain and hypovolemia, intense thirst, minimal urine output, shivering as a result of heat loss or anxiety, and adynamic ileus. Unconsciousness or altered mental status is not usually the result of a burn, but rather smoke inhalation or head trauma. Complications may include dysrhythmias, airway obstruction, and acute tubular necrosis and renal failure.

Table 19	Burn Unit Referral Criteria*

Burn injuries that should be referred to a burn unit include the following:
1. Partial-thickness burns greater than 10% total body surface area (TBSA)
2. Burns that involve the face, hands, feet, genitalia, perineum, or major joints
3. Third-degree burns in any age group
4. Electrical burns, including lightning injury
5. Chemical burns
6. Inhalation injury
7. Burn injury in patients with pre-existing medical disorders that could complicate management, prolong recovery, or affect mortality
8. Any patients with burns and concomitant trauma (e.g., fractures) in which the burn injury poses the greatest risk of morbidity or mortality. In such cases, if the trauma poses the greater immediate risk, the patient may be initially stabilized in a trauma center before being transferred to a burn unit
9. Burn injury in patients who will require special social, emotional, or long-term rehabilitative intervention

Source: Guidelines for the operations of burn units. In American College of Surgeons, Committee on Trauma: Resources for optimal care of the injured patient, 1999. Available at www.ameriburn.org.
* Guidelines from the American Burn Association.

- *Acute phase:* Partial-thickness wounds form eschar. When eschar is removed, reepithelialization begins at wound margins and appears as red or pink scar tissue. Wound closure and healing usually occur within 10 to 14 days. Separation of eschar from full-thickness wounds takes longer, and these wounds require surgical debridement and skin grafting for healing. Wound infection is a serious complication. Survival is directly related to prevention of wound contamination that can progress to bacteremia and sepsis. Other complications include acute transient neurologic reactions, including extreme disorientation and delirium, contractures, Curling's ulcer, and stress diabetes.
- *Rehabilitative phase:* Mature healing occurs over 6 to 24 months. New scar tissue will shorten, causing a contracture if adequate range of motion (ROM) is not performed. The healing site, which is extremely sensitive to trauma, may itch. Complications are skin and joint contractures and hypertrophic scarring.

Diagnostic Studies
- Serum electrolytes, especially sodium (Na⁺) and potassium (K⁺), to monitor shifts
- Chest x-ray, arterial blood gases (ABGs), and sputum for inhalation injury
- Urine output and specific gravity to evaluate fluid replacement and detect acute tubular necrosis and/or renal ischemia
- Complete blood count (CBC) to detect anemia and immunologic response to injury
- White blood cell (WBC) count and wound cultures if infection is suspected

Collaborative Care
Burn management can be classified into three phases: emergent (resuscitative), acute, and rehabilitative (Table 20). *Emergent* (resuscitative) phase is the period of time required to resolve immediate problems resulting from burn injury. This phase may last from burn onset to 5 or more days, but it usually lasts 24 to 48 hours. This phase begins with fluid loss and edema and continues until fluid mobilization and diuresis begin.

Acute phase begins with mobilization of extracellular fluid and subsequent diuresis. The acute phase is concluded when the burned area is completely covered or when the wounds are healed. This may take weeks or many months.

Rehabilitation phase begins when the burn wound is covered with skin or healed and the patient is capable of assuming some self-care activity. This can occur as early as 2 weeks to as long as 2 or 3 months after the injury.

Nursing Management
Goals
The patient with a burn injury will resume self-care activities, experience no contractures or infection, maintain a positive nitrogen balance with weight loss limited to no more than 10%, express satisfaction with pain control, and verbalize realistic rehabilitation goals.

See NCP 25-1 for the burn patient, Lewis and others, *Medical-Surgical Nursing,* edition 7, pp. 494 to 496.

Nursing Diagnoses
- Risk for deficient fluid volume
- Acute pain
- Self-care deficits
- Risk for infection
- Disturbed body image
- Imbalanced nutrition: less than body requirements

Table 20   Phases of Burn Management

Emergent Phase	Acute Phase	Rehabilitation Phase
Airway Management ■ Early endotracheal intubation as necessary with or without ventilatory assistance. ■ Bronchoscopy to evaluate lower respiratory tract. ■ Humidified air or oxygen. **Fluid Therapy** ■ Determine fluid needs with formulas based on extent of burn. ■ Begin IV fluid replacement. ■ Insert urinary catheter. ■ Monitor urinary output. **Wound Care** ■ Assess extent of burns. ■ Start hydrotherapy or wound cleansing. ■ Debride as necessary. ■ Administer tetanus toxoid or tetanus antitoxin. **Pain and Anxiety** ■ Assess and manage pain and anxiety.	**Fluid Therapy** ■ Continue replacing fluids, depending on patient's response. **Wound Care** ■ Continue hydrotherapy/cleansing. ■ Assess wound daily, and adjust dressing protocols as necessary. ■ Observe for complications. ■ Continue debridement (if necessary). ■ Continue to assess and treat pain and anxiety. ■ Provide temporary homografts. ■ Provide permanent autografts. ■ Care for donor sites. **Nutritional Therapy** ■ Continue to assess diet to support wound healing. **Physical/Occupational Therapy** ■ Range-of-motion program. ■ Assess need for splints and anticontracture positioning. ■ Teach patient and family about physical and psychologic aspects of care.	**Physical/Occupational Therapy** ■ Encourage and assist patient in resuming self-care. ■ Prevent or minimize contractures (surgery, physical/occupational therapy, splinting, or pressure garments). ■ Discuss possible reconstructive surgery. ■ Prepare for discharge home or transfer to rehabilitation facility.

B

Nursing Interventions
- Emergent phase: Assess adequacy of airway management and fluid therapy, provide pain medication and wound care, and offer support to patient and family.
- Acute phase: Wound care, fluid therapy, comfort, hygiene measures, and ROM exercises continue. A critical function is pain assessment and management.
- Rehabilitative phase: Responsibility is shared among the health care team to return the patient to optimal functioning.

▼ **Patient and Family Teaching**
- Describe to the patient and family the burn injury process and the expected signs and symptoms related to phases of burn management.
- Explain therapeutic interventions, precautionary measures, gowning and hand washing, and institution visiting policy to elicit cooperation and decrease anxiety.
- Teach the patient to watch for injuries to new skin.
- Instruct the patient and family about the signs and symptoms of infection so early treatment can be initiated.
- Teach family members how to perform dressing changes to ensure proper technique and increase their sense of control.
- Emphasize the importance of exercise and appropriate physical therapy to the patient and family. Plan a daily program with the patient, and offer appropriate resources to provide a continuing activity program as needed.
- Help the patient and family in setting realistic future expectations because anticipatory guidance decreases anxiety and inaccurate perceptions. The patient and family will need anticipatory guidance to know what to expect physiologically as well as psychologically during recovery.
- Assist the patient and family to establish contact with family and patient support groups, such as the Phoenix Society *(www.phoenix-society.org)*.

CARDIOMYOPATHY

Description
Cardiomyopathy (CMP) constitutes a group of diseases that directly affect the structural or functional ability of the myocardium. A diagnosis of CMP is based on the patient's clinical manifestations and diagnostic noninvasive and invasive cardiac procedures.

CMP can be classified as primary or secondary:
- Primary CMP includes those conditions in which the etiology of the heart disease is unknown. The heart muscle in this instance is the only portion of the heart involved, and other cardiac structures are unaffected.
- In secondary CMP the cause of the myocardial disease is known and is secondary to another disease process. Common causes of secondary CMP are coronary artery disease (CAD), myocarditis, hypertension, cardiotoxic agents (alcohol, cocaine), valve disease, and metabolic and autoimmune disorders.

CMP has also been classified into three general types: *dilated, hypertrophic,* and *restrictive*. Each of these types has its own pathogenesis, clinical presentation, and treatment protocols (Table 21). All types of CMP can lead to cardiomegaly and heart failure (HF) and are the leading cause for heart transplants.

Dilated Cardiomyopathy

Pathophysiology. Dilated cardiomyopathy is the most common type of CMP and is characterized by diffuse inflammation and rapid degeneration of myocardial fibers, resulting in ventricular dilation without hypertrophy.
- Dilated CMP often follows an infectious myocarditis. Other common causes include alcohol and cocaine, hypertension, and CAD.

Clinical Manifestations. The patient may have signs and symptoms of HF, including fatigue, dyspnea at rest, paroxysmal nocturnal dyspnea, and orthopnea. Dry cough, abdominal bloating, and anorexia may occur as the disease progresses. Signs can include S_3, S_4, pulmonary crackles, edema, pallor, hepatomegaly, and jugular venous distention. The patient may also have murmurs, dysrhythmias, or systemic embolism.

Diagnostic Studies. A diagnosis is made on the basis of patient history and ruling out other conditions that cause HF.
- Doppler echocardiography provides the basis for the diagnosis of dilated CMP and distinguishes dilated CMP from other structural abnormalities.
- Chest x-ray may show cardiomegaly with pulmonary hypertension and pleural effusions.
- Electrocardiogram (ECG) may reveal dysrhythmias with conduction disturbances.
- Serum levels of b-type natriuretic peptide (BNP) are elevated in the presence of HF.
- Cardiac catheterization and coronary angiography are used to rule out CAD and evaluate cardiac output.

Table 21   Characteristics of Cardiomyopathies

	Dilated	Hypertrophic	Restrictive
Major Manifestations	Fatigue, weakness, palpitations, dyspnea	Exertional dyspnea, fatigue, angina, syncope, palpitations	Dyspnea, fatigue
Cardiomegaly	Moderate to marked	Mild to moderate	Mild
Contractility	Decreased	Increased or decreased	Normal or decreased
Valvular Incompetence	Atrioventricular valves, particularly mitral	Mitral valve	Atrioventricular valves
Dysrhythmias	Sinoatrial tachycardia, atrial and ventricular dysrhythmias	Atrial and ventricular dysrhythmias	Atrial and ventricular dysrhythmias
Cardiac Output	Decreased	Normal or decreased	Normal or decreased
Outflow Tract Obstruction	None	Increased	None

Nursing and Collaborative Management. Interventions focus on controlling HF by enhancing myocardial contractility and decreasing afterload (similar to treatment for chronic HF).

- Nitrates and loop diuretics are used to decrease preload, and angiotensin-converting enzyme (ACE) inhibitors are used to reduce afterload.
- β-Adrenergic blockers and aldosterone antagonists are used to control the neurohormonal stimulation that occurs in HF.
- Digitalis is used to treat atrial fibrillation but with caution because these patients are susceptible to digoxin toxicity.
- Antidysrhythmics and anticoagulants are used as indicated.
- Drug therapy, nutritional therapy, and cardiac rehabilitation may help alleviate symptoms of HF and improve cardiac output (CO).
- A patient with secondary dilated CMP must be treated for the underlying disease process. For example, the patient with alcohol-induced dilated CMP must abstain from all alcohol intake.
- The patient with terminal end-stage CMP may require cardiac transplantation.
- Patients with dilated CMP are very ill people with a grave prognosis who need expert nursing care. The patient's family must learn cardiopulmonary resuscitation (CPR) and how to access emergency care in their neighborhood.
- Nursing care should focus on monitoring the patient's response to medications and observing for signs and symptoms of worsening HF, dysrhythmias, and embolic formation.

Hypertrophic Cardiomyopathy

Pathophysiology. Hypertrophic cardiomyopathy (HCM), is asymmetric myocardial hypertrophy without ventricular dilation. HCM occurs less commonly than dilated CMP and is more common in men than in women. It is usually diagnosed in young adulthood and is often seen in active, athletic individuals.

- The primary defect of HCM is diastolic dysfunction caused by left ventricular stiffness. Decreased ventricular filling and obstruction to outflow result in decreased CO.

Clinical Manifestations. Patients are often asymptomatic. The most common symptom is dyspnea, which is caused by an elevated left ventricular diastolic pressure. Other manifestations of HCM include fatigue, angina, syncope, and dysrhythmias.

- Common dysrhythmias include atrial fibrillation, ventricular tachycardia, and ventricular fibrillation. Any of these dysrhythmias may lead to syncope or sudden cardiac death (SCD).

Diagnostic Studies. Clinical findings on examination may be unremarkable.

- Echocardiogram is the primary diagnostic tool revealing the classic feature of HCM, which is LV hypertrophy; the echocardiogram may also demonstrate wall motion abnormalities and diastolic dysfunction.
- ECG findings usually indicate ventricular hypertrophy, ST-T wave abnormalities, prominent Q waves, and ventricular and atrial dysrhythmias.

Nursing and Collaborative Management. The goal of therapy is to improve ventricular filling by reducing ventricular contractility and relieving LV outflow obstruction. This can be accomplished with the use of β-adrenergic blockers or calcium channel blockers.

- Antidysrhythmics are used to control dysrhythmias. An alternative treatment for ventricular dysrhythmias may be an implantable defibrillator.
- Atrioventricular pacing can reduce the degree of outflow obstruction by causing the septum to move away from the left ventricular wall.
- Patients with severe symptoms refractory to therapy with marked obstruction to aortic outflow may be candidates for surgical treatment (ventriculomyotomy and myectomy) of their hypertrophied septum. Most patients have good symptomatic improvement after surgery and improved exercise tolerance.
- An alternative to surgery to reduce symptoms is alcohol-induced, percutaneous transluminal septal myocardial ablation (PTSMA) in which alcohol is used to cause ischemia and septal wall myocardial infarction. Ablation of the septal wall decreases the obstruction to flow, and the patient's symptoms decrease.

Nursing interventions focus on relieving symptoms, observing for and preventing complications, and providing emotional and psychologic support.

- Teaching should focus on helping the patients to adjust their lifestyle to avoid strenuous activity and dehydration. Any activity or procedure that causes an increase in systemic vascular resistance (thus increasing obstruction to forward blood flow) is dangerous for this patient and should be avoided.

Restrictive Cardiomyopathy

Pathophysiology. Restrictive cardiomyopathy is the least common of cardiomyopathic conditions. It is a disease of the heart muscle that impairs diastolic filling and stretch.

- A number of pathologic processes may be involved, including myocardial fibrosis, hypertrophy, and infiltration, which produce stiffness of the ventricular wall.
- The ventricles are resistant to filling and therefore demand high diastolic filling pressures to maintain CO.

Clinical Manifestations. Classic symptoms of restrictive CMP are fatigue, exercise intolerance, and dyspnea on exertion.

- Other manifestations include angina, orthpnea, syncope, palpations, and signs of HF.

Diagnostic Studies. Chest x-ray may be normal or show cardiomegaly with pleural effusions and pulmonary congestion.

- ECG may reveal tachycardia at rest. The most common dysrhythmias are atrial fibrillation or atrioventricular blocks.
- ECG may reveal a left ventricle that is normal size with a thickened wall, a slightly dilated right ventricle, and dilated atria.
- Endomyocardial biopsy, CT scan, and nuclear imaging may be helpful in a definitive diagnosis.

Nursing and Collaborative Management. Currently, no specific treatment for restrictive CMP exists. Interventions are aimed at improving diastolic filling and the underlying disease process. Treatment includes conventional therapy for HF and dysrhythmias. Heart transplant may also be a consideration.

Nursing care is similar to the care of a patient with HF. As in the treatment of patients with HCM, patients should be taught to avoid situations that impair ventricular filling, such as strenuous activity, dehydration, and increases in systemic vascular resistance.

CARPAL TUNNEL SYNDROME

Description
Carpal tunnel syndrome (CTS) is a condition caused by compression of the median nerve where it enters the hand through the narrow carpal tunnel located at the wrist. The condition is often due to pressure from trauma or edema caused by inflammation of a tendon (tenosynovitis), neoplasm, rheumatoid arthritis, or soft tissue masses such as ganglia.

- This syndrome is associated with hobbies or occupations that require continuous wrist movement (e.g., butchers, computer operators, musicians, painters, carpenters, bowlers, knitters).

Clinical Manifestations
Manifestations include weakness (especially of the thumb), burning pain and numbness, impaired sensation in the distribution

of the median nerve, and clumsiness in performing fine hand movements. Numbness and tingling may awaken the patient at night.

- Holding the wrist in acute flexion for 60 seconds will
  produce tingling and numbness over the distribution of the
  median nerve, palmar surface of the thumb, index finger,
  middle finger, and part of the ring finger. This is known as
  a positive Phalen's sign.
- In late stages there is atrophy of the thenar muscles around
  the base of the thumb resulting in recurrent pain and eventual dysfunction of the hand.

Nursing and Collaborative Management

Prevention of carpal tunnel syndrome involves educating employ-
ees and employers to identify risk factors. Ergonomic modifications of workstations and body positions and frequent breaks from
repetitive wrist movment should be made. Adaptive devices such
as wrist splints may be worn to relieve pressure on the median
nerve. Special keyboard pads are available for computer operators
to help prevent CTS or a worsening of symptoms if present.

Therapy is directed toward relieving the underlying cause of the
nerve compression. Stopping the aggravating movement and
placing the hand and wrist at rest by immobilizing them in a hand
splint can usually relieve early symptoms. Injection of a corticosteroid drug directly into the carpal tunnel may provide short-term
(up to 6 months) relief.

- Because of impaired sensation, the patient should be
  instructed to avoid hazards such as extremes in heat and
  cold to prevent thermal injury.
- If the problem continues, the median nerve may have to be
  surgically decompressed by longitudinal division of the
  transverse carpal ligament. Endoscopic carpal tunnel
  release is a surgical procedure in which decompression is
  done through a small puncture site.
- If surgery is performed, the neurovascular status of the
  hand should be evaluated regularly. The patient should be
  instructed in assessments to perform at home, because
  surgery is done on an outpatient basis.

CATARACTS

Description

A cataract is an opacity within the crystalline lens of one or both
eyes, causing a gradual decline in vision. Cataracts are the third

leading cause of preventable blindness and the most common cause of self-declared visual disability in the United States. Approximately 50% of people in the United States between 65 and 74 years old have some degree of cataract formation. Cataract removal is the most common surgical procedure for people in the United States older than 65 years. Congenital cataracts are relatively common, occurring in 1 of every 250 newborns.

C

Pathophysiology

Although most cataracts are age related (senile cataracts), they can be associated with other factors, including blunt or penetrating trauma, congenital factors (e.g., maternal rubella), radiation or ultraviolet (UV) light exposure, certain drugs such as systemic corticosteroids or long-term topical corticosteroids, and ocular inflammation. The patient with diabetes mellitus tends to develop cataracts at a younger age than does a patient without diabetes.

- In senile cataract formation, altered metabolic processes within the lens cause water accumulation and alterations in the fiber structure of the lens. These changes affect lens transparency causing vision changes.

Clinical Manifestations

- The patient may complain of decreased vision, abnormal color perception, and glare that worsens at night.
- Visual decline is gradual, but the rate of cataract development varies from patient to patient.
- Secondary glaucoma may also occur if the enlarging lens causes increased intraocular pressure.

Diagnostic Studies

- Opacity directly observable by ophthalmoscopic or slit lamp microscopic examination
- Visual acuity measurement
- Glare testing
- Keratometry and A-scan ultrasound if surgery is planned

Collaborative Care

The presence of a cataract does not necessarily indicate a need for surgery. For many patients the diagnosis is made long before they actually decide to have surgery. Currently, there is no available treatment to "cure" cataracts other than surgical removal. If the cataract is not removed, the patient's vision will continue to deteriorate.

- Helpful palliative measures include a change in eyeglass prescription, strong reading glasses or magnifiers, an increased amount of light for reading, and avoidance of nighttime driving.

- Surgery may be performed to remove the source of visual impairment when the patient's decreasing vision interferes with normal activities such as driving, reading, and watching television. Removal of the lens may also be medically necessary in patients with increased intraocular pressure and diabetic retinopathy. In these cases the goals of surgery include management of intraocular pressure and visualization of the retina. Surgical treatment can involve lens removal (e.g., phacoemulsification, extracapsular extraction) and correction (e.g., intraocular lens implantation and contact lenses). Almost all patients have an intraocular lens implanted at the time of cataract extraction.

Nursing Management

Goals

Preoperatively, the patient will make informed decisions and experience minimal anxiety. Postoperatively, the patient will understand and comply with therapy, maintain an acceptable level of physical and emotional comfort, and remain free of infection and other complications.

Nursing Diagnoses

- Self-care deficits
- Anxiety
- Risk for infection
- Risk for injury

Nursing Interventions

For the patient who chooses not to have surgery, suggest vision enhancement techniques and a modification of activities and lifestyle to accommodate visual deficits.

For the patient who elects surgery, provide information, support, and reassurance about the surgical and postoperative experience to reduce or alleviate patient anxiety. Inform all patients that they will not have depth perception until their patch is removed (usually within 24 hours).

- Postoperatively, offer mild analgesics for slight scratchiness or mild eye pain. The physician needs to be notified if severe pain, increased or purulent drainage, increased redness, or decreased visual acuity is present.

▼ Patient and Family Teaching

- Written and verbal discharge teaching should include postoperative eye care, activity restrictions, medications, follow-up visit schedule, and signs of possible complications (Table 22).
- The patient's family should be included in the instruction, since some patients may have difficulty with self-care activities,

Table 22	Patient and Family Teaching Guide: After Eye Surgery

Teach patient or patient and family:
- Proper hygiene and eye care techniques to ensure that medications, dressings, and/or surgical wound are not contaminated during necessary eye care
- Signs and symptoms of infection, and when and how to report those to allow early recognition and treatment of possible infection
- Importance of complying with postoperative restrictions on head positioning, bending, coughing, and Valsalva maneuver to optimize visual outcomes and prevent increased intraocular pressure
- How to instill eye medications using aseptic techniques and to comply with prescribed eye medication routine to prevent infection
- How to monitor pain, take prescribed medication for pain as directed, and to report pain not relieved by prescribed medications
- Importance of continued follow-up as recommended to maximize potential visual outcomes

From American Society of Ophthalmic Registered Nurses: *Core curriculum for ophthalmic nursing,* ed 2, Dubuque, Iowa, 2004, Kendall/Hunt Publishing.

especially if vision in the unoperated eye is poor. Provide an opportunity for the patient and family to present return demonstrations of any necessary self-care activities.
- Suggest ways for the patient and family to modify activities and environment to maintain a level of safe functioning for patients with delayed visual correction. Suggestions may include getting assistance with steps, removing area rugs and other potential obstacles, preparing meals for freezing before surgery, and obtaining audio books for diversion until visual acuity improves.

CELIAC DISEASE (SPRUE)

Description
Until recently, celiac disease was considered a relatively rare intestinal disease that began in childhood and was accompanied by symptoms of diarrhea, malabsorption, and malnutrition. It is now

known that it is a common disease that occurs at all ages and can affect multiple body systems besides its primary site in the intestines. *Celiac sprue* and *gluten-sensitive enteropathy* are other names for celiac disease.

Celiac disease should not be confused with *tropical sprue,* a chronic disorder acquired in tropical areas that is characterized by progressive disruption of jejunal and ileal tissue resulting in nutritional difficulties. Tropical sprue is treated with folic acid and tetracycline.

Incidence is thought to be anywhere from 1 in 1500 to 1 in 133 people. The mean age at diagnosis of celiac disease is the mid-40s, and diagnosis is made most often during screening of high-risk groups. High-risk groups include first- or second-degree relatives of someone with celiac disease and people with disorders associated with the disease.

Pathophysiology

Three factors are necessary for the development of celiac disease: a genetic predisposition, gluten ingestion, and an immune-mediated response.

- About 90% of patients with celiac disease have human leukocyte antigen (HLA) allele HLA-DQ2, and the other 10% have HLA-DQ8. However, HLA type does not appear to influence the disease severity, and not everyone with these genetic markers develops the disease.
- Tissue destruction that occurs with celiac disease is the result of chronic inflammation activated by the ingestion of gluten found in wheat, rye, and barley. A portion of poorly digested gluten, called the *gliadin fraction,* stimulates antibodies that activate release of cytokines. The cytokines destroy the microvilli and brush border of the small intestine, decreasing the amount of surface area available for nutrient absorption. Malabsorption can be so severe that the person develops malnutrition and wasting.
- The inflammation lasts as long as gluten ingestion continues. Unabated chronic inflammation can lead to lymphoma, and adenocarcinoma of the small intestine is also associated with celiac disease.
- Treatment with a lifelong, gluten-free diet halts the process.

Clinical Manifestations

Adults with celiac disease have different symptoms than the classic symptoms observed in infants (foul-smelling diarrhea, abdominal distention, failure to thrive).

- Some people have no symptoms, and the disease is discovered only during screening.
- Diarrhea occurs in less than half of all patients with celiac disease.
- Atypical symptoms, such as osteoporosis, dental enamel hypoplasia, iron and folate deficiencies, peripheral neuropathy, and reproductive problems, may occur.
- Celiac disease is also associated with other autoimmune diseases, particularly rheumatoid arthritis, type 1 diabetes mellitus, and thyroid disease.

Diagnostic Studies

- Histologic examination of biopsy specimens from duodenum and proximal small intestine can confirm a diagnosis of celiac disease.
- Biopsy specimens show flattened mucosa and noticeable losses of villi.
- Serologic testing for IgA tissue transglutaminase antibody and other serologic testing may be used but can result in both false-positive and false-negative findings.

Celiac disease should be ruled out during a diagnostic workup of inflammatory bowel disease, since the symptoms are similar. Many people seek treatment for nonspecific complaints for years before celiac disease is diagnosed.

Nursing and Collaborative Management

Because early diagnosis and treatment can prevent complications such as lymphoma, osteoporosis, and possibly other autoimmune diseases, screening for celiac disease should be encouraged for close relatives of patients known to have the disease, young patients with decreased bone density, and those with anemias of unknown cause.

- Celiac disease is treated with lifelong avoidance of dietary gluten from wheat, barley, rye, and oats (oats do not contain gluten but can become contaminated with gluten during milling).
- Gluten in food additives, perservatives, and stablizers must also be avoided.
- In patients with refractory celiac disease who do not respond to the gluten-free diet alone, corticosteroids may be used.

▼ **Patient and Family Teaching**
- Maintenance of a gluten-free diet is difficult. The patient needs to know where to purchase gluten-free products and may need financial assistance because of the increased cost of gluten-free products.

- Referral of the patient and family members to the Celiac Sprue Association is helpful for recipes and suggestions for maintaining a gluten-free diet.
- Patients need continuous encouragement and motivation to continue the gluten-free diet to prevent recurrence of intestinal damage and development of complications.

CERVICAL CANCER

Description
The number of deaths from cervical cancer has fallen steadily over the last 40 years. This is due to earlier and better diagnosis with widespread use of the Pap test. In addition to cancer, the Pap test detects precancerous changes. By treating precancerous lesions, progression to cervical cancer can be prevented.
- An increased risk of cervical cancer is associated with low socioeconomic status, early sexual activity (before 17 years old), multiple sexual partners, infection with human papillomavirus (HPV), immunosuppression, and smoking.

Precancerous changes are asymptomatic, which highlights the importance of routine screening. Noninvasive cervical cancer is four times more common than invasive cervical cancer and peaks in women in their early 30s. The average age for women with invasive cervical cancer is 50 years.

A vaccine is now available that reduces the incidence of both cervical-related neoplasia and cervical cancer due to infection from HPV (types 16 and 18).

Pathophysiology
The progression from normal cervical cells to dysplasia and on to cervical cancer appears to be related to repeated injuries to the cervix. The progression occurs slowly over years rather than months. There is a strong relationship between certain subtypes of HPV and cervical cancer.

Clinical Manifestations
Early cervical cancer is generally asymptomatic, but leukorrhea and intermenstrual bleeding eventually occur.
- A vaginal discharge that is usually thin and watery becomes dark and foul smelling as the disease advances.
- Vaginal bleeding is initially only spotting, but as the tumor enlarges, it becomes heavier and more frequent.

- Pain is a late symptom and is followed by weight loss, anemia, and cachexia.

Diagnostic Studies

- Pap test, colposcopy, and biopsy are performed for diagnostic purposes.
- The stage of cervical cancer determined by biopsy guides its treatment (see Table 54-11, Lewis and others, *Medical-Surgical Nursing,* edition 7, p. 1401).

Collaborative Care

Treatment is guided by tumor stage, patient's age, and patient's general health state. Four procedures can preserve fertility, an important consideration for younger women.

1. Conization may be the only therapy needed for noninvasive cervical cancer if analysis of removed tissue indicates that a wide area of normal tissue surrounds the excised tissue
2. Laser treatments can be used, in which a directed infrared beam is used to destroy abnormal tissue
3. Cautery
4. Cryosurgery

Invasive cancer of the cervix is treated with surgery, chemotherapy, and radiation as single treatments or in combination.

- Surgical procedures commonly carried out include hysterectomy, radical hysterectomy, and, rarely, pelvic exenteration (Table 23). Radiation may be external (e.g., cobalt) or internal (e.g., cesium or radium). Standard radiation treatment is 4 to 6 weeks of external radiation followed by one or two treatments with internal implants. Cisplatin-based chemotherapy regimens have shown benefit for patients with cancer spread beyond the cervix.

Nursing Management: Cervical Cancer and Other Cancers of the Female Reproductive System

In addition to cervical cancer, malignant tumors of the female reproductive system can be found in the endometrium, ovaries, vagina, and vulva. Management of the patient with any cancer of the female reproductive system includes many similar interventions.

Goals

The patient with a malignant tumor of the female reproductive system will actively participate in treatment decisions, achieve satisfactory pain and symptom management, recognize and report problems promptly, maintain preferred lifestyle as long as possible, and continue to practice cancer detection strategies.

| Table 23 | Surgical Procedures Involving the Female Reproductive System |

Type of Surgery	Description
Hysterectomy	
Total hysterectomy	Removal of uterus and cervix
Total abdominal hysterectomy and bilateral salpingo-oophorectomy (TAH-BSO; panhysterectomy)	Removal of uterus, cervix, fallopian tubes, and ovaries
Vulvectomy	
Simple vulvectomy	Excision of vulva and wide margin of skin
Radical vulvectomy	Excision of tissue from anus to few centimeters above symphysis pubis (skin, labia majora and minora, and clitoris) with superficial and deep lymph node dissection
Vaginectomy	Removal of vagina
Pelvic exenteration	Radical hysterectomy, total vaginectomy, removal of bladder with diversion of urinary system and resection of bowel with colostomy

Nursing Diagnoses
- Anxiety
- Acute pain
- Disturbed body image
- Ineffective sexuality patterns
- Grieving

Nursing Interventions
Through their contact with women in a variety of settings, nurses can teach women the importance and value of the cervical cancer vaccine and of routine screening for cancers of the reproductive system. Cancer can be prevented from occurring when screening reveals precancerous conditions of the vulva, cervix, or endometrium. Also, routine screening increases the chance that a cancer will be identified in its early stage. Nurses can assist women in viewing immunization and routine cancer screening as important self-care activities.

- Educating women about risk factors for cancers of the reproductive system is also important. Limiting sexual activity
during adolescence, using condoms, having fewer sexual
partners, and not smoking reduce the risk of cervical cancer.

Hysterectomy. Preoperatively, the patient is prepared for surgery
with the standard perineal or abdominal preparation. A vaginal
douche and enemas may be given according to surgeon preference.
The bladder should be emptied before the patient is sent to the
operating room. An indwelling catheter is often inserted.

After surgery the patient who has had a hysterectomy will have
an abdominal dressing (abdominal hysterectomy) or a sterile perineal pad (vaginal hysterectomy) (see NCP 54-1 for care of a patient
after a total abdominal hysterectomy, Lewis and others, *Medical-
Surgical Nursing,* edition 7, p. 1398).

- The dressing should be observed frequently for any sign of
bleeding during the first 8 hours after surgery. A moderate
amount of serosanguineous drainage on the perineal pad is
expected after a vaginal hysterectomy.
- Urinary retention may occur postoperatively because of temporary bladder atony resulting from edema or nerve trauma.
An indwelling catheter may be used for 1 or 2 days to maintain bladder drainage and prevent strain on the suture line.
- Food and fluids may be restricted if the patient is nauseated.
A rectal tube may be prescribed to relieve abdominal flatus.
Ambulation is encouraged.
- Special care must be taken to prevent the development of
deep vein thrombosis (DVT). Frequent position changes
and avoidance of high Fowler's position minimize blood
flow stasis and pooling. Leg exercises to promote circulation and the use of compression stockings or elastic ban-
dages are also helpful.

The loss of the uterus may bring about grief responses similar
to any great personal loss. The ability to bear children is central
to society's image of being a female. Eliciting the woman's feelings and concerns about her surgery provides needed information
to give understanding care.

The patient should be prepared for what to expect after surgery
(e.g., she will not menstruate). Teaching should include specific
activity restrictions. Intercourse should be avoided until the wound
is healed (about 4 to 6 weeks). If a vaginal hysterectomy is performed, the woman needs to know that there may be a temporary
loss of vaginal sensation.

- Physical restrictions are limited for a short time. Heavy
lifting should be avoided for 2 months. Activities that may
increase pelvic congestion, such as dancing and brisk

walking, should be avoided for several months, whereas activities such as swimming may be both physically and mentally helpful.

Salpingectomy and Oophorectomy. Postoperative care of the woman who has undergone removal of a fallopian tube (salpingectomy) or an ovary (oophorectomy) is similar to that for any patient having abdominal surgery. When both ovaries are removed (bilateral oophorectomy), surgical menopause results. Symptoms are similar to those of regular menopause but may be more severe because of the sudden withdrawal of hormones. To counter this, hormone replacement therapy may be initiated in the early postoperative period.

Pelvic Exenteration. When other forms of therapy are ineffective in stopping cancer spread and no metastases have been found outside the pelvis, pelvic exenteration may be performed. Although different types are done, this radical surgery usually involves removal of the uterus, ovaries, fallopian tubes, vagina, bladder, urethra, and pelvic lymph nodes. In some situations, the descending colon, rectum, and anal canal may also be removed. Postoperative care involves that of a patient who has had a radical hysterectomy, an abdominal perineal resection, and an ileostomy or colostomy. Physical, emotional, and social adjustments to life on the part of the woman and her family are great. There are urinary or fecal diversions in the abdominal wall, a reconstructed vagina, and the onset of menopausal symptoms.

CHLAMYDIAL INFECTION

Description

Chlamydia trachomatis is a gram-negative bacterium recognized as a genital pathogen responsible for a variety of illnesses.

- Different strains of *C. trachomatis* are responsible for urogenital infections (e.g., nongonococcal urethritis [NGU] in men and cervicitis in women), ocular trachoma, and lymphogranuloma venereum.
- In the United States and Canada, chlamydial infections are the most commonly reported sexually transmitted disease (STD).

Risk factors include women and adolescents, new or multiple sex partners, sex partners who have had multiple partners, history of STDs and cervical ectopy, coexisting STDs, and inconsistent or incorrect use of a condom.

- Chlamydial infections are a major contributor to pelvic inflammatory disease, ectopic pregnancy, infertility among women, and NGU in men.
- Chlamydial infections are closely associated with gonococcal infections, making clinical differentiation difficult.
- Because of the high prevalence of asymptomatic infections in both men and women, screening of high-risk populations is needed to identify those infected.

Clinical Manifestations

As with gonorrhea, chlamydial infections result in a superficial mucosal infection that can become more invasive.

- Symptoms may be absent or minor in most infected women and many men.
- Signs and symptoms that may occur in men include urethritis (dysuria, urethral discharge), epididymitis (unilateral scrotal pain, swelling, tenderness, fever), and proctitis (rectal discharge and pain during defecation).
- Signs and symptoms that may be found in women include cervicitis (mucopurulent discharge and hypertrophic ectopy [area that is edematous and bleeds easily]), urethritis (dysuria and frequent urination), dyspareunia (painful intercourse), bartholinitis (purulent exudate), and pelvic inflammatory disease (abdominal pain, nausea, vomiting, fever, abnormal vaginal bleeding, and menstrual abnormalities). A large number of women with chlamydial cervicitis have been found to have a male partner with NGU.

Complications often develop from poorly managed, inaccurately diagnosed, or undiagnosed chlamydial infections.

- Infection in men may result in epididymitis with possible infertility and reactive arthritis.
- Women may develop pelvic inflammatory disease leading to chronic pelvic pain and infertility.

Diagnostic Studies

Chlamydial infections in men can be diagnosed by excluding gonorrhea. The most common diagnostic tests include direct fluorescent antibody (DFA) test, enzyme immunoassay (EIA), and DNA amplification. These tests do not require special handling of specimens, are easier to perform than cell cultures, and can be used with urine samples rather than urethral and cervical swabs. DNA amplification test is the most sensitive diagnostic method available.

Collaborative Care

Chlamydial infections respond to treatment with doxycycline (Vibramycin), 100 mg twice per day for 7 days, or azithromycin

(Zithromax), 1 g in a single dose. Alternative regimens include erythromycin, ofloxacin (Floxin), or levofloxacin (Levaquin).

- Follow-up care should include advising the patient to return if symptoms persist or recur, treating sex partners, and encouraging the use of condoms during all sexual contacts.

Nursing Management
See Nursing Management: Sexually Transmitted Diseases, p. 564.

CHOLELITHIASIS/CHOLECYSTITIS

Description
The most common disorder of the biliary system is *cholelithiasis* (stones in the gallbladder). *Cholecystitis* (inflammation of the gallbladder) is usually associated with cholelithiasis. The stones may be lodged in the neck of the gallbladder or in the cystic duct. Cholecystitis may be acute or chronic, with these conditions also occurring together.

- The incidence of cholelithiasis is higher in women, especially multiparous women, and persons over 40 years old.
- Other predisposing factors for gallbladder disease are sedentary lifestyle, familial tendency, and obesity.
- Gallbladder disease is more common in whites than in Asian Americans and African Americans. There is an especially high incidence in the Native American population, particularly in the Navaho and Pima tribes.

Pathophysiology
The actual cause of gallstones is unknown. Cholelithiasis develops when the balance that keeps cholesterol, bile salts, and calcium in solution is altered so that precipitation of these substances occurs. Conditions that upset this balance include infection and disturbances in the metabolism of cholesterol. Mixed cholesterol stones, which are predominantly cholesterol, are the most common gallstones.

The stones may remain in the gallbladder or migrate to the cystic duct or common bile duct. They cause pain as they pass through the ducts and may lodge in the ducts and produce an obstruction. Stasis of bile in the gallbladder can lead to cholecystitis.

Cholecystitis is most commonly associated with obstruction resulting from gallstones or biliary sludge. Cholecystitis without obstruction from stones can occur as a result of trauma, extensive burns, prolonged immobility and fasting, and prolonged parenteral nutrition. Bacteria reaching the gallbladder by the vascular or lymphatic route or chemical irritants in the bile can also produce cholecystitis. *Escherichia coli,* streptococci, and salmonellae are the most common causative bacteria. Other etiologic factors include adhesions, neoplasms, anesthesia, and opioids.

- During an acute attack of cholecystitis the gallbladder is edematous and hyperemic. It may be distended with bile or pus. The cystic duct is also involved and may become occluded.
- The wall of the gallbladder becomes scarred after an acute attack. Decreased functioning occurs if large amounts of tissue are fibrosed.

Clinical Manifestations

Cholelithiasis may produce severe symptoms or none at all. Many patients have "silent cholelithiasis." Severity of symptoms depends on whether the stones are stationary or mobile and whether obstruction is present.

- When a stone is lodged in the ducts or when stones are moving through the ducts, spasms may result. This sometimes produces severe pain, which is termed *biliary colic.* The pain can be accompanied by tachycardia, diaphoresis, and prostration. The severe pain may last up to 1 hour, and when it subsides there is residual tenderness in the right upper quadrant.
- The attacks of pain frequently occur 3 to 6 hours after a heavy meal or when the patient lies down.
- When total obstruction occurs, symptoms related to bile blockage are manifested; these include steatorrhea, pruritus, dark amber urine, bleeding tendencies, and jaundice.

Cholecystitis manifestations may vary from indigestion to moderate to severe pain, leukocytosis, fever, and jaundice. Initial symptoms include indigestion and pain and tenderness in the right upper quadrant, which may be referred to the right shoulder and scapula. Pain may be acute and is accompanied by restlessness, diaphoresis, and nausea and vomiting.

- Symptoms of chronic cholecystitis include a history of fat intolerance, dyspepsia, heartburn, and flatulence.

Complications

Complications of cholecystitis include gangrenous cholecystitis, subphrenic abscess, pancreatitis, *cholangitis* (inflammation of

biliary ducts), biliary cirrhosis, fistulas, and rupture of the gallbladder, which can produce bile peritonitis. Many of the same
complications can occur from cholelithiasis, including cholangitis,
carcinoma, and peritonitis.

Diagnostic Studies

- Ultrasonography diagnoses gallstones.
- Endoscopic retrograde cholangiopancreatography (ERCP)
  allows for visualization of the gallbladder, cystic duct, common hepatic duct, and common bile duct. Bile taken during
  ERCP is sent for culture to identify any possible infecting
  organism.
- Percutaneous transhepatic cholangiography may be used to
  diagnose obstructive jaundice and to locate stones within the
  bile ducts.
- Laboratory studies may demonstrate liver function test abnormalities, elevated serum enzymes and pancreatic enzymes,
  increased white blood cell (WBC) count, elevated direct and
  indirect bilirubin levels, and urinary bilirubin.

Collaborative Care

During an acute episode of cholecystitis the focus is on control of
pain, control of possible infection with antibiotics, and maintenance of fluid and electrolyte balance. Treatment is mainly supportive and symptomatic.

- If nausea and vomiting are severe, gastric decompression
  may be used to prevent further gallbladder stimulation. Anticholinergics to decrease secretions (which prevents biliary
  contraction) and counteract smooth muscle spasms may be
  administered. Analgesics are given to decrease pain.

Cholelithiasis is most commonly treated by means of ERCP.
Standard ERCP techniques will clear stones from the biliary tree
in approximately 90% of patients. This procedure allows for visualization of the biliary system as well as the placement of stents
and sphincterotomy (papillotomy) if warranted. Endoscopic
sphincterotomy is especially effective in removing common bile
duct stones.

If the stone is too large to pass through the duct, the endoscopist
can crush the stone (mechanical lithotripsy). In approximately
10% of patients, nonstandard management, including mechanical,
electrohydraulic, or laser lithotripsy, will be needed. Other options
for cholelithiasis include cholesterol solvents such as methyl tertiary tributyl ester (MTBE), oral drugs that dissolve stones, endoscopic sphincterotomy, extracorporeal shock wave lithotripsy
(ESWL), and surgery.

Supportive treatment, similar to that given for cholecystitis, may also be necessary.

- If stones cause an obstruction, additional treatment consists of replacement of fat-soluble vitamins, administration of bile salts to facilitate digestion and vitamin absorption, and a low-fat diet.

Surgical intervention for cholelithiasis is frequently indicated and may consist of one of several procedures.

- Cholecystectomy is often the preferred surgical procedure. Most cholecystectomies are now performed laparoscopically. In this procedure the gallbladder is removed through one of four small punctures in the abdomen. Most patients experience minimal postoperative pain and are discharged the day of surgery or the day after. In most cases they are able to resume normal activities and return to work after a few days.

Drug therapy for gallbladder disease includes analgesics, anticholinergics (antispasmodics, such as atropine), fat-soluble vitamins, and bile salts. Morphine may be used initially for pain management. Therapy with ursodeoxycholic acid (UDCA), ursodiol (Actigall), and chenodeoxycholic acid (CDCA, chenodiol, Chenix) may be used to dissolve small, radiolucent stones in patients who are poor surgical risks.

Nutritional therapy for cholelithiasis and cholecystitis is a low-fat diet, which decreases stimulation of the gallbladder. If obesity is a problem, a reduced-calorie diet is indicated.

Nursing Management
Goals
The patient with gallbladder disease will have relief of pain and discomfort, no postoperative complications, and no recurrent attacks of cholecystitis or cholelithiasis.
Nursing Diagnoses
- Acute pain
- Ineffective therapeutic management regimen
Nursing Interventions
Nursing objectives for the patient undergoing conservative therapy include relieving pain, relieving nausea and vomiting, providing comfort and emotional support, maintaining fluid and electrolyte balance and nutrition, making accurate assessments for effectiveness of treatment, and observing for complications.

The patient with cholecystitis or cholelithiasis is frequently experiencing severe pain; medications ordered to relieve pain should be given as required before the pain becomes more severe.

The nurse should observe for signs of obstruction of the ducts by stones, including jaundice; clay-colored stools; dark, foamy urine; steatorrhea; fever; and increased WBC count.

Postoperative nursing care after a laparoscopic cholecystectomy includes monitoring for complications such as bleeding, making the patient comfortable, and preparing the patient for discharge.

A common problem after a laparoscopic cholecystectomy is referred pain to the shoulder because of the CO_2 that was not released or absorbed by the body. CO_2 can irritate the phrenic nerve and the diaphragm, causing some difficulty breathing.

- Placing the patient in Sims' position (left side with right knee flexed) helps move the gas pocket away from the diaphragm. Deep breathing should be encouraged, along with movement and ambulation.
- There is usually minimal pain that can be relieved by nonsteroidal antiinflammatory drugs (NSAIDs) or codeine.

▼ **Patient and Family Teaching**

- When the patient is on conservative therapy, dietary teaching is usually necessary. The diet is usually low in fat, and sometimes a weight-reduction diet is also recommended. The patient may need to take fat-soluble vitamin supplements.
- Instructions should be provided regarding observations the patient should make indicating obstruction (stool and urine changes, jaundice, and pruritus).

CHRONIC FATIGUE SYNDROME

Description

Chronic fatigue syndrome (CFS) is a disorder characterized by debilitating fatigue and a variety of associated complaints. Immune abnormalities are frequently present.

- CFS affects women more often than men and occurs in all ethnic and socioeconomic groups. Prevalence of this syndrome is difficult to determine because of the lack of validated diagnostic tests, but it can have a devastating impact on the lives of patients and their families.

Pathophysiology

Despite numerous attempts to determine the etiology and pathology of CFS, the precise mechanisms remain unknown. There are many theories about the etiology of CFS.

- Neuroendocrine abnormalities have been implicated involving a hypofunction of the HPA (hypothalamic-pituitary-adrenal) axis and HPG (hypothalamic-pituitary-gonadal) axis, which together regulate the stress response and reproductive hormone levels.
- Several microorganisms have been investigated as etiologic agents, including herpes viruses (e.g., Epstein Barr [EBV], cytomegalovirus [CMV]), retroviruses, enteroviruses, *Candida albicans,* and mycoplasma).
- Because cognitive deficits such as decreased memory, attention, and concentration occur in many of the patients, it has been proposed that CFS is due to changes in the central nervous system.

Clinical Manifestations

It is often difficult to distinguish between CFS and fibromyalgia syndrome (FMS) because many clinical features are similar (Table 24).

In about half of the cases, CFS develops insidiously, or the patient may have intermittent episodes that gradually become chronic.

- Incapacitating fatigue is the most common symptom that causes the patient to seek health care. Associated symptoms (Table 25) may fluctuate in intensity over time.
- The patient may become angry and frustrated with the inability of health care providers to diagnose a problem. The disorder may have a major impact on work and family responsibilities. Some individuals may even need help with activities of daily living.

Diagnostic Studies

Physical examination and diagnostic studies can be used to rule out other possible causes of the patient's symptoms. No laboratory test can diagnose CFS or measure its severity. The Centers for Disease Control and Prevention (CDC) have helped develop diagnostic criteria based on the patient's symptoms (see Table 25). In general, CFS remains a diagnosis of exclusion.

Nursing and Collaborative Management

Because there is no definitive therapy for CFS, supportive management is essential. The patient should be informed about what is known about the disease and all complaints should be taken seriously.

- Nonsteroidal antiinflammatory drugs (NSAIDs) can be used to treat headaches, muscle and joint aches, and fever.

Table 24	Commonalities Between Fibromyalgia Syndrome and Chronic Fatigue Syndrome
Occurrence	Previously healthy, young and middle-aged women
Etiology (theories)	Infectious trigger, dysfunction in HPA axis, alteration in CNS
Clinical manifestations	Malaise and fatigue, cognitive dysfunction, headaches, sleep disturbances, depression, anxiety, fever, generalized musculoskeletal pain
Course of disease	Variable—intensity of symptoms fluctuates over time
Diagnosis	No definitive laboratory tests or joint and muscle examinations; mainly a diagnosis of exclusion
Collaborative care	Treatment symptomatic and may include antidepressant drugs such as amitriptyline (Elavil) and fluoxetine (Prozac); other measures: heat, massage, regular stretching, biofeedback, stress management, and relaxation training; patient and family teaching essential

CNS, Central nervous system; *HPA*, hypothalamic-pituitary-adrenal axis.

Antihistamines and decongestants can be used to treat allergic symptoms. Tricyclic antidepressants (e.g., doxepin [Sinequan], amitriptyline [Elavil]) and selective serotonin reuptake inhibitors (e.g., fluoxetine [Prozac], paroxetine [Paxil]) can improve mood and sleep disorders.
- Total rest is not advised, because it can potentiate the self-image of being an invalid. On the other hand, strenuous exertion can exacerbate the exhaustion. Therefore it is important to plan a carefully graduated exercise program.
- Behavioral therapy may be used to promote a positive outlook, as well as improve overall disability, fatigue, and other symptoms.

CFS does not appear to progress. Although most patients recover or at least improve over time, they experience substantial occupational and psychosocial impairments and loss, including the social

Table 25	Diagnostic Criteria for Chronic Fatigue Syndrome*

Major Criteria
- Unexplained, persistent, or relapsing chronic fatigue that is of new and definite onset (not lifelong)
- Fatigue is not due to ongoing exertion
- Fatigue is not substantially alleviated by rest
- Fatigue results in substantial reduction in occupational, educational, social, or personal activities

Minor Criteria
- Substantial impairment in short-term memory or concentration
- Sore throat
- Tender cervical or axillary lymph nodes
- Muscle pain
- Multijoint pain without joint swelling or tenderness
- Headaches of a new type, pattern, or severity
- Unrefreshing sleep
- Postexertional malaise lasting more than 24 hours

Adapted from Fukuda K et al (International Chronic Fatigue Syndrome Study Group): The chronic fatigue syndrome: a comprehensive approach to its definition and study, *Ann Intern Med* 121:953, 1994.
* For a diagnosis to be made, the patient must fulfill all the major criteria plus four or more of the minor criteria. Each minor criterion must have persisted or recurred during 6 or more consecutive months of illness and must not have predated the fatigue. These criteria were prepared by the Centers for Disease Control and Prevention, National Institutes of Health, and International Chronic Fatigue Syndrome Study Group.

pressure and isolation from being characterized as lazy or "crazy."

CHRONIC OBSTRUCTIVE PULMONARY DISEASE: EMPHYSEMA AND CHRONIC BRONCHITIS

Description

Chronic obstructive pulmonary disease (COPD) is a disease state characterized by the presence of airway obstruction that is not fully reversible. The limited airflow is usually progressive and is associated with an abnormal inflammatory response of the lungs to noxious particles or gases, primarily cigarette smoke. The term *chronic obstructive pulmonary disease* encompasses two types of obstructive airway diseases, *chronic bronchitis* and *emphysema*.

- Chronic bronchitis is the presence of chronic productive cough for 3 months in each of 2 consecutive years in a patient in whom other causes of chronic cough have been excluded.
- Emphysema is an abnormal permanent enlargement of the air spaces distal to the terminal bronchioles, accompanied by destruction of their walls and without obvious fibrosis.
- Patients with COPD may have a predominance of one of these conditions, but the conditions usually coexist, and COPD is considered one disease state in terms of management.

More than 11 million persons in the United States have emphysema and chronic bronchitis. COPD is the fourth leading cause of death in the United States.

Etiology
Cigarette smoking is the major risk factor for developing COPD.

- The irritating effect of cigarette smoke causes hyperplasia of cells, which subsequently results in increased mucous production. Hyperplasia reduces airway diameter and increases the difficulty in clearing secretions. Smoking reduces ciliary activity and produces abnormal dilation of the distal air space with destruction of alveolar walls.
- COPD can develop independently of cigarette smoking if a person has intense or prolonged exposure to various dusts, vapors, irritants, or fumes in the workplace.
- High levels of urban air pollution are harmful to persons with existing lung diease, but the effect of outdoor air pollution as a risk factor for COPD appears to be small compared with the effect of cigarette smoking.
- Severe recurring respiratory tract infections impair normal defense mechanisms, making the bronchioles and alveoli more susceptible to injury and intensifying the pathologic destruction of lung tissue.

A form of hereditary primary emphysema is related to a deficiency of α_1-antitrypsin (AAT) that normally has an inhibitory effect on proteolytic enzymes. Emphysema results when lysis of lung tissues by proteolytic enzymes from neutrophils and macrophages occurs because of AAT deficiency. Although this emphysema accounts for only 1% to 2% of COPD cases in the United States, smoking greatly exacerbates the disease process in these patients.

Some degree of emphysema is common in the lungs of older persons, even nonsmokers. Aging results in changes in the lung structure, thoracic cage, and respiratory muscles. However, clinically significant emphysema is usually not caused by aging alone.

Pathophysiology

The pathogenesis of COPD is complex and involves many mechanisms, but the primary process is inflammation that affects the airways, lung parenchyma, and pulmonary vasculature.

- The inflammatory process starts with inhalation of noxious particles (e.g., cigarette smoke) that causes the release of inflammatory mediators that damage lung tissue. Airways become inflamed, resulting in enlarged mucus-secreting glands and an increased number of goblet cells. This results in excess mucus production (or chronic bronchitis).

- Small bronchi and bronchioles are remodeled and become fibrotic because of scar tissue formation as a result of repeated cycles of injury and repair of the airway walls.

- Destruction of the lung parenchyma is thought to be due to an imbalance of proteinases/antiproteinases that occurs as a result of inflammation. Emphysema results from this damage.

- One type of emphysema, called *centrilobular,* involves dilation and destruction of the respiratory bronchioles and is most commonly seen in upper lobes in mild disease.

- The second type of emphysema, *panlobular,* involves destruction of the alveolar ducts, alveolar sacs, and respiratory bronchioles. It is most prominent in the lower lobes and is seen with α_1-antitrypsin (a proteinase inhibitor) deficiency.

The basic elastin structure of the parenchyma is destroyed, and there is no pull or traction on the walls of the bronchioles. The bronchioles tend to collapse on expiration, and air is trapped in the distal alveoli, resulting in hyperinflation and overdistention of the alveoli. In COPD the lungs can be inflated easily but can only partially deflate.

- Pulmonary vascular changes result as inflammatory cells infiltrate the smooth muscle of the blood vessels, causing thickening. Capillaries are lost with the alveoli, and because air can move into the lung but perfusion of gases is impaired, a ventilation/perfusion imbalance occurs. In severe cases, collagen is deposited in the pulmonary vessels, leading to pulmonary hypertension and cor pulmonale.

The pathophysiologic changes of COPD result in the following characteristic disease manifestations: hypersecretion of mucus, dysfunction of the cilia, airflow limitation and hyperinflation of the lungs, gas exchange abnormalities, pulmonary hypertension, and cor pulmonale.

Some patients with COPD may also have asthma, and some patients with asthma may develop fixed or irreversible airflow obstruction. However, pathologically the types of inflammatory cells are quite different between COPD and asthma. Table 29-17 in Lewis and others, *Medical-Surgical Nursing,* edition 7, p. 635 compares the clinical features and diagnostic results of asthma and COPD.

Clinical Manifestations

Clinical manifestations of COPD typically develop slowly around 50 years of age after 20 pack-years of cigarette smoking.

- The earliest symptom is an intermittent cough that usually occurs in the morning with the expectoration of small amounts of sticky mucus resulting from bouts of coughing. Later in the disease, the cough is present every day, usually with increasing amounts of mucus.
- Dyspnea is often progressive and usually occurs with exertion. In late stages of COPD, dyspnea may be present at rest.
- As increasing amounts of air are trapped, the diaphragm becomes flattened and the anteroposterior diameter of the chest increases, forming the typical "barrel chest."
- During physical examination a prolonged expiratory phase of respiration, wheezes, or decreased breath sounds are noted in all lung fields. The patient may assume a tripod position, use pursed-lip breathing, and use accessory muscles of respiration.
- Hypoxemia and hypercapnia may develop later in the disease. The bluish red color of the skin results from polycythemia and cyanosis. Polycythemia develops as a result of increased production of red blood cells secondary to the body's attempt to compensate for chronic hypoxemia.
- The person with advanced COPD frequently experiences weight loss and anorexia, for reasons not well understood.

Complications

Cor pulmonale is hypertrophy of the right side of the heart, with or without heart failure, resulting from pulmonary hypertension. In COPD, pulmonary hypertension is caused primarily by constriction of pulmonary vessels in response to alveolar hypoxia, with acidosis further potentiating vasoconstriction. Increased pulmonary vascular resistance is also caused by inflammatory-induced vascular remodeling, increased viscosity of the blood from polycythemia, and reduction in the pulmonary capillary bed. When pulmonary hypertension develops, the pressure on the right side of the heart must increase to push blood into the lungs. Eventually, right-sided heart failure develops (see Cor Pulmonale, p. 149).

Exacerbations of COPD are "flares" in the status of disease and are signaled by an increase in the patient's usual dyspnea, cough, and/or sputum. Other complaints include malaise, insomnia, fatigue, depression, confusion, or decreased exercise tolerance. The primary causes of exacerbations are tracheobronchial infection and air pollution. The most common organisms causing exacerbations are *Haemophilus influenzae, Moraxella catarrhalis,* and *Streptococcus pneumoniae.* Exacerbations are managed with bronchodilators, oral systemic corticosteroids, antibiotics, and supplemental oxygen therapy.

Acute respiratory failure may occur in patients with severe COPD who have exacerbations (see Acute Respiratory Distress Syndrome, p. 13). Respiratory failure may also be precipitated by cor pulmonale, failure to take respiratory medications, use of respiratory depressants such as sedatives and opioids, or carbon dioxide narcosis.

Peptic ulcer and gastroesophageal reflux disease (GERD) occur frequently in patients with COPD (see Peptic Ulcer Disease, p. 480, and Gastroesophageal Reflux Disease, p. 242). These occurrences are partly explained by hypersecretion of gastric acid resulting from increased arterial CO_2 and decreased arterial O_2 tension. This occurs only in patients who chronically retain CO_2. GERD may aggravate respiratory symptoms.

Depression and **anxiety** are other common complications of COPD. The prevalence of depression may be four times more frequent in patients with COPD than in the general population. Anxiety can complicate respiratory compromise and may precipitate dyspnea and hyperventilation. Treatment consists of cognitive and behavioral psychotherapy and/or pharmacotherapy.

Diagnostic Studies

The diagnosis of COPD is confirmed by spirometry and can be classified as at risk, mild, moderate, severe, and very severe.

- The forced expiratory volume/forced vital capacity (FEV_1/FVC) <70% establishes the diagnosis of COPD, and the severity of obstruction (FEV_1) determines the stage of COPD.
- Chest x-ray is seldom diagnostic unless bullous emphysema is present.
- Serum α_1-antitrypsin levels may be decreased in emphysema.
- Electrocardiogram (ECG) may be normal or indicate right ventricular failure from cor pulmonale.

- Sputum culture and sensitivity are done if exacerbation is present.
- Arterial blood gases (ABGs) in later stages usually indicate low PaO_2, elevated $PaCO_2$, decreased or low normal pH, and increased bicarbonate (HCO_3^-) levels.

Collaborative Care

The primary goals of care for the patient with COPD are to prevent disease progression, relieve symptoms and improve exercise tolerance, prevent and treat complications, promote patient participation in care, prevent and treat exacerbations, and improve quality of life and reduce mortality.

- The patient with COPD should have a pneumococcal and influenza virus vaccine yearly and avoid environmental or occupational irritants.
- Exacerbations of COPD should be treated as soon as possible. Often the best indication of the presence of a respiratory infection is the increasing quantity, viscosity, or purulence of sputum. Some patients are given a prescription for a 7- to 10-day supply of antibiotics and are instructed to begin taking them at the first signs of change in sputum.
- Cessation of cigarette smoking in any stage of COPD is the single most effective intervention to reduce the risk of developing COPD and stop the progression of the disease. Smoking cessation techniques are discussed in Lewis and others, *Medical-Surgical Nursing,* edition 7, pp. 170 to 174, and in Tables 12-4, 12-5, and 12-6, pp. 171 to 173.
- Bronchodilator drug therapy is often helpful in relieving symptoms. Although patients with COPD do not respond as dramatically as those with asthma to bronchodilator therapy, a reduction in dyspnea and an increase in FEV_1 are usually achieved. Bronchodilator drugs commonly used are β_2-adrenergic agonists, anticholinergic agents, and methylxanthines. Inhaled corticosteroids may be helpful for patients with severe COPD. Medications are given in a stepwise fashion (Table 26). Drug therapy for COPD is discussed in Table 29-7, Lewis and others, *Medical-Surgical Nursing,* edition 7, pp. 618 to 620.
- Long-term O_2 therapy improves survival, exercise tolerance, cognitive performance, and sleep in hypoxemic patients. The goal of O_2 administration is to supply the patient with adequate O_2 to maximize the O_2-carrying ability of the blood. O_2 may be prescribed for continuous use, only at night, or with exercise (see Oxygen Therapy, p. 734).

Table 26 Therapy at Each Stage of COPD

Stage 0 At Risk	Stage 1 Mild COPD	Stage 2 Moderate COPD	Stage 3 Severe COPD	Stage 4 Very Severe COPD
Avoidance of risk factor or factors; influenza vaccination				
	Add short-acting bronchodilator when needed			
		Add regular treatment with one or more long-acting bronchodilators		
		Add pulmonary rehabilitation		
			Add inhaled corticosteroids if repeated exacerbations	
				Add long-term oxygen if chronic respiratory failure Consider surgical treatments

Adapted from Global Initiative for Chronic Obstructive Lung Disease (GOLD) Workshop report. Available at www.goldcopd.org.
COPD, Chronic obstructive pulmonary disease.

- Respiratory and physical therapy activities include breathing retraining, effective cough techniques, chest physiotherapy, and aerosol-nebulization therapy (see Lewis and others, *Medical-Surgical Nursing,* edition 7, pp. 646 to 649 for further information on respiratory care). These therapies often require a collaborative effort among nurses, respiratory therapists, and physical therapists.
- Nutritional therapy is directed toward helping the patient with COPD maintain a body mass index between 21 and 25 kg/m^2. Weight loss and malnutrition are common in the patient with severe emphysematous COPD. To decrease dyspnea and conserve energy, the patient should rest at least 30 minutes before eating, use the bronchodilator before meals, and select foods that can be prepared in advance. The patient should eat five or six small, frequent meals to avoid feelings of bloating and early satiety when eating.

Surgical Therapy

Three different surgical procedures have been used in severe COPD. One type of surgery is *lung volume reduction surgery* (LVRS), in which about 30% of the most diseased lung tissue is removed. The rationale for this type of surgery is that by reducing the size of the hyperinflated emphysematous lungs, there is decreased airway obstruction and increased room for the remaining normal alveoli to function.

Another surgical procedure is a bullectomy (removal of bullae) in emphysematous patients who have large bullae (dilated air spaces within the lungs). This operation is rarely performed because only a small percentage of patients have large bullae.

A third surgical procedure is lung transplantation. COPD patients are the largest group of patients on waiting lists for lung transplantation. In appropriately selected patients with COPD, lung transplantation prolongs life, improves functional capacity, and enhances quality of life.

Nursing Management

Goals

The patient with COPD will have prevention of disease progression, ability to perform activities of daily living (ADLs) and improved exercise tolerance, relief from symptoms, no complications related to COPD, knowledge and ability to implement a long-term treatment regimen, and overall improved quality of life.

See NCP 29-2 for the patient with chronic obstructive pulmonary disease, Lewis and others, *Medical-Surgical Nursing,* edition 7, pp. 651 to 653.

Nursing Diagnoses
- Ineffective airway clearance
- Impaired gas exchange
- Imbalanced nutrition: less than body requirements
- Insomnia
- Risk for infection

Nursing Interventions
- The nurse is in an important position to dramatically reduce the incidence of COPD by advocating smoking cessation in all smokers and working to prevent smoking in adolescents.
- Other preventive measures to maintain healthy lungs include avoiding or controlling exposure to pollutants and irritants, early detection of small airway disease, and early diagnosis and treatment of respiratory tract infections. Patients with COPD should maintain influenza and pneumococcal vaccines and avoid exposure to large crowds in peak periods for influenza.
- The patient with COPD will require acute intervention for complications such as pneumonia, cor pulmonale, and acute respiratory failure. Once the crisis in these situations has been resolved, the nurse can assess the degree and severity of the underlying respiratory problem. The information obtained will help to plan nursing care.

▼ **Patient and Family Teaching**

The most important aspect in long-term care of the patient with COPD is education (Table 27).

- Pulmonary rehabilitation should be recommended for all patients with symptomatic COPD. The components of pulmonary rehabilitation include physical therapy (e.g., bronchial hygiene, exercise conditioning, breathing retraining, energy conservation), nutrition, and education and other topics such as smoking cessation, environmental factors, health promotion, psychologic counseling, and vocational rehabilitation.
- Energy conservation is an important component in COPD rehabilitation. Exercise training of the upper extremities may improve function and reduce dyspnea. Alternative energy-saving practices for ADLs and scheduled rest periods should be planned.
- Walking is the best physical exercise for the COPD patient. Coordinated walking with slow, pursed-lip breathing without breath holding is a difficult task that requires conscious effort and frequent reinforcement. The nurse should walk with the patient, giving verbal reminders when necessary regarding breathing (inhalation and exhalation) and steps. The patient should be encouraged to walk 15 to 20

Table 27	Patient and Family Teaching Guide: Chronic Obstructive Pulmonary Disease (COPD)

Teaching Topic

What is COPD?
- Basic anatomy and physiology of lung
- Basic pathophysiology of COPD
- Signs and symptoms of COPD, respiratory infection, heart failure

Breathing Retraining
- Pursed-lip breathing

Energy Conservation Techniques
- Pacing and pursing (pacing activity and using pursed-lip breathing with activities)

Medications
- Types (include mechanism of action)
    Methylxanthines
    β_2-Adrenergic agonists
    Corticosteroids
    Anticholinergics
    Antibiotics
- Establishing medication schedule

Correct Use of Metered-Dose Inhaler, Spacer, and Nebulizer Home Oxygen
- Explanation of rationale for use
- Guide for home O_2 use

Psychosocial and Emotional Issues
- Concerns about interpersonal relationships
    Dependency
    Intimacy
- Problems with emotions
    Depression
    Anxiety
    Panic
- Effects of medications
- Support and rehabilitation groups

COPD Management Plan
- Focusing on self-management
- Knowing usual signs/symptoms
- Need to report changes
- Cause of flare-ups
- Recognition of signs and symptoms of respiration infection, heart failure
- Yearly follow-up

Healthy Nutrition
- Strategies to lose weight (if overweight)
- Strategies to gain weight (if underweight)

minutes per day with gradual increases, using O_2 if necessary.

- Patients should be informed that modifying but not abstaining from sexual activity can also contribute to a healthy psychologic well-being. Using an inhaled bronchodilator before sexual activity can help ventilation.

- Adequate sleep is extremely important. The patient who is a restless sleeper, snores, stops breathing while asleep, and has a tendency to fall asleep during the day may need to be tested for sleep apnea.

- Healthy coping is often the most difficult task for a patient with COPD. People with COPD frequently have to deal with many lifestyle changes that may involve decreased ability to care for themselves, decreased energy for social activities, and loss of a job. Support groups at local chapters of the American Lung Association, hospitals, and clinics may be helpful.

CIRRHOSIS

Description

Cirrhosis is a chronic progressive disease of the liver characterized by extensive degeneration and destruction of liver parenchymal cells. It is the fourth leading cause of death in persons between 35 and 54 years of age, and the highest incidence occurs between the ages of 40 and 60 years. The four types of cirrhosis, in order of incidence, are as follows:

1. Alcoholic (previously Laënnec's) cirrhosis, also called portal or nutritional cirrhosis, is usually associated with alcohol abuse. The first change in the liver from excessive alcohol intake is an accumulation of fat in the liver cells. Uncomplicated fatty changes in the liver are potentially reversible if the person stops drinking alcohol.

2. Postnecrotic cirrhosis is a complication of viral, toxic, or idiopathic hepatitis. Broad bands of scar tissue form within the liver.

3. Biliary cirrhosis is associated with chronic biliary obstruction and infection. There is diffuse fibrosis of the liver with jaundice as the main feature.

4. Cardiac cirrhosis results from long-standing, severe, right-sided heart failure in patients with cor pulmonale, constrictive pericarditis, and tricuspid insufficiency.

Pathophysiology
In cirrhosis, the liver cells attempt to regenerate following cell damage and necrosis, but the regenerative process is disorganized, resulting in abnormal blood vessel and bile duct structure. Eventually the irregular, disorganized regeneration, poor cellular nutrition, and hypoxia caused by inadequate blood flow and scar tissue result in decreased liver function.

- Approximately 20% of patients with chronic hepatitis C and 10% to 20% of those with chronic hepatitis B will develop cirrhosis.

Clinical Manifestations
The onset of cirrhosis is usually insidious. Occasionally there is an abrupt onset of symptoms.

- Early manifestations include anorexia, dyspepsia, flatulence, nausea and vomiting, and change in bowel habits (diarrhea or constipation). In addition, fever, lassitude, abdominal pain, slight weight loss, and enlargement of the liver and spleen may occur.
- Later manifestations may be severe and result from liver failure and portal hypertension. Jaundice, peripheral edema, and ascites develop gradually. Other late symptoms include skin lesions, hematologic disorders, endocrine disturbances, and peripheral neuropathies. In advanced stages the liver becomes small and nodular. (See Fig. 44-6, Lewis and others, *Medical-Surgical Nursing*, edition 7, p. 1104, for systemic manifestations of cirrhosis.)
- *Jaundice* occurs as a result of the decreased ability of the liver to conjugate and excrete bilirubin (hepatocellular jaundice).
- *Skin lesions* such as *spider angiomas* that occur on the nose, cheeks, upper trunk, and neck and a redness of the palms of the hands known as *palmar erythema* result from an increase in circulating estrogen because the liver cannot metabolize steroid hormones.
- *Hematologic disorders* such as anemia, leukopenia, and thrombocytopenia result from overactivity of an enlarged spleen, and coagulation problems result from the liver's inability to produce prothrombin and other coagulation factors.
- *Endocrine imbalances* result because adrenocortical hormones, estrogen, and testosterone cannot be metabolized and inactivated by the damaged liver. Men lose masculine sex characteristics as a result of increased estrogen levels and amenorrhea may occur in women. Sodium and water

retention and potassium loss occur as a result of hyperaldosteronism.

- *Peripheral neuropathy* probably results from a deficiency of thiamine, folic acid, and cobalamin.

Complications

Major complications are portal hypertension with resultant esophageal varices, peripheral edema and ascites, hepatic encephalopathy (coma), and hepatorenal syndrome.

Portal hypertension and *esophageal varices* result because of structural liver changes from cirrhosis; there is compression and destruction of the portal and hepatic veins and sinusoids. Pathophysiologic changes resulting from portal hypertension include the development of collateral circulation in an attempt to reduce high portal pressure and also to reduce increased plasma volume and lymphatic flow.

- Common areas where collateral channels form are the lower esophagus (anastomosis of the left gastric vein and azygos veins), anterior abdominal wall, parietal peritoneum, and rectum.
- Varicosities may develop in areas where collateral and systemic circulations communicate, resulting in esophageal and gastric varices, caput medusae (ring of varices around the umbilicus), and hemorrhoids.

Esophageal varices are a complex of tortuous veins at the end of the esophagus, which are enlarged and swollen as a result of portal hypertension. They are a common complication, occurring in two thirds to three fourths of all patients with cirrhosis. These collateral vessels contain little elastic tissue and are quite fragile. They tolerate high pressure poorly, and the result is distended veins that bleed easily.

- Bleeding esophageal varices are the most life-threatening complication of cirrhosis.
- Varices rupture and bleed in response to ulceration and irritation. Factors producing ulceration and irritation include alcohol ingestion; swallowing of poorly masticated food; ingestion of coarse food; acid regurgitation from the stomach; and increased intraabdominal pressure caused by nausea, vomiting, straining at stool, coughing, sneezing, or lifting heavy objects.
- Patients may have melena or hematemesis. There may be slow oozing or massive bleeding, which is a medical emergency.

Peripheral edema results from decreased colloidal osmotic pressure from impaired liver synthesis of albumin and increased portocaval pressure from portal hypertension. Peripheral edema occurs as ankle and presacral edema.

Ascites is the accumulation of serous fluid in the peritoneal or abdominal cavity. When blood pressure (BP) is elevated in the liver, as occurs in cirrhosis, proteins move from the blood vessels by way of larger pores of the sinusoids (capillaries) into the lymph space. When the lymphatic system is unable to carry off excess proteins and water, proteins leak through the liver capsule into the peritoneal cavity. A second mechanism of ascites formation is hypoalbuminemia and decreased colloidal oncotic pressure resulting from the inability of the liver to synthesize albumin. A third mechanism of ascites, hyperaldosteronism, results when aldosterone is not metabolized by damaged hepatocytes, which causes increased renal reabsorption of sodium and water.

- Ascites is manifested by abdominal distention with weight gain. If ascites is severe, the umbilicus may be everted. Abdominal striae with distended abdominal wall veins may also be present.
- The patient has signs of dehydration (e.g., dry tongue and skin, sunken eyeballs, muscle weakness), with a decrease in urinary output.
- Hypokalemia is common and is due to an excessive loss of potassium from hyperaldosteronism and the use of diuretic therapy to treat ascites.

Hepatic encephalopathy is a frequent neuropsychiatric manifestation of liver disease. It is considered a terminal complication. Encephalopathy can occur in any condition in which liver damage causes ammonia to enter the systemic circulation without liver detoxification.

- The main pathogenic agents appear to be nitrogenous ammonia and aromatic amino acids. When blood is shunted past the liver by way of collateral anastomoses or the liver is unable to convert ammonia to urea, large quantities of ammonia remain in the systemic circulation. Ammonia crosses the blood-brain barrier and produces neurologic toxic manifestations.
- A number of factors may precipitate hepatic encephalopathy mostly because they increase the amount of circulating ammonia, including gastrointestinal (GI) hemorrhage, constipation, infection, hypokalemia, hypovolemia, dehydration, and metabolic alkalosis.
- Hepatic encephalopathy is manifested by changes in neurologic and mental responsiveness, ranging from sleep disturbance to lethargy to deep coma. A characteristic symptom is *asterixis* (flapping tremor), a rapid flexion and extension

movement of the hands when the arms and hands are held stretched out.

Hepatorenal syndrome is a serious complication of cirrhosis. It is characterized by functional renal failure with advancing azotemia, oliguria, and intractable ascites.

- There is no structural abnormality of the kidneys. The etiology is complex, but the final common pathway is usually portal hypertension along with liver decompensation that results in splanchnic and systemic vasodilation and decreased arterial blood volume. As a result, renal vasoconstriction occurs and renal failure follows.
- This syndrome frequently follows diuretic therapy, GI hemorrhage, or paracentesis. It can be reversed by liver transplant.

Diagnostic Studies

- Liver function studies demonstrate an elevation in alkaline phosphatase, aspartate aminotransferase (AST), alanine aminotransferase (ALT), and γ-glutamyl transferase (GGT).
- Liver biopsy (percutaneous needle) and scan are done.
- Prothrombin time is prolonged.
- Serum albumin and protein levels are decreased, and bilirubin and globulin are increased.
- Differential analysis of ascitic fluid is done.

Collaborative Care

Although there is no specific therapy for cirrhosis, certain measures can be taken to promote liver cell regeneration and prevent or treat complications.

- Rest is significant in reducing metabolic demands of the liver and allowing for recovery of liver cells. At various times during the progress of cirrhosis, rest may have to take the form of complete bed rest.

Management of ascites is focused on sodium restriction (250 to 500 mg/day for severe ascites), diuretic therapy (e.g., a potassium-sparing diuretic combined with a loop diuretic), and fluid removal (paracentesis) for those patients with impaired respiration or abdominal pain. Peritoneovenous shunt insertion provides for the continuous reinfusion of ascitic fluid into the venous system. Transjugular intrahepatic portosystemic shunt (TIPS) is also used to alleviate ascites.

The main therapeutic goal related to esophageal varices is avoidance of bleeding and hemorrhage. The patient who has esophageal varices should avoid ingesting alcohol, aspirin, and irritating foods. Upper respiratory infections should be treated promptly, and coughing should be controlled. For patients who have not bled from esophageal varices, prophylactic treatment with nonselective β blockers (e.g., propranolol [Inderal]) has been shown to reduce the risk of bleeding, as well as bleeding-related deaths.

- Management related to bleeding esophageal varices includes the use of the somatostatin analog octreotide (Sandostatin), vasopressin (VP), nitroglycerin (NTG), β-adrenergic blockers, balloon tamponade, sclerotherapy, ligation of varices, and TIPS therapy.
- Supportive measures during an acute variceal bleed include administration of fresh frozen plasma and packed red blood cells (RBCs), vitamin K (AquaMEPHYTON), and histamine blockers such as cimetidine (Tagamet). Neomycin or lactulose (Cephulac) administration may be started to prevent hepatic encephalopathy from the breakdown of blood and the release of ammonia in the intestine.

The goal of management in hepatic encephalopathy is the reduction of ammonia formation. This consists mainly of protein restriction and reduction of ammonia formation in the intestines. Lactulose (Cephulac) discourages bacterial growth, traps ammonia in the gut, and expels ammonia from the colon. Constipation should be prevented with cathartics and enemas to decrease bacterial action.

- Treatment of hepatic encephalopathy also involves controlling GI bleeding and removing blood from the GI tract to decrease protein in the intestine. Electrolyte and acid-base imbalances and infections should also be treated.

Additional Management

A number of medications may be used to treat symptoms and complications of advanced liver disease (see Table 44-16, Lewis and others, *Medical-Surgical Nursing,* edition 7, p. 1110). Specific nutritional therapy varies with the degree of liver damage and the danger of encephalopathy; generally, the diet is high in calories and carbohydrates with sodium restricted. Protein restriction is rarely justified in patients with persistent hepatic encephalopathy because malnutrition is a more serious clinical problem than hepatic encephalopathy for many of these patients.

Liver transplantation should be considered in patients with recurring hepatic encephalopathy and end-stage liver disease. Transplantation depends on a number of factors, including the cause of the cirrhosis and other systemic medical problems.

Nursing Management

Goals

The patient with cirrhosis will have relief of discomfort, have minimal to no complications (ascites, esophageal varices, hepatic encephalopathy), and return to as normal a lifestyle as possible.

See NCP 44-2 for the patient with cirrhosis, Lewis and others, *Medical-Surgical Nursing,* edition 7, pp. 1112 to 1113.

Nursing Diagnoses/Collaborative Problems

- Imbalanced nutrition: less than body requirements
- Impaired skin integrity
- Ineffective breathing pattern
- Risk for infection
- Acute/chronic confusion
- Dysfunctional family processes
- Potential complication: hemorrhage
- Potential complication: hepatic encephalopathy

Nursing Interventions

Prevention and early treatment of cirrhosis must focus on the primary etiology.

- Alcoholism needs to be treated; adequate nutrition, especially for the alcoholic and other individuals at risk for cirrhosis, is essential to promote liver regeneration.
- Acute hepatitis must be identified and treated early so that it does not progress to chronic hepatitis.
- Biliary disease must be treated so that stones do not cause obstruction and infection.
- The underlying cause (e.g., chronic lung disease) of right-sided heart failure must be treated so that the heart failure does not lead to cirrhosis.

The focus of acute nursing interventions is on conserving the patient's strength. Rest enables the liver to restore itself. Complete bed rest may not always be necessary.

- Anorexia, nausea and vomiting, pressure from ascites, and poor eating habits all create problems in the maintenance of an adequate intake of nutrients. Nursing measures relating to nutrition for patients with hepatitis also apply, including oral hygiene and between-meal nourishment.
- The patient's physiologic response to cirrhosis should be assessed, including the presence and progression of jaundice, any pruritus, and urine and stool color.
- Accurate recordings of intake and output, daily weights, and measurements of extremities and abdominal girth help in the ongoing assessment of edema.

- When the patient is taking diuretics, the serum levels of sodium, potassium, chloride, and bicarbonate should be monitored.
- A semi-Fowler's or Fowler's position allows for maximal respiratory efficiency when dyspnea is a problem. Pillows can be used to support arms and chest and may increase patient comfort and ability to breathe.
- Meticulous skin care is essential because edematous tissues are subject to breakdown. An alternating air pressure mattress or other special mattress should be used. A turning schedule (minimum of every 2 hours) must be adhered to rigidly. The abdomen may be supported with pillows.
- When a paracentesis is done, have the patient void immediately before the procedure to prevent puncture of the bladder. After the procedure, monitor for hypovolemia and electrolyte imbalances, and check the dressing for bleeding and leakage.
- If the patient has esophageal varices, monitor for signs of bleeding from varices, such as hematemesis and melena. If hematemesis occurs, the nurse should assess the patient for hemorrhage, call the physician, and be ready to assist with treatments to control bleeding. The patient will be admitted to the intensive care unit (ICU).
- The focus of care with hepatic encephalopathy is on sustaining life and assisting with measures to reduce the formation of ammonia. Factors that are known to precipitate coma should be controlled as much as possible.

▼ **Patient and Family Teaching**

The patient and family need to understand the importance of continuous health care and medical supervision. They should be taught symptoms of complications and when to seek medical attention.

- Measures to achieve and maintain remission should be encouraged, including proper diet, rest, avoidance of potentially hepatotoxic over-the-counter drugs such as acetaminophen, and abstinence from alcohol.
- Provide information regarding community support programs such as Alcoholics Anonymous for help with alcohol abuse.
- Other health teaching should include instruction about adequate rest periods, how to detect early signs of complications, skin care, drug therapy precautions, observation for bleeding, and protection from infection.
- Counseling information regarding sexual problems may be needed.

- Referral to a community or home health nurse may be helpful to ensure adequate patient compliance with prescribed therapy.

COLORECTAL CANCER

C

Description
Colorectal cancer (cancer of the colon and rectum) is the third most common form of cancer and the second leading cause of cancer-related death in the United States. Because symptoms do not appear until the disease is quite advanced, regular screening is necessary to detect precancerous lesions. Eighty-five percent of colorectal cancers arise from adenomatous polyps that can be detected and removed from the colon by colonscopy.

Pathophysiology
The causes of colorectal cancer remain unclear. It may occur at any age but is most prevalent over the age of 50 years. Major risk factors include increasing age, family or personal history of colorectal cancer, colorectal polyps, and inflammatory bowel disease. Hereditary diseases account for 5% to 10% of cases, and certain lifestyle factors are also associated with colorectal cancer.
- Obesity, smoking, alcohol, and a large intake of red meat increase the risk.
- Physical exercise and a diet with large amounts of fruits, vegetables, and grains may decrease the risk.
- Nonsteroidal antiinflammatory drugs (NSAIDs) (e.g., aspirin) and hormone replacement therapy in women also seem to decrease the risk.

Adenocarcinoma is the most common type of colorectal cancer. Most colorectal cancers appear to arise from adenomatous polyps. All tumors tend to spread through the walls of the intestine and into the lymphatic system. Since venous blood leaving the colon and rectum flows through the portal vein and the inferior rectal vein, the liver and lung are common sites of metastasis. The cancer can also spread directly into adjacent structures and can obstruct the bowel.

Clinical Manifestations
Most people with colorectal cancer have hematochezia (passage of blood through the rectum) or melena (black, tarry stools), abdominal pain, and/or changes in bowel habits. Manifestations

are usually nonspecific or do not appear until the disease is advanced. Cancer on the right side of the colon has manifestations that differ from those on the left side of the colon.

- Rectal bleeding, the most common symptom of colorectal cancer, is most often seen with left-sided lesions. Other manifestations of left-sided lesions include alternating constipation and diarrhea, change in stool caliber (narrow, ribbonlike), and sensation of incomplete evacuation. Obstruction symptoms appear earlier with left-sided lesions because lesions in the descending colon and rectum tend to progressively constrict the lumen.
- Cancers on the right side are usually asymptomatic. Vague abdominal discomfort or crampy, colicky abdominal pain may be present. Iron deficiency anemia and occult bleeding lead to weakness and fatigue.

Diagnostic Studies
- Digital rectal examination (DRE)
- Colonoscopy: the screening procedure of choice to examine the entire colon, obtain biopsy specimens, remove polyps, and detect colorectal lesions
- Fecal occult blood tests
- Complete blood count (CBC) and liver function tests when diagnosis confirmed by colonoscopy and biopsy
- Computed tomography (CT) scan or magnetic resonance imaging (MRI) of abdomen and pelvis to detect liver or other metastases
- Carcinoembryonic antigen (CEA) serum test to follow progress of patient after surgery

Collaborative Care
- Prognosis and treatment correlate with pathologic staging of the disease. Two staging systems are used, including the TNM staging system and the Duke's classification system (see Tables 43-27 and 43-28 in Lewis and others, *Medical-Surgical Nursing*, edition 7, pp. 1066 and 1067). The TNM sytem is currently the preferred system (see p. 796). As with other cancers, prognosis worsens with greater size and depth of tumor, lymph node involvement, and metastasis.

Surgical Therapy
Surgical goals include complete resection of the tumor with adequate margins of healthy tissue, a thorough exploration of the abdomen to detect spread, removal of all lymph nodes that drain the cancer area, restoration of bowel continuity so that normal bowel function will return, and prevention of surgical complications.

- Polypectomy during colonoscopy can be used to resect colorectal cancer in situ and is considered successful when the resected margin of the polyp is free of cancer, the cancer is well differentiated, and there is no apparent lymphatic or blood vessel involvement.
- The optimal procedure is *bowel resection* of the affected tissue with reanastomosis of the remaining healthy segments.
- Abdominal-perineal resection is most often performed when the cancer is located within 5 cm of the anus. In the abdominal-perineal resection, an abdominal incision is made, and the proximal sigmoid is brought through the abdominal wall to form a permanent colostomy. The distal sigmoid, rectum, and anus are removed through a perineal incision.
- Sphincter-sparing procedures are performed for the patient with early disease. In these procedures a local resection is performed and anal sphincters are left intact.
- Once the cancer has spread to distant sites (e.g., liver, lungs, ovaries), surgery is palliative.

Radiation Therapy and Chemotherapy

Radiation may be used postoperatively as an adjunct to colon resection and chemotherapy or as a palliative measure for patients with advanced lesions. As a palliative measure, it helps to reduce the tumor size and provide symptomatic relief.

Chemotherapy is recommended when the patient has positive lymph nodes at the time of surgery or has metastatic disease. Chemotherapy is used both as an adjuvant therapy after colon resection, as well as primary treatment for nonresectable colorectal cancer (see Chemotherapy, p. 712). At present, the combination of 5-fluorouracil (5-FU) plus leucovorin and irinotecan (Camptosar) is approved as first-line chemotherapy for patients with metastatic colorectal cancer. Additional treatment protocols include the use of 5-FU and levamisole (Ergamisol) with or without leucovorin (Wellcovorin). For patients who are not considered appropriate candidates for this triple therapy, either leucovorin-modulated 5-FU (Orzel) or capecitabine (Xeloda) is used as an acceptable alternative first-line treatment. New agents being examined for adjuvant therapy of colorectal cancer include oxaliplatin (Eloxatin) and raltitrexed (Tomudex).

Two monoclonal antibodies are used for targeted therapy for colon cancer. Cetuximab (Erbitux) targets epidermal growth factor receptor, and bevacizumab (Avastin) prevents the formation of new blood vessels. These drugs can be used alone or in conjunction with other chemotherapeutic agents.

Nursing Management

Goals

The patient with colorectal cancer will have normal bowel elimination patterns, quality of life appropriate to disease progression, relief of pain, and feelings of comfort and well-being.

Nursing Diagnoses

- Diarrhea or constipation
- Acute pain
- Fear
- Ineffective coping

Nursing Interventions

Screening recommendations from the American Cancer Society for colorectal cancer in a person who has no established risk factors include a digital rectal examination and a fecal occult blood test or fecal immunochemical test yearly, a double-contrast enema every 5 years, a sigmoidoscopy every 5 years, or a colonoscopy every 10 years starting at the age of 50 years. All positive findings are followed up with colonoscopy.

- For high-risk patients, colorectal cancer screening should begin earlier and be repeated more often.

Preoperative Care. Nursing care for patients with a colon resection is similar to the care of the patient having a laparotomy (see Abdominal Pain, Acute, p. 3). The patient who undergoes an abdominal-perineal resection will have a permanent ostomy and closure of the anus. These patients will likely need intense emotional support to cope with their prognosis and the radical change in body appearance and function. The patient should be taught that side-to-side positioning will be necessary postoperatively.

Postoperative Care. After an abdominal-perineal resection, there are two surgical wounds and a stoma. The resection of the colon results in an abdominal incision, and an incision is made in the perineum to remove the lower colon and anus.

- Management of the perineal incision differs depending on the type of wound. Three techniques are used: (1) packing of the entire open wound, (2) partial closure with Penrose drains for open drainage, and (3) primary closure of the perineal wound with closed-suction drainage of the pelvic cavity.
- A patient who has open and packed wounds requires meticulous care. During the immediate postoperative period the perineal dressing is reinforced and changed frequently because drainage can be profuse for several hours after surgery. All drainage is carefully assessed for the amount, color, and consistency; drainage is usually serosanguineous. The perineal wound is usually irrigated with a normal

saline solution when the dressings are changed until the patient is able to take warm sitz baths for 10 to 20 minutes three or four times per day to assist in tissue debridement.

■ The nurse should examine all perineal wounds regularly and record bleeding, excessive drainage, and unusual odor. In addition the nurse should observe for signs of edema, erythema, fever, and elevated white blood cell (WBC) count.

■ The patient may experience pain and itching in and around the wound. Antipruritic agents and sitz baths are usually ordered. Use of a pressure-reducing chair cushion provides comfort when sitting. Sitting on a toilet for prolonged periods is discouraged until the perineal wound is well healed.

■ The perineal wound may not be completely healed before discharge. After discharge the patient is usually seen by the health care provider, home health nurse, and enterostomal therapist in an outpatient clinic. The wound is usually irrigated and debrided. The nurse should report drainage because it may also indicate the presence of a foreign body, fistula, osteomyelitis, or rectal tissue not removed during surgery. The patient and significant others are taught management of the wound and the procedure to take a sitz bath at home.

■ Sexual dysfunction is a possible complication of an abdominal-perineal resection and should be included in the plan of care. The enterostomal therapy nurse can often provide correct and factual information concerning sexual dysfunction.

■ Psychologic support for patient as well as for family is important. The recovery period is long, and the possibility of recurrence of cancer is always present.

■ The patient and family should be aware of all community services available for assistance.

CONJUNCTIVITIS

Description

Conjunctivitis is an inflammation or infection of the conjunctiva. Conjunctivitis may be caused by bacteria or viruses, and inflammation can result from exposure to allergens or chemical irritants (including cigarette smoke). The tarsal conjunctiva (lining of the lid's interior surface) may become inflamed as a result of a long-term foreign body in the eye, such as a contact lens or an ocular prosthesis. See Table 28 for a comparison of the clinical manifestations and management of the different types of conjunctivitis.

Table 28 Types of Conjunctivitis

Description	Clinical Manifestations	Management
Bacterial		
Acute bacterial conjunctivitis (pinkeye); more common in children and most commonly caused by *Staphylococcus aureus*	Irritation, tearing, redness, mucopurulent drainage; rapid spread from one eye to the other	Usually self-limiting but antibiotic drops will shorten course; prevent spread with careful hand washing and use of individual or disposable towels
Viral		
Caused by many different viruses; adenovirus conjunctivitis contracted by direct contact with infected person and in contaminated swimming pools	Tearing, foreign body sensation, redness, mild photophobia; usually mild and self-limiting but can be severe with increased discomfort and subconjunctival hemorrhaging	Treatment usually palliative; topical corticosteroids provide temporary relief if patient is severely symptomatic but have no benefit in outcome; antiviral drops ineffective; good hygiene practices encouraged

Chlamydial
Chlamydia trachomatis (serotypes A-C) causes trachoma, a chronic conjunctivitis that is a major cause of blindness worldwide and is spread through hands and flies; adult inclusion conjunctivitis (AIC) caused by *Chlamydia trachomatis* (serotypes D-K) and is increasing with the increase in sexually transmitted chlamydial infections

Mucopurulent ocular discharge, irritation, redness, lid swelling; AIC does not lead to blindness as does trachoma

Antibiotic therapy usually effective for both trachoma and AIC; patients with AIC have a high risk of concurrent chlamydial genital infection and other sexually transmitted diseases; instruction about the ocular condition and sexual implications of condition necessary

Allergic
Conjunctivitis may develop in response to exposure to pollens, animal dander, ocular solutions, contact lenses, or other allergens

Itching (defining symptom), burning, redness, tearing, and white or clear exudate; severe responses cause significant swelling that may cause ballooning of the conjunctiva beyond eyelids

Artificial tears to dilute allergen and wash from eye; effective topical medications include antihistamines and corticosteroids; instruction to avoid allergen if known

C

CONSTIPATION

Description

Constipation is a decrease in the frequency of bowel movements from what is normal for the individual; hard, difficult-to-pass stool; a decrease in stool volume; and/or retention of feces in the rectum. Normal bowel elimination may vary from three times per day to once every 3 days.

- Frequently constipation may be due to insufficient dietary fiber, inadequate fluid intake, decreased physical activity, and ignoring the urge to defecate. Many medications, especially opioids, cause constipation. Constipation occurs with many diseases that slow gastrointestinal (GI) transit, such as diabetes mellitus, Parkinson's disease, and multiple sclerosis. Depression and stress can also result in constipation. Long-term laxative use causes *cathartic colon syndrome,* resulting in a dilated and atonic colon that does not empty without the laxative.

Clinical Manifestations

Constipation may vary from a chronic discomfort to an acute event mimicking an acute abdomen. Clinical manifestations are presented in Table 29.

- Hemorrhoids are the most common complication of chronic constipation. They result from venous engorgement resulting from repeated Valsalva maneuvers (straining) and venous compression from hard impacted stool (see Hemorrhoids, p. 293).
- Diverticulosis is another potential complication of chronic constipation (see Diverticulitis/Diverticulosis, p. 194).

Table 29	Clinical Manifestations of Constipation
Abdominal distention	Increased rectal pressure
Abdominal pain	Nausea
Anorexia	Palpable mass
Decreased frequency of bowel movements	Stone or rock-shaped stool
	Stool with blood
Hard, dry stool	Straining
Headache	Tenesmus
Increased flatulence	

- In the presence of obstipation (fecal impaction secondary to constipation), colonic perforation may occur. Perforation, which is life threatening, causes abdominal pain, nausea, vomiting, fever, and an elevated white blood cell (WBC) count.

Diagnostic Studies

A thorough history and physical examination should be performed so the underlying cause can be identified.

- Abdominal x-rays, barium enema, colonoscopy, sigmoidoscopy, and anorectal manometry may be helpful in the diagnosis.
- In severe constipation, anorectal manometry, GI tract transit studies, and sigmoidoscopic rectal biopsies may be performed.

Collaborative Care

Most cases of constipation can be managed with diet therapy, including fiber and fluids, and an exercise program. Laxatives and enemas may be used to treat acute constipation but are used cautiously because overuse leads to chronic constipation.

- Milder laxatives that may be used include daily bulk-forming preparations that work like dietary fiber and do not cause dependence and stool-softening agents. Osmotic agents and stimulants are more potent and more likely to cause dependence (see Table 43-8 in Lewis and others, *Medical-Surgical Nursing,* edition 7, p. 1042). Tegaserod (Zelnorm), a serotonergic drug, has recently been approved for the management of chronic constipation and constipation associated with irritable bowel syndrome.
- Enemas are fast acting and beneficial in the immediate treatment of constipation but should be limited for long-term treatment. Soapsuds enemas produce inflammation of colon mucosa, tap water enemas can lead to water intoxication, and sodium phosphate enemas may cause electrolyte imbalances in some patients.
- Biofeedback therapy may benefit patients who are constipated as a result of anismus (uncoordinated contraction of the anal sphincter during straining).
- The patient with severe constipation related to a motility or mechanical disorder may require more intensive treatment. In a patient with unrelenting constipation, a subtotal colectomy with ileorectal anastomosis is the procedure of choice.

Many patients experience an improvement in their symptoms when they increase their intake of dietary fiber and fluids. Dietary fiber adds to the stool bulk directly and by attracting water. The diet should include a fluid intake of at least 3 L/day unless contraindicated by cardiac or renal disease. Increasing fiber intake without increasing fluids may predispose the patient to impaction or obstruction.

Nursing Management
Goals
The patient with constipation will increase dietary intake of fiber and fluids; increase physical activity; have passage of soft, formed stools; and not have any complications, such as bleeding hemorrhoids.
Nursing Diagnosis
- Constipation
Nursing Interventions
Interventions should be based on the assessment and symptoms of the patient.
- Proper position is important when defecating. For a patient in bed, the head of the bed should be elevated as high as the patient can tolerate. For the person who can sit on a toilet, a footstool may be placed in front of toilet. Placing feet on a footstool promotes flexion of the hips, which assists in defecation.
- The patient with poor muscle tone should be encouraged to exercise the abdominal muscles and can be taught to contract abdominal muscles several times each day. Sit-ups and straight leg raises can also be used to improve abdominal muscle tone.

▼ Patient and Family Teaching
- Teach the patient the importance of dietary measures to prevent constipation. Emphasis should be placed on maintenance of a high-fiber diet, increased fluid intake, and a regular exercise program.
- The patient should be taught to establish a regular time to defecate and to not suppress the urge to defecate. In many persons the urge to defecate occurs after breakfast because of stimulation of the gastrocolic reflex.
- The patient should be discouraged from using laxatives and enemas to achieve fecal elimination.

COR PULMONALE

Description

Cor pulmonale is enlargement of the right ventricle (RV) secondary to diseases of the lung, thorax, or pulmonary circulation. Pulmonary hypertension is usually a preexisting condition in the individual with cor pulmonale. Cor pulmonale may be present with or without overt cardiac failure.

- The most common cause of cor pulmonale is chronic obstructive pulmonary disease (COPD) (see p. 121). Almost any disorder that affects the respiratory system can cause cor pulmonale.

Clinical Manifestations

Manifestations include dyspnea, chronic productive cough, wheezing respirations, retrosternal or substernal pain, and fatigue.

- If heart failure accompanies cor pulmonale, additional manifestations will also be found, such as peripheral edema, weight gain, distended neck veins, full, bounding pulse, and enlarged liver.
- A chest x-ray will show an enlarged RV and pulmonary artery.

Collaborative Care

Management is directed at treating the underlying pulmonary problem that precipitated the heart problem. Long-term, low-flow oxygen (O_2) therapy is used to correct hypoxemia and reduce vasoconstriction in chronic states of respiratory disorders.

- If fluid, electrolyte, and acid-base imbalances are present, they must be corrected.
- Diuretics and a low-sodium diet will help to decrease the plasma volume and the load on the heart.
- Bronchodilator therapy is indicated if the underlying respiratory problem is due to an obstructive disorder.
- Although digoxin use is controversial, studies have confirmed that it has a modest inotropic effect on the failing right ventricle in chronic cor pulmonale.
- Theophylline may help because of its weak inotropic effect on the heart.
- Other treatments include those for pulmonary hypertension and include vasodilator therapy, calcium channel blockers, and anticoagulants.

- When medical treatment fails, lung transplantation may be an option.

Long-term management of cor pulmonale resulting from COPD is similar to that described for COPD (see p. 128). Continuous low-flow O_2 during sleep, exercise, and small, frequent meals may allow the patient to feel better and be more active.

CORONARY ARTERY DISEASE

Description
Coronary artery disease (CAD) is a type of blood vessel disorder that is included in the general category of atherosclerosis. Atherosclerosis is derived from two Greek words: *athero,* meaning "fatty mush," and *skleros,* meaning "hard." Atherosclerosis is often referred to as "hardening of the arteries." Although this condition can occur in any artery in the body, the atheromas (fatty deposits) have a preference for coronary arteries.

- Arteriosclerotic heart disease, cardiovascular heart disease, ischemic heart disease, coronary heart disease, and CAD are synonymous terms used to describe this disorder.
- Cardiovascular disease is the major cause of death in the United States. CAD is the most common type of cardiovascular disease and accounts for the majority of these deaths.
- Patients with CAD may be asymptomatic or develop *chronic stable angina.*
- More serious manifestations of CAD include *unstable angina (UA)* and *myocardial infarction (MI).* These manifestations are termed *acute coronary syndrome (ACS).*

Figure 2 illustrates the relationships among the clinical manifestations of CAD.

Pathophysiology
Atherosclerosis is the major cause of CAD. It is characterized by a focal deposit of cholesterol and lipids, primarily within the arterial intimal wall. Plaque formation is the result of complex interactions between components of the blood and the elements forming the vascular wall. Inflammation and endothelial injury play a central role in the development of atherosclerosis.

- The endothelial lining can be injured as a result of tobacco use, hyperlipidemia, hypertension, diabetes, hyperhomocystinemia, and infection (e.g., *Chlamydia pneumoniae,* herpes) causing a local inflammatory response.

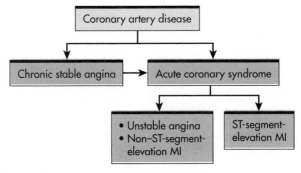

Fig. 2. Relationships among coronary artery disease, chronic stable angina, and acute coronary syndrome. *MI,* Myocardial infarction.

- C-reactive protein (CRP), a nonspecific marker of inflammation, is increased in many patients with CAD and can trigger rupture of plaques and promote uptake of low-density lipoprotein (LDL) into the endothelial lining.
- CAD takes many years to develop. When it becomes symptomatic, the disease process is usually well advanced. Stages of development in atherosclerosis are (1) fatty streak, (2) fibrous plaque resulting from smooth muscle cell proliferation, and (3) complicated lesion.

Figure 34-2, Lewis and others, *Medical-Surgical Nursing,* edition 7, p. 786 illustrates the progression of atherosclerosis.

Risk factors for CAD can be categorized as nonmodifiable and modifiable (Table 30).

Risk factors in different populations may vary, and studies continue to identify additional factors (e.g., lipoprotein-associated phospholipase A_2 [an inflammatory enzyme] and coronary artery calcification) that are associated with an increased risk of CAD.

Clinical Manifestations

The three major clinical manifestations of CAD include chronic stable angina, acute coronary syndrome, and sudden cardiac death. These conditions result from myocardial ischemia that occurs when the demand for myocardial oxygen exceeds the ability of the coronary arteries to supply the heart with oxygen. The primary reason for insufficient blood flow is narrowing of coronary arteries by atherosclerosis.

- Angina, or chest pain, is the clinical manifestation of reversible myocardial ischemia.

| Table 30 | Risk Factors for Coronary Artery Disease |

Nonmodifiable	Modifiable
Age Gender (men more than women until 60 yr of age) Ethnicity (whites more than African Americans) Genetic predisposition and family history of heart disease	**Major** Serum lipids: elevated triglycerides and LDL cholesterol; decreased HDL cholesterol* Hypertension: ≥130/85* Tobacco use Physical inactivity Obesity: waist circumference >102 cm (>39.8 inches) in men and >88 cm (>34.3 inches) in women* **Contributing** Diabetes mellitus Fasting blood sugar >110 mg/dl* Psychologic states Homocysteine levels Stressful lifestyle

HDL, High-density lipoprotein; LDL, low-density lipoprotein.
* Three or more of these risk factors meet the criteria for metabolic syndrome as defined by the National Heart, Lung, and Blood Institute and American Heart Association.

- Chronic stable angina refers to chest pain that occurs intermittently over a long period with the same pattern of onset, duration, and intensity of symptoms (see Chronic Stable Angina, p. 44).
- When ischemia is prolonged and not immediately reversible, acute coronary syndrome (ACS) develops (see Acute Coronary Syndrome, p. 6). ACS encompasses the following spectrum:
  - Unstable angina (UA): chest pain that is new in onset, occurs at rest, or has a worsening pattern, and represents an emergency
  - Non–ST-segment-elevation myocardial infarction (NSTEMI): irreversible myocardial cell death caused by deterioration of an atherosclerotic plaque and lesion *partially* occluded by a thrombus
  - ST-segment-elevation myocardial infarction (STEMI): irreversible myocardial cell death caused by deteriora-

tion of an atherosclerotic plaque and lesion *totally* occluded by a thrombus

Diagnostic Studies

- Chest x-ray to detect cardiac enlargement, cardiac calcifications, and pulmonary congestion
- 12-lead electrocardiogram (ECG)
- Serum lipid levels to screen for positive risk factors
- Treadmill exercise testing to detect ST-segment and T-wave changes that indicate ischemia with exercise
- Ambulatory 24- to 48-hour ECG monitoring to identify silent ischemia
- Nuclear imaging studies to determine myocardial perfusion
- Positron emission tomography (PET) to identify and quantify ischemia and infarction
- Angiography studies for visualization of coronary arteries to help determine treatment and prognosis
- Echocardiography with exercise to diagnose coronary artery stenosis

See Chapter 32 and Table 32-7 for a discussion of these studies, including nursing considerations, in Lewis and others, *Medical-Surgical Nursing,* edition 7, pp. 752 to 755.

Collaborative Care

Management of CAD involves modification of risk factors to prevent, modify, or retard the progression of the disease.The risk of CAD can be decreased by maintaining an ideal body weight, getting adequate physical exercise, reducing intake of saturated fats, and avoiding tobacco use. The FITT formula (**F**requency, **I**ntensity, **T**ype, and **T**ime) is designed to improve physical fitness, and the Therapeutic Lifestyle Changes Diet is recommended to reduce LDL cholesterol levels and maintain ideal body weight. Specific diet recommendations and plans are presented in Tables 34-4 and 34-5 in Lewis and others, *Medical-Surgical Nursing,* edition 7, p. 793. Drug therapy for elevated cholesterol may be started if serum cholesterol levels are elevated after 6 months of diet therapy.

Drug Therapy

Various drugs are available to treat hyperlipidemia. The statin drugs are the most widely used and studied lipid-lowering drugs. Examples include lovastatin (Mevacor), pravastatin (Pravachol), simvastatin (Zocor), fluvastatin (Lescol), atorvastatin (Lipitor), and rosuvastatin (Crestor). These drugs inhibit the synthesis of cholesterol in the liver by blocking hydroxy-methyl-glutaryl coenzyme A (HMG-CoA) reductase. These drugs primarily lower low-density lipoprotein (LDL) cholesterol and also cause an increase in high-density lipoprotein (HDL). Niacin (Nicobid), a water-soluble B vitamin, also interferes with the synthesis of LDL and triglyceride levels.

Fibric acid derivatives such as clofibrate (Atromid-S) and gemfibrozil (Lopid) are effective in lowering very low-density lipoprotein (VLDL) levels and triglycerides, while increasing HDL levels. Drugs that increase lipoprotein removal by increasing conversion of cholesterol to bile acids include cholestyramine (Questran), colestipol (Colestid), and colesevelam (Welchol) and are commonly used. Ezetimibe (Zetia) inhibits the absorption of dietary and biliary cholesterol across the intestinal wall and may be combined with a statin to promote greater reductions in LDL.

- Drug therapy for hyperlipidemia is likely to be prolonged, perhaps continuing for a lifetime. It is essential that diet modification be used to minimize the need for drug therapy. The patient must fully understand the rationale and goals of treatment as well as any medication side effects.

Antiplatelet therapy with low-dose aspirin is recommended for people at risk for CAD unless contraindicated (e.g., history of GI bleeding). For people who are aspirin intolerant, clopidogrel (Plavix) can be considered.

Nursing Management

In both the acute care setting and the community, the nurse should identify persons at high risk for CAD. Risk screening involves obtaining personal and family health histories. Environmental factors, such as eating habits, type of diet, and level of exercise, are also assessed. A psychosocial history is included to determine smoking habits, alcohol ingestion, type A behaviors, recent life-stressing events, and presence of negative psychologic states (e.g., anxiety, depression, hopelessness). The place and type of work can provide information on activity, exposure to pollutants or chemicals, and emotional stress associated with employment.

- The nurse should identify patient attitudes and beliefs about health and illness. This information can give some indication of how disease and lifestyle changes may affect the patient and can reveal possible misconceptions about heart disease.
- Knowledge of the patient's educational background is frequently helpful in deciding at what level to beginteaching.
- Once a high-risk person is identified, preventive measures can be taken. Risk factors such as age, gender, and genetic

inheritance cannot be modified. However, the person with any of these risk factors can modify the risk of CAD by controlling or changing the additive effects of modifiable risk factors.

- Persons who have modifiable risk factors need to be encouraged and motivated to make changes in their lifestyle to reduce their risk of heart disease. For highly motivated persons, knowing how to reduce this risk may be the only information needed to get them to make changes.

CROHN'S DISEASE

Description
Crohn's disease is an autoimmune disorder that, along with ulcerative colitis, is referred to as *inflammatory bowel disease* (IBD). See Inflammatory Bowel Disease, p. 352 for the discussion of the disorder.

CUSHING SYNDROME

Description
Cushing syndrome is a spectrum of clinical abnormalities caused by excess corticosteroids, particularly glucocorticoids. Several conditions can cause Cushing syndrome; the most common cause is iatrogenic administration of exogenous corticosteroids (e.g., prednisone). *Cushing disease* is specifically caused by an adrenocorticotropic hormone (ACTH)–secreting pituitary tumor.

- Other causes of Cushing syndrome include adrenal tumors and ectopic ACTH production by tumors outside the hypothalamic-pituitary-adrenal axis (usually in the lung or pancreas).

Clinical Manifestations
Manifestations can be seen in most body systems and are related to excess levels of corticosteroids (see Table 50-13, Lewis and others, *Medical-Surgical Nursing,* edition 7, p. 1313). Although manifestations of glucocorticoid excess usually predominate, symptoms of mineralocorticoid and androgen excess may also be seen.

- Corticosteroid excess causes pronounced changes in physical appearance. Weight gain, the most common feature, results from accumulation of adipose tissue in the trunk, face, and cervical neck area. Transient weight gain from sodium and water retention may be present because of the mineralocorticoid effects of cortisol. Glucose intolerance occurs because of cortisol-induced insulin resistance and increased gluconeogenesis by the liver.
- Protein wasting is caused by the catabolic effects of cortisol on peripheral tissue. Muscle wasting leads to muscle weakness, especially in the extremities. Loss of bone protein matrix leads to osteoporosis with pathologic fractures (e.g., vertebral compression fractures) and bone and back pain. Loss of collagen makes the skin weaker, thinner, and easier to bruise.
- Mineralocorticoid excess may cause hypertension, whereas adrenal androgen excess may cause pronounced acne, virilization in women, and feminization in men.

Clinical presentation, as revealed by the history and physical examination, is the first indication of Cushing syndrome. Of particular importance are a combination of centripedal obesity; "moon facies" (fullness of face); purplish red striae on abdomen, breast, or buttocks; menstrual disorders in women; and unexplained hypokalemia.

Diagnostic Studies

- Plasma cortisol levels may be elevated with loss of diurnal variation.
- Plasma ACTH levels may be low, normal, or elevated depending on the underlying problem.
- Twenty-four–hour urine collection results in 50 to 100 mcg of free cortisol; high-dose dexamethasone suppression test may be done for borderline urine results.
- Complete blood count (CBC) findings indicate granulocytosis, lymphopenia, and eosinopenia.
- Other findings on diagnostic tests associated with, but not diagnostic of, Cushing syndrome include hyperglycemia, hypokalemia, glycosuria, hypercalciuria, and osteoporosis.
- Computed tomography (CT) scan and magnetic resonance imaging (MRI) are done for tumor localization.

Collaborative Care

The primary goal is to normalize hormone secretion. The standard treatment for a pituitary adenoma is transsphenoidal hypophysectomy. Adrenalectomy is indicated for adrenal tumors or hyperplasia. Patients with ectopic ACTH-secreting tumors are managed by treating the neoplasm. Occasionally, bilateral adrenalectomy is necessary.

- In cases when surgery is contraindicated, treatment with mitotane (Lysodren) may be used. This drug suppresses cortisol production, alters peripheral metabolism of cortisol, and decreases plasma and urine steroid levels by actually destroying adrenocortical cells. The action of this drug results in a "medical adrenalectomy."
- Metyrapone, ketoconazole (Nizoral), and aminoglutethimide (Cytadren) may be used to inhibit cortisol synthesis.

If Cushing syndrome has developed during the course of prolonged administration of corticosteroids, one or more of the following alternatives may be tried: (1) gradual discontinuance of corticosteroid therapy, (2) reduction of corticosteroid dose, and (3) conversion to an alternate-day regimen.

Nursing Management
Goals
The patient with Cushing syndrome will experience relief of symptoms with no serious complications, maintain a positive self-image, and actively participate in the therapeutic plan.

See the nursing care plan for the patient with Cushing syndrome, *http://evolve.elsevier.com/Lewis/medsurg.*

Nursing Diagnoses
- Risk for infection
- Imbalanced nutrition: more than body requirements
- Situational low self-esteem
- Impaired skin integrity

Nursing Interventions
Because the therapy for Cushing syndrome has many side effects, the focus of assessment is on the signs and symptoms of hormone and drug toxicity and on complicating conditions (e.g., cardiovascular disease, diabetes mellitus, and infection). Daily nursing assessment includes the following:

- Vital signs, glucose monitoring, and daily weights (gain possibly indicating volume excess)
- Signs and symptoms of infection, especially pain, loss of function, and purulent drainage, because other signs such as fever and redness may be minimal or absent
- Signs of abnormal thromboembolic phenomena, such as sudden chest pain, dyspnea, and tachypnea

Another important focus of nursing care is emotional support. Changes in appearance, such as centripetal obesity, multiple bruises, hirsutism in females, and gynecomastia in males, can be distressing. The nurse can help by offering respect and unconditional acceptance. The patient can be reassured that the physical changes and much of the emotional lability will resolve when hormone levels return to normal.

If treatment involves surgical removal of a pituitary adenoma, an adrenal tumor, or one or both adrenal glands, nursing care will have an additional focus on preoperative and postoperative care. Surgery on glands poses risks beyond those of other types of operations. Because glands are highly vascular, the risk of hemorrhage is increased. Manipulation of glandular tissue during surgery may release large amounts of hormone into the circulation, producing marked fluctuations in metabolic processes affected by these hormones (e.g., hypertension, susceptibility to infection).

Preoperative Care. Before surgery, hypertension and hyperglycemia need to be controlled, with hypokalemia corrected by diet and potassium supplements; a high-protein meal plan helps correct protein depletion.

Preoperative teaching depends on the type of surgical approach planned (hypophysectomy or adrenalectomy) but should include information regarding postoperative care the patient should anticipate.

- In the postoperative period (for both open and laparoscopic adrenalectomy), patients will likely have a nasogastric (NG) tube, urinary catheter, intravenous (IV) therapy, central venous pressure monitoring, and sequential compression devices to prevent emboli.

Postoperative Care. Because of hormone fluctuations, the patient's blood pressure (BP), fluid balance, and electrolyte levels tend to be unstable after surgery. High doses of corticosteroids (hydrocortisone) are administered IV during surgery and for several days afterward to ensure adequate responses to the stress of the procedure.

- Any rapid or significant changes in BP, respirations, or heart rate (HR) should be reported.
- Fluid intake and output should be monitored carefully and assessed for potential imbalance.
- If corticosteroid dosage is tapered too rapidly after surgery, acute adrenal insufficiency may develop. Vomiting, increased weakness, dehydration, and hypotension may indicate hypocortisolism. In addition, the patient may complain of painful joints, pruritus, or peeling skin and may experience severe emotional disturbances.

The nurse must constantly be alert for signs of corticosteroid imbalance. After surgery the patient is usually maintained on bed rest until the BP stabilizes. The nurse must also be alert for subtle signs of postoperative infections. Meticulous care must be used when changing the dressing and during any other procedures that necessitate access to body cavities, circulation, or areas under skin.

▼ **Patient and Family Teaching**

Discharge instructions are based on the patient's lack of endogenous cortisol and resulting inability to react to stressors physiologically.

- Patients should wear Medic-Alert bracelets at all times and carry medical identification and instructions in a wallet or purse. Exposure to extremes of temperature, infections, and emotional disturbances should be avoided as much as possible.
- Stress may produce or precipitate acute adrenal insufficiency because the remaining adrenal tissue cannot meet an increased hormonal demand. Many patients can be taught to adjust their corticosteroid replacement therapy in accordance with stress levels.
- If the patient cannot adjust his or her own medication or if weakness, fainting, fever, or nausea and vomiting occur, the patient should notify the health care provider for a possible adjustment in corticosteroid dosage.
- Lifetime replacement therapy is required by many patients, but it may take several months to satisfactorily adjust the hormone dose.

CYSTIC FIBROSIS

Description

Cystic fibrosis (CF) is an autosomal recessive, multisystem disease characterized by altered function of the exocrine glands involving primarily the lungs, pancreas, and sweat glands.

The severity and progression of the disease vary from person to person. With early diagnosis and improvements in therapy, the prognosis has been significantly improved. The median predicted survival in 1970 was 16 years, and in 2004 it was 35 years of age. Approximately 12% of adults with CF live past age 40 years.

Pathophysiology

CF results from mutations in a gene located on chromosome 7 that produces a protein called CF transmembrane regulator (CFTR).

CFTR normally regulates sodium and chloride channels in the lining of the exocrine portion of particular organs, such as airways, pancreatic duct, sweat gland duct, and reproductive tract. Mutations in the CFTR gene alter this protein in such a way that the channel is blocked.

- Cells that line the passageways of the lungs, pancreas, and other organs produce abnormally thick, sticky mucus that adheres to the lumen of the ducts. The glands distal to the duct eventually undergo fibrosis.
- The hallmark of respiratory involvement is its effect on the airways. Thick secretions obstruct bronchioles and lead to air trapping and hyperinflation of the lungs. The stasis of mucus provides an excellent growth medium for bacteria and causes chronic airway infections that are difficult to eradicate. Lung disorders include chronic bronchiolitis and bronchitis that eventually lead to bronchiectasis, blebs, large cysts, and hemoptysis from erosion of pulmonary arteries.
- Pancreatic insufficiency is caused primarily by mucus plugging the pancreatic duct and its branches, which results in fibrosis of the acinar glands of the pancreas. Because pancreatic digestive enzymes cannot reach the intestine, malabsorption of fat, protein, and fat-soluble vitamins occurs.
- Fat malabsorption results in steatorrhea, and protein malabsorption results in failure to grow and gain weight.
- Diabetes mellitus may occur if the islets of Langerhans become fibrotic.
- Patients with CF secrete normal volumes of sweat but are unable to absorb sodium chloride from sweat as it moves through the sweat duct. Therefore they excrete 4 times the normal amount of sodium and chloride in sweat. This abnormality rarely affects the health of the person, but it is useful in diagnosis of CF.

Clinical Manifestations

Manifestations vary depending on the disease severity. Early childhood signs are failure to grow, clubbing, persistent cough with mucous production, tachypnea, and large, frequent bowel movements.

- In the adult, the first symptom is frequent cough that becomes persistent and produces viscous, purulent sputum.
- Over time exacerbations become frequent, bronchiectasis develops, and the recovery of lost lung function is less complete, ultimately leading to respiratory failure.

Diagnostic Studies
- Sweat chloride test (pilocarpine iontophoresis method) measures sweat production and sodium and chloride concentrations.
- Chest x-ray, pulmonary function tests, and fecal analysis for fat are used to support the diagnosis.

Collaborative Care
- The objectives of therapy are to promote clearance of secretions, control infection in the lungs, and provide adequate nutrition. Management of pulmonary problems is focused on relieving airway obstruction and controlling infection. Drainage of thick bronchial mucus is assisted by aerosol and nebulization treatments that liquefy mucus and facilitate coughing.
- Airway clearance techniques include chest physiotherapy (CPT), positive expiratory pressure (PEP) devices, and high-frequency chest wall oscillation systems.
- Aerobic exercise also seems to be effective in clearing airways. Early intervention with antibiotics for lung infection is useful, with long courses of antibiotics generally prescribed.

Management of pancreatic insufficiency includes pancreatic enzyme replacement (e.g., lipase, Pancrease, Cotazym-S, and Creon) administered before each meal and snack. A high-calorie, high-protein diet and multivitamins are recommended. Fat-soluble vitamins need to be supplemented. Added dietary salt is indicated whenever sweating is excessive, such as during hot weather, in the presence of fever, or from intense physical activity.

Lung transplantation has resulted in significant improvement of pulmonary function.

Nursing Management
Goals
The patient with CF will have adequate airway clearance, reduced risk factors associated with respiratory infections, adequate nutritional support to maintain appropriate body mass index (BMI), the ability to perform activities of daily living (ADLs), no complications related to CF, and active participation in planning and implementing a therapeutic regimen.
Nursing Diagnoses
- Ineffective airway clearance
- Ineffective breathing pattern
- Impaired gas exchange
- Imbalanced nutrition: less than body requirements
Nursing Interventions
The nurse can assist young adults to gain independence by helping them assume responsibility for their care and for their vocational

or school goals. For a couple considering children, genetic counseling may be suggested.

▼ **Patient and Family Teaching**
- Sexuality is an important issue that should be discussed with the young adult. Delayed or irregular menstruation is not uncommon. There may also be delayed development of secondary sex characteristics, such as breasts in girls, or prolonged short stature in boys.
- Home management of CF includes an aggressive plan of postural drainage with percussion and vibration, aerosol-nebulization therapy, and breathing retraining.
- The patient is taught controlled coughing techniques, deep breathing exercises, and progressive exercise conditioning, such as a bicycling program.

DIABETES INSIPIDUS

Description

Diabetes insipidus (DI) is associated with a deficiency of production or secretion of antidiuretic hormone (ADH) or a decreased renal response to ADH. The decrease in ADH results in fluid and electrolyte imbalances caused by increased urinary output and increased plasma osmolality. Depending on the cause, DI may be transient or a lifelong condition.

There are several classifications of DI. *Central DI* (also known as *neurogenic DI*) occurs when any organic lesion of the hypothalamus, infundibular stem, or posterior pituitary interferes with ADH synthesis, transport, or release.

Nephrogenic DI describes conditions in which there is adequate ADH, but there is a decreased response to ADH in the kidney. Lithium is one of the most common causes of drug-induced nephrogenic DI.

Psychogenic DI, a less common condition, is associated with excessive water intake. This can be caused by a structural lesion in the thirst center or a psychiatric disorder.

Clinical Manifestations

The primary characteristic of DI is excretion of large quantities of urine (5 to 20 L/day) with a very low specific gravity and urine osmolality. Serum osmolality is elevated as a result of hypernatremia caused by pure water loss in the kidney.

- Most patients compensate for fluid loss by drinking great amounts of water (polydipsia) so that serum osmolality is normal or only moderately elevated. The patient may be fatigued from nocturia and may experience generalized weakness.

- Central DI usually occurs suddenly with excessive fluid loss. Central DI that results from head trauma is usually self-limiting and improves with treatment of the underlying problem. DI following cranial surgery is more likely to be permanent.
- Although the clinical manifestations of nephrogenic DI are similar, the onset and amount of fluid losses are less dramatic than with central DI.
- If oral fluid intake cannot keep up with urinary losses, severe fluid volume deficit results. This is manifested by weight loss, poor tissue turgor, hypotension, tachycardia, constipation, and shock.
- The patient also shows central nervous system (CNS) manifestations ranging from irritability and mental dullness to coma. These symptoms are related to rising serum osmolality and hypernatremia.

Diagnostic Studies

Because DI may be central, nephrogenic, or dipsogenic in origin, identification of the cause is the initial step.

- A complete history and physical examination are done. Psychogenic DI is associated with overhydration and hypervolemia, rather than the dehydration and hypovolemia that are often seen in other forms of DI.
- A water deprivation test is usually done to confirm the diagnosis of central DI.

Collaborative Care

Determining and treating the primary cause are central to the collaborative management of DI. The therapeutic goal is the maintenance of fluid and electrolyte balance.

- In acute DI, hypotonic saline or dextrose 5% in water is administered IV, titrated to replace urinary output.
- In central DI, hormone replacement is necessary; desmopressin (DDAVP), an analog of ADH, is administered orally, IV, or as a nasal spray.
- Other drugs available for ADH replacement include aqueous vasopressin (Pitressin), vasopressin tannate, and lysine vasopressin (Diapid); chlorpropamide (Diabinese) may be used to potentiate the action of ADH and stimulate endogenous ADH release.

- Treatment for nephrogenic DI revolves around dietary measures (low-sodium diet) and thiazide diuretics.

Nursing Management

Care of the patient with DI is based on early detection, adequate hydration, and patient teaching.

- Fluids must be replaced orally or IV, depending on the patient's condition and ability to drink copious amounts of fluids. Adequate fluids should be kept at the bedside.
- If IV glucose is used, serum glucose should be monitored because hyperglycemia and glucosuria can lead to osmotic diuresis, which increases the fluid volume deficit.
- Accurate records of intake and output, urine specific gravity, and daily weights are mandatory in the assessment of fluid volume status.

▼ Patient and Family Teaching

- The patient who requires long-term ADH replacement needs instruction in self-management.
- Headache, nausea, and other signs of hyponatremia may indicate DDAVP overdosage, whereas failure to improve may indicate underdosage. Any of these symptoms should be reported. Patients taking DDAVP should also be instructed to monitor their weight daily to detect fluid loss or gain.

DIABETES MELLITUS

Description

Diabetes mellitus (DM) is a multisystem disease related to abnormal insulin production, impaired insulin utilization, or both. DM is a serious health problem throughout the world. Diabetes is the leading cause of end-stage renal disease, adult blindness, and nontraumatic lower limb amputations; it is a major contributing factor in heart disease and stroke. Current theories link the causes of diabetes, singly or in combination, to genetic, autoimmune, viral, and environmental factors (e.g., stress). Regardless of its cause, diabetes is primarily a disorder of glucose metabolism related to absent or insufficient insulin supplies or poor utilization of the insulin that is available.

- The two most common types of diabetes are classified as type 1 or type 2 DM (Table 31). Gestational diabetes, prediabetes, and secondary diabetes are other classifications of diabetes commonly seen in clinical practice.

Table 31	Characteristics of Type 1 and Type 2 Diabetes Mellitus

Type 1 Diabetes Mellitus	Type 2 Diabetes Mellitus
Age at onset More common in young persons but can occur at any age	Usually age 35 yr or older but can occur at any age Incidence increasing in children
Type of onset Signs and symptoms abrupt, but disease process may be present for several years	Insidious, may go undiagnosed for years
Prevalence Accounts for 5%-10% of all types of diabetes	Accounts for 90% of all types of diabetes
Environmental factors Virus, toxins	Obesity, lack of exercise
Primary defect Absent or minimal insulin production	Insulin resistance, decreased insulin production over time, and alterations in production of adipokines
Islet cell antibodies Often present at onset	Absent
Endogenous insulin Minimal or absent	Possibly excessive; adequate but delayed secretion or reduced utilization; secretions diminish over time
Nutritional status Thin, catabolic state	Obese or possibly normal
Symptoms Thirst, polyuria, polyphagia, fatigue, weight loss	Frequently none, fatigue, recurrent infections
Ketosis Prone at onset or during insulin deficiency	Resistant except during infection or stress
Nutritional therapy Essential	Essential
Insulin Required for all	Required for some
Vascular and neurologic complications Frequent	Frequent

D

Type 1 Diabetes Mellitus

Formerly known as "juvenile onset" or "insulin-dependent" diabetes, type 1 DM most often occurs in people who are less than 30 years old, with a peak onset between 11 and 13 years.

Pathophysiology. Type 1 diabetes is the end result of a long-standing process where the body's own T cells attack and destroy pancreatic β cells. In addition, autoantibodies to the islet cells cause a reduction of 80% to 90% of β-cell function before hyperglycemia and other manifestations occur (Fig. 3).

- A genetic predisposition and exposure to a virus are factors that may contribute to the pathogenesis of type 1 diabetes.

Type 1 diabetes is associated with a long preclinical period. Islet cell autoantibodies responsible for β-cell destruction are present for months to years before onset of symptoms. Manifestations

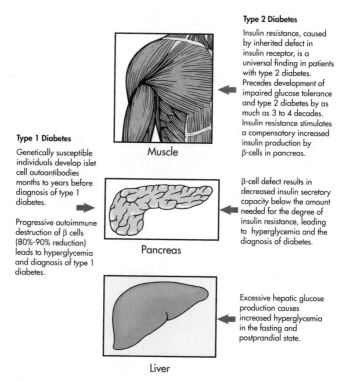

Type 2 Diabetes

Insulin resistance, caused by inherited defect in insulin receptor, is a universal finding in patients with type 2 diabetes. Precedes development of impaired glucose tolerance and type 2 diabetes by as much as 3 to 4 decades. Insulin resistance stimulates a compensatory increased insulin production by β-cells in pancreas.

Muscle

β-cell defect results in decreased insulin secretory capacity below the amount needed for the degree of insulin resistance, leading to hyperglycemia and the diagnosis of diabetes.

Pancreas

Type 1 Diabetes

Genetically susceptible individuals develop islet cell autoantibodies months to years before diagnosis of type 1 diabetes.

Progressive autoimmune destruction of β cells (80%-90% reduction) leads to hyperglycemia and diagnosis of type 1 diabetes.

Excessive hepatic glucose production causes increased hyperglycemia in the fasting and postprandial state.

Liver

Fig. 3. Altered mechanisms in type 1 and type 2 diabetes.

develop when the person's pancreas can no longer produce insulin. Once this occurs, the onset of symptoms is usually rapid.

- The patient usually has a history of recent and sudden weight loss, as well as the classic symptoms of *polydipsia* (excessive thirst), *polyuria* (frequent urination), and *polyphagia* (excessive hunger).
- The individual with type 1 diabetes requires a supply of insulin from an outside source (*exogenous insulin*), such as an injection, in order to sustain life. Without insulin, the patient develops *diabetic ketoacidosis* (DKA), a life-threatening condition resulting in metabolic acidosis.

Prediabetes

Prediabetes, also known as *impaired glucose tolerance* (IGT) or *impaired fasting glucose,* is a condition in which fasting blood glucose levels are higher than normal (>100 mg/dl) but not high enough for a diagnosis of diabetes (>126 mg/dl). People with pre-diabetes usually do not have symptoms, but if no preventive measures are taken, they will usually develop type 2 diabetes within 10 years. Maintaining a healthy weight, exercising regularly, and eating a healthy diet have all been found to reduce the risk of developing diabetes in people with prediabetes.

Type 2 Diabetes Mellitus

Type 2 DM is the more prevalent type of diabetes, accounting for more than 90% of patients with diabetes. Type 2 diabetes usually occurs in people older than 35 years, with 80% to 90% of patients being overweight at the time of diagnosis. However, type 2 diabetes is now being seen in children as a result of childhood obesity. Type 2 DM has a tendency to run in families and probably has a genetic basis.

- Native Americans and Alaska Natives have the highest rate of type 2 diabetes in the world. Hispanic groups that share genes with the Native American populations, such as Mexican Americans, also have high rates.

Pathophysiology. In type 2 DM, the pancreas usually continues to produce some endogenous (self-made) insulin. However, the insulin that is produced either is insufficient for the body's needs or is poorly utilized by the tissues. The presence of endogenous insulin is the major pathophysiologic distinction between type 1 and type 2 diabetes.

- Obesity is believed to be the most powerful risk factor, and genetic mutations that lead to insulin resistance and a higher risk for obesity have been found in many people with type 2 DM.

Four major metabolic abnormalities play a role in the development of type 2 DM.

- The first factor is *insulin resistance,* which is a condition in which body tissues do not respond to the action of insulin. This is due to insulin receptors that are either unresponsive to the action of insulin or insufficient in number. Entry of glucose into the cell is impeded, resulting in hyperglycemia.
- A second factor is a marked decrease in the ability of the pancreas to produce insulin as the β cells become fatigued from the compensatory overproduction of insulin or when β-cell mass is lost.
- A third factor is inappropriate glucose production by the liver. Instead of properly regulating the release of glucose in response to blood levels, the liver does so in a haphazard way that does not correspond to the body's needs at the time.
- A fourth factor is alteration in the production of hormones and cyokines by adipose tissue (adipokines). Adipokines appear to play a role in glucose and fat metabolism and likely contribute to pathophysiology of type 2 DM.

Another factor related to diabetes is *metabolic syndrome,* a cluster of abnormalities that act synergistically to greatly increase the risk for cardiovascular disease and diabetes. It is characterized by insulin resistance, elevated insulin levels, high levels of triglycerides, decreased levels of high-density lipoproteins (HDLs), increased levels of low-density lipoproteins (LDLs), and hypertension. Some risk factors for metabolic syndrome include central obesity, sedentary lifestyle, urbanization, and ethnicities such as Native Americans and Hispanic Americans. See Metabolic syndrome, p. 409.

Disease onset in type 2 DM is usually gradual. The person may go for many years with undetected hyperglycemia that might produce few, if any, symptoms. If the patient with type 2 DM has marked hyperglycemia (e.g., 500 to 1000 mg/dl [27.6 to 55.1 mmol/L]), a sufficient endogenous insulin supply may prevent DKA from occurring. However, osmotic fluid and electrolyte loss related to hyperglycemia may become severe and lead to hyperosmolar coma.

Clinical Manifestations
Type 1 DM
Because the onset of type 1 DM is rapid, the initial manifestations are usually acute. The osmotic effect of glucose produces the manifestations of polydipsia and polyuria. Polyphagia is a consequence of cellular malnourishment when insulin deficiency pre-

vents utilization of glucose for energy. Weight loss, weakness, and fatigue may also be experienced.

Type 2 DM

Manifestations of type 2 DM are often nonspecific, including fatigue, recurrent infections, prolonged wound healing, and visual changes.

Acute Complications

The acute problems of DKA and hyperosmolar hyperglycemic nonketotic syndrome (HHNS) coma result from hyperglycemia and insufficient insulin. A problem that may arise from too much insulin or an excessive dose of an oral antidiabetes agent (OA) is *hypoglycemia* (also referred to as insulin reaction or low blood glucose). It is important for the health care provider to be able to distinguish between hyperglycemia and hypoglycemia because hypoglycemia can constitute a serious threat and requires immediate attention. Table 32 compares hypoglycemia and hyperglycemia.

Diabetic Ketoacidosis. DKA, also referred to as diabetic acidosis and diabetic coma, is caused by a profound deficiency of insulin and is characterized by hyperglycemia, ketosis, acidosis, and dehydration. Precipitating factors include illness and infection, inadequate insulin dosage, undiagnosed type 1 DM, poor self-management, and neglect.

- DKA is most likely to occur in type 1 diabetes but may be seen in type 2 in conditions of severe illness or stress when the extra demand for insulin cannot be met by the pancreas.
- Manifestations of DKA include dehydration signs (e.g., poor skin turgor, dry mucous membranes), tachycardia, orthostatic hypotension with a weak and rapid pulse, vomiting, Kussmaul respirations, and a sweet fruity odor of acetone on the breath.

Hyperosmolar Hyperglycemic Syndrome. Hyperosmolar hyperglycemic syndrome (HHS) is a life-threatening syndrome that can occur in the patient with DM who is able to produce enough insulin to prevent DKA but not enough to prevent severe hyperglycemia, osmotic diuresis, and extracellular fluid depletion. The main difference between HHS and DKA is that the patient with HHS usually has enough circulating insulin so that ketoacidosis does not occur.

- HHS often occurs in the older adult patient with type 2 diabetes and is often related to impaired thirst sensation and/or a functional inability to replace fluids. There is usually a history of inadequate fluid intake, increasing mental depression, and polyuria.

| Table 32 | Comparison of Hyperglycemia and Hypoglycemia |

Hyperglycemia	Hypoglycemia
Manifestations*	
Elevated blood glucose[†]	Blood glucose <70 mg/dl (<3.9 mmol/L)
Increase in urination	Cold, clammy skin
Increase in appetite followed by lack of appetite	Numbness of fingers, toes, mouth
Weakness, fatigue	Rapid heartbeat
Blurred vision	Emotional changes
Headache	Headache
Glycosuria	Nervousness, tremors
Nausea and vomiting	Faintness, dizziness
Abdominal cramps	Unsteady gait, slurred speech
Progression to DKA or HHS	Hunger
	Changes in vision
	Seizures, coma
Causes	
Illness, infection	Alcohol intake without food
Corticosteroids	Too little food—delayed, omitted, inadequate intake
Too much food	
Too little or no diabetes medication	Too much diabetic medication
	Too much exercise without compensation
Inactivity	Diabetes medication or food taken at wrong time
Emotional, physical stress	
Poor absorption of insulin	Loss of weight without change in medication
	Use of β blockers interfering with recognition of symptoms

DKA, Diabetic ketoacidosis; HHS, hyperosmolar hyperglycemic syndrome; OA, oral agent.
* There is usually a gradual onset of symptoms in hyperglycemia and a rapid onset in hypoglycemia.
[†] Specific clinical manifestations related to elevated levels of blood glucose vary according to the patient.

Table 32	Comparison of Hyperglycemia and Hypoglycemia—cont'd

Hyperglycemia	Hypoglycemia
Treatment	
Physician's attention	Immediate ingestion of 15-20 g of simple carbohydrates
Continuance of diabetes medication as ordered	Ingestion of another 15-20 g of simple carbohydrates in 15 min if no relief obtained
Checking blood glucose frequently; checking urine for ketones; recording results	Contacting of health care provider if no relief obtained
Hourly drinking of fluids	Discussion with health care provider about medication dosage
Preventive Measures	
Taking prescribed dose of medication at proper time	Taking prescribed dose of medication at proper time
Accurate administration of insulin/OA	Accurate administration of insulin/OA
Maintenance of diet	Ingestion of all recommended foods at proper time
Maintenance of good personal hygiene	Provision of compensation for exercise
Adherence to sick day rules when ill	Ability to recognize and know symptoms and treat them immediately
Checking of blood for glucose as ordered	Carrying of simple carbohydrates
Contacting of physician regarding ketonuria	Education of friends, family, fellow employees about symptoms and treatment
Wearing of diabetic identification	Checking blood glucose as ordered
	Wearing medical alert (diabetic) identification

D

Hypoglycemia. Hypoglycemia, or low blood glucose, occurs when there is too much insulin in proportion to available glucose in the blood. This causes the blood glucose level to drop to <70 mg/dl (<3.9 mmol/L).

- Manifestations include confusion, irritability, diaphoresis, tremors, hunger, weakness, and visual disturbances. Untreated hypoglycemia can progress to loss of consciousness, seizures, coma, and death.

Chronic Complications

Chronic complications are primarily those of end-organ disease damage to the large and small blood vessels from chronic hyperglycemia. *Angiopathy,* or blood vessel disease, is estimated to account for the majority of deaths in patients with diabetes. These chronic blood vessel problems are divided into two categories: macrovascular complications and microvascular complications.

Macrovascular complications are diseases of the large- and medium-sized blood vessels that occur with greater frequency and with an earlier onset in people with diabetes. It is essentially atherosclerotic vascular disease that affects the cerebral, cardiac, and peripheral vessels. The development of macrovascular disease seems to be promoted by the altered lipid metabolism common to diabetes and may be delayed by tight glucose control. *Insulin resistance syndrome,* an association of insulin resistance, hypertension, elevated very-low-density lipoprotein (VLDL), and decreased HDL, reflects the role of insulin resistance in dyslipidemia.

Microvascular complications are specific to diabetes and result from thickening of the vessel membranes in the capillaries and arterioles in response to chronic hyperglycemia. Although microangiopathy can be found throughout the body, the areas most noticeably affected are the eyes (retinopathy), kidneys (nephropathy), and skin (dermopathy).

- *Diabetic retinopathy* is the leading cause of visual disability and blindness in persons with long-standing uncontrolled diabetes. *Nonproliferative retinopathy* is the most common form and is characterized by capillary microaneurysms, retinal swelling, and hard exudates. Macular edema may result as plasma leaks from macular blood vessels. As the disease progresses to *proliferative retinopathy,* abnormal, fragile blood vessels that are predisposed to leak grow in the retina, causing severe vision loss. Laser photocoagulation is used as treatment of the retinopathy.
- *Diabetic nephropathy* is the leading cause of chronic kidney disease in the United States. Tight blood glucose control is critical to the prevention and delay of diabetic nephropathy.

In addition, aggressive blood pressure management is indicated for all patients with DM because hypertension significantly accelerates the progression of diabetic nephropathy. Annual microalbuminuria (MAU) and creatinine tests are recommended for early detection of nephropathy.

Neuropathy is nerve damage that occurs because of the metabolic derangements associated with DM and is seen equally in type 1 and type 2 diabetes. Two major categories of diabetic neuropathy are *sensory neuropathy,* which affects the peripheral nervous sytem, and *autonomic neuropathy,* which can affect nearly all body systems.

- The most common form of sensory neuropathy is distal symmetric neuropathy, which affects the hands or feet bilaterally. Characteristics include loss of sensation, abnormal sensations, pain, and paresthesias. The pain, which is often described as burning, cramping, crushing, or tearing, is usually worse at night. The paresthesias may be associated with tingling, burning, and itching.
- Autonomic neuropathy can lead to hypoglycemic unawareness, bowel incontinence and diarrhea, and urinary retention. Delayed gastric emptying (gastroparesis), a complication of autonomic neuropathy, can produce nausea, vomiting, esophageal reflux, and persistent feelings of fullness. Sexual function can be affected, and cardiovascular abnormalities, such as postural hypotension and resting tachycardia, can occur.

Control of blood glucose is the only treatment for diabetic neuropathy. It is effective in many but not all cases. Drug therapy may be used to treat neuropathic symptoms, particularly pain.

Diagnostic Tests

The diagnosis of diabetes can be made through one of three methods that is confirmed on a subsequent day.

- Fasting plasma glucose level ≥126 mg/dl (≥7 mmol/L)
- Random plasma glucose level ≥200 mg/dl (≥11.1 mmol/L) plus manifestations of DM
- Two-hour oral glucose tolerance test (OGTT) level ≥200 mg/dl (≥11.1 mmol/L) with a glucose load of 75 g

Other diagnostic tests are used to evaluate glucose control and monitor for complications of diabetes.

- Glycosylated hemoglobin (hemoglobin A1C), lipid profile, blood urea nitrogen (BUN), serum creatinine, and electrolytes, thyroid-stimulating hormone (TSH)
- Urine for complete urinalysis, microalbuminuria, glucose, and acetone

- Neurologic and funduscopic examination
- Electrocardiogram (ECG), blood pressure (BP), and monitoring of weight
- Doppler scan to determine the presence and degree of peripheral vascular disease
- Foot (podiatric) examination

Collaborative Care

The goals of DM management are to reduce symptoms, promote well-being, prevent and manage acute complications of hyperglycemia, and delay the onset and progression of long-term complications. Nutrition, drug therapy, exercise, and self-monitoring of blood glucose are the tools used in the management of DM. The two major types of glucose-lowering agents (GLAs) used in the treatment of diabetes are insulin and OAs. For the majority of people, drug therapy is necessary.

Drug Therapy: Insulin

Exogenous insulin is needed when a patient has inadequate insulin to meet specific metabolic needs. People with type 1 diabetes require exogenous insulin to survive. People with type 2 diabetes, who are usually controlled with diet, exercise, and/or OAs, may require exogenous insulin during periods of severe stress, such as illness or surgery. When patients with type 2 diabetes cannot maintain satisfactory blood glucose levels, exogenous insulin will be added to the management plan.

Human insulin derived from bacteria or yeast cells using recombinant DNA technology is the basis for a variety of types of insulin used today. All insulins start with regular insulin as a base, and by adding zinc, acetate buffers, and protamine to insulin in various ways, the onset of activity, peak, and duration times can be manipulated (Table 33). The specific properties of each type of insulin are matched with the patient's diet and activity.

Examples of insulin regimens ranging from one to four injections per day are presented in Table 49-4 in Lewis and others, *Medical-Surgical Nursing,* edition 7, p. 1261.

- The exogenous insulin regimen that most closely mimics endogenous insulin production is a basal-bolus regimen that uses rapid and short-acting (bolus) insulin before meals and long-acting (basal) background insulin once per day.
- Combination insulin therapy involves the mixing of short- or rapid-acting insulin with an intermediate-acting insulin to provide both mealtime and basal coverage with one injection. Premixed formulas are available for this regimen, but optimal blood glucose control is not as likely because there is less flexibility in dosing.

Table 33	Drug Therapy: Types of Insulin
Classification	**Examples, Clarity of Solution**
Rapid-acting insulin	lispro (Humalog), clear aspart (Novolog), clear glulisine (Apidra), clear
Short-acting insulin	regular (Humulin R, Novolin R, ReliOn R), clear
Intermediate-acting insulin	NPH (Humulin N, Novolin N, ReliOn N), cloudy
Long-acting insulin	glargine (Lantus), clear detemir (Levemir), clear
Combination therapy (premixed)	NPH/regular 70/30* (Humulin 70/30, Novolin 70/30, ReliOn 70/30), cloudy NPH/regular 50/50* (Humulin 50/50), cloudy lispro protamine/lispro 75/25* (Humalog Mix 75/25), cloudy aspart protamine/aspart 70/30* (Novolog Mix 70/30), cloudy

D

* These numbers refer to percentages of each type of insulin.

Because insulin is inactivated by gastric juices, it cannot be taken orally. Previously, injection was the only route of administration approved for self-administration, but inhaled insulin is now available for use. Other alternate delivery methods include an insulin pump and intensive insulin therapy.

- Continuous SC insulin infusion uses an insulin pump, a small battery-operated device that resembles a standard paging device in size and appearance. Every 2 or 3 days the insertion site is changed and the pump is refilled with insulin and reprogrammed. A major advantage of the pump is the potential for tight glucose control.
- An alternative to the insulin pump is intensive insulin therapy, which consists of multiple daily insulin (MDI) injections together with frequent self-monitoring of blood glucose.

Nursing Care Related to Insulin Therapy. Nursing responsibilities for the patient receiving insulin include proper administration, assessment of patient's response to insulin therapy, and education of the patient regarding administration of, adjustment to, and side effects of insulin.

- Assessment of the patient who is new to insulin must include an evaluation of his or her ability to manage this therapy safely. This includes the ability to understand the interaction of insulin, diet, and activity and to be able to recognize and treat appropriately the symptoms of hypoglycemia.
- The patient or significant other also must be able to prepare and inject the insulin (see Table 49-5, Lewis and others, *Medical-Surgical Nursing,* edition 7, p. 1262). If the patient or family lacks the skills to prepare insulin, additional resources are needed to assist the patient.
- Follow-up evaluation of the patient who has been using insulin therapy includes inspection of insulin sites for lipodystrophy (atrophy of subcutaneous tissue) and other reactions, a review of the insulin preparation and injection technique, a history pertaining to the occurrence of hypoglycemic episodes, and the patient's method for handling hypoglycemic episodes.
- A review of the patient's record of urine and blood glucose tests is also important in assessing overall glycemic control.

Drug Therapy: Oral Agents

OAs are not insulin, but they work on the three defects of type 2 diabetes: insulin resistance, decreased insulin production, and increased hepatic glucose production. OAs may be used in combination with agents from other classes or with insulin to achieve blood glucose targets.

Currently six classes of oral medications are used in the treatment of type 2 diabetes:

- *Sulfonylureas* increase insulin production from the pancreas and include glipizide (Glucotrol, Glucotrol XL), glyburide (Micronase, DiaBeta, Glynase), and glimepiride (Amaryl).
- *Meglitinides* also increase insulin production from the pancreas, but they are more rapidly absorbed and eliminated than the sulfonylureas, decreasing the potential for hypoglycemia. Meglitinides include repaglinide (Prandin) and nateglinide (Starlix).
- *Biguanides* primarily reduce glucose production by the liver, but they also enhance insulin sensitivity and improve glucose transport into cells. Metformin (Glucophage) is a currently used biguanide that is also prepared in combination with glyburide (Glucovance), with rosiglitazone (Avandamet), and with glipizide (Metaglip).
- α-*Glucosidase inhibitors* slow down the absorption of carbohydrate in the small intestine. Acarbose (Precose) and miglitol (Glyset) are the available drugs in this class.

- *Thiazolidinediones* improve insulin sensitivity, transport, and utilization at target tissues. These agents include pioglitazone (Actos) and rosiglitazone (Avandia).
- *Dipeptidyl peptidase-4 (DDP-4) inhibitors* slow the inactivation of incretin hormones. Incretin hormones are released by the intestines throughout the day but levels increase in response to a meal. This class of drugs includes sitagliptin (Januvia) and vildagliptin (Galvus).

Nursing Care Related to Oral Agents. Nursing responsibilities for the patient taking OAs are similar to those for the patient taking insulin. Proper administration, assessment of patient's use of and response to OAs, and education of the patient and family are all part of the nurse's role.

- The nurse's assessment can be invaluable in determining the most appropriate OA for a patient. The assessment includes the patient's mental status, eating habits, home environment, attitude toward diabetes, and medication history.
- The patient needs to understand the importance of diet and activity plans.
- The patient also needs to know that medication to control blood glucose helps prevent serious long- and short-term complications of diabetes.
- In addition, the patient should be instructed to contact a health care provider if periods of illness or extreme stress occur. During such a period, insulin therapy may be required to prevent or treat hyperglycemic symptoms and avoid a hyperglycemic emergency.

Drug Therapy: Other Agents

Pramlintide (Symlin) is a synthetic analog of human amylin, a hormone secreted by the β cells of the pancreas. When taken concurrently with insulin, it works to control diabetes by slowing gastric emptying, reducing postprandial glucagon secretion, and increasing satiety. It must be administered subcutaneously and cannot be mixed with insulin.

Exenatide (Byetta) is a synthetic peptide that stimulates the release of insulin from the pancreatic β cells. It suppresses glucagon secretions from pancreatic α cells, reduces food intake by increasing satiety, and slows gastric emptying. It is an adjunct therapy for patients with type 2 diabetes and must be administered subcutaneously.

Nutritional Therapy

Nutritional therapy is the cornerstone of diabetes care. Today there is no one "diabetic" diet. Recent guidelines from the American

Diabetes Association indicate that within the context of an overall healthy eating plan, a person with DM can eat the same foods as a person who does not have diabetes. This means that the same principles of good nutrition that apply to the general population also apply to the person with diabetes. The USDA MyPyramid summarizes and illustrates nutritional guidelines and nutrient needs (see Fig. 40-1 and Table 40-1 in Lewis and others, *Medical-Surgical Nursing,* edition 7, pp. 949 to 950).

- *Type 1 diabetes.* Meal planning should be based on the individual's usual food intake, with insulin therapy integrated into the usual eating and exercise patterns. For patients using conventional, fixed insulin regimens, day-to-day consistency in timing and amount of food eaten is important. Patients using rapid-acting insulin can make adjustments in dosage before meals based on current blood glucose level and the carbohydrate content of the meal. Intensified insulin therapy, such as multiple daily injections or the use of an insulin pump, allows considerable flexibility in food selection and can be adjusted for deviations from usual eating and exercise habits.

- *Type 2 diabetes.* The emphasis for nutritional therapy in type 2 DM should be placed on achieving glucose, lipid, and BP goals. Weight loss usually improves glycemic control. Weight loss is best attempted by a moderate decrease in calories and an increase in calorie expenditure (regular exercise). The nutrient balance of the diet of the diabetic patient is essential to maintenance of blood glucose levels. Amounts of carbohydrates, the glycemic index of carbohydrates, types and amounts of fats, amounts of protein, and use of alcohol must be considered when planning meals. (See Table 49-9 for nutritional therapy for type 1 and type 2 diabetes, Lewis and others, *Medical-Surgical Nursing,* edition 7, p. 1268.)

Because of the complexity of nutrition issues, it is recommended that a registered dietitian with expertise in diabetes management and a diabetes nurse educator be members of the treatment team. Diet teaching by the dietitian or nurse should include the patient's family and significant others whenever possible. It is most effective to direct teaching efforts to the person who will be cooking.

Management of Acute Complications
Diabetic Ketoacidosis

- Because the fluid imbalance of DKA is potentially life threatening, the initial goal of therapy is to establish IV access and begin fluid and electrolyte replacement.

- Early potassium replacement is essential because hypokalemia is a significant cause of unnecessary and avoidable death during treatment of DKA.
- IV insulin administration is directed toward correcting hyperglycemia and hyperketonemia. Initially a bolus of insulin is delivered, followed by continuous infusion.

Hyperosmolar Hyperglycemic Syndrome

- Laboratory values in HHS include blood glucose >400 mg/dl (>22.25 mmol/L) and a marked increase in serum osmolality. The increased osmolality produces more severe neurologic manifestations, such as somnolence, coma, and seizures.
- HHS constitutes a medical emergency and has a high mortality rate. Therapy is similar to that for DKA except that HHS requires greater fluid replacement (see Table 33).
- Regular insulin is given by IV bolus, followed by an infusion.
- Electrolytes are monitored and replaced as needed. Vital signs, intake and output, tissue turgor, laboratory values, and cardiac monitoring are assessed to monitor the efficacy of fluid and electrolyte replacement.

Hypoglycemia

- At the first sign of hypoglycemia, the blood glucose should be checked if possible. If it is below 70 mg/dl (3.9 mmol/L), the patient should immediately begin treatment for hypoglycemia. If monitoring equipment is not available, hypoglycemia should be assumed and treatment should be initiated.
- Hypoglycemia is treated by ingesting 15 to 20 g of a simple (fast-acting) carbohydrate, such as 4 to 6 ounces of fruit juice or regular soft drink, or 8 ounces of low-fat milk. Overtreatment with large quantities of quick-acting carbohydrates, such as a whole candy bar, should be avoided so that rapid fluctuation to hyperglycemia does not occur.
- Blood glucose should be checked about 15 minutes following the initial teatment, and treatment should be repeated if the blood glucose remains below 70 mg/dl (3.9 mmol/L).
- Once the blood glucose is greater than 70 mg/dl (3.9 mmol/L) and symptoms have improved, the patient should eat a snack to prevent hypoglycemia from recurring. Good snacks include peanut butter and cheese and crackers.
- If there is little improvement in the patient's condition after two or three doses of 15 g of simple carbohydrate or if the patient is not alert enough to swallow, 1 mg of glucagon may be administered by intramuscular (IM) or subcutaneous (SC) injection.
- Once acute hypoglycemia has been reversed, the nurse should explore with the patient the reasons why the situation devel-

D

oped. This assessment may indicate a need for additional education of the patient and family to avoid future episodes of hypoglycemia. The danger of hypoglycemic reactions must be stressed because memory and learning impairment can result from repeated episodes of severe hypoglycemia.

Nursing Management

Goals

The patient with DM will be an active participant in the management of the diabetes regimen; experience few or no episodes of acute hyperglycemic emergencies or hypoglycemia; maintain blood glucose levels at normal or near normal levels; prevent, minimize, or delay the occurrence of chronic complications of diabetes; and adjust lifestyle to accommodate a diabetes regimen with a minimum of stress.

See NCP 49-1 for the patient with diabetes, Lewis and others, *Medical-Surgical Nursing,* edition 7, pp. 1273 to 1274.

Nursing Diagnoses

- Ineffective therapeutic regimen management
- Imbalanced nutrition: more than body requirements
- Risk for injury
- Risk for peripheral neurovascular dysfunction
- Powerlessness

Nursing Interventions

The role of the nurse in health promotion and maintenance relates to the identification, monitoring, and education of the patient at risk for the development of DM. Acute situations involving the patient with diabetes include hypoglycemia, DKA, and HHS, but the major goal of patient care is to enable the patient to reach an optimal level of independence in self-care activities.

Exercise. Regular, consistent exercise is considered an essential part of diabetes and prediabetes management. Exercise increases insulin receptor sites in the tissue and can have a direct effect on lowering the blood glucose levels. It also contributes to weight loss, which also decreases insulin resistance. Regular exercise may also delay long-term complications by reducing triglyceride and LDL cholesterol levels, increasing HDL, reducing BP, and improving circulation. Information about exercise and diabetes that is important for both the patient and the health care provider is provided in the patient and family teaching guide (see Table 49-11, Lewis and others, *Medical-Surgical Nursing,* edition 7, p. 1269).

Blood Glucose Monitoring. Patient self-monitoring of blood glucose (SMBG) enables the patient to make self-management decisions regarding diet, exercise, and medication. SMBG is also important for detecting episodic hyperglycemia and hypoglycemia.

Patients with type 1 DM typically test 4 times per day (before meals and at bedtime). Those using an insulin pump may test more frequently. Patients with type 2 DM will have more variable and individualized testing regimens. Testing may be more frequent for all persons with diabetes to determine the effects of exercise on glucose levels, in the event of illness, or when hypoglycemia is suspected.

- The nurse involved in this aspect of management should anticipate a close working relationship with patients as they refine their techniques and learn appropriate decision making about managing their diabetes.

Management of Acute Illness and Surgery. Emotional and physical stress can increase blood glucose levels and result in hyperglycemia. Acute illness (even minor), injury, and surgery may evoke a counterregulatory hormone response resulting in hyperglycemia.

- Patients with diabetes who are ill should continue with the regular meal plan while increasing the intake of noncaloric fluids, such as broth, water, diet gelatin, and other decaffeinated beverages. They should also continue taking oral agents and insulin as prescribed and check blood glucose at least every 4 hours. If the glucose is >240 mg/dl (>13.3 mmol/L), urine should be tested for ketones every 3 to 4 hours. Moderate to large ketone levels should be reported to the health care provider.
- If illness causes the patient to eat less than normal, OAs and insulin should be taken as prescribed while supplementing food intake with carbohydrate-containing fluids. The health care provider should be notified promptly if the patient is unable to keep any fluids or fluid down.
- Adjustments in the diabetes regimen during the intraoperative period can be planned to ensure glycemic control. The patient is given IV fluids and insulin immediately before, during, and after surgery when there is no oral intake. The type 2 DM patient receiving OAs usually has them discontinued 48 hours before surgery and is treated with insulin during the surgical period.
- The nurse caring for an unconscious surgical patient receiving insulin must be alert for hypoglycemic signs, such as sweating, tachycardia, and tremors. The nurse should be aware that blood glucose monitoring must also be done frequently.

Ambulatory and Home Care. Successful management of diabetes requires ongoing interaction among the patient, family, and the health care team. It is important that a diabetes nurse educator be involved in the care of the patient and family.

A diagnosis of diabetes affects the patient in many profound ways. Patients with diabetes must continually contend with life-style choices that affect the food they eat, the activities they engage in, and demands on their time and energy. In addition, they face the potential of developing the devastating complications of this disease. Careful assessment of what it means to the patient to have diabetes should be the starting point of patient teaching. The nurse can help patients make adjustments by displaying a supportive and nonjudgmental attitude.

Personal hygiene is an important practice by the patient with DM. The potential for microvascular complications and infections requires diligent skin and dental hygiene practices on the part of the patient. Routine care should include tooth brushing and flossing and regular bathing, with particular emphasis given to foot care. If cuts, scrapes, or burns occur, they should be treated promptly and monitored carefully. If the injury does not begin to heal within 24 hours or if signs of infection develop, the health care provider should be notified immediately.

▼ Patient and Family Teaching

The goals of diabetes self-management education are to enable the patient to become the most active participant in his or her care. Patients who actively manage their diabetes care have better outcomes than those who do not. For this reason, an educational approach that facilitates informed decision making on the part of the patient is widely advocated. Guidelines for patient and family teaching for management of diabetes are in Table 34.

- The patient should be instructed to carry medical identification at all times indicating diabetes. An identification card can supply valuable information, such as the name of the health care provider and the type and dose of insulin or OA.

- The major educational objective is a level of self-management appropriate to the individual patient. Ideally, the patient should be taught about the disease and encouraged to achieve self-management with guidance only from the health care provider.

- A knowledgeable patient should be able to make minor adjustments in insulin dosage and diet prescription to compensate for special circumstances, such as illness or increased exercise.

- Not all patients with diabetes are capable of self-management. If the patient is not able to manage the disease, a family member may be able to assume this role. If the patient or family cannot make decisions related to diabetes management, the nurse may identify appropriate resources

Table 34	Patient and Family Teaching Guide: General Guidelines for Management of Diabetes Mellitus

Do	Do Not
Blood Glucose	
■ Monitor your blood glucose at home and record results in a log	■ Skip doses of your insulin, especially when you are sick
■ Take your insulin or OA as prescribed	■ Run out of insulin
■ Obtain a hemoglobin A1C blood test every 3-6 mo as an indicator of your long-term blood glucose control	■ Enroll in a fad diet
	■ Rub the area where insulin was administered
■ Carry some form of glucose at all times so you can treat hypoglycemia quickly	
■ Instruct family members in the use of glucagon administration in case of emergencies caused by hypoglycemia	
Exercise	
■ Learn how exercise and food affect your blood glucose levels	■ Forget that exercise will lower your blood glucose level
■ Begin a medically supervised exercise program	■ Exercise if your blood glucose levels are very elevated; this may lead to a temporary worsening of your blood glucose levels
Diet	
■ Follow your diet, eating regular meals at regular times	■ Drink excessive amounts of alcohol because this may lead to unpredictable low blood glucose reactions
■ Eat slowly and chew food thoroughly	
■ Choose foods low in saturated fats	■ Eat fried foods
■ Limit the amount of alcohol you drink	
■ Learn your cholesterol level	

OAs, Oral agents.

Continued

D

Table 34	Patient and Family Teaching Guide: General Guidelines for Management of Diabetes Mellitus—cont'd

Do	Do Not
Other Guidelines	
▪ Obtain an annual eye examination by an ophthalmologist	▪ Smoke
	▪ Apply hot or cold directly to your feet
▪ Obtain an annual urine test for protein	▪ Go barefoot
▪ Examine your feet at home	▪ Ignore the symptoms of hypoglycemia and hyperglycemia
▪ Wear comfortable, well-fitting shoes to help prevent foot injury; break in new shoes gradually	▪ Put baby oil or lotion between your toes
▪ Always carry identification that says you have diabetes	
▪ Have other medical problems treated, especially high BP	
▪ Know the symptoms of hypoglycemia and hyperglycemia	
▪ Quit smoking	

BP, Blood pressure.

outside the family. These resources can assist the patient and family in outlining a feasible treatment program that meets their capabilities.

DIARRHEA

Description
Diarrhea is not a disease but a symptom. The term is commonly used to denote an increase in stool frequency or volume and an increase in stool looseness.

▪ Causes can be divided into the general classifications of decreased fluid absorption, increased fluid secretion, motility disturbances, or a combination of these. Causes of diar-

Table 35	Causes of Diarrhea

Decreased Fluid Absorption
- Oral intake of poorly absorbable solutes (e.g., laxatives)
- Maldigestion and malabsorption (e.g., maldigestion of fat with pancreatitis, poorly absorbed bile salts in terminal ileum disease)
- Mucosal damage (e.g., tropical sprue, celiac disease, inflammatory bowel disease, ischemic bowel disease, radiation injury)
- Intestinal enzyme deficiencies (e.g., lactase)
- Decreased surface area (e.g., intestinal resection)
- Osmotic diarrhea (candy, gum, sorbitol, laxatives)

Increased Fluid Secretion
- Infections: bacterial endotoxins, viral agents, and parasitic agents (see Table 37)
- Hormonal: vasoactive intestinal polypeptide secretion from adenoma of the pancreas; gastrin secretion caused by Zollinger-Ellison syndrome; calcitonin secretion from carcinoma of the thyroid
- Tumor: villous adenoma

Motility Disturbances
- Irritable bowel syndrome: ↑ visceral sensitivity and transit
- Diabetic enteropathy: ↑ transit secondary to peripheral neuropathy
- Gastrectomy: ↑ transit as a result of dumping syndrome

rhea are listed in Table 35, and specific causes of acute infectious diarrhea are listed in Table 36.

Clinical Manifestations

Diarrhea may be acute or chronic. *Acute* diarrhea most commonly results from infection. Bacterial or viral infection of the intestine may result in explosive watery diarrhea, *tenesmus* (spasmodic contraction of the anal sphincter with pain and persistent desire to defecate), and abdominal cramping pain. Perianal skin irritation may also develop.

- Systemic manifestations include fever, nausea, vomiting, and malaise. Leukocytes, blood, and mucus may be present in the stool, depending on the causative agent (see Table 37).
- Acute diarrhea is often self-limiting in the adult, with symptoms continuing until the irritant or causative agent is excreted.

Diarrhea is considered chronic when it persists for at least 4 weeks. Severe chronic diarrhea produces life-threatening

Table 36   Causes of Acute Infectious Diarrhea

	Onset	Duration	Symptoms and Signs
Viral			
Rotavirus, Norwalk	18-24 hr	24-48 hr	Explosive, watery diarrhea; nausea; vomiting; abdominal cramps
Bacterial			
Escherichia coli	6-24 hr	3-4 days	Four or five loose stools per day, nausea, malaise, low-grade fever
Enterohemorrhagic *E. coli* (O157:H7)	8-24 hr	4-9 days	Bloody diarrhea, severe cramping, fever
Shigella	24 hr	7 days	Watery stools containing blood and mucus, tenesmus, urgency, severe cramping, fever
Salmonella	6-48 hr	2-5 days	Watery diarrhea, nausea, vomiting, abdominal cramps, fever
Staphylococcal (toxin from *S. aureus*)	30 min–7 hr	24-48 hr	Diarrhea, abdominal cramping, vomiting, nausea
Campylobacter species	24 hr	<7 days	Profuse, watery diarrhea; malaise; nausea; abdominal cramps; low-grade fever
Clostridium perfringens	8-24 hr	24 hr	Watery diarrhea, abdominal cramps, vomiting (rare)
Clostridium difficile	4-9 days after start of antibiotics	24 hr	Associated with antibiotic treatment; symptoms range from mild, watery diarrhea to severe abdominal pain, fever, leukocytosis, leukocytes in stool
Parasitic			
Giardia lamblia	1-3 wk	Few days to 3 mo	Sudden onset; malodorous, explosive, watery diarrhea; flatulence; epigastric pain and cramping; nausea
Entamoeba histolytica	4 days	Weeks to months	Frequent soft stools with blood and mucus (in severe cases, watery stools), flatulence, distention, abdominal cramps, fever, leukocytes in stool
Cryptosporidium	2-10 days	1-6 mo	Watery diarrhea, nausea, vomiting, abdominal cramps, weight loss in AIDS

AIDS, Acquired immunodeficiency syndrome.

dehydration, electrolyte disturbances (e.g., hypokalemia), and acid-base imbalances (metabolic acidosis).

- Malabsorption and malnutrition are also sequelae of chronic diarrhea.

Diagnostic Studies

An accurate diagnosis requires a thorough history, physical examination, and laboratory testing.

- A history of travel, medication use, diet, previous surgery, and interpersonal contacts, as well as family history, should be obtained.
- Blood tests may identify anemia, elevated white blood cell (WBC) count, iron and folate deficiencies, and abnormal electrolyte levels.
- Increased hemoglobin, hematocrit, and blood urea nitrogen (BUN) levels suggest fluid deficits.
- Stools are examined for blood, mucus, WBCs, and parasites. Stool cultures may help in identifying infectious organisms.
- In a patient with chronic diarrhea, measurement of stool electrolytes, pH, and osmolality may help to determine whether diarrhea is related to decreased fluid absorption or increased fluid secretion (secretory diarrhea).
- Measurement of stool fat and undigested muscle fibers may indicate fat and protein malabsorption conditions, including pancreatic insufficiency.
- Colonoscopy may be used to examine mucosa and to obtain specimens for examination.
- Upper and lower barium studies may be helpful in detecting mucosal disease.

Collaborative Care

Treatment is based on the cause and is aimed at replacing fluids and electrolytes and resolving the diarrhea. Oral solutions containing glucose and electrolytes (e.g., Gatorade, Pedialyte) may be sufficient to replace losses from mild diarrhea. In severe diarrhea, parenteral administration of fluids, electrolytes, vitamins, and nutrition is warranted.

Once the cause has been determined, antidiarrheal agents may be given to coat and protect mucous membranes, absorb irritating substances, inhibit gastrointestinal (GI) motility, decrease intestinal secretions, and decrease central nervous system (CNS) stimulation to the GI tract.

- Antiperistaltic agents are not given to a patient who has infectious diarrheal syndromes because of the potential for

prolonging exposure to the infectious agent. Regardless of the cause, antidiarrheal medications should only be given for a short period.
■ Antibiotics are reserved for treating specific bacterial organisms. Antibiotics can cause diarrhea by altering normal bowel flora.

Nursing Management: Acute Infectious Diarrhea
Goals
The patient with diarrhea will not transmit the microorganism causing the infectious diarrhea, will cease having diarrhea and resume normal bowel patterns, will have normal fluid and electrolyte and acid-base balance, will have normal nutritional status, and will have no perianal skin breakdown.

See NCP 43-1 for the patient with acute infectious diarrhea, Lewis and others, *Medical-Surgical Nursing,* edition 7, p. 1039.

Nursing Diagnoses
■ Diarrhea
■ Deficient fluid volume
■ Impaired skin integrity

Nursing Interventions
All cases of acute diarrhea should be considered infectious until the cause is known.
■ Hand washing is the most important measure in the prevention of the transfer of microorganisms. Hands should be washed before and after contact with each patient and when body fluids of any kind are handled.
■ Patients with *Clostridium difficile* should be placed in a private room, and gloves and gowns should be worn for all care.

▼ Patient and Family Teaching
■ Patients should be taught the principles of hygiene, infection control precautions, and potential dangers of an illness that is infectious to themselves and others.
■ Proper handling, cooking, and storage of food should be discussed with patients suspected of having infectious diarrhea.

DISLOCATION AND SUBLUXATION

Description
A *dislocation* is a severe injury of the ligamentous structures that surround a joint. It results in the complete displacement or separa-

tion of joint articular surfaces. A *subluxation* is a partial or incomplete displacement of the joint surface. Manifestations of a subluxation are similar to those of a dislocation but are less severe. Treatment of a subluxation is similar to that of a dislocation, but subluxation requires less healing time.

Dislocations characteristically result from overwhelming forces transmitted to the joint that cause a disruption of the soft tissues. Joints most frequently dislocated in the upper extremity include the thumb, elbow, and shoulder. In the lower extremity, the hip is vulnerable to dislocation occurring as a result of severe trauma, often associated with motor vehicle accidents.

D

Clinical Manifestations

The most obvious manifestation of a dislocation is deformity. For example, if a hip is dislocated, the limb is shorter and often externally rotated on the affected side.

- Additional manifestations include local pain, tenderness, loss of function of the injured part, and swelling of soft tissues in the region of the joint.

Complications of a dislocated joint are open joint injuries, avascular necrosis (bone cell death as a result of inadequate blood supply), intraarticular fractures, fracture-dislocation, and damage to adjacent neurovascular tissue.

Diagnostic Studies

- X-ray studies determine extent of displacement of the involved structures.
- Joint aspiration determines the presence of blood or fat cells. Fat cells in the aspirate indicate a probable intraarticular fracture.

Collaborative Care

Dislocation requires prompt attention. The longer the joint remains unreduced, the greater the possibility of avascular necrosis. Compartment syndrome may also occur and is associated with significant vascular injury. The hip joint is particularly susceptible to avascular necrosis.

The first goal of management is to realign the dislocated portion of the joint in its original anatomic position. This can be accomplished by a closed reduction, which may be performed with the patient under local or general anesthesia. In some situations, surgical open reduction may be necessary.

- After reduction, the extremity is usually immobilized by bracing, splinting, taping, or using a sling to allow the torn ligaments and capsular tissue time to heal.

Nursing Management

Nursing care is directed toward relief of pain and support and protection of the injured joint. After the joint has been reduced and immobilized, motion is usually restricted.

- A carefully regulated rehabilitation program can prevent fracture instability and joint dysfunction.
- An exercise program with gentle range of motion slowly and methodically restores the joint to its original range of motion without causing another dislocation.
- Activity restrictions of the affected joint may be imposed to decrease the risk of repeatedly dislocating the joint.

DISSEMINATED INTRAVASCULAR COAGULATION

Description

Disseminated intravascular coagulation (DIC) is a serious bleeding and thrombotic disorder. It results from abnormally initiated and accelerated clotting. Subsequent decreases in clotting factors and platelets may lead to uncontrollable hemorrhage. The term *DIC* can be misleading because it suggests that blood is clotting. The paradox of this condition is that profuse bleeding results from depletion of platelets and clotting factors. DIC is always caused by an underlying disease; the underlying disease must be treated for DIC to resolve.

Pathophysiology

DIC is an abnormal response of the normal clotting cascade stimulated by a disease process or disorder. The diseases and disorders known to predispose patients to DIC are major physiologic assaults and include shock, septicemia, abruptio placentae, severe head injury, heat stroke, and pulmonary emboli.

- DIC can occur as an acute, catastrophic condition, or it may exist at a subacute or chronic level. Each condition may have one or multiple triggering mechanisms to start the clotting cascade.

Initially in DIC, a stimulus such as an injury or a malignant tumor causes release of tissue factor, and normal coagulation mechanisms are enhanced. Intravascular thrombin is produced, and it catalyzes the conversion of fibrinogen to fibrin and enhances platelet aggregation. There is widespread fibrin and platelet deposition in capillaries and arterioles, resulting in thrombosis. Excessive clotting activates the fibrinolytic system, which in turn breaks down newly formed clots, creating fibrin-split (fibrin-degradation) products (FSPs), which inhibit normal blood clotting. Ultimately the blood loses its ability to form a stable clot at injury sites, which predisposes the patient to hemorrhage.

  ▪ Chronic DIC is most commonly seen in patients with long-standing illnesses such as malignant disorders or autoimmune diseases.

Clinical Manifestations

There is no well-defined sequence of events in acute DIC. Bleeding in a person with no previous history or obvious cause should be questioned because it may be one of the first manifestations of acute DIC. Other nonspecific manifestations include weakness, malaise, and fever. There are both bleeding and thrombotic manifestations in DIC (Fig. 4).

  ▪ Bleeding manifestations of DIC are multifactorial and result from consumption and depletion of platelets and coagulation factors. Manifestations include petechiae, oozing blood, tachypnea, hemoptysis, tachycardia, hypotension, bloody stools, hematuria, dizziness, headache, changes in mental status, and bone and joint pain.
  ▪ Thrombotic manifestations are a result of fibrin or platelet deposition in the microvasculature. Manifestations include ischemic tissue necrosis, acute respiratory distress syndrome (ARDS), cardiovascular and electrocardiogram (ECG) changes, kidney damage, and paralytic ileus.

Diagnostic Studies

  ▪ Prolonged prothrombin time and partial thromboplastin time
  ▪ Prolonged activated partial thromboplastin time and thrombin time
  ▪ Reduced fibrinogen, antithrombin III (AT III), and platelets
  ▪ Elevated FSPs and elevated D-dimers (cross-linked fibrin fragments)
  ▪ Reduced levels of factors V, VII, VIII, X, and XIII

Collaborative Care

It is important to diagnose DIC quickly, institute therapy that will resolve the underlying causative disease or problem, and provide supportive care. Treatment of DIC remains controversial and under investigation as researchers determine how to suitably manage this dangerous syndrome. It is imperative that the nurse

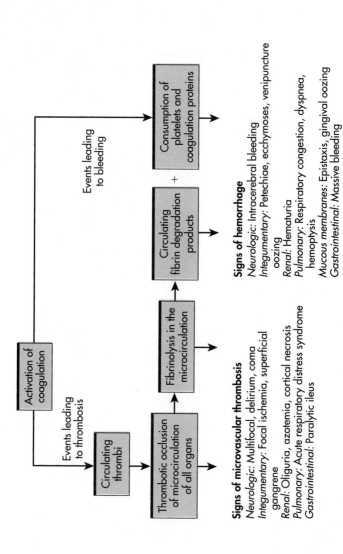

Signs of microvascular thrombosis
Neurologic: Multifocal, delirium, coma
Integumentary: Focal ischemia, superficial gangrene
Renal: Oliguria, azotemia, cortical necrosis
Pulmonary: Acute respiratory distress syndrome
Gastrointestinal: Paralytic ileus

Signs of hemorrhage
Neurologic: Intracerebral bleeding
Integumentary: Petechiae, ecchymoses, venipuncture oozing
Renal: Hematuria
Pulmonary: Respiratory congestion, dyspnea, hemoptysis
Mucous membranes: Epistaxis, gingival oozing
Gastrointestinal: Massive bleeding

Fig. 4. The sequence of events that occur during disseminated intravascular coagulation (DIC).

maintain an ongoing awareness of current modes of therapy. Diagnosing and treating the primary disease process are essential to the resolution of DIC. Depending on its severity, a variety of different methods are used to provide supportive and symptomatic management of DIC.

- If chronic DIC is diagnosed in a patient who is not bleeding, no therapy for DIC is necessary. Treatment of the underlying disease may be sufficient to reverse DIC (e.g., antineoplastic therapy when DIC is due to malignancy).
- When the patient with DIC is bleeding, therapy is directed toward providing support with necessary blood products while treating the primary disorder. Blood products are administered on the basis of specific component deficiencies to patients who have serious bleeding, are at high risk for bleeding (e.g., surgery), or require invasive procedures. Platelets are given to correct thrombocytopenia, cryoprecipitate replaces factor VIII and fibrinogen, and fresh-frozen plasma (FFP) replaces all clotting factors except platelets and provides a source of antithrombin.
- A patient with manifestations of thrombosis is often treated by anticoagulation with heparin or low-molecular-weight heparin. Use of heparin in the treatment of DIC remains controversial. Antithrombin III (AT III, ATnativ), a cofactor of heparin that becomes depleted during DIC, is sometimes useful in fulminant DIC, although it increases the risk of bleeding.
- A recombinant human activated protein C (drotrecogin alfa [Xigris]) has been shown to have both anticoagulant and antiinflammatory effects and has reduced the relative risk of death from sepsis.
- Hirudin, a thrombin inhibitor and neutralizer, is being studied as a blocker of the abnormal coagulation process.
- Although used in the past, epsilon aminocaproic acid (EACA, Amicar) is generally contraindicated because of its ability to inhibit fibrinolysis and enhance thrombosis.

Therapy will stabilize a patient, prevent exsanguination or massive thrombosis, and permit institution of definitive therapy to treat the underlying cause.

Nursing Management
Nursing Diagnoses
- Ineffective tissue perfusion
- Acute pain
- Decreased cardiac output
- Anxiety

Nursing Interventions
Nurses must be alert to the possible development of DIC. The
nurse must remember that because DIC is secondary to an underlying disease, appropriate care for managing the causative problem
must be provided while providing supportive care related to the
manifestations of DIC.

- Nursing care for the patient with thrombocytopenia is
  appropriate for the patient with DIC (see Thrombocytopenic Purpura, p. 635).
- Early detection of bleeding, both occult and overt, must be
  a primary goal. The patient is assessed for signs of external
  bleeding (e.g., petechiae, oozing at intravenous [IV] or
  injection sites) and signs of internal bleeding (e.g., changes
  in mental status, increasing abdominal girth, pain).
- Any sites of bleeding are carefully monitored for continued
  bleeding. Tissue damage should be minimized and the
  patient protected from additional foci of bleeding.
- An additional nursing responsibility is to administer blood
  products correctly. Infusing cryoprecipitate or FFP is
  similar to giving other blood products.

DIVERTICULITIS/DIVERTICULOSIS

Description
A *diverticulum* is a saccular dilation or outpouching of the mucosa
through the circular smooth muscle of the intestinal wall. Clinically, diverticular disease covers a spectrum from asymptomatic,
uncomplicated diverticulosis to diverticulitis with complications
such as perforation, abscess, fistula, and bleeding. Multiple non-
inflamed diverticula are present with *diverticulosis. Diverticulitis*
is an infection of the diverticular sacs that is thought to be caused
by obstruction with fecal matter. In diverticulitis, inflammation of
the diverticula occurs that can result in perforation of one or more
diverticula. Diverticula may occur at any point within the gastrointestinal (GI) tract but are most commonly found in the sigmoid
colon.

- Diverticular disease is a common GI disorder that affects
  50% of the population by the age of 80 years. Most cases
  are asymptomatic.

Pathophysiology
The etiology of diverticulosis of the ascending colon is unknown,
but diverticula in the sigmoid colon are thought to be associated

with high luminal pressures from a deficiency in dietary fiber and perhaps combined with a loss of muscle mass and collagen with the aging process. The disease is more prevalent in Western populations that consume diets low in fiber and high in refined carbohydrates, and it is virtually unknown in areas of the world, such as rural Africa, where high-fiber diets are consumed.

- When diverticula form, the smooth muscle of the colon wall becomes thickened. Lack of dietary fiber slows transit time, and more water is absorbed from the stool, making it more difficult to pass through the lumen. Decreased stool size raises intraluminal pressure, thus promoting diverticula formation.

- Diverticulitis results from retention of stool and bacteria in the diverticulum, forming a hardened mass called a *fecalith*. This causes inflammation and usually small perforations.

Clinical Manifestations and Complications

The majority of patients with diverticulosis have no symptoms. Those with symptoms typically have abdominal pain or changes in bowel habits but no symptoms of inflammation. Approximately 15% of patients with diverticulosis progress at some point to acute diverticulitis.

In patients with diverticulitis, abdominal pain is localized over the involved area of the colon. The most common symptoms of diverticulitis in the sigmoid colon include left lower quadrant abdominal pain, fever, leukocytosis, and sometimes a palpable abdominal mass. Elderly patients with diverticulitis are frequently afebrile, with little, if any, abdominal tenderness.

Complications of diverticulitis include perforation with peritonitis, abscess and fistula formation, bowel obstruction, ureteral obstruction, and bleeding. Bleeding can be extensive but usually stops spontaneously. Diverticulitis is the most common cause of lower GI hemorrhage.

Diagnostic Studies

- Complete blood count (CBC), urinalysis, and fecal occult blood test
- Flat and upright x-rays of the abdomen
- Ultrasound and computed tomography (CT) scan with contrast to confirm diagnosis and evaluate severity
- Barium enema to determine narrowing or obstruction of the colonic lumen
- Colonoscopy to rule out polyps or lesions

Barium enemas and colonoscopy should not be performed on patients suspected of having or known to have acute diverticulitis because of the possibility of perforation and peritonitis.

Collaborative Care

Diverticular disease may be prevented by a high-fiber diet composed primarily of fruits and vegetables with a decreased intake of fat and red meat. Risk may also be decreased by high levels of physical activity, and weight reduction is recommended for obese persons. When diverticular disease is present, a high-fiber diet is also recommended, although its benefits are unclear.

In acute diverticulitis, the goal of treatment is to allow the colon to rest and the inflammation to subside. The patient is kept on nothing by mouth (NPO) status and bed rest and is given parenteral fluids. The white blood cell (WBC) count is monitored, and the patient is observed for signs of peritonitis. In acute diverticulitis, broad-spectrum antibiotic therapy is required.

- Surgery is reserved for patients with complications such as an abscess or obstruction that cannot be managed medically. The usual surgical procedures involve resection of the involved colon with either a primary anastomosis if adequate bowel cleansing is feasible or a temporary diverting colostomy. The colostomy is reanastomosed after the colon is healed.

Nursing Management

Patients with diverticular disease should be taught to avoid increased intraabdominal pressure because it may precipitate an attack.

- Factors that increase intraabdominal pressure are straining at stool, vomiting, bending, lifting, and tight, restrictive clothing.

When an acute attack subsides, the patient gradually resumes diet and activity.

- Oral fluids progressing to a semisolid diet are allowed. Ambulation is also permitted. At this stage the patient needs to be observed for a recurrent attack.
- If the patient has a bowel resection or colostomy, nursing care is the same as for these procedures.
- The patient should be provided with a full explanation of the condition. Patients who understand the disease process well and adhere to the prescribed regimen are less likely to experience an exacerbation of the disease and its complications.

DYSMENORRHEA

Description

Dysmenorrhea is cramping abdominal pain or discomfort associated with menstrual flow. The degree of pain and discomfort varies with the individual. Two types of dysmenorrhea exist: *primary,* when no pathologic finding exists, and *secondary,* when a pelvic disease is the underlying cause.

- Approximately 50% of all women experience dysmenorrhea, making it one of the most common gynecologic problems.

D

Pathophysiology

Primary dysmenorrhea is not a disease; rather it is caused by either an excess of or an increased sensitivity to prostaglandin $F_{2\alpha}$ ($PGF_{2\alpha}$). Primary dysmenorrhea begins in the few years after menarche, typically with the onset of regular ovulatory cycles.

- With the onset of menses, degeneration of the endometrium releases prostaglandin. Prostaglandins increase myometrial contractions and constriction of small endometrial blood vessels, with consequent tissue ischemia and increased sensitization of the pain receptors resulting in menstrual pain.

Secondary dysmenorrhea occurs most commonly in persons in their 30s and 40s. Secondary dysmenorrhea is due to pelvic diseases such as endometriosis, chronic pelvic inflammatory disease (PID), and uterine leiomyomas (fibroids).

Clinical Manifestations

Primary dysmenorrhea starts 12 to 24 hours before the onset of menses. The pain is most severe the first day of menses and rarely lasts more than 2 days.

- Characteristic manifestations include lower cramping abdominal pain that is colicky in nature, frequently radiating to the lower back and upper thighs. The abdominal pain is often accompanied by nausea, diarrhea, loose stools, fatigue, headache, and light-headedness.

Secondary dysmenorrhea usually occurs after the woman has experienced problem-free periods for some time. The pain, which may be unilateral, is generally more constant in nature and continues for a longer time than primary dysmenorrhea.

- Depending on the cause, symptoms such as *dyspareunia* (painful intercourse), painful defecation, or irregular bleeding may occur at times other than menstruation.

Collaborative Care

Evaluation begins with distinguishing primary from secondary dysmenorrhea. A complete health history with special attention to menstrual and gynecologic history should be obtained. A pelvic examination is also done.

- If the pelvic examination is normal and the history reveals an onset shortly after menarche with symptoms only associated with menses, the probable diagnosis is primary dysmenorrhea.
- If any cause or etiology for the pain is evident, the diagnosis is secondary dysmenorrhea. Further evaluation of the cause would then be indicated.

Nondrug treatment for primary dysmenorrhea includes heat applied to the lower abdomen or back and exercise. Regular exercise is thought to be beneficial because it may reduce endometrial hyperplasia and subsequently reduce prostaglandin production.

Drug therapy involves nonsteroidal antiinflammatory drugs (NSAIDs), such as naproxen (Naprosyn), which have an antiprostaglandin activity. NSAIDs are started at the first sign of menses and continued every 4 to 8 hours for the duration of the usual discomfort.

- Oral contraceptives may also be used to decrease dysmenorrhea by reducing endometrial hyperplasia.

Nursing Management

- The nurse should instruct the woman that during acute pain, relief may be obtained by lying down for short periods, drinking hot beverages, applying heat to the abdomen, taking warm tub baths, and taking NSAIDs for analgesia.
- The nurse can also suggest noninvasive pain-relieving practices, such as distraction and guided imagery.
- Other health care measures that can decrease discomfort include maintenance of proper nutritional habits, avoidance of constipation, maintenance of good body mechanics, and avoidance of stress and overfatigue, particularly during the time preceding menstrual periods.
- Staying active and interested in activities may also help.
- Education and supportive therapy can provide women with a foundation for coping with this common occurrence and increase feelings of control and self-reliance.

DYSRHYTHMIAS

Description

Dysrhythmias are abnormal cardiac rhythms. Prompt assessment of abnormal cardiac rhythms and the patient's response to the rhythm is critical. Disorders of impulse formation can initiate dysrhythmias. A pacemaker from a site other than the sinoatrial (SA) node may be discharged in two ways. If the SA node discharges more slowly than a secondary pacemaker, electrical discharges from the secondary pacemaker may passively "escape" and discharge automatically at its intrinsic rate. Secondary pacemakers can also originate when they discharge more rapidly than the SA node. *Triggered beats* (early or late) may come from an *ectopic focus* (area outside the normal conduction pathway) in the atria, atrioventricular (AV) node, or ventricles. Discharge from an ectopic focus can replace the normal SA stimulus, resulting in a dysrhythmia.

- Dysrhythmias occur as the result of various abnormalities and disease states. The cause of a dysrhythmia influences the treatment of the patient. Common causes of dysrhythmias are presented in Table 37. Table 38 presents a systematic approach to assessing a cardiac rhythm.

Table 37	Common Causes of Dysrhythmias

Cardiac Conditions

Accessory pathways	Myocardial cell degeneration
Cardiomyopathy	Myocardial infarction
Conduction defects	Valve disease
Heart failure	

Other Conditions

Acid-base imbalances	Electrolyte imbalances (e.g.,
Alcohol	hypokalemia,
Caffeine, tobacco	hypocalcemia)
Connective tissue disorders	Emotional crisis
Drug effects (e.g., antidysrhythmia drugs, stimulants, β-adrenergic blockers) or toxicity	Herbal supplements
	Hypoxia, shock
	Metabolic conditions (e.g., thyroid dysfunction)
Electric shock	Near-drowning
	Poisoning

Table 38	Systematic Approach to Assessing Cardiac Rhythm

Recommended Approach
1. Note the P wave. Is it upright or inverted? Is there one for every QRS?
2. Evaluate the atrial rhythm. Is it regular or irregular?
3. Calculate the atrial rate.
4. Measure the duration of the PR interval. Is it normal or prolonged?
5. Evaluate the ventricular rhythm. Is it regular or irregular?
6. Calculate the ventricular rate.
7. Measure the duration of the QRS complex. Is it normal or prolonged?
8. Assess the ST segment. Is it isoelectric, elevated, or depressed?
9. Measure the duration of the QT interval. Is it normal or prolonged?
10. Note the T wave. Is it upright or inverted?

Questions to Then Consider
1. What is the dominant rhythm and/or dysrhythmia?
2. What is the clinical significance of the findings?
3. What is the treatment for the particular rhythm?

Types of Dysrhythmias

Examples of electrocardiogram (ECG) tracings of common dysrhythmias are presented in Figs. 36-11 to 36-19, Lewis and others, *Medical-Surgical Nursing*, edition 7, pp. 850 to 855. The characteristics of common dysrhythmias are described in the Reference Appendix on p. 779.

Sinus Bradycardia. This condition occurs when the SA node discharges at a rate of <60 beats/min. It may be a normal sinus rhythm in aerobically trained athletes or during sleep. It also occurs in response to carotid sinus massage, Valsalva maneuver, hypothermia, increased intraocular pressure, increased vagal tone, and the administration of parasympathomimetic drugs. Disease states associated with sinus bradycardia are hypothyroidism, increased intracranial pressure, obstructive jaundice, and inferior wall myocardial infarction (MI).

- Clinical significance depends on how the patient tolerates bradycardia hemodynamically. Signs of symptomatic bradycardia include pale, cool skin; hypotension; weakness; angina; dizziness or syncope, confusion, or disorientation; and shortness of breath.

- Treatment consists of administration of atropine for patients with symptoms. Pacemaker therapy may be required.

Sinus Tachycardia. This dysrhythmia involves a discharge rate >100 beats per minute from the SA node as a result of vagal inhibition or sympathetic stimulation. Sinus tachycardia is associated with physiologic and psychologic stressors, such as exercise, fever, pain, hypotension, hypovolemia, anemia, hypoxia, hypoglycemia, myocardial ischemia, heart failure (HF), hyperthyroidism, anxiety, and fear. It can also be an effect of drugs such as epinephrine, norepinephrine, caffeine, theophylline, nifedipine (Procardia), or hydralazine (Apresoline). Pseudoephedrine (Sudafed) found in many over-the-counter cold remedies can also cause tachycardia.

- Clinical significance depends on the patient's tolerance of the increased heart rate (HR). The patient may have symptoms of dizziness, dyspnea, and hypotension. Angina or an increase in infarction size may accompany persistent sinus tachycardia in the patient with an acute MI.
- If possible, treatment is based on the underlying cause (e.g., pain, hypovolemia, hyperthyroidism). In certain settings, intravenous (IV) adenosine (Adenocard) and β-adrenergic blockers (e.g., metoprolol [Lopressor]) may be used to reduce heart rate and decrease myocardial oxygen (O_2) consumption.

Premature Atrial Contraction (PAC). PAC occurs as a result of contractions originating from an ectopic focus in the atrium in a location other than the SA node. The impulse originates in the left or right atrium and travels across the atria by an abnormal pathway, creating a distorted P wave. At the AV node it may be stopped (nonconducted PAC), delayed (lengthened PR interval), or conducted normally. If the impulse moves through the AV node, in most cases it is conducted normally through the ventricles. In a normal heart, a PAC can result from emotional stress or physical fatigue or from the use of caffeine, tobacco, or alcohol. A PAC can also result from hypoxia, electrolyte imbalances, and disease states such as hyperthyroidism, chronic obstructive pulmonary disease (COPD), and heart disease, including coronary artery disease (CAD) and valvular disease.

- HR varies with the underlying rate and frequency of PAC, and the rhythm is irregular.
- Isolated PACs are not significant in persons with healthy hearts. In persons with heart disease, PACs may warn of or initiate more serious dysrhythmias (e.g., supraventricular tachycardia).

- Treatment depends on patient symptoms. Withdrawal of sources of stimulation such as caffeine may be warranted. β-Adrenergic blockers may also be used to decrease PACs.

Paroxysmal Supraventricular Tachycardia (PSVT). PSVT is a dysrhythmia originating in an ectopic focus anywhere above the bifurcation of the bundle of His. Paroxysmal refers to an abrupt onset and termination. Some degree of AV block may be present. In the normal heart PSVT is associated with overexertion, emotional stress, deep inspiration, and stimulants such as caffeine and tobacco. PSVT is also associated with rheumatic heart disease, Wolff-Parkinson-White (WPW) syndrome (conduction by way of accessory pathways), digitalis intoxication, CAD, and cor pulmonale.

- HR is 100 to 300 beats/min, and rhythm is regular.
- Clinical significance depends on symptoms and HR. A prolonged episode and HR >180 beats/min may precipitate a decreased cardiac output (CO), resulting in hypotension, dyspnea, and myocardial ischemia.
- Treatment includes vagal stimulation induced by carotid massage or Valsalva maneuver. IV adenosine (Adenocard) is the first drug of choice to convert PSVT to a normal sinus rhythm. IV β-adrenergic blockers, calcium channel blockers (e.g., diltiazem [Cardizem]), digoxin (Lanoxin), and amiodarone (Cordarone) can also be used.

Atrial Flutter. This condition is an atrial tachydysrhythmia identified by recurring, regular, sawtooth-shaped flutter waves that originate from a single ectopic focus in the right atrium. Atrial flutter rarely occurs in a normal heart. It is associated with CAD, hypertension, mitral valve disorders, pulmonary embolus, chronic lung disease, cor pulmonale, cardiomyopathy, hyperthyroidism, and the use of drugs such as digoxin, quinidine, and epinephrine.

- Atrial rate is 250 to 350 beats/min. Ventricular rate varies according to conduction ratio. In 2:1 conduction, ventricular rate is typically about 150 beats/min. Atrial and ventricular rhythms are usually regular.
- High ventricular rates can decrease CO and cause serious consequences such as HF.
- Primary goal in treatment is to slow ventricular response by increasing AV block. Drugs used to control ventricular rate include calcium channel blockers and β-adrenergic blockers. Antidysrhythmic drugs used to convert atrial flutter to sinus rhythm or maintain sinus rhythm include amiodarone (Cordarone), propafenone (Rythmol), procainamide (Pronestyl), ibutilide (Corvert), and flecainide (Tambocor). Electrical cardioversion may be used to convert

atrial flutter to sinus rhythm in an emergency situation. Radiofrequency catheter ablation is increasingly being used to cure atrial flutter. Warfarin (Coumadin) is used to prevent stroke from embolization in patients with atrial flutter of greater than 48 hours' duration.

Atrial Fibrillation. This condition is a total disorganization of atrial electrical activity because of multiple ectopic foci. Effective atrial contraction does not occur. It is the most common dysrhythmia in the United States and Canada. The dysrhythmia may be chronic or intermittent and usually occurs in the patient with underlying heart disease. It is also associated with thyrotoxicosis, alcohol intoxication, caffeine use, electrolyte disturbances, stress, and cardiac surgery.

- Atrial rate may be as high as 350 to 600 beats/min. Ventricular rate can vary from 50 to 180 beats/min. Atrial rhythm is chaotic, and ventricular rhythm is usually irregular.
- Atrial fibrillation can often result in a decrease in CO because of ineffective atrial contractions and rapid ventricular response. Thrombi may form in atria as a result of ineffective atrial contraction. Warfarin is used to prevent a stroke.
- The goal of treatment is a decrease in ventricular response to <100 beats/min and prevention of cerebral embolic events. Drugs used for rate control include calcium channel blockers, β-adrenergic blockers, and digoxin. Antidysrhythmic drugs used for cardioversion to and maintenance of sinus rhythm include amiodarone, propafenone, flecainide, procainamide, and ibutilide. Cardioversion may be used to convert atrial fibrillation to normal sinus rhythm after a period of anticoagulation therapy.

First-Degree AV Block. In this type of AV block every impulse from the atria is conducted to the ventricles, but the duration of AV conduction is prolonged. After the impulse moves through the AV node, it is usually conducted normally through the ventricles. First-degree AV block is associated with MI, CAD, rheumatic fever, hyperthyroidism, vagal stimulation, and drugs such as digoxin, β-adrenergic blockers, calcium channel blockers, and flecainide.

- HR is normal, and rhythm is regular.
- First-degree AV block may be a precursor of higher degrees of AV block.
- There is no treatment for first-degree AV block.

Second-Degree AV Block, Type I (Mobitz I, Wenckebach). A type I, second-degree AV block is characterized by gradual lengthening of the PR interval. It occurs because of an AV conduction

time that is prolonged until an atrial impulse is nonconducted and
a QRS complex is dropped. Once a ventricular beat is dropped,
the cycle repeats itself with progressive lengthening of PR intervals until another QRS complex is dropped. Type I AV block may
result from use of digoxin or β-adrenergic blockers and is also
associated with CAD. It is usually the result of myocardial ischemia or infarction. It is usually transient and well tolerated.
However, it may be a warning signal of an impending significant
AV conduction disturbance.

- The rhythm appears in a pattern of grouped beats.
- If the patient is symptomatic, atropine is used to increase
  HR or a temporary pacemaker may be needed, especially
  if the patient has an acute MI.

Second-Degree Heart Block, Type II (Mobitz II). In this type of
heart block, the P wave is nonconducted without progressive ante-
cedent PR lengthening; this almost always occurs when a bundle
branch block is present. On conducted beats, the PR interval is
constant. In a second-degree heart block a certain number of
impulses from the sinus node are not conducted to the ventricles.
This occurs in ratios of 2:1, 3:1, and so on when there are two P
waves to one QRS complex, three P waves to one QRS complex,
and so on. It may occur with varying ratios. Type II AV block almost
always occurs in the His-Purkinje system and is associated with
rheumatic heart disease, CAD, anterior MI, and digitalis toxicity.

- Atrial rate is usually normal. Ventricular rate depends on
  intrinsic rate and degree of AV block. Sinus rhythm is
  regular, but ventricular rhythm may be irregular.
- Type II AV block often progresses to third-degree AV block
  and is associated with a poor prognosis.
- Reduced HR may result in decreased CO with subsequent
  hypotension and myocardial ischemia.
- Type II AV block is an indication for therapy with a permanent pacemaker.
- Treatment before insertion of a permanent pacemaker
  involves the use of a temporary pacemaker (see Pacemakers, p. 740).

Third-Degree AV Heart Block (Complete Heart Block). This
condition constitutes one form of AV dissociation in which no
impulses from the atria are conducted to the ventricles. The atria
are stimulated and contract independently of the ventricles. Ventricular rhythm is an escape rhythm, and focus may be above or
below the bifurcation of the bundle of His. This rhythm is associated with severe heart disease, including CAD, MI, myocarditis,
cardiomyopathy, and some systemic diseases such as amyloidosis
and progressive systemic sclerosis (scleroderma).

- Atrial rate is usually a sinus rate of 60 to 100 beats/min. Ventricular rate depends on the site of the block. If it is in the AV node, the rate is 40 to 60 beats/min, and if it is in the Purkinje system, it is 20 to 40 beats/min. Atrial and ventricular rhythms are regular but asynchronous.
- Third-degree AV block almost always results in reduced CO with subsequent ischemia and heart failure.
- A temporary transvenous or transcutaneous pacemaker is used until a permanent pacemaker can be inserted. Use of drugs such as atropine, epinephrine, isoproterenol, and dopamine is a temporary measure to increase HR and support blood pressure (BP) before pacemaker insertion (see Pacemakers, p. 740).

D

Premature Ventricular Contractions (PVCs). These contractions originate in an ectopic focus in the ventricles. PVCs are a premature occurrence of the QRS complex, which is wide and distorted in shape. PVCs that are initiated from different foci appear different in shape from each other and are termed *multifocal PVCs.* When every other beat is a PVC, it is called *ventricular bigeminy.* When every third beat is a PVC, it is called *ventricular trigeminy.* Two consecutive PVCs are called *couplets.* Three consecutive PVCs are called *triplets. Ventricular tachycardia* occurs when there are three or more consecutive PVCs. When a PVC falls on the T wave of a preceding beat, the *R on T phenomenon* occurs and is considered to be dangerous because it may precipitate ventricular tachycardia or ventricular fibrillation. PVCs are associated with stimulants such as caffeine, alcohol, nicotine, epinephrine, isoproterenol, and digoxin. They are also associated with electrolyte imbalances, hypoxia, fever, exercise, and emotional stress. Disease states associated with PVCs include MI, mitral valve prolapse, HF, and CAD.

- HR varies according to the intrinsic rate and the number of PVCs. Rhythm is irregular because of premature beats.
- PVCs are usually a benign finding in a patient with a normal heart. In heart disease, PVCs may reduce CO and precipitate angina and HF. PVCs in CAD or acute MI represent ventricular irritability.
- Assessment of the patient's hemodynamic status is important to determine if treatment with drug therapy is indicated. Drugs that should be considered include β-adrenergic blockers, procainamide, amiodarone, or lidocaine (Xylocaine).

Ventricular Tachycardia. This dysrhythmia is a run of three or more PVCs that occurs when an ectopic focus or foci fire repetitively and the ventricle takes control as the pacemaker. Different forms of ventricular tachycardia exist. The appearance of ventricular tachycardia is an ominous sign. It is considered to be a life-threatening dysrhythmia because of decreased CO and the possibility of deterioration of ventricular tachycardia to ventricular fibrillation, which is a lethal dysrhythmia. Ventricular tachycardia is associated with MI, CAD, significant electrolyte imbalances, cardiomyopathy, mitral valve prolapse, long QT syndrome, digitalis toxicity, and central nervous system disorders. The dysrhythmia has also been observed in patients who have no evidence of cardiac disease.

- The ventricular rate is 150 to 250 beats/min. Atria may also be depolarized by the ventricles in a retrograde fashion.
- If the patient is hemodynamically stable and has monomorphic VT (QRS complexes have same shape, size, and direction) with preserved left ventricular function, then IV procainamide, sotalol (Betapace), amiodarone, or lidocaine is used. If the patient is unstable or has poor left ventricular function, amiodarone or lidocaine is given followed by cardioversion.
- If VT is polymorphic (QRS complexes change from one shape, size, or direction over a series of beats) with normal baseline QT interval, any one of the following medications are used: β-adrenergic blockers, lidocaine, amiodarone, procainamide, or sotalol (Betapace). Cardioversion is used when drug therapy is ineffective.
- Ventricular tachycardia without a pulse is treated in the same manner as ventricular fibrillation. A rapid defibrillation attempt is performed.

Ventricular Fibrillation. This condition is a severe derangement of the heart rhythm characterized on the ECG by irregular undulations of varying contour and amplitude. This represents the firing of multiple ectopic foci in the ventricle. Mechanically, the ventricle is simply "quivering," and no effective contraction or CO occurs. Ventricular fibrillation occurs in acute MI and myocardial ischemia and in chronic diseases such as CAD and cardiomyopathy. It may occur during cardiac pacing or cardiac catheterization procedures because of catheter stimulation of the ventricle. It may also occur with coronary reperfusion after fibrinolytic therapy. Other clinical associations are accidental electrical shock, hyperkalemia, hypoxemia, acidosis, and drug toxicity.

- HR is not measurable. Rhythm is irregular and chaotic.
- Ventricular fibrillation results in an unresponsive, pulseless, and apneic state. If not rapidly treated, the patient will die.
- Treatment consists of immediate initiation of cardiopulmonary resuscitation (CPR) and initiation of advanced cardiac

life support (ACLS) measures with the use of defibrillation and definitive drug therapy.

ENCEPHALITIS

Description
Encephalitis, a serious, sometimes fatal, acute inflammation of the brain, is usually caused by a virus. Many different viruses have been implicated in encephalitis; some of them are associated with certain seasons of the year and are endemic to certain geographic areas. Ticks and mosquitoes transmit epidemic encephalitis, whereas nonepidemic encephalitis may occur as a complication of measles, chickenpox, or mumps.

- Herpes simplex virus (HSV) encephalitis is the most common form of nonepidemic viral encephalitis. Cytomegalovirus encephalitis is one of the common complications in patients with acquired immunodeficiency syndrome (AIDS).
- The first outbreak of West Nile virus encephalitis in North America occurred in 1999 and has spread across the country. Four thousand to 5000 cases are reported each year. The incubation period of West Nile virus is from 2 to 14 days, and most cases involve only mild flulike symptoms. However, about 1 in 150 infections will result in severe neurologic disease.

Clinical Manifestations and Diagnostic Studies
The onset of the infection is typically nonspecific, with fever, headache, nausea, and vomiting. It can be acute or subacute. Signs of encephalitis appear on day 2 or 3 and may vary from minimal alterations in mental status to coma.

- Almost any central nervous system (CNS) abnormality can occur, including hemiparesis, tremors, seizures, cranial nerve palsies, personality changes, memory impairment, and amnesia.
- West Nile virus should be strongly considered in adults older than 50 years who develop encephalitis or meningitis in summer or early fall. The best diagnostic test for West Nile virus is a blood test that detects viral RNA.
- Diagnostic findings related to viral encephalitis are shown in Table 39.

Table 39   Comparison of Cerebral Inflammatory Conditions

	Meningitis	Encephalitis	Brain Abscess
Causative Organisms	Bacteria (*Streptococcus pneumoniae, Neisseria meningitidis*, group B streptococcus, viruses, fungi)	Bacteria, fungi, parasites, herpes simplex virus (HSV), other viruses (e.g., West Nile virus)	Streptococci, staphylococci through bloodstream
CSF			
Pressure (normal, 60-150 mm H₂O)	Increased	Normal to slight increase	Increased
WBC count (normal, 0-8/µl)	Bacterial: >1000/µl (mainly PMN) Viral: 25-500/µl (mainly lymphocytes)	<500/µl, PMN (early), lymphocytes (later)	25-300/µl (PMN)
Protein (normal, 15-45 mg/dl [0.15-0.45 g/L])	Bacterial: >500 mg/dl Viral: 50-500 mg/dl	Slight increase	Normal

Glucose (normal, 45-75 mg/dl [2.5-4.2 mmol/L])	Bacterial: decreased Viral: normal or low	Normal	Low or absent
Appearance	Bacterial: turbid, cloudy Viral: clear or cloudy	Clear	Clear
Diagnostic Studies	CT scan, Gram stain, smear, culture, PCR*	CT scan, EEG, MRI, PET, PCR, IgM antibodies to virus in serum or CSF	CT scan
Treatment	Antibiotics, dexamethasone, supportive care, prevention of ↑ ICP	Supportive care, prevention of ↑ ICP, acyclovir (Zovirax) for HSV	Antibiotics, incision and drainage, supportive care

E

CSF, Cerebrospinal fluid; CT, computed tomography; EEG, electroencephalogram; ICP, intracranial pressure; IgM, immunoglobulin M; MRI, magnetic resonance imaging; PET, positron emission tomography; PCR, polymerase chain reaction; PMN, polymorphonuclear cells; WBC, white blood cell.
* PCR is used to detect viral RNA or DNA.

Collaborative and Nursing Management
Management is symptomatic and supportive. Initially many patients require intensive care. Acyclovir (Zovirax) and vidarabine suspension (Vira-A) are used to treat HSV encephalitis. For maximal benefit, antiviral agents must be started before the onset of coma.

- Prophylactic treatment with antiseizure drugs may be used in severe cases of encephalitis.

ENDOCARDITIS, INFECTIVE

Description
Infective endocarditis (IE), previously known as *bacterial endocarditis,* is an infection of the endocardial surface of the heart. Inflammation from IE affects the cardiac valves because they are contiguous with the endocardium.

Classification
Two forms of IE, subacute and acute, have been described.

- The subacute form typically affects those with preexisting valve disease and has a clinical course that may extend over months.
- In contrast, the acute form typically affects those with healthy valves and presents as a rapidly progressive illness.

Although this classification system has been used historically and may be conceptually useful, clinicians prefer to classify IE based on the cause or site of involvement.

Pathophysiology
The most common causative agents, *Staphylococcus aureus* and *Streptococcus viridans,* are bacterial. Other pathogens include fungi and viruses. Newly identified pathogens that are difficult to cultivate (e.g., *Baronella, Tropheryma whipplei*) and resistant organisms (e.g., methicillin-resistant *S. aureus*) also cause IE.

IE occurs when blood flow turbulence within the heart allows the causative organism to infect previously damaged valves or other endothelial surfaces. This can occur in individuals with underlying cardiac conditions. The principal risk factors for IE are prior endocarditis, prosthetic valves, acquired valvular disease, and cardiac lesions. A variety of invasive procedures (e.g., intravenous [IV] drug abuse, proliferation of intravascular device placement, and renal dialysis) also can allow large numbers of organisms to enter the bloodstream and trigger the infectious process.

Vegetations, the primary lesions of infective endocarditis, consist of fibrin, leukocytes, platelets, and microbes that adhere to the valve surface or endocardium. The loss of portions of this vegetation into the circulation results in embolization. Systemic embolization occurs from left-sided heart vegetation, progressing to organ (particularly kidney, spleen, and brain) and limb infarction. Right-sided heart lesions embolize to the lungs.

The infection may spread locally to cause damage to valves or their supporting structures. This results in dysrhythmias, valvular incompetence, and eventual invasion of the myocardium leading to heart failure (HF), sepsis, and heart block.

Clinical Manifestations

The clinical manifestations are nonspecific and can involve multiple organ systems. Low-grade fever occurs in more than 90% of patients with endocarditis.

Nonspecific manifestations that may accompany fever include chills, weakness, malaise, fatigue, and anorexia. Arthralgias, myalgias, abdominal discomfort, back pain, weight loss, headache, and clubbing of fingers may occur in subacute forms of endocarditis.

Vascular manifestations include splinter hemorrhages (black longitudinal streaks) that may occur in the nail beds. Petechiae, as a result of fragmentation and microembolization of vegetative lesions, are common in the conjunctivae, lips, buccal mucosa, and palate and over the ankles, feet, and antecubital and popliteal areas. *Osler's nodes* (painful, tender, red or purple, pea-size lesions) may be found on the fingertips or toes. *Janeway's lesions* (flat, painless, small, red spots) may be found on the palms and soles. Funduscopic examination may reveal hemorrhagic retinal lesions called *Roth's spots.*

- Onset of a new murmur is frequently noted, with the aortic and mitral valves most commonly affected.

Clinical manifestations secondary to embolization in various body organs may also be present: (1) embolization to the spleen may result in sharp, left upper quadrant pain and splenomegaly, local tenderness, and abdominal rigidity; (2) embolization to the kidneys may cause pain in the flank, hematuria, and azotemia; (3) emboli may lodge in the small peripheral blood vessels of the arms and legs and cause gangrene; (4) embolization to the brain may result in hemiplegia, ataxia, aphasia, visual changes, and change in the level of consciousness; and (5) pulmonary emboli may occur in right-sided endocarditis.

Diagnostic Studies

A recent health history should be obtained with inquiry made regarding any recent dental, urologic, surgical, or gynecologic procedures including normal or abnormal obstetric delivery. Previous history of heart disease, recent cardiac catheterization, cardiac surgery, intravascular device placement, renal dialysis, and infections (e.g., skin, respiratory, or urinary tract) should be documented.

- Two blood cultures drawn 30 minutes apart will be positive in more than 90% of patients.
- A mild leukocytosis (white blood cell count ranging from 10,000 to 11,000/µl (10 to 11 × 10⁹/L).
- Erythrocyte sedimentation rate (ESR) and C-reactive protein (CRP) levels may be elevated.
- Chest x-ray is used to detect an enlarged heart.
- Echocardiography can detect vegetation on valves.
- Electrocardiogram (ECG) may show first- or second-degree heart block because the valves lie in close proximity to the atrioventricular (AV) node.
- Cardiac catheterization may be used to evaluate valve functioning.

Collaborative Care

Prophylactic Treatment

Antibiotic prophylaxis is recommended for patients with specific cardiac conditions before they undergo certain dental or surgical procedures.

- High cardiac risk conditions that need prophylaxis include prosthetic heart valves, history of endocarditis, surgically constructed systemic-pulmonary shunts, and pacemakers.
- Specific antibiotic regimens are recommended for dental, respiratory tract, gastrointestinal (GI), and genitourinary (GU) procedures.

Drug Therapy

Accurate identification of the infecting organism is the key to successful treatment. Complete eradication of the organisms clustered within the valvular vegetations generally takes weeks to achieve, and relapses are common. Initially patients are hospitalized and IV antibiotic therapy is started. Table 37-5 Lewis and others, *Medical-Surgical Nursing,* edition 7, p. 869 outlines specific regimens for outpatient drug therapy.

- The patient's antibiotic serum levels should be monitored periodically. Subsequent blood cultures may be done to evaluate the effectiveness of antibiotic therapy. Blood cultures that remain positive indicate inadequate or inappropriate antibiotic administration, aortic root or myocardial abscess, or the wrong diagnosis (e.g., an infection elsewhere).
- Fever may persist for several days after treatment has been started and is treated with aspirin, acetaminophen, fluids, and rest.

■ Complete bed rest is usually not indicated unless the temperature remains elevated or there are signs of heart damage.

The results of drug therapy alone are generally poor in patients with fungal endocarditis and prosthetic valve endocarditis. Early valve replacement followed by prolonged drug therapy is recommended in these situations.

Nursing Management

Goals

The patient with IE will have normal or baseline cardiac function, perform activities of daily living without fatigue, and understand the therapeutic regimen to prevent recurrence of endocarditis.

See NCP 37-1 for the patient with infective endocarditis, Lewis and others, *Medical-Surgical Nursing,* edition 7, pp. 870 to 871.

Nursing Diagnoses

■ Hyperthermia
■ Decreased cardiac output
■ Activity intolerance
■ Deficient knowledge

Nursing Interventions

The incidence of IE can be decreased by identifying individuals who are at risk for the development of endocarditis. Assessment of the patient's history and an understanding of the disease process are crucial for planning and implementing appropriate health maintenance strategies.

IE generally requires treatment with antibiotics for 4 to 6 weeks. After initial treatment in the hospital, the patient may continue treatment in the home setting if hemodynamically stable and compliant. Patients who receive outpatient IV antibiotics will require vigilant home nursing care.

■ Fever, chronic or intermittent, is a common early sign. Frequent assessment of body temperature is important because persistent, prolonged temperature elevations may mean that drug therapy is ineffective.

■ The patient needs adequate periods of physical and emotional rest. Bed rest may be necessary when fever is present or there are complications (e.g., heart damage). Otherwise the patient may ambulate and perform moderate activity.

■ Laboratory data should be monitored to determine the effectiveness of long-term, high-dose antibiotic therapy. IV lines should be monitored for patency, and antibiotics should be given when scheduled. The patient should be monitored continuously for undesirable reactions to drugs.

■ To prevent problems because of immobility, the patient should wear elastic compression gradient stockings; perform range-of-motion (ROM) exercises; and turn, cough, and deep breathe every 2 hours.

- The patient may experience anxiety and fear associated with the illness. The nurse must recognize this problem and implement strategies to help reduce the patient's fears and anxieties.

Patients with active endocarditis are at risk for life-threatening complications such as cerebral emboli and pulmonary edema. Adequacy of the home environment in terms of in-home companions and hospital access must be determined for successful management.

- After therapy is completed in either the home or hospital setting, management focuses on teaching the patient about the nature of the disease and on reducing the risk of reinfection.

▼ **Patient and Family Teaching**

- Once therapy has been completed, the patient should be instructed about symptoms that may indicate recurrent infection, such as fever, fatigue, malaise, and chills. If any of these symptoms occur, the patient should be aware of the importance of notifying the health care provider.
- The patient must be instructed about the need for prophylactic antibiotic therapy before any invasive procedure is performed.
- Explain to the patient the relationship of follow-up care, good nutrition, and early treatment of common infections (e.g., colds) to maintain good health.

ENDOMETRIAL CANCER

Description

Cancer of the endometrium is the most common gynecologic malignancy, accounting for nearly 50% of female genital tract neoplasms. However, it has a relatively low mortality, with a survival rate of 94% if the cancer has not spread at the time of diagnosis. About 25% of cases of endometrial cancer are diagnosed before menopause. The average age at the time of diagnosis is 61 years.

- The major risk factor for endometrial cancer is estrogen, especially unopposed estrogen. Additional risk factors include increasing age, nulliparity, late menopause, obesity, smoking, and diabetes mellitus (DM). Pregnancy and oral contraceptives are protective factors.

Pathophysiology

This type of cancer arises from the endometrial lining. The precursor may be a hyperplastic state that progresses to invasive carcinoma. Hyperplasia occurs when estrogen is not counteracted by progesterone. Direct extension develops into the cervix and through the uterine serosa. As invasion of the myometrium occurs, regional lymph nodes, including the paravaginal and paraaortic, become involved. Hematogenous metastases develop concurrently. The usual sites of metastases are the lung, bone, liver, and eventually the brain. Endometrial cancer grows slowly, metastasizes late, and is amenable to therapy if diagnosed early.

Clinical Manifestations

- The first symptom is abnormal uterine bleeding, usually in postmenopausal women. Because perimenopausal women have sporadic periods for a time, it is important that this sign not be ignored or automatically blamed on menopause.
- Pain occurs late in the disease process, and other symptoms that may arise are related to metastasis to other organs.

Diagnostic Studies

Endometrial biopsy is the primary diagnostic procedure for endometrial cancer.
- Endometrial biopsy can be done on an outpatient basis and involves obtaining endometrial tissue from the uterus. Occurrence of spotting or unexpected bleeding in a postmenopausal woman mandates obtaining a tissue sample to exclude endometrial cancer.
- The Pap test is not a reliable diagnostic tool for endometrial cancer, but it can rule out cervical cancer.

Collaborative Care

Treatment is a total hysterectomy and bilateral salpingo-oophorectomy with lymph node biopsies. Surgery may be followed by radiation, either to the pelvis or abdomen externally or intravaginally, to decrease local recurrence. Treatment of advanced or recurrent disease is difficult. Progesterone hormonal therapy (e.g., megestrol [Megace]) is the treatment of choice when the progesterone receptor status is positive and the tumor is well differentiated. Tamoxifen (Novaldex) is also effective in women with advanced or recurrent endometrial cancer. Chemotherapy is considered when progesterone therapy is unsuccessful. Agents used include doxorubicin (Adriamycin), cisplatin (Platinol), 5-fluorouracil (5-FU), carboplatin (Paraplatin), and paclitaxel (Taxol).

Nursing Management: Cancers of the Female Reproductive Tract

See Cervical Cancer, p. 108.

ENDOMETRIOSIS

Description

Endometriosis is the presence of normal endometrial tissue in sites outside the endometrial cavity. The most frequent sites are in or near the ovaries, uterosacral ligaments, and uterovesical peritoneum. However, endometrial tissues can be found in many other locations, such as the stomach, lungs, intestines, and spleen.

- The endometrial tissue responds to hormones of the ovarian cycle and undergoes a mini–menstrual cycle similar to uterine endometrium.
- Endometriosis is found in approximately 7% of women of reproductive age.

The etiology of endometriosis is unknown. A widely held view is that retrograde menstrual flow passes through the fallopian tubes, carrying viable endometrial tissues into the pelvis and attaching to various sites.

Clinical Manifestations

A wide range of symptoms and severity exists. The magnitude of a woman's symptoms does not necessarily correlate with the clinical extent of her endometriosis.

- The most common symptoms are secondary dysmenorrhea, infertility, pelvic pain, dyspareunia, and irregular bleeding.
- Less common symptoms include backache, painful bowel movements, and dysuria.
- Symptoms may or may not correspond to the woman's menstrual cycles. With menopause, estrogen is no longer produced in the ovaries, which may lead to the disappearance of symptoms.
- When a cyst ruptures, the pain may be acute and the resulting irritation promotes the formation of adhesions, which fix the affected area to another pelvic structure. The adhesions may become severe enough to cause a bowel obstruction or painful micturition. Adhesions involving the uterus, fallopian tubes, or ovaries may result in infertility.

Diagnostic Studies

Diagnosis is frequently confirmed by patient history and the palpation of firm nodular lumps in the adnexa on bimanual examination. Laparoscopic examination is necessary for a definitive diagnosis.

Collaborative Care

Treatment is influenced by a patient's age, desire for pregnancy, symptom severity, and the extent and location of the disease. When symptoms are not disruptive, a "watch and wait" approach is used.

Drug Therapy

Drug therapy is used to control symptoms. Drugs are selected to inhibit estrogen production by the ovary so that the endometrial tissue will shrink. The various drugs used imitate a state of pregnancy or menopause.

- Continuous use (for 9 months) of combined progestin and estrogen causes regression of endometrial tissue. Ovulation is suppressed, and pseudopregnancy (hyperhormonal amenorrhea) is produced by progestin agents such as medroxyprogesterone (Depo-Provera).
- Another approach to hormonal treatment is danazol (Danocrine), a synthetic androgen that inhibits the anterior pituitary. The drug produces a pseudomenopause (ovarian suppression), with atrophy of ectopic endometrial tissue. Subjective relief of symptoms is noted within 6 weeks of danazol use.
- Another class of drugs used is gonadotropin-releasing hormone (GnRH) agonists, such as leuprolide acetate (Lupron) and nafarelin (Synarel). These drugs cause a hypoestrogenic state resulting in amenorrhea.

Surgical Therapy

The only cure for endometriosis is surgical removal of all the endometrial implants. Surgical therapy may be conservative or definitive. *Conservative surgery* to confirm the diagnosis or to remove implants involves removal or destruction of endometrial implants and lysing or excision of adhesions by means of laparoscopic laser surgery and laparotomy.

- For women wishing to get pregnant, conservative surgical therapy is used to remove implants that may block the fallopian tube. Adhesions are removed from the tubes, ovaries, and pelvic structures.

Definitive surgery involves removal of the uterus, tubes, ovaries, and as many endometrial implants as possible. Each woman should be actively involved in making the decision about preserving part or all of her ovaries if surgically possible. Her feelings about maintaining her cyclic ovarian function need to be explored.

Nursing Management

- Education of the patient and reassurance that a health-threatening situation does not exist may permit her to accept a conservative and progressive treatment. Nurses need to assist patients to understand the drugs ordered to treat their condition.
- Psychologic support may be needed for the patient experiencing severe disabling pain, sexual difficulties secondary to dyspareunia, and infertility.
- If conservative surgery is the treatment selected, nursing care is similar to general preoperative and postoperative care of a patient undergoing laparotomy (see Abdominal Pain, Acute, p. 3).
- If definitive surgery is planned, nursing care is similar to the patient undergoing an abdominal hysterectomy. (See NCP 54-1 for the patient undergoing an abdominal hysterectomy, Lewis and others, *Medical-Surgical Nursing,* edition 7, p. 1398.)

ESOPHAGEAL CANCER

Description

Esophageal cancer is a rare malignant neoplasm. However, it is a growing concern in that it has had a 200% increase in incidence in the past 10 years in the United States. The 5-year prognosis for esophageal cancer is poor because it is rarely diagnosed in the early stages.

- The percentage of esophageal cancers that are adenocarcinomas ranges from 30% to 70%, with the remainder being squamous cell carcinoma.
- Approximately 1 in 200 cases of Barrett's esophagus, a metaplastic change in esophageal mucosa associated with gastroesophageal reflux disease (GERD), progresses to esophageal cancer.

Pathophysiology

Although the cause of esophageal cancer is unknown, smoking and excessive alcohol intake are important risk factors. Diets that are low in fruits and vegetables and certain minerals and vitamins may increase the risk of this cancer. Patients with a history of achalasia, a condition in which there is delayed emptying of the lower esophagus, are at greater risk for squamous cell cancer. Other risk factors include exposure to lye, asbestos, and types of metals.

- The malignant tumor usually appears as an ulcerated lesion. It may have advanced to this stage before symptoms appear.
- The majority of tumors are located in the middle and lower portions of the esophagus. The tumor may penetrate the muscular layer and extend outside the esophageal wall.
- Tumor obstruction of the esophagus occurs in the later stages.

Clinical Manifestations

The onset of symptoms is usually late in relation to the extent of the tumor.

- Progressive dysphagia is the most common symptom and may be expressed as a substernal feeling that food is not passing. Initially dysphagia occurs only with meat, then with soft foods, and eventually with liquids.
- Pain develops late and is described as occurring in the substernal, epigastric, or back areas and usually increases with swallowing. The pain may radiate to the neck, jaw, ears, and shoulders.
- If the tumor is in the upper third of the esophagus, symptoms such as sore throat, choking, and hoarseness may occur. Weight loss is fairly common.
- When esophageal stenosis is severe, regurgitation of blood-flecked esophageal contents is common.

Complications may include hemorrhage from cancer eroding through the esophagus and into the aorta. Esophageal perforation into the lung or trachea may also develop. The liver and lung are common metastatic sites.

Diagnostic Studies

- Barium swallow with fluoroscopy may demonstrate esophageal narrowing at the tumor site.
- Esophagoscopy with biopsy is needed to make a definitive diagnosis.
- Endoscopic ultrasonography detects tumor invasion into the muscle layer.
- Bronchoscopic examination detects malignant involvement of the trachea or lung.
- Computed tomography (CT) scan and magnetic resonance imaging (MRI) assess extent of the disease.

Collaborative Care

Treatment depends on tumor location and whether metastasis has occurred. The best results may be obtained with a combination of surgery, chemotherapy, and radiation. In some patients, concurrent radiation and chemotherapy are used to slow the progression of esophageal cancer before surgery.

If the tumor is in the cervical section (upper third) of the esophagus, radiation is usually indicated. A tumor in the lower third of the esophagus is usually resected surgically. Dilation may be used to relieve dysphagia and allow for improved nutrition.

- Palliative therapy consists of restoration of the swallowing function and maintenance of nutrition and hydration. Obstruction can be relieved by dilation, stent placement, or both. Laser therapy or vaporization of the tumor by means of endoscopy may be used in combination with dilation.

Nutritional Therapy

After esophageal surgery, parenteral fluids are given. When fluids are allowed after bowel sounds have returned and the patient is able to swallow, 30 to 60 ml of water is given hourly, with gradual progression to small, frequent, bland meals. The patient should be in an upright position to prevent fluid regurgitation. Symptoms of food intolerance include vomiting and abdominal distention. A gastrostomy may be performed for the purpose of feeding the patient and reducing aspiration.

Nursing Management

Goals

The patient with esophageal cancer will have relief of symptoms including pain and dysphagia, achieve optimal nutritional intake, understand the prognosis of the disease, and experience a quality of life appropriate to disease progression.

Nursing Diagnoses

- Imbalanced nutrition: less than body requirements
- Chronic pain
- Risk for aspiration
- Deficient fluid volume
- Anxiety
- Grieving

Nursing Interventions

In addition to general preoperative teaching and preparation, particular attention is given to the patient's nutritional needs. Many patients are poorly nourished because of the inability to ingest adequate amounts and fluids. Meticulous oral care is essential. Teaching should include information about chest tubes (if a thoracic approach is used), intravenous (IV) lines, nasogastric

(NG) tube, gastrostomy feeding, turning, coughing, and deep breathing.

Postoperative care should include assessment of drainage; maintenance of the NG tube; oral and nasal care; and prevention of respiratory complications by turning, coughing, and deep breathing, incentive spirometry every 2 hours, and placing the patient in a semi-Fowler's position to prevent gastric reflux and aspiration.

Many patients require long-term follow-up care after surgery for esophageal cancer. The patient may undergo chemotherapy and radiation treatment after surgery. The patient needs encouragement and assistance in maintaining adequate nutrition. The patient may need a permanent feeding gastrostomy. The patient usually has fears and anxieties about a diagnosis of cancer.

- The nurse should know what the physician has told the patient regarding the prognosis and then provide appropriate counseling. Some communities have resource groups consisting of persons with cancer who can serve as support systems.
- Referral to a home health nurse may be necessary for continued care of the patient (e.g., gastrostomy teaching and follow-up wound care).

▼ **Patient and Family Teaching**
- Health promotion includes follow-up evaluation and care for patients diagnosed with GERD, and hiatal hernia.
- Patients diagnosed with Barrett's esophagus should be monitored because this is considered a premalignant condition.
- Health counseling should focus on the elimination of smoking and excessive alcohol intake.
- The patient should be encouraged to have regular physical examinations and seek medical attention for any esophageal problems, especially dysphagia.
- Maintenance of good oral hygiene and dietary habits (intake of fresh fruits and vegetables) may be helpful.

FIBROCYSTIC BREAST CHANGES

Description

Fibrocystic changes in the breast constitute the most frequently occurring breast disorder. These changes include the development of excess fibrous tissue, hyperplasia of the epithelial lining of the mammary ducts, proliferation of mammary ducts, and cyst formation. Fibrocystic changes occur most frequently in women between

35 and 50 years old but often begin in women as young as 20 years old.

Fibrocystic changes most commonly occur in women with premenstrual abnormalities, nulliparous women, women with a history of spontaneous abortion, nonusers of oral contraceptives, and women with early menarche and late menopause.

Pathophysiology

- The cause of fibrocystic changes is thought to be heightened responsiveness of breast parenchyma and stroma to circulating estrogen and progesterone.
- Fibrocystic changes produce pain by nerve irritation from connective tissue edema and by fibrosis from nerve pinching.
- Masses or nodularities can appear in both breasts and are often found in the upper, outer quadrants; they usually occur bilaterally.
- Symptoms of fibrocystic changes often are exacerbated in the premenstrual phase and subside after menstruation.

Clinical Manifestations

Manifestations of fibrocystic breast changes include one or more palpable lumps that are usually round, well delineated, and freely movable within the breast. There may be accompanying discomfort ranging from tenderness to pain.

- The lump usually increases in size and perhaps in tenderness before menstruation. Cysts may enlarge or shrink rapidly.
- Nipple discharge associated with fibrocystic breasts is often milky, watery-milky, yellow, or green.
- Pain and nodularity often increase over time but tend to subside after menopause unless high doses of estrogen replacement are used.

Nursing and Collaborative Management

With the initial discovery of a discrete mass in the breast, aspiration or surgical biopsy may be indicated. A wait of 7 to 10 days may be planned if the nodularity is recurrent to note changes as the menstrual cycle changes.

- An excisional biopsy should be done if no fluid is found on aspiration, if the fluid that is found is hemorrhagic, or if a residual mass remains. This surgery is performed in an office or day surgery unit with the patient under local anesthesia.

Many types of treatment have been suggested for a fibrocystic condition. These approaches include diet restrictions of sodium and methylxanthines, such as coffee and chocolate; therapeutic measures such as analgesics, diuretics, vitamin E therapy, hormone therapy, and antiestrogen therapy (danazol [Danocrine]); and stress reduction if it is a contributing factor in breast discomfort. The benefit of most of these treatments has not been proven, but many women report less discomfort with their use.

▼ **Patient and Family Teaching**

The role of the nurse in the care of the patient with fibrocystic breast changes is primarily one of teaching. A woman should be told that she may expect recurrences of the cysts in one or both breasts until menopause and that cysts may enlarge or become painful just before menstruation. In addition, these women should be reassured that cysts do not "turn into" cancer.

- The woman with cystic changes should be encouraged to return regularly for follow-up examinations. She should also be taught breast self-examination (BSE) to self-monitor the problem. Any new lumps should be evaluated, and changes in symptoms should be reported and investigated.

FIBROMYALGIA SYNDROME

F

Description

Fibromyalgia syndrome (FMS) is a chronic disorder characterized by widespread, nonarticular musculoskeletal pain and fatigue with multiple tender points. People with FMS also typically experience nonrestorative sleep, morning stiffness, irritable bowel syndrome, and anxiety. FMS occurs 6 times more frequently in women than men, but it affects persons of all ages and ethnic groups. FMS and chronic fatigue syndrome (CFS) share many commonalities (see Table 24, p. 120).

Pathophysiology

Although the etiology and pathophysiologic mechanisms of FMS are not clearly understood, there is general agreement that FMS is a disorder of central processing with neuroendocrine/neu-rotransmitter dysregulation. The patient with FMS has multiple physiologic abnormalities, including increased levels of substance P in the spinal cord, low levels of blood flow to the thalamus, dysfunction of the hypothalamic-pituitary-adrenal (HPA) axis, low levels of serotonin and tryptophan, and abnormalities in cyto-kine function.

- Serotonin and substance P play a role in mood regulation, sleep, and pain perception. Changes in the HPA axis can lead to depression and a decreased response to stress.

- A recent viral illness or Lyme disease may serve as an infectious trigger in susceptible persons.

Clinical Manifestations

Clinical manifestations overlap with those of CFS. The patient experiences a widespread burning pain that worsens and improves through the course of a day. It is often difficult for the patient to discriminate if pain occurs in the muscles, joints, or soft tissues.

- Head or facial pain often results from stiff or painful neck and shoulder muscles. This pain can accompany temporomandibular joint dysfunction. Nonrestorative sleep and resulting fatigue are typical. Physical examination characteristically reveals point tenderness at 11 or more of 18 identified sites (see Fig. 65-14, Lewis and others, *Medical-Surgical Nursing,* edition 7, p. 1728).
- Cognitive effects range from difficulty concentrating to memory lapses and a feeling of being overwhelmed when dealing with multiple tasks. Many individuals report migraine headaches, depression, and anxiety.
- Numbness or tingling in the hands or feet (paresthesia) often accompanies FMS. Restless legs syndrome is also common.
- Irritable bowel syndrome with manifestations of diarrhea or constipation, abdominal pain, and bloating can occur, in addition to symptoms of overactive bladder.

Diagnostic Studies

A definitive diagnosis is often difficult to establish. Laboratory results serve to rule out other suspected disorders based on the patient's history and physical examination.

- Occasionally a low antinuclear antibody (ANA) titer is seen, but it is not considered diagnostic.
- Muscle biopsy may reveal a nonspecific moth-eaten appearance or fiber atrophy.

The American College of Rheumatology classifies an individual as having FMS if two criteria are met: (1) pain is experienced in 11 of the 18 tender points on palpation and (2) the patient has a history of widespread pain for at least 3 months. Up to 70% of all patients with FMS also meet criteria for a diagnosis of CFS.

Collaborative Care

Treatment is symptomatic and requires a high level of patient motivation. The nurse can play a key role in teaching the patient to be an active participant in the therapeutic regimen. Rest can help pain, aching, and tenderness. Analgesics, such as acetamino-phen (Tylenol), and nonsteroidal antiinflammatory drugs (NSAIDs) (e.g., tramadol [Ultram]) are effective for some patients.

Stress, fatigue, and sleep disturbances can be helped by taking a low-dose tricyclic antidepressant, such as amitriptyline. The skeletal muscle relaxant cyclobenzaprine (Flexeril) is also used to treat sleep disturbances. Benzodiazepines (e.g., diazepam [Valium], alprazolam [Xanax]) combined with low doses of ibu-profen (Motrin, Advil) are used to treat anxiety and the muscle spasms that affect FMS patients. Selective serotonin reuptake inhibitor antidepressants (e.g., sertraline [Zoloft], paroxetine [Paxil]) tend to be reserved for FMS patients who are also suffer-ing from depression.

Nursing and Collaborative Management
Because of the chronic nature of FMS and the need to maintain an ongoing rehabilitation program, the patient needs consistent support from the nurse. Massage is often combined with ultra-sound or the application of alternating heat and cold packs to soothe tense, sore muscles and increase blood circulation.

- Gentle stretching can be performed by a physical therapist or practiced by the patient at home to relieve muscle tension and spasm.
- Dietitians often urge FMS patients to limit their consump-tion of sugar, caffeine, and alcohol because these substances have been shown to be muscle irritants.
- Pain and the related symptoms of FMS can cause significant stress. There is also some indication that these patients simply do not handle stress well. Effective relaxation strate-gies include biofeedback, guided imagery, and autogenic training. Psychologic counseling (individual or group) may also prove beneficial for the FMS patient.

FLAIL CHEST

Description
Flail chest results from multiple rib fractures causing instability of the chest wall. Flail chest may occur with pneumothorax, hemo-thorax, and tension pneumothorax.

Pathophysiology
The unstable chest wall at the flail area cannot provide the bony structure necessary to maintain bellows action and ventilation.

The affected (flail) area moves paradoxically to the intact portion of the chest during respiration. During inspiration the affected portion is sucked in, and during expiration it bulges out.

- This paradoxic chest movement prevents adequate ventilation of the lung in the injured area. The underlying lung may have a pulmonary contusion aggravating hypoxemia.
- Associated pain, fractures, and lung injury give rise to an alteration in breathing pattern and hypoxia.

Clinical Manifestations
Flail chest is usually apparent on visual examination of the unconscious patient.

- Manifestations include rapid, shallow respirations and tachycardia.
- A flail chest may not be initially apparent in the conscious patient as a result of splinting of the chest wall. The patient moves air poorly, and movement of the thorax is asymmetric and uncoordinated.

Diagnostic Studies
- Crepitus at rib fractures
- Chest x-ray and arterial blood gases (ABGs)

Collaborative Care
Initial therapy consists of airway management, adequate ventilation, supplemental oxygen (O_2) therapy, careful administration of intravenous (IV) solutions, and pain control. Definitive therapy is to reexpand the lung and ensure adequate oxygenation. Although many patients can be managed without the use of mechanical ventilation, a short period of intubation and ventilation may be necessary until the diagnosis of the lung injury is complete. Lung parenchyma and fractured ribs will heal with time.

FRACTURE

Description
A fracture is a disruption or break in the continuity of the structure of bone. Traumatic injuries account for the majority of fractures, although some fractures are secondary to a disease process (pathologic fractures). Fractures are described and classified according to (1) type, (2) communication or noncommunication with the external environment, and (3) location of the fracture. Illustrations

of the various classifications of fractures can be found in Figs. 63-6, 63-7, and 63-8 in Lewis and others, *Medical-Surgical Nursing,* edition 7, p. 1636.

Fractures are also described as stable or unstable. A *stable fracture* occurs when a piece of the periosteum is intact across the fracture and either external or internal fixation has rendered the fragments stationary. Stable fractures are usually transverse, spiral, or greenstick. An *unstable fracture* is grossly displaced during injury and is a site of poor fixation. Unstable fractures are usually comminuted (having several breaks in the bone) or oblique (having a slanted fracture of the shaft).

Stages of Fracture Healing

Bone goes through a reparative process of self-healing (called *union*) that occurs in the following stages:

1. *Fracture hematoma.* When a fracture occurs, bleeding and edema create a hematoma, which surrounds the ends of the fragments.
2. *Granulation tissue.* Active phagocytosis absorbs the products of local necrosis. The hematoma changes into granulation tissue (consisting of new blood vessels, fibroblasts, and osteoblasts), which produces a new bony substance called *osteoid* during days 3 to 14 after injury.
3. *Callous formation.* As calcium, phosphorus, and magnesium are deposited in the osteoid, an unorganized network of bone called *callus* is formed that is woven about the fracture parts. Callus usually begins to appear by the end of the second week after injury. Evidence of callous formation can be verified by x-ray.
4. *Ossification.* Ossification of the callus occurs from 3 weeks to 6 months after fracture and continues until the fracture has healed. Callous ossification will prevent movement at the fracture site when bones are gently stressed. During this stage the patient may be allowed limited mobility or the cast may be removed.
5. *Consolidation.* As the callus continues to develop, the distance between bone fragments diminishes and eventually closes. This stage is called *consolidation,* and ossification continues. It can be equated with radiographic union.
6. *Remodeling.* Excess bone cells are absorbed, and union is completed. Gradual return of the injured bone to its preinjury structural strength and shape occurs. Bone remodels in response to physical stress. Initially stress is provided through exercise. Weight bearing is gradually introduced. This phase can occur up to 1 year after injury.

Clinical Manifestations

The patient's history indicates injury associated with numerous signs and symptoms, including immediate localized pain, decreased function, and inability to bear weight or use the affected part. The patient guards and protects the extremity against movement. The fracture may not be accompanied by obvious bone deformity.

Complications

The majority of fractures heal without complications. If death occurs after a fracture, it is usually the result of damage to underlying organs and soft tissue or from complications of the fracture or injury. For a summary of the complications of fracture healing, see Table 63-5, Lewis and others, *Medical-Surgical Nursing,* edition 7, p. 1638.

- Direct complications include problems with bone union, avascular necrosis, and bone infection.
- Indirect complications are associated with blood vessel and nerve damage resulting in conditions such as compartment syndrome, venous thrombosis, and fat embolism syndrome. A discussion of these complications is in Lewis and others, *Medical-Surgical Nursing,* edition 7, pp. 1649 to 1651. Hypovolemic shock may also occur (see Shock, p. 565).
- Although most musculoskeletal injuries are not life threatening, open fractures or fractures accompanied by severe blood loss and fractures that damage vital organs (e.g., the lung or bladder) are medical emergencies requiring immediate attention.

Diagnostic Studies

- History and physical examination
- X-ray examination

Collaborative Care

The goals of treatment are anatomic realignment of bone fragments (reduction), immobilization to maintain realignment, and restoration of function of the injured part.

Fracture Reduction

Closed reduction is a nonsurgical, manual realignment of bones to their previous anatomic position. Traction and countertraction are manually applied to bone fragments to restore position, length, and alignment.

- Closed reduction is usually performed with the patient under local or general anesthesia. After reduction, the injured part is immobilized by casting, traction, external fixation, splints, or orthoses (braces) to maintain alignment until healing occurs.

Open reduction is correction of bone alignment through a surgical incision. It may include internal fixation of the fracture with the use of wire, screws, pins, plates, intramedullary rods, or nails.

- Open reduction with internal fixation (ORIF) facilitates early ambulation, which decreases the risk of complications related to prolonged immobility and promotes fracture healing. If ORIF is used for intraarticular fractures, early initiation of range of motion of the joint is indicated. Machines that provide continuous passive motion (CPM) to various joints are now available.

Traction devices can be used to reduce a fracture or dislocation by applying a pulling force on the fractured extremity while countertraction pulls in the opposite direction. The two most common types of traction are skin traction and skeletal traction.

- Skin traction is generally used for short-term treatment (48 to 72 hours) until skeletal traction or surgery is possible. Tape, boots, or slings are applied directly to the skin to maintain alignment, assist in reduction, and help diminish muscle spasms in the injured part.
- Skeletal traction, generally in place for longer periods, is used to align injured bones and joints. It provides a long-term pull that keeps injured bones and joints aligned. Skeletal traction requires the insertion of a pin or wire into the bone to which the pull is applied.

Fracture alignment depends on correct positioning and alignment of the patient while traction forces remain constant. For extremity traction to be effective, forces must be pulling in the opposite direction *(countertraction)* to prevent the patient from sliding to the end or side of the bed.

- Countertraction is commonly supplied by the patient's body weight or may be augmented by elevating the end of the bed.

Fracture Immobilization

External fixation of fractures is achieved by a cast or an external fixator. Casting is a common treatment after closed reduction has been performed. It allows the patient to perform many normal activities of daily living (ADLs) while providing sufficient immobilization to ensure stability (see Casts, p. 710).

An *external fixator* is a metal device composed of metal pins that are inserted into the bone and attached to external rods to stabilize the fracture while it heals. It can be used to apply traction, to immobilize reduced fragments when the use of a cast or traction is not appropriate, or to compress fracture fragments. The external fixator is attached directly to the bones by percutaneous pins or wires. Assessment for pin loosening and infection is critical. Infection signaled by exudate, redness, tenderness, and pain may require removal of the device.

Internal fixation devices are surgically inserted at the time of realignment. Examples of internal fixation devices include pins, plates, and screws. Biologically inert devices such as titanium, stainless steel, or Vitallium are used to realign and maintain bony fragments. Proper alignment is evaluated by x-ray studies at regular intervals.

Other Therapy

Patients with fractures experience varying degrees of pain associated with muscle spasms that result from edema and nerve injury following muscle injury.

- Central and peripheral muscle relaxants, such as carisoprodol (Soma), cyclobenzaprine (Flexeril), or methocarbamol (Robaxin), may be prescribed for relief of pain associated with muscle spasms.

To ensure optimal soft tissue and bone healing, proper nutrition is necessary.

- The patient's diet must include ample protein (e.g., 1 g/kg body weight), vitamins (especially B, C, and D), and calcium, phosphorus, and magnesium.

Nursing Management

Goals

The patient with a fracture will have physiologic healing with no associated complications, obtain satisfactory pain relief, and achieve maximal rehabilitation potential.

See NCP 63-1 for the patient with a fracture, Lewis and others, *Medical-Surgical Nursing,* edition 7, pp. 1644 to 1645.

Nursing Diagnoses

- Impaired physical mobility
- Risk for peripheral neurovascular dysfunction
- Acute pain
- Ineffective therapeutic regimen management

Nursing Interventions

Patients with fractures may be treated in an emergency department or physician's office and released to home care, or they may require hospitalization. Specific nursing measures depend on the type of treatment used and setting in which the patient is placed.

Preoperative Management. If surgical intervention is required to treat the fracture, patients will need preoperative preparation. In addition to the usual preoperative nursing measures, the nurse should inform patients of the type of immobilization device that will be used and the expected activity limitations.

- Proper skin preparation is an important part of preoperative preparation. The aim of skin preparation is to clean the skin and remove debris and hair to reduce the possibility of infection.
- Patients must be assured that their needs will be met by the nursing staff until they can again meet their own needs. Assurance that pain medication will be available if needed is often beneficial.

Postoperative Management. Frequent neurovascular assessments of the affected extremity are necessary to detect subtle changes. Any limitations of movement or activity related to turning, positioning, and extremity support should be monitored closely.

- Pain and discomfort can be minimized through proper alignment and positioning.
- Dressings or casts should be carefully observed for any overt signs of bleeding or drainage. A significant increase in the size of the drainage area should be reported.
- If a wound drainage system is in place, the patency of the system and the volume of drainage should be regularly assessed. Whenever the contents of a drainage system are measured or emptied, the nurse should use sterile technique to avoid contamination.

If the patient is immobilized as a result of the fracture, the nurse must plan care to prevent complications of immobility.

- Constipation can be prevented by increased activity, maintenance of a high fluid intake, and a diet high in bulk and roughage. If these measures are not effective in maintaining the patient's normal bowel pattern, stool softeners, laxatives, or suppositories may be necessary. Maintaining a regular time for elimination despite bed rest is effective in promoting regularity.
- Renal calculi can develop as a result of bone demineralization caused by immobilization. Unless contraindicated, a fluid intake of 2500 ml/day is recommended. Cranberry juice or ascorbic acid (500 mg/day) may be recommended to acidify the urine and prevent calcium precipitation.
- Rapid deconditioning of the circulatory system can occur as a result of bed rest, resulting in orthostatic hypotension and decreased lung capacity. Unless contraindicated, these effects can be diminished by permitting the patient to sit on the side of the bed, allowing the lower limbs

to dangle over the bedside, and performing standing transfers.

- Patients must also be assessed for deep vein thrombosis (DVT) and pulmonary emboli resulting from venous stasis.

▼ **Patient and Family Teaching**

Because many fractures are cast in an outpatient setting, the patient often requires only a short hospitalization or none at all. Therefore patient education is an important nursing responsibility to prevent complications. In addition to specific instructions for cast care (see Casts, p. 710) and recognition of complications, the nurse should encourage the patient to contact the clinic or care provider should questions arise. The nurse should validate patient understanding of these instructions before discharge from the clinic or hospital.

For further information on rehabilitation management of fractures, including the use of assistive devices such as walkers and crutches, see Lewis and others, *Medical-Surgical Nursing,* edition 7, pp. 1648 to 1649), and also the specific types of fractures discussed in this *Companion.*

FRACTURE, HIP

Description

Hip fractures are common in older adults. In adults older than 65 years, hip fractures occur more often in women than in men because of osteoporosis. It is estimated that 10% to 20% of patients who experience a hip fracture will die within 1 year of the injury because of medical complications caused by the fracture or the resulting immobility. Many older adults with a hip fracture develop disabilities necessitating long-term care.

A fracture of the hip refers to a fracture of the proximal third of the femur, which extends up to 5 cm below the lesser trochanter.

- Fractures that occur within the hip joint capsule are called *intracapsular fractures.* Intracapsular fractures (femoral neck) are further identified by a name derived from specific locations: capital, subcapital, and transcervical. These fractures are often associated with osteoporosis and minor trauma.
- *Extracapsular fractures* occur below the joint capsule and are termed *intertrochanteric* if they occur in a region between the greater and lesser trochanter. They are termed *subtrochanteric* if they occur in the region below the lesser

trochanter. Extracapsular fractures are usually caused by severe direct trauma or a fall.

Clinical Manifestations
Manifestations of a hip fracture are external rotation, muscle spasm, shortening of the affected extremity, and severe pain and tenderness in the region of the fracture site. Displaced femoral neck fractures cause serious disruption of the blood supply to the femoral head, which can result in avascular necrosis.

Collaborative Care
Surgical repair is the preferred method of managing intracapsular and extracapsular hip fractures. Surgical treatment permits the patient to be out of bed sooner and decreases the risk of major complications. Initially the affected extremity may be temporarily immobilized by Buck's traction until the patient's physical condition is stabilized and surgery can be performed. Buck's traction relieves painful muscle spasms.

- Intracapsular fractures are usually repaired with the use of an endoprosthesis to replace the femoral head. Extracapsular fractures are repaired using fixed nail plates, sliding nail plates, intramedullary devices, and replacement prostheses. The principles of patient care for these procedures are similar.

Nursing Management
Preoperative Management. Because older adults are most prone to hip fractures, chronic health problems (e.g., diabetes mellitus, hypertension, arthritis) must often be considered when planning treatment. Surgery may be delayed for a brief time until the patient's general health is stabilized.

- Before surgery, severe muscle spasms can increase pain. Appropriate analgesics or muscle relaxants, comfortable positioning unless contraindicated, and properly adjusted traction can help manage spasms.
- The patient should be taught the method and frequency for exercising the unaffected leg and both arms. The patient should also be encouraged to use the overhead trapeze bar and opposite side rail to assist in changing positions. A physical therapist can begin to teach bed and chair transfers.
- The family should be informed about the patient's weight-bearing status after surgery. Plans for discharge begin as the patient enters the hospital, since the length of postoperative stay is only a few days.

Postoperative Management. Initial management of a patient after open reduction and internal fixation (ORIF) of a hip fracture is similar to that for any older surgical patient and includes monitoring vital signs and intake and output, supervising respiratory activities such as deep breathing and coughing, giving pain medication cautiously, and observing the dressing and incision for signs of bleeding and infection. Specific nursing interventions for the orthopedic surgical patient are presented in NCP 63-2, Lewis and others, *Medical-Surgical Nursing,* edition 7, pp. 1647 to 1648.

In the early postoperative period there is potential for neurovascular impairment. The nurse should assess the patient's extremity for motor function, temperature and color, sensation, distal pulses, capillary refill, edema, and pain.

- Edema is alleviated by elevation of the leg whenever the patient is in a chair.
- Pain resulting from poor alignment of the affected extremity can be prevented by keeping pillows (or an abductor splint) between the knees when the patient is turning to either side. Sandbags and pillows are also used to prevent external rotation.

Ambulation usually begins the first or second postoperative day. The nurse in collaboration with the physical therapist monitors the patient's ambulation status for proper crutch walking or use of the walker. The patient must be able to safely demonstrate the use of crutches or a walker before discharge.

If the hip fracture has been treated by insertion of a femoral-head prosthesis, measures to prevent dislocation must always be used (Table 40). If the hip fracture is treated by pinning, dislocation precautions are not necessary.

- The patient and family must be fully aware of positions and activities that predispose the patient to dislocation (>90 degrees of flexion, adduction, or internal rotation). Many daily activities may reproduce these positions (e.g., putting on shoes and socks, crossing legs or feet while seated, assuming side-lying position incorrectly, standing up or sitting down while the body is flexed relative to the chair, sitting on low seats—especially low toilet seats).
- Until the soft tissue surrounding the hip has healed sufficiently to stabilize the prosthesis, these activities must be avoided, usually for at least 6 weeks.
- Sudden severe pain, a lump in the buttock, limb shortening, and extreme external rotation indicate prosthesis dislocation. This requires a closed reduction or open reduction to realign the femoral head in the acetabulum.

The nurse should place a large pillow between the patient's legs when turning, keep leg abductor splints on the patient except when bathing, avoid extreme hip flexion, and avoid turning the patient on the affected side until it is approved by the surgeon.

Table 40	Patient and Family Teaching Guide: Femoral-Head Prosthesis

Do Not
- Force hip into greater than 90 degrees of flexion (e.g., sitting in low chairs or toilet seats)*
- Force hip into adduction
- Force hip into internal rotation
- Cross legs
- Put on own shoes or stockings until 8 wk after surgery without adaptive device (e.g., long-handled shoehorn or stocking helper)
- Sit on chairs without arms to aid rising to a standing position*

Do
- Use toilet elevator on toilet seat*
- Place chair inside shower or tub and remain seated while washing
- Use pillow between legs for first 8 wk after surgery when lying on "good" side or when supine*
- Keep hip in neutral, straight position when sitting, walking, or lying
- Notify surgeon if severe pain, deformity, or loss of function occurs*
- Inform dentist of presence of prosthesis before dental work so that prophylactic antibiotics can be given

* These precautions may also apply after a hip pinning.

The nurse assists both the patient and family in adjusting to the restrictions and dependence imposed by the hip fracture. Depression can easily occur, but creative nursing care and awareness of the problem can do much to prevent it.

- The patient and family may need to be informed about community referral services that can assist in the postdischarge rehabilitation phase.
- Hospitalization averages 4 days. Patients frequently require care in a subacute unit, skilled nursing facility, or rehabilitation facility for a few weeks before returning home.

FRACTURE, HUMERUS

Fractures involving the shaft of the humerus are a common injury among young and middle-aged adults. Clinical manifestations are an obvious displacement of the humeral shaft, shortened extremity, abnormal mobility, and pain.

- Major complications are radial nerve injury and vascular injury to the brachial artery as a result of laceration, transection, or muscle spasm.

Treatment for a fracture of the humerus depends on the location and displacement of the fracture.

- Nonoperative treatment may include a hanging arm cast, shoulder immobilizer, or the sling and swathe, which is a type of immobilization that prevents glenohumeral movement.

When these devices are used, the head of the bed should be elevated to assist gravity in reducing the fracture. The arm should be allowed to hang freely when the patient is sitting and standing.

Nursing care should include measures to protect the axilla and prevent skin maceration by placing lightly powdered absorption pads in the axilla and changing them twice daily or as needed.

- Skin or skeletal traction may also be used for purposes of reduction and immobilization.
- During the rehabilitative phase an exercise program geared toward improving strength and motion of the injured extremity is extremely important. This program should include assisted motion of the hands and fingers. The shoulder can also be exercised to prevent stiffness if the fracture is stable.

FRACTURE, MANDIBLE

A fracture of the mandible may result from trauma to the face or jaws and may be simple, with no bone displacement, or it may involve loss of tissue and bone. Surgery consists of immobilization, usually by wiring the lower jaw to the upper jaw with wires or rubber bands (intermaxillary fixation). When teeth are missing or if there is bone displacement, other forms of fixation, such as metal arch bars in the mouth or insertion of a pin in the bone, may be needed.

Postoperative care should focus on a patent airway, oral hygiene, communication, pain management, and adequate nutrition. Two major potential problems in the immediate postoperative period are airway obstruction and aspiration of vomitus.

- A wire cutter or scissors (for rubber bands) must be taped to the head of the bed and sent with the patient on all appointments and examinations away from the bedside. The wires or bands should be cut only as a last resort in case of an emergency.

- If the patient begins to vomit or choke, the nurse should try to clear the mouth and airway with suctioning and positioning. A nasogastric tube may help prevent aspiration and vomiting and may be used later as a feeding tube.

Oral hygiene is an extremely important part of nursing care.

- The mouth should be rinsed after each meal and snack with warm normal saline solution or water and inspected several times per day with a flashlight and tongue depressor.

Ingestion of adequate nutrients is a challenge because the diet must be liquid. Liquid protein supplements may be helpful for improving nutritional status.

- The low-bulk, high-carbohydrate diet and the intake of air through the straw create a problem with constipation and flatus. Ambulation, prune juice, and bulk-forming laxatives may help relieve these problems.

The patient is usually discharged with the wires in place. Discharge teaching should include oral care, techniques of handling secretions, diet, how and when to use wire cutters, and when to notify the health care provider for concerns and problems.

FRACTURE, PELVIS

Although only a small percentage of all fractures are pelvic fractures, this type of injury is associated with the highest mortality rate. Preoccupation with associated injuries at the time of a traumatic event may result in an oversight of pelvic injuries.

- Pelvic fractures may cause serious intraabdominal injury, such as paralytic ileus, hemorrhage, and laceration of the urethra, bladder, or colon. Patients may survive the initial pelvic injury, only to die from complications such as sepsis or deep venous thrombosis.
- Pelvic fractures are diagnosed by x-ray. They can range in severity from benign to life threatening depending on the mechanism of injury and associated vascular insult.
- Physical examination demonstrates local swelling, tenderness, deformity, unusual pelvic movement, and ecchymosis on the abdomen.

Treatment depends on the severity of the injury. Bed rest for stable pelvic fractures is maintained from a few days to 6 weeks.

More complex fractures may be treated with pelvic sling traction, skeletal traction, hip spica casts, external fixation, open reduction, or a combination of these methods. Open reduction and internal fixation of a pelvic fracture may be necessary if the fracture is displaced.

- Extreme care in handling or moving the patient is important to prevent serious injury from a displaced fracture fragment. Because a pelvic fracture can damage other organs, assessment of bowel and urinary tract function and assessment of distal neurovascular status are important nursing activities for this patient.
- The patient should be turned only when the health care provider specifically orders it. Back care is provided while the patient is raised from the bed, either by independent use of the trapeze or with adequate assistance.
- Weight bearing on the affected side should be avoided until healing is complete.
- If the pelvic fracture is nondisplaced, the patient is usually allowed to ambulate using a walker or crutches to distribute the weight bearing between the upper and lower extremities.

GASTRITIS

Description
Gastritis, an inflammation of the gastric mucosa, is one of the most common problems affecting the stomach. Gastritis may be acute or chronic and may be diffuse or localized.

Pathophysiology
Gastritis is the result of a breakdown in the normal gastric mucosal barrier. The mucosal barrier normally protects the stomach tissue from autodigestion by hydrochloric (HCl) acid and the enzyme pepsin. When the barrier is broken, HCl acid diffuses back into the mucosa. This acid back-diffusion results in tissue edema, disruption of capillary walls with plasma lost into the gastric lumen, and possible hemorrhage.

Causes of gastritis are listed in Table 41. Three important risk factors for gastritis are ulcerogenic drugs (especially nonsteroidal antiinflammatory drugs [NSAIDs]), *Helicobacter pylori* infection, and an autoimmune condition.

- Corticosteroids and NSAIDs inhibit the synthesis of prostaglandins that are protective to the gastric mucosa. This leaves the mucosa more susceptible to injury.

Table 41	Causes of Gastritis

Drugs	**Pathophysiologic Conditions**
Aspirin	Burns
Corticosteroid drugs	Large hiatal hernia
Nonsteroidal antiinflammatory drugs	Physiologic stress
	Reflux of bile and pancreatic secretions
Diet	Renal failure (uremia)
Alcohol	Sepsis
Spicy, irritating food	Shock
Microorganisms	**Other Factors**
Helicobacter pylori	Endoscopic procedures
Salmonella	Nasogastric suction
Staphylococcus organisms	Psychologic stress
Environmental Factors	
Radiation	
Smoking	

- Alcohol can cause acute damage to the gastric mucosa ranging from localized injury of superficial epithelial cells to desquamation and destruction of the mucosa.
- *H. pylori* is capable of promoting the breakdown of the gastric mucosal barrier, given certain "triggers" or conditions. *H. pylori* infection is an important cause of chronic gastritis.
- Autoimmune atrophic gastritis is a form of chronic gastritis that affects both the fundus and the body of the stomach and is associated with an increased risk of gastric cancer.

Clinical Manifestations

- Symptoms of *acute gastritis* include anorexia, nausea and vomiting, epigastric tenderness, and a feeling of fullness. Hemorrhage is commonly associated with alcohol abuse and at times may be the only symptom. Acute gastritis is self-limiting, lasting from a few hours to a few days, with complete healing of mucosa expected.
- Manifestations of chronic gastritis are similar to those of acute gastritis. Some patients have no symptoms directly associated with the gastric lesion. However, when the acid-secreting cells are lost or do not function as a result of atrophy, the source of intrinsic factor is lost and cobalamin (vitamin B_{12}) cannot be absorbed in the ileum, resulting in pernicious anemia.

Diagnostic Studies

Diagnosis of acute gastritis is most often based on a history of drug
and alcohol use. The diagnosis of chronic gastritis may be delayed
or completely missed because symptoms are nonspecific.

- Endoscopic examination with biopsy to obtain a definitive
  diagnosis
- Breath, urine, serum, stool, or gastric tissue biopsy and
  analysis for *H. pylori*
- Complete blood count (CBC) to possibly demonstrate
  anemia from blood loss or lack of intrinsic factor
- Stools tested for occult blood
- Gastric analysis to determine achlorhydria associated with
  severe atrophic gastritis
- Serum tests for antibodies to parietal cells and intrinsic
  factor (IF)

Collaborative Care

Eliminating the cause and preventing or avoiding it in the future
are generally all that are needed to treat acute gastritis. The plan
of care is supportive and similar to that described for nausea and
vomiting.

- During the acute phase, bed rest, nothing by mouth (NPO),
  and intravenous (IV) fluids may be prescribed. Fluids and
  electrolytes lost through vomiting and occasional diarrhea
  are replaced. Antiemetics are often given for nausea and
  vomiting. In severe cases a nasogastric (NG) tube may be
  used, either for lavage of the precipitating agent from the
  stomach or with suctioning to keep the stomach empty and
  free of noxious stimuli.
- Clear liquids are resumed when acute symptoms have subsided, with gradual reintroduction of solid, bland foods.
- Antacids are used for relief of abdominal discomfort,
  and H$_2$-histamine receptor (H$_2$R) blockers (e.g., ranitidine
  [Zantac], cimetidine [Tagamet]) or proton pump inhibitors
  (PPIs) (e.g., omeprazole [Prilosec], lansoprazole [Prevacid])
  will reduce gastric HCl acid secretion.

Treatment of chronic gastritis focuses on evaluating and eliminating the specific cause.

- Currently antibiotic combinations are used to eradicate
  infection with *H. pylori*.
- For the patient with pernicious anemia, lifelong injections
  of cobalamin are needed.

The patient undergoing treatment for chronic gastritis may have
to adapt to lifestyle changes and strictly adhere to medication

regimens. An interdisciplinary team approach in which the physician, nurse, dietitian, and pharmacist provide consistent information and support may increase patient success in making these alterations.

GASTROENTERITIS

Gastroenteritis is an inflammation of the mucosa of the stomach and small intestine. The condition may be attributed to infectious agents, chemical toxins, or miscellaneous conditions such as food allergies or drug reactions. Most cases are self-limiting and do not require hospitalization. However, older adults and chronically ill patients may be unable to consume sufficient fluids orally to compensate for fluid loss.

Clinical manifestations include nausea, vomiting, diarrhea, abdominal cramping, and distention. Fever, leukocytosis, and blood or mucus in the stool may be present.

Until vomiting has ceased, the patient should be on nothing by mouth (NPO) status. If dehydration has occurred, intravenous (IV) replacement of fluids may be necessary. As soon as they can be tolerated, fluids containing glucose and electrolytes (e.g., Pedialyte) should be given. Accurate monitoring of intake and output is important for successful replacement of lost fluid.

If the causative agent is identified, appropriate antibiotic, antimicrobial, or antiinfective medication is given. Strict medical asepsis and enteric precautions should be instituted when indicated.

Symptomatic nursing care is given for nausea, vomiting, and diarrhea (see Nausea and Vomiting, p. 426, and Diarrhea, p. 184). The nurse should assess complaints of pain, vomiting, and diarrhea because gastroenteritis is often confused with appendicitis.

- The patient should be instructed in the importance of proper food handling and preparation of food to prevent infections such as salmonellosis and trichinosis.
- The importance of rest and increased fluid intake should be stressed.
- To allay patient apprehension, the nurse should explain that gastroenteritis usually runs an acute course with no sequelae.

GASTROESOPHAGEAL REFLUX DISEASE

Description

Gastroesophageal reflux disease (GERD) is not a disease but a syndrome produced by conditions that result in the reflux of gastric secretions into the lower esophagus. GERD is the most common upper gastrointestinal (GI) problem in adults.

Predisposing conditions include hiatal hernia, incompetent lower esophageal sphincter (LES), decreased esophageal clearance, and decreased gastric emptying.

Pathophysiology

In GERD, the acidic gastric secretions that reflux up into the lower esophagus result in esophageal irritation and inflammation (esophagitis). In addition, the presence of the gastric enzyme pepsin and intestinal enzymes such as trypsin and bile salts are also corrosive to the esophageal mucosa. The degree of inflammation depends on the amount of acid refluxed, as well as on the ability of the esophagus to clear the acid (esophageal clearance).

Clinical Manifestations

- Heartburn (pyrosis), caused by irritation of the esophagus by secretions, is the most common clinical manifestation. Heartburn is described as a burning, tight sensation that appears intermittently beneath the lower sternum and spreads upward to the throat or jaw. It may occur following ingestion of food or drugs that decrease the LES pressure or directly irritate the esophageal mucosa.
- Regurgitation (the effortless return of material from the stomach into the esophagus or mouth) is another fairly common manifestation. It is often described as hot, bitter, or sour liquid coming into the throat or mouth.
- Gastric symptoms include early satiety, postmeal bloating, and nausea and vomiting related to delayed gastric emptying.

Complications

Complications are related to the effects of gastric acid on the esophageal mucosa. As a result of repeated gastric acid exposure and esophagitis, there may be scar tissue formation and decreased distensibility of the esophagus resulting in esophageal stricture and dysphagia. *Barrett's esophagus,* a precancerous lesion that increases the patient's risk for esophageal cancer, may also occur.

- The potential for pulmonary complications (pneumonia) exists secondary to aspiration of gastric contents into the pulmonary system. Other respiratory complications include cough, bronchospasm, laryngospasm, asthma, and chronic bronchitis.
- Dental erosion may result from acid reflux into the mouth.

Diagnostic Studies

Diagnostic studies help determine the cause of the GERD.
- Barium swallow determines if there is protrusion of the upper part of the stomach into the esophagus.
- Endoscopy is useful in assessing LES competence and extent of inflammation (if present), potential scarring, and strictures.
- Biopsy and cytologic specimens can be taken to differentiate stomach and esophageal cancer from Barrett's esophagus (see Esophageal Cancer, p. 218).
- High-dose proton pump inhibitor (PPI) treatment for 2 weeks may be used as a first step in the diagnosis of GERD. If GERD is present, PPI treatment should result in a marked reduction or elimination of symptoms.

Collaborative Care

The patient is taught to avoid those factors that aggravate symptoms. Particular attention is given to diet and other medications that may affect the LES, acid secretion, or gastric emptying. Patients who smoke are encouraged to stop.

Food can aggravate symptoms. No specific diet is necessary, but food causing reflux should be avoided. High-fat foods decrease the rate of gastric emptying. Foods that decrease LES pressure, such as chocolate, coffee, and tea, should be avoided because they predispose to reflux. Small, frequent meals are advised. Fluids should be taken between rather than with meals to reduce gastric distention. Late evening meals and nocturnal snacking should be avoided. Weight reduction is recommended if the patient is obese.

Drug therapy focuses on improving LES function, increasing esophageal clearance, decreasing volume and acidity of reflux, and protecting esophageal mucosa. There are two approaches to drug therapy:

The *step-up approach* begins with antacids to neutralize gastric acid and over-the-counter (OTC) H_2-histamine receptor (H_2R) blockers. This approach then steps up, increasing to prescription H_2R blockers and finally, PPIs. The *step-down approach* involves starting with a PPI and over time titrating down to prescription

H_2R blockers and finally, OTC H_2R blockers and antacids. More recently as-needed (prn) PPIs are being used more frequently.

- H_2R blockers (e.g., cimetidine [Tagamet], ranitidine [Zantac], famotidine [Pepcid], and nizatidine [Axid]) are available in OTC and prescription formulations.
- PPIs (e.g., omeprazole [Prilosec], esomeprazole [Nexium]) also decrease HCl acid secretion. PPIs may also help decrease the incidence of esophageal strictures. Omeprazole is available as an OTC preparation.

Surgical therapy may be necessary if conservative therapy fails, a hiatal hernia is present, or complications such as stenosis, chronic esophagitis, and bleeding exist. The objective of surgery is to restore gastroesophageal integrity. In these procedures the fundus of the stomach is wrapped around the lower portion of the esophagus to reinforce and repair the defective barrier.

- Laparoscopically performed Nissen and Toupet fundoplications are common antireflux surgeries that have reduced complications and overall morbidity, as well as the cost of hospitalization.
- Three types of endoscopic procedures are currently used to increase the integrity of the LES, provide barriers, and reinforce the LES: endoscopic intraluminal valvuloplasty,

Table 42	Patient and Family Teaching Guide: Gastroesophageal Reflux Disease (GERD)

The following are teaching guidelines for the patient and family:
1. Explain the rationale for a high-protein, low-fat diet.
2. Encourage the patient to eat small, frequent meals to prevent gastric distention.
3. Explain the rationale for avoiding alcohol, smoking (causes an almost immediate, marked decrease in LES pressure), and beverages that contain caffeine.
4. Teach the patient not to lie down for 2 to 3 hours after eating, wear tight clothing around the waist, or bend over (especially after eating).
5. Have patient avoid eating within 3 hours of bedtime.
6. Encourage the patient to sleep with head of bed elevated on 4- to 6-inch blocks (gravity fosters esophageal emptying).
7. Teach information regarding drugs including rationale for their use and common side effects.
8. Discuss strategies for weight reduction if appropriate.
9. Encourage patient and family to share concerns about lifestyle changes and living with a chronic problem.

LES, Lower esophageal sphincter.

endoscopic radiofrequency therapy, and endoscopic injection or implantation of foreign material.

Nursing Management

Nursing care for the patient who is having acute symptoms consists mainly of teaching and encouraging the patient to follow the necessary regimen found in the teaching guide provided in Table 42.

- Postoperative care focuses on concerns related to prevention of respiratory complications, maintenance of fluid and electrolyte balance, and prevention of infection. Laparoscopic procedures reduce the risk of respiratory complications. Only fluids are given initially, and solids are added gradually so that the stomach is not overdistended.

GLAUCOMA

Description

Glaucoma is a group of disorders characterized by increased intraocular pressure (IOP) and the consequences of elevated pressure, including optic nerve atrophy and peripheral visual field loss. The presence of glaucoma is directly related to the balance or imbalance of aqueous humor.

- Glaucoma is the second leading cause of permanent blindness in the United States and the leading cause of blindness among African Americans.

Pathophysiology

Increased IOP results when the rate of aqueous production (inflow) is greater than aqueous reabsorption (outflow). If the pressure remains elevated, permanent visual damage may begin. Outflow of aqueous humor can be decreased by several mechanisms.

- Primary open-angle glaucoma (POAG) represents 90% of the cases of primary glaucoma. In POAG, the aqueous outflow is decreased in the trabecular meshwork. The increased pressure affects the nerve tissue of the optic disc, causing ischemia, and the patient begins to lose peripheral vision.
- In primary angle-closure glaucoma (PACG), the mechanism reducing the outflow of aqueous humor is angle closure. The lens usually bulges forward because of age-related changes, blocking aqueous outflow. Angle closure

may also occur as a result of pupil dilation in the patient with anatomically narrow angles. This condition can be acute, subacute, or chronic.

- In secondary glaucoma, increased IOP results from other ocular or systemic conditions that may block the outflow channels in some way, such as trauma and ocular neoplasms.

Clinical Manifestations

- PAOG develops slowly with no symptoms of pain or pressure. The patient usually does not notice gradual visual field loss until peripheral vision is severely compromised (tunnel vision).
- Acute angle-closure glaucoma causes symptoms of sudden, excruciating pain in or around the eye that is often accompanied by nausea and vomiting. Visual symptoms include seeing colored halos around lights, blurred vision, and ocular redness. The acute pressure rise may cause corneal edema, giving the cornea a frosted appearance.
- Manifestations of subacute or chronic angle-closure glaucoma appear gradually. The patient who has had a previous unrecognized episode of subacute angle-closure glaucoma might report a history of blurred vision, colored halos around lights, ocular redness, or eye or brow pain.

Diagnostic Studies

- IOP with tonometry.
- Visual acuity measurement and visual field perimetry.
- In open-angle glaucoma, slit-lamp microscopy reveals a normal angle. In angle-closure glaucoma, a markedly narrow or flat anterior chamber angle, an edematous cornea, and a fixed, moderately dilated pupil are noticed. Gonioscopy allows better visualization of the anterior chamber angle.
- Ophthalmoscopy (direct and indirect) is done to check for optic disc cupping.

Collaborative Care

If not recognized and treated, glaucoma may cause blindness that could have been prevented in most patients. The primary focus of therapy is to keep the IOP low enough to prevent the patient from developing optic nerve damage leading to severe and permanent visual loss. Specific therapies vary with the type of glaucoma.

- In chronic open-angle glaucoma, initial drug therapy can include β-adrenergic receptor blocking agents, α-adrenergic agents, cholinergic agents (miotics), and carbonic anhydrase inhibitors (hyperosmotic agents).

- When medications are not effective or are not used as prescribed, surgical options include argon laser trabeculoplasty
(ALT), trabeculectomy, or surgical placement of a tube to
shunt aqueous humor from the anterior chamber.
- Acute angle-closure glaucoma is an ocular emergency that
requires immediate interventions, including miotics and
oral or intravenous (IV) hyperosmotic agents. Laser peripheral iridotomy or surgical iridectomy is necessary for long-
term treatment and prevention of subsequent episodes.
- Secondary glaucoma is managed by treating the underlying
problem and using antiglaucoma drugs.

Nursing Management
Nursing management focuses on the chronicity of this disease and
the fact that visual impairment is preventable in most patients with
proper therapeutic management.
Goals
The patient with glaucoma will have no progression of visual
impairment, understand the disease process and rationales for
therapy, comply with all aspects of therapy (including medication
administration and follow-up care), and have no postoperative
complications.
Nursing Diagnoses
- Acute pain
- Self-care deficits
- Noncompliance
- Risk for injury
Nursing Interventions
- The patient with acute angle-closure glaucoma requires immediate medication to lower the IOP. This patient may be uncomfortable, and nursing comfort interventions may include
darkening the environment, applying cool compresses to the
patient's forehead, and providing a quiet and private space. Most
surgical procedures for glaucoma are outpatient procedures.
- The patient needs encouragement to follow therapy recommendations, including information about the disease processes,
normal course of the condition, and treatment options that
include the rationale underlying each option.
▼ **Patient and Family Teaching**
See Table 22, Patient and Family Teaching: After Eye Surgery,
p. 105.
- Because loss of vision from glaucoma is preventable, it is
important to teach patients about risk factors of glaucoma
and stress the importance of its early detection and
treatment.

- The patient should know that the incidence of glaucoma increases with age and that a comprehensive ophthalmologic examination is invaluable in identifying persons with glaucoma or at risk for developing glaucoma.
- All persons between the ages of 40 and 64 years should be instructed to have an ophthalmologic examination every 2 to 4 years and every 1 to 2 years for persons age 65 years or older. African Americans should have examinations more often because of the increased incidence and more aggressive course of glaucoma.
- The patient with glaucoma should be provided with information about prescribed antiglaucoma drugs.

GLOMERULONEPHRITIS

Glomerulonephritis is an inflammation of renal glomeruli caused by immunologic processes. It affects both kidneys equally and is the third leading cause of renal failure in the United States. Two types of antibody-induced injury can initiate glomerular damage.

- In the first type, antibodies have specificity for antigens within the glomerular basement membrane (GBM). The mechanism that causes a person to develop autoantibodies against its GBM is not known.
- In the second type of immune process, antibodies react with circulating nonglomerular antigens and are randomly deposited as immune complexes along the GBM. Bacterial products appear to be important in poststreptococcal glomerulonephritis. Viral agents have been recognized in rare cases of glomerulonephritis that develop after hepatitis B or C and rubella (measles).
- All forms of immune complex disease are characterized by an accumulation of antigen, antibody, and complement in the glomeruli. Immune complexes activate complement; complement activation results in release of chemotactic factors that attract inflammatory mediators; and glomerular injury results.

Clinical manifestations of glomerulonephritis include varying degrees of hematuria (ranging from microscopic to gross) and urinary excretion of various formed elements, including red blood cells (RBCs), white blood cells (WBCs), and casts. Proteinuria and elevated blood urea nitrogen (BUN) and serum creatinine levels are other manifestations.

In most cases, recovery from the acute illness is complete. If progressive involvement occurs, the result is destruction of renal tissue and marked renal insufficiency.

- The patient's history provides important information related to glomerulonephritis. It is necessary to assess exposure to drugs, immunizations, microbial infections, and viral infections such as hepatitis.
- It is also important to evaluate the patient for more generalized conditions involving immune disorders, such as systemic lupus erythematosus and systemic progressive sclerosis (scleroderma).

GLOMERULONEPHRITIS, ACUTE POSTSTREPTOCOCCAL

G

Description

Acute poststreptococcal glomerulonephritis (APSGN) is most common in children and young adults, but all age-groups can be affected. It develops 5 to 21 days after an infection of the pharynx or skin (e.g., streptococcal sore throat, impetigo) by certain nephrotoxic strains of group A β-hemolytic streptococci. Antibodies are produced to the streptococcal antigen, and tissue injury occurs as the antigen-antibody complexes are deposited in the glomeruli and complement is activated.

More than 95% of patients with APSGN recover completely or improve rapidly with conservative management. Chronic glomerulonephritis develops in 5% to 15% of the affected persons, and irreversible renal failure occurs in less than 1% of patients.

Clinical Manifestations

Manifestations appear as a variety of signs and symptoms, which may include generalized body edema, hypertension, oliguria, hematuria with a smoky or rusty appearance, and proteinuria. Fluid retention occurs as a result of decreased glomerular filtration.

- Edema initially appears in low-pressure tissues, such as the eyes (periorbital edema), but later progresses to involve the total body as ascites or peripheral edema in the legs.

- Smoky urine indicates bleeding in the upper urinary tract. The degree of proteinuria varies with the severity of the glomerulonephropathy.
- Hypertension results from increased extracellular fluid volume.
- The patient may have abdominal or flank pain. At times the patient has no symptoms, and the problem is found on routine urinalysis.

Diagnostic Studies
- Determination of the presence or history of group A β-hemolytic streptococci throat or skin infection is important in diagnosis.
- Urinalysis reveals significant numbers of erythrocytes. Erythrocyte casts are highly suggestive of acute glomerulonephritis. Proteinuria may be mild to severe.
- Complete blood count (CBC), blood urea nitrogen (BUN), serum creatinine, and albumin assess extent of renal impairment.
- Decreased complement levels indicate an immune-mediated response.
- Antistreptolysin O (ASO) titers demonstrate an immune response to *Streptococcus*.
- Renal biopsy may be performed to confirm the diagnosis.

Collaborative Care
Management focuses on symptomatic relief.
- Rest is recommended until the signs of glomerular inflammation (proteinuria, hematuria) and hypertension subside.
- Edema is treated by restricting sodium and fluid intake and by administering diuretics.
- Severe hypertension is treated with antihypertensive drugs.
- Dietary protein intake may be restricted if there is evidence of an increase in nitrogenous wastes (e.g., elevated BUN).
- Antibiotics should be given only if streptococcal infection is still present. Corticosteroids and cytotoxic drugs have not been shown to be of value.

Nursing Management
One of the most important ways to prevent the development of APSGN is to encourage early diagnosis and treatment of sore throats and skin lesions. If streptococci are found in the culture, treatment with appropriate antibiotic therapy (usually penicillin) is essential. The patient must be encouraged to take the full course of antibiotics to ensure that the bacteria have been eradicated.

- Good personal hygiene is an important factor in preventing the spread of cutaneous streptococcal infections.

GLOMERULONEPHRITIS, CHRONIC

Chronic glomerulonephritis is a syndrome that reflects the end stage of glomerular inflammatory disease. Most types of glomerulonephritis and nephrotic syndrome can eventually lead to chronic glomerulonephritis.

The syndrome is characterized by proteinuria, hematuria, and the slow development of the uremic syndrome as a result of decreasing renal function. Chronic glomerulonephritis progresses insidiously toward renal failure over a few years to as many as 30 years.

- Chronic glomerulonephritis is often found coincidentally when an abnormality on a urinalysis or elevated blood pressure (BP) is detected. It is common to find that the patient has no recollection or history of acute nephritis or any renal problems. A renal biopsy may be performed to determine the exact cause and nature of the glomerulonephritis. Ultrasound and computed tomography (CT) scan are preferred diagnostic measures.

Treatment is supportive and symptomatic. Hypertension and urinary tract infections (UTIs) should be treated vigorously. Protein and phosphate restrictions may slow the rate of progression of renal failure (see Kidney Disease, Chronic, p. 372).

GONORRHEA

Description
Gonorrhea is the second most frequently occurring sexually transmitted disease (STD). Overall cases of gonorrhea declined from 1975 to 1997 but have been increasing since 1999.

- Gonorrhea rates are highest in adolescents of all racial and ethnic groups, in people living in the southeastern United States, and among minorities.
- Most states have enacted laws that permit examination and treatment of minors without parental consent.

Pathophysiology

Gonorrhea is caused by *Neisseria gonorrhoeae,* a gram-negative diplococcus. Mucosa with columnar epithelium is susceptible to gonococcal infection. This tissue is present in the genitalia (urethra in men, cervix in women), rectum, and oropharynx.

- The disease is spread by direct physical contact with an infected host, usually during sexual activity (vaginal, oral, or anal).
- Neonates can develop a gonococcal infection during delivery from an infected mother.
- Indirect transmission is rare because the delicate gonococcus is easily killed by drying, heating, or washing with an antiseptic.
- Incubation period is 3 to 8 days. The disease confers no immunity to subsequent reinfection.
- Gonococcal infection elicits an inflammatory response, which, if left untreated, leads to formation of fibrous tissue and adhesions. This fibrous scarring is subsequently responsible for many complications such as strictures and tubal abnormalities, which can lead to tubal pregnancy, chronic pelvic pain, and infertility.

Clinical Manifestations

Men. The initial site of infection in men is usually the urethra.

- Symptoms of urethritis consist of dysuria and profuse, purulent urethral discharge developing 2 to 5 days after infection. Painful or swollen testicles may also occur.
- Men generally seek medical assistance early in the disease because their symptoms are usually obvious and distressing. It is unusual for men with gonorrhea to be asymptomatic.

Women. Many women who contract gonorrhea are asymptomatic or have minor symptoms that are often overlooked, making it possible for them to remain a source of infection.

- A few women may complain of vaginal discharge, dysuria, or frequency of urination. Changes in menstruation may be a symptom, but these changes are often disregarded by the woman.
- After the incubation period, redness and swelling occur at the site of contact, which is usually the cervix or urethra. A purulent exudate often develops with a potential for abscess formation.
- The disease may remain local or can spread by direct tissue extension to the uterus, fallopian tubes, and ovaries.

Although the vulva and vagina are uncommon sites for a gonorrheal infection, they may become involved when little or no estrogen is present, such as in prepubertal girls and postmenopausal women.

Anorectal gonorrhea may be present and is usually caused by anal intercourse. Symptoms may include soreness, itching, and discharge.

- Most patients with rectal infections and infections in the throat have few symptoms. A small percentage of individuals develop gonococcal pharyngitis resulting from orogenital sexual contact. When the gonococcus can be demonstrated by culture, individuals of either gender are infectious to their sexual partners.

Complications

Because men often seek treatment early in the course of the disease, they are less likely to develop complications. Complications that do occur in men are prostatitis, urethral strictures, and sterility from orchitis or epididymitis.

Because women who are free of symptoms seldom seek treatment, complications are more common and usually constitute the reason for seeking medical attention. Pelvic inflammatory disease (PID), Bartholin's abscess, ectopic pregnancy, and infertility are the main complications in women.

- A small percentage of infected persons, mainly women, may develop a disseminated gonococcal infection (DGI). In DGI the appearance of skin lesions, fever, arthralgia, or arthritis usually causes the patient to seek medical help.

Diagnostic Studies

- For men, a presumptive diagnosis of gonorrhea is made if there is a history of sexual contact with an infected individual followed within a few days by a urethral discharge. Typical clinical manifestations combined with a positive finding in a gram-stained smear of discharge from the penis gives an almost certain diagnosis.
- A culture is indicated for men whose smears are negative in the presence of strong clinical evidence. Cultures of the discharge or secretion can provide definitive diagnosis after incubation for 24 to 48 hours.
- Making a diagnosis in women is difficult because most women are symptom free. A culture must be performed to confirm the diagnosis.

- Gonococcal tests are now available that can test both *N. gonorrhoeae* and *Chlamydia trachomatis* with one cervical or urethral specimen. These nonculture tests include nucleic acid amplification tests (NAAT), enzyme immunoassays (EIAs), and direct fluorescent antibody (DFA) tests.
- A ligase chain reaction (LCR) assay can also detect both *N. gonorrhoeae* and *C. trachomatis.* This technique uses DNA amplification and has a high rate of sensitivity and specificity. The test can be performed on urine, vaginal fluid or discharge, or urethra secretions.

Collaborative Care

Because of a short incubation period and high infectivity, treatment is instituted without awaiting culture results, even in the absence of signs or symptoms.

Treatment of gonorrhea in the early stage is curative. The most common treatment for gonorrhea is a single intramuscular (IM) dose of ceftriaxone (Rocephin). Other medications that may be used include cefixime (Suprax), ciprofloxacin (Cipro), ofloxacin (Floxin), or levofloxacin (Levaquin). The high frequency (up to 20% in men and 40% in women) of coexisting chlamydial and gonococcal infections has led to the addition of azithromycin (Zithromax) or doxycycline (Vibramycin) to the treatment regimen. Patients with coexisting syphilis are likely to be cured by the same drugs.

- All sexual contacts of patients with gonorrhea must be treated to prevent reinfection after resumption of sexual relations. The "ping-pong" effect of reexposure, treatment, and reinfection can cease only when infected partners are treated simultaneously.
- The patient should be counseled to abstain from sexual intercourse and alcohol during treatment. Sexual intercourse allows the infection to spread and can retard complete healing as a result of vascular congestion. Alcohol has an irritating effect on the healing urethral walls.
- Men should be cautioned against squeezing the penis to look for further discharge.
- All patients should return to the treatment center for a repeat culture at designated times to determine the effectiveness of treatment.
- Reinfection, rather than treatment failure, is the main cause of infections identified after treatment has ended.

Nursing Management

See Nursing Management: Sexually Transmitted Diseases, p. 564.

Gout

Description

Gout is caused by an increase in uric acid production, underexcretion of uric acid by the kidneys, or increased intake of foods containing purines, which are metabolized to uric acid by the body. Characteristic deposits of monosodium urate crystals occur in articular, periarticular, and subcutaneous tissues. Joint involvement includes recurrent attacks of acute arthritis.

Gout may be classified as primary or secondary. In *primary gout,* a hereditary error of purine metabolism leads to overproduction or retention of uric acid. Primary gout occurs predominantly in middle-aged men and is very rare in premenopausal women. *Secondary gout* may be related to another acquired disorder, or it may be the result of medications known to inhibit uric acid excretion. Secondary gout may also be caused by drugs that increase the rate of cell death, such as the chemotherapeutic agents used in treating cancers.

Pathophysiology

G

Uric acid is the major end product of purine catabolism and is primarily excreted by the kidneys. Hyperuricemia may be the result of increased purine synthesis, decreased renal excretion, or both.

- A high dietary intake of purine alone has little effect on uric acid levels. Hyperuricemia may result from prolonged fasting or excessive drinking because of increased production of keto acids, which inhibit uric acid excretion.

Clinical Manifestations

In the acute phase, gouty arthritis may occur in one or more joints. Affected joints may appear dusky or cyanotic and are extremely tender. Inflammation of the great toe (*podagra*) is the most common initial problem. Other joints affected are the midtarsal area of the foot, ankle, knee, wrist, and the olecranon bursa.

- Acute gouty arthritis is usually precipitated by events such as trauma, surgery, alcohol ingestion, or systemic infection. Onset of symptoms is usually rapid, with swelling and pain peaking within several hours, often accompanied by a low-grade fever.
- Individual attacks usually subside, treated or untreated, in 2 to 10 days. The affected joint returns entirely to

normal, and patients are often free of symptoms between attacks.

Chronic gout is characterized by multiple joint involvement and deposits of sodium urate crystals *(tophi)*. These are typically seen in the synovium, subchondral bone, olecranon bursa, and vertebrae; along tendons; and in the skin and cartilage. Tophi are generally noted only many years after the onset of the disease.

Chronic inflammation may result in joint deformity, and cartilage destruction may predispose the joint to secondary osteoarthritis. Tophaceous deposits may be large and unsightly and may perforate overlying skin, producing draining sinuses that often become secondarily infected. Excessive uric acid excretion may lead to urinary tract stone formation. Pyelonephritis associated with intrarenal sodium urate deposits and obstruction may contribute to renal disease.

The severity of gouty arthritis is variable. The clinical course may consist of infrequent mild attacks or multiple severe episodes associated with a slowly progressive disability.

Diagnostic Studies
- Joint aspiration to check for the presence of monosodium urate monohydrate crystals in the synovial fluid.
- Serum uric acid levels are usually elevated.
- Twenty-four–hour urine collection for uric acid levels determines whether the patient undersecretes or overproduces uric acid.
- X-rays in chronic disease identify tophi as eroded areas in the bone.

Collaborative Care
Goals for care include termination of an acute attack through the use of an antiinflammatory agent such as colchicine, with nonsteroidal antiinflammatory drugs (NSAIDs) for pain management. Future attacks are prevented by a maintenance dose of allopurinol (Zyloprim), weight reduction if necessary, and possible avoidance of alcohol and high-purine foods (red and organ meats). Treatment is also aimed at preventing formation of uric acid kidney stones and other associated conditions, such as hypertriglyceridemia and hypertension.

Drug Therapy
Acute gouty arthritis is treated with colchicine and NSAIDs. Intraarticular injection of corticosteroids may be helpful in treating acute gout.

- Aspirin inactivates the effect of uricosurics, resulting in urate retention, and should be avoided while patients are taking uricosuric drugs (e.g., probenecid [Benemid]). Acetaminophen can be used safely if analgesia is required.
- Adequate urine volume must be maintained to prevent precipitation of uric acid in the renal tubules. Allopurinol, which blocks production of uric acid, is particularly useful in patients with uric acid stones or renal impairment, in whom uricosuric drugs may be ineffective or dangerous.
- Febuxostat, a selective inhibitor of xanthine oxidase, is a drug that can reduce serum uric acid in persons with chronic gout.

Regardless of which drugs are used to treat gout, serum uric acid levels must be checked regularly to monitor treatment effectiveness.

Nutritional Therapy
Dietary restrictions may include limiting the use of alcohol and foods high in purine. However, medication can generally control gout without necessitating these changes. Obese patients should be instructed in a weight-reduction program.

Nursing Management
Nursing intervention is directed at supportive care of the inflamed joints.

- Bed rest may be appropriate, with affected joints properly immobilized. Limitation of motion and the degree of pain should be assessed.
- Special care is taken to avoid causing pain to an inflamed joint by careless handling. Involvement of a lower extremity may require the use of a cradle or footboard to protect the painful area from the weight of bedclothes.

▼ **Patient and Family Teaching**
The patient and family should understand that hyperuricemia and gouty arthritis are chronic problems that can be controlled with careful adherence to a treatment program.

- Thorough explanations should be given concerning the importance of drug therapy and the need for periodic determination of serum uric acid levels.
- The patient should be able to demonstrate knowledge of precipitating factors that may cause an attack, including overindulgence in purine-containing foods and alcohol, starvation (fasting), medication use (e.g., aspirin, diuretics), and major medical events (e.g., surgery, myocardial infarction).

GUILLAIN-BARRÉ SYNDROME

Description
Guillain-Barré syndrome is an acute, rapidly progressing, and potentially fatal form of polyneuritis. It is also called *postinfectious polyneuropathy* and *ascending polyneuropathic paralysis*. This disorder affects the peripheral nervous system and results in loss of myelin and edema and inflammation of the affected nerves. With adequate supportive care, 85% to 95% of these patients recover completely.

Pathophysiology
The etiology is unknown, but it is believed to be a cell-mediated immunologic reaction directed at the peripheral nerves. The syndrome is frequently preceded by immune system stimulation from a viral infection, trauma, surgery, viral immunization (e.g., swine flu vaccine), or human immunodeficiency virus (HIV). *Campylobacter jejuni,* found in gastroenteritis, is the most recognized organism associated with Guillain-Barré syndrome. These stimuli are thought to cause an alteration in the immune system, resulting in sensitization of T lymphocytes to the patient's myelin and subsequent myelin damage. Demyelination occurs, and the transmission of nerve impulses is stopped or slowed down. Muscles innervated by the damaged peripheral nerves undergo denervation and atrophy.
- In the recovery phase, remyelination occurs slowly and returns in a proximal to distal pattern.

Clinical Manifestations
Symptoms usually develop 1 to 3 weeks after an upper respiratory or gastrointestinal (GI) infection.
- Weakness of the lower extremities (evolving more or less symmetrically) occurs over hours to days to weeks, usually peaking about day 14. Distal muscles are more severely affected.
- Paresthesia (numbness and tingling) is frequent, and paralysis usually follows in the extremities. Hypotonia and areflexia are common, persistent symptoms. Sensory loss is variable, with deep sensation more affected than superficial sensations.
- Autonomic nervous system dysfunction is usually seen in patients with severe muscle involvement and respiratory muscle paralysis. The most dangerous autonomic dysfunc-

tions include orthostatic hypotension, hypertension, and abnormal vagal responses (bradycardia, heart block, and asystole).
- Other autonomic dysfunctions include bowel and bladder dysfunction, facial flushing, and diaphoresis.
- Patients may also have syndrome of inappropriate anti-diuretic hormone (SIADH) secretion (see Syndrome of Inappropriate Antidiuretic Hormone, p. 612).
- Progression of Guillain-Barré syndrome to include the lower brainstem involves the facial, abducens, oculomotor, hypoglossal, trigeminal, and vagus cranial nerves. This involvement manifests itself through facial weakness, extra-ocular eye movement difficulties, dysphagia, and facial paresthesia.
- Pain is a common finding; the pain can be categorized as paresthesias, muscular aches and cramps, and hyper-esthesias. Pain appears to be worse at night. Opioids may be indicated for those experiencing severe pain. Pain may lead to a decrease in appetite and interfere with sleep.

The most serious complication is respiratory failure, which occurs as paralysis progresses to the nerves that innervate the thoracic area. Respiratory infections or urinary tract infections (UTIs) may occur. Fever is generally the first sign of infection, and treatment is directed at the infecting organism. Immobility from the paralysis can cause problems such as paralytic ileus, muscle atrophy, deep vein thrombosis, pulmonary emboli, skin breakdown, and orthostatic hypotension.

Diagnostic Studies
Diagnosis is based primarily on patient history and clinical signs.
- Cerebrospinal fluid is normal or has a low protein content initially, but after 7 to 10 days it shows a greatly elevated protein level (700 mg/dl [7 g/L]).
- Electromyographic (EMG) and nerve conduction studies are markedly abnormal (showing reduced nerve conduction velocity) in affected extremities.

Collaborative Care
Management is aimed at supportive care, particularly ventilatory support, during the acute phase.
- Plasmapheresis is used in the first 2 weeks. In patients with severe disease treated within 2 weeks of onset, there is a distinct reduction in length of stay, length of time on venti-lator, and time required to resume walking.

- Intravenous (IV) administration of high-dose immunoglobulin (Sandoglobulin) has been as effective as plasmapheresis and has the advantage of immediate availability and
  increased safety. After 3 weeks past disease onset, plasmapheresis and immunoglobin therapies have little value.
- Corticosteroids appear to have little effect on the disease
  prognosis or duration.

Nutritional intake is compromised during the acute phase. The
patient may experience difficulty swallowing because of cranial
nerve involvement. As a result, the patient's nutritional status,
including body weight, serum albumin levels, and calorie counts,
must be evaluated a regular intervals.

- Mild dysphagia can be managed by placing the patient in
  an upright position and flexing the head forward during
  feeding. For more severe dysphagia, tube feedings may be
  required. Later in the course of the disease, motor paralysis
  or weakness affects the ability to self-feed.

Autonomic dysfunction is common and usually takes the form
of bradycardia. Orthostatic hypotension secondary to muscle
atony may occur in severe cases.

- Vasopressor agents and volume expanders may be needed
  to treat low BP.

Nursing Management
Goals
The patient with Guillain-Barré syndrome will maintain adequate
ventilation, be free from aspiration, be free of pain or have pain
controlled, maintain an acceptable method of communication,
maintain adequate nutritional intake, and return to usual physical
functioning.
Nursing Diagnoses
- Impaired spontaneous ventilation
- Risk for aspiration
- Acute pain
- Impaired verbal communication
- Fear
- Self-care deficits
Nursing Interventions
The objective of care is to support the body systems until the patient
recovers. Respiratory failure and infection are serious threats.

- Monitoring vital capacity and arterial blood gases (ABGs)
  is essential. A tracheostomy or endotracheal intubation may
  be done so that the patient can be mechanically ventilated
  (see Tracheostomy, p. 746, and Artificial Airways: Endotracheal Tubes, p. 693).

- Whether the patient has an endotracheal tube or tracheostomy, meticulous suctioning technique is needed to prevent infection. Thorough bronchial hygiene and chest physiotherapy help clear secretions and prevent respiratory deterioration.
- If fever develops, sputum cultures should be obtained to identify the pathogen. Appropriate antibiotic therapy is then initiated.

Monitoring blood pressure (BP) and cardiac rate and rhythm is also important during the acute phase because transient cardiac dysrhythmias have been reported.

A communication system must be established with the use of the patient's available abilities. This is extremely difficult if the disease progresses to involvement of cranial nerves; at the peak of a severe episode the patient may be incapable of communicating.

- The nurse must explain all procedures before doing them and reassure the patient that muscle function will return.

Urinary retention is common for a few days. Intermittent catheterization is preferred to an indwelling catheter to avoid UTIs. However, for the acutely ill patient receiving a large volume of fluids (>2.5 L/day), indwelling catheterization may be safer to reduce overdistention of a temporarily flaccid bladder and to prevent vesicoureteral reflux.

Physical therapy is indicated early to help prevent problems related to immobility. Passive range-of-motion (ROM) exercises and attention to body position help maintain function and prevent contractures.

Nutritional needs must be met in spite of possible problems associated with gastric dilation, paralytic ileus, and aspiration potential if the gag reflex is lost.

- The nurse should note drooling and other difficulties with secretions, which may indicate an inadequate gag reflex.
- Initially tube feedings or parenteral nutrition may be used to ensure adequate caloric intake. Fluid and electrolyte therapy must be monitored carefully to prevent electrolyte imbalances.

HEAD INJURY

Description

Head injury includes any trauma to the scalp, skull, or brain. The term *head trauma* refers primarily to craniocerebral trauma, which includes an alteration in consciousness no matter how brief. Deaths from head trauma occur at three time points after injury: immediately after injury, within 2 hours of injury, and approximately 3 weeks after injury. The majority of deaths occur immediately after the injury, either from the direct head trauma or massive hemorrhage and shock. Progressive worsening of cerebral edema or internal bleeding may cause death within a few hours of the trauma. Immediate notation of changes in neurologic status and surgical intervention are critical in the prevention of deaths at this point. Deaths occurring 3 weeks or more after the injury result from multisystem failure.

Types of Head Injuries

Scalp Lacerations. Because the scalp contains many blood vessels with poor constrictive abilities, even relatively small lacerations can bleed profusely. The major complications of scalp lesions are blood loss and infection.

Skull Fractures. Fractures frequently occur with head trauma. Fractures may be closed or open, depending on the presence of a scalp laceration or extension of the fracture into the air sinuses or dura.

- Type and severity of a skull fracture depend on the velocity, momentum, and direction of the injuring agent, and the site of impact. Specific manifestations of a skull fracture are generally associated with the location of the injury (see Table 57-7, Lewis and others, *Medical-Surgical Nursing,* edition 7, p. 1482).

Major potential complications of skull fracture are intracranial infections and hematoma, as well as meningeal and brain tissue damage.

Minor Head Trauma

- Concussion is a sudden transient head injury associated with a disruption in neural activity and a change in the level of consciousness (LOC). The patient may not lose total consciousness. Signs include a brief disruption in LOC, amnesia for the event (retrograde amnesia), and headache. Manifestations are generally of short duration.
- Postconcussion syndrome is seen anywhere from 2 weeks to 2 months after the concussion. Symptoms include persistent headache, lethargy, behavior changes, decreased short-term memory, and changes in intellectual ability.

Although concussion is generally considered benign and usually resolves spontaneously, the symptoms may be the beginning of a more serious, progressive problem. At the time of discharge it is important to give the patient and family instructions for observation and accurate reporting of symptoms or changes in neurologic status.

Major Head Trauma. Contusions and lacerations are injuries that involve severe brain trauma. Contusions and lacerations are generally associated with closed injuries.

- A *contusion* is a bruising of brain tissue with a potential for the development of areas of necrosis, hemorrhage, and edema. A contusion frequently occurs at the site of a fracture. Contusions or lacerations may occur both at the site of the direct impact of the brain on the skull *(coup)* and at a secondary area of damage on the opposite side away from injury *(contrecoup)*, leading to multiple contused areas. Patient prognosis depends on the amount of bleeding around the contusion site, which can range from minimal to severe. Neurologic assessment demonstrates focal findings as well as generalized findings. Seizures are a common complication.
- *Lacerations* involve actual tearing of brain tissue and often occur with compound fractures and penetrating injuries. Tissue damage is severe, and surgical repair of the laceration is impossible because of the texture of the brain tissue. If bleeding is deep into the brain parenchyma, focal and generalized signs are noted.

When major head trauma occurs, many delayed responses are seen, including hemorrhage, hematoma formation, seizures, and cerebral edema (see Increased Intracranial Pressure, p. 344, and Seizure Disorders, p. 556).

- Prognosis is generally poor for the person with a large intracerebral hemorrhage. Subarachnoid hemorrhage and intraventricular hemorrhage can also occur secondary to head trauma.

Complications

Epidural Hematoma. An epidural hematoma results from bleeding between the dura and inner surface of the skull. An epidural hematoma is a neurologic emergency and is usually associated with a linear fracture crossing a major artery in the dura, causing a tear. It can have a venous or an arterial origin.

- Venous epidural hematomas are associated with a tear of the dural venous sinus and develop slowly.
- With arterial hematomas, the middle meningeal artery lying under the temporal bone is frequently torn. Because this is an arterial hemorrhage, the hematoma develops rapidly.

Manifestations typically include unconsciousness, with a brief lucid interval followed by a decrease in LOC. Other symptoms may be headache, nausea and vomiting, or focal findings. Rapid surgical intervention is needed to prevent cerebral herniation.

Subdural Hematoma. A subdural hematoma occurs from bleeding between the dura mater and the arachnoid layer of the meningeal covering of the brain. A subdural hematoma usually results from injury to the brain substance and its parenchymal vessels. A subdural hematoma is usually venous in origin, with slow development of the hematoma, but rapid development can occur if the hematoma is of arterial origin. Subdural hematomas may be acute, subacute, or chronic (see Table 57-8, Lewis and others, *Medical-Surgical Nursing,* edition 7, p. 1484).

- An *acute subdural hematoma* manifests signs within 48 hours of the injury. Manifestations are similar to those associated with brain tissue compression in increased intracranial pressure (ICP) (see Increased Intracranial Pressure, p. 344). The patient appears drowsy and confused, and the ipsilateral pupil dilates and becomes fixed if ICP is significantly increased.

- A *subacute subdural hematoma* usually occurs within 2 to 14 days of the injury. After the initial bleeding, a subdural hematoma may appear to enlarge over time as the breakdown products of the blood draw fluid into the subdural space to maintain isotonicity.

- A *chronic subdural hematoma* develops over weeks or months after a seemingly minor head injury. Peak incidence is in the sixth and seventh decades of life when a larger subdural space is available as a result of brain atrophy. The presenting complaints are focal symptoms, rather than signs of increased ICP.

Intracerebral Hematoma. An *intracerebral hematoma* occurs from bleeding within the parenchyma. It usually occurs within the frontal and temporal lobes, possibly from the rupture of intracerebral vessels at the time of injury.

Diagnostic Studies

- Skull x-rays to rule out skull fracture; cervical spine x-rays to rule out spinal trauma often associated with head injury
- Computed tomography (CT) scan: best diagnostic test to evaluate for craniocerebral trauma
- Magnetic resonance imaging (MRI), positron emission therapy (PET), and evoked potential studies to assist in diagnosis and differentiation of head injuries
- Transcranial Doppler studies to measure cerebral blood flow and velocity

Collaborative Care

Emergency management of the patient with head injury includes measures to prevent secondary injury by treating cerebral edema and managing increased ICP (see Table 57-9, Lewis and others, *Medical-Surgical Nursing,* edition 7, p. 1484). The principal treatment of head injuries is timely diagnosis and surgery if necessary. For the patient with a concussion or contusion, observation and management of increased ICP are primary management strategies.

- The treatment of skull fractures is usually conservative. For depressed fractures and fractures with loose fragments, a craniotomy is necessary to elevate depressed bone and remove free fragments. If large amounts of bone are destroyed, the bone may be removed (craniectomy) and a cranioplasty will be needed at a later time (see the section on cranial surgery, Lewis and others, *Medical-Surgical Nursing,* edition 7, pp. 1491 to 1493).

- In cases of large acute subdural and epidural hematomas or those associated with significant neurologic impairment, the blood must be removed. A craniotomy is generally performed to visualize the bleeding vessels so that bleeding can be controlled. Burr hole openings may be used in an extreme emergency for more rapid decompression, followed by a craniotomy to stop all bleeding. A drain is generally placed postoperatively for several days to prevent any reaccumulation of blood.

Nursing Management

Goals

The patient with an acute head injury will maintain adequate cerebral oxygenation and perfusion; remain normothermic; achieve control of pain and discomfort; be free from infection; and attain maximal cognitive, motor, and sensory function.

Nursing Diagnoses/Collaborative Problems

- Ineffective tissue perfusion (cerebral)
- Hyperthermia
- Acute pain
- Impaired physical mobility
- Anxiety
- Potential complication: increased ICP

Nursing Interventions

One of the best ways to prevent head injuries is to prevent car and motorcycle accidents.

- The nurse can be active in campaigns that promote driving safety and can speak to driver education classes regarding

the dangers of unsafe driving and of driving after drinking alcohol and using drugs.
- The use of seat belts in cars and the use of helmets for riding on motorcycles are the most effective measures for increasing survival after accidents.
- The nurse should also teach younger children about safety precautions for bicycle riding, skateboarding, and snow and contact sports.

The general goal of nursing management of the head-injured patient is to maintain cerebral oxygenation and perfusion and prevent secondary cerebral ischemia. Surveillance or monitoring for changes in neurologic status is critically important because the patient's condition may deteriorate rapidly, necessitating emergency surgery.
- The nurse should explain the need for frequent neurologic assessments to both the patient and family.
- Behavioral manifestations associated with head injury can result in a frightened, disoriented patient who is combative and resists help.

The Glasgow Coma Scale (GCS) is useful in assessing the LOC (see Glasgow Coma Scale, p. 783). Indications of a deteriorating neurologic state, such as a decreasing LOC or lessening of motor strength, should be reported.

The major focus of nursing care for the brain-injured patient relates to increased ICP (see Increased Intracranial Pressure: Nursing Management, p. 349).
- Loss of the corneal reflex may necessitate administering lubricating eyedrops or taping the eyes shut to prevent abrasion.
- Periorbital ecchymosis and edema disappear spontaneously, but cold and, later, warm compresses provide comfort and hasten the process.
- Diplopia can be relieved by use of an eye patch.
- Hyperthermia can result in increased metabolism, cerebral blood flow, cerebral blood volume, and ICP. Increased metabolic waste also produces further cerebral vasodilation. The nurse should attempt to maintain normothermia in the head-injured patient.
- If cerebrospinal fluid (CSF) rhinorrhea or otorrhea occurs, the nurse should inform the physician immediately and elevate the head of the bed to decrease the CSF pressure. A loose collection pad may be placed under the nose or over the ear. The patient should be cautioned not to sneeze or blow the nose.

- Nausea and vomiting may be a problem and can be alleviated by antiemetic medication.
- Headache can usually be controlled with aspirin or small doses of codeine.

If the patient's condition deteriorates, intracranial surgery may be necessary. A burr-hole opening or craniotomy may be indicated, depending on the underlying injury. The patient is often unconscious before surgery, making it necessary for a family member to sign the consent form for surgery. This is a difficult and frightening time for the patient's family and requires sensitive nursing management. Suddenness of the situation makes it especially difficult for the family to cope.

Once the condition has stabilized, the patient is usually transferred for acute rehabilitation management. As with any craniocerebral problem, there may be chronic problems related to motor and sensory deficits, communication, memory, and intellectual functioning.

- Many of the principles of nursing management of the patient with a stroke are appropriate (see Stroke, p. 598). Outward appearance is not a good indicator of how well the patient will function in the home or work environment.

Progressive recovery may continue for 6 months or more before a plateau is reached and a prognosis for recovery can be made. Specific nursing management depends on residual deficits. In all cases the family must be given special consideration. They need to understand what is happening and taught appropriate interaction patterns.

- The family often has unrealistic expectations of the patient as the coma begins to recede. The nurse needs to prepare the family for the emergence of the patient from coma and must explain that mental and emotional changes often occur after head injuries and can be the most incapacitating problems.
- Family members, particularly spouses, go through role transition as the role changes from one of spouse to that of caregiver.

HEAD AND NECK CANCER

Description

Although head and neck cancer is not common, disability is great because of the potential loss of voice, disfigurement, and social consequences. Most head and neck cancers occur at age 50 years or older after prolonged use of tobacco and alcohol. Other risk factors include consumption of a diet poor in fruits and vegetables and infection by the human papillomavirus (HPV). Males are affected two to five times more often than women.

Clinical Manifestations

Early signs of upper airway cancers vary with tumor location. Cancer of the oral cavity may be a painless growth in the mouth, an ulcer that does not heal, or a change in the fit of dentures. Pain is a late symptom that may be aggravated by acidic food.

Cancers of the oropharynx, hypopharynx, and supraglottic larynx are almost always squamous cell carcinomas, rarely produce early symptoms, and are usually diagnosed in later stages.

- The patient may complain of persistent unilateral sore throat or otalgia (ear pain). Hoarseness may be a symptom of early laryngeal cancer. Some patients experience a change in voice quality or what may feel like a lump in the throat.
- Oral leukoplakia (white patch) or erythroplakia (red patch) may be seen and should be noted for later biopsy. Both leukoplakia and carcinoma in situ (localized to a defined area) may precede invasive carcinoma by many years.
- There may be thickening of the normally soft and pliable oral mucosa.
- Late stages of head and neck cancer have easily detectable signs and symptoms, including pain, dysphagia, decreased mobility of the tongue, airway obstruction, and cranial neuropathies.

Diagnostic Studies

- If lesions are suspected, upper airways may be examined using an indirect laryngoscopy or a flexible nasopharyngoscope. The larynx and vocal cords are visually inspected for lesions and tissue mobility.
- A computed tomography (CT) scan or magnetic resonance imaging (MRI) may be performed to detect local and regional spread.
- Multiple biopsy specimens are obtained to determine the extent of the disease.

Collaborative Care

Using diagnostic information obtained, a decision will be made about the stage of the disease based on tumor size (T), number and location of involved nodes (N), and extent of metastasis (M). TNM staging classifies the disease as stage I to stage IV and guides treatment (see p. 796).

- Approximately one third of patients have stage I or II highly confined lesions at diagnosis. These patients can undergo surgery or radiation therapy with the goal of cure.
- Advanced lesions of the larynx are treated by a total laryngectomy in which the entire larynx and preepiglottic region are removed and a permanent tracheostomy is performed (see Tracheostomy, p. 746). Radical neck dissection frequently accompanies total laryngectomy. Depending on the extent of involvement, extensive dissection and reconstruction may be performed.
- The patient may refuse surgery for advanced lesions because of the extent of the procedure and the potential risk to the patient. In this situation, external radiation therapy may be used as the sole treatment or in combination with chemotherapy.

Nutritional Therapy

After radical neck surgery, the patient may be unable to take in nutrients through the normal route of ingestion.

- Because of swelling and difficulty swallowing postoperatively, tube feedings are usually given through a nasogastric, nasointestinal, or gastrostomy tube that was placed during surgery (see Tube Feeding, p. 751).
- When the patient can swallow, small amounts of water are given with the patient in high Fowler's position. If the patient chokes, suctioning may be necessary to prevent aspiration.
- Swallowing problems should be anticipated when the patient resumes eating. Swallowing can be enhanced by thickening liquids through the use of a commercially available thickening agent (Thick-It).
- If radiation therapy is used, good nutrition is important to provide calories and protein for tissue repair.

Nursing Management

Goals

The patient with head or neck cancer will have a patent airway, no complications related to therapy, adequate nutritional intake, minimal to no pain, the ability to communicate, and an acceptable body image.

See NCP 27-2 for the patient having total laryngectomy or radical neck surgery, Lewis and others, *Medical-Surgical Nursing,* edition 7, pp. 554 to 556.

Nursing Diagnoses
- Anxiety
- Ineffective airway clearance
- Ineffective tissue perfusion
- Imbalanced nutrition: less than body requirements
- Impaired verbal communication
- Disturbed body image
- Acute pain
- Ineffective therapeutic regimen management

Nursing Interventions

Development of head and neck cancer is closely related to personal habits, primarily prolonged tobacco and alcohol use. The nurse should include information about these risk factors in health teaching.

- If cancer has been diagnosed, smoking cessation is still important because the patient who continues to smoke during radiation therapy has lower rates of response and survival.
- Radiation therapy may be used in the treatment of early tumors. The nurse should suggest interventions to reduce the side effects of radiation therapy to the head and neck.

Preoperative care for radical neck surgery should include explanations of postoperative measures relating to communication and feeding. For procedures that involve a laryngectomy, teaching should include information about expected changes in speech. The nurse or speech pathologist should demonstrate means of communicating without speech. This approach assists in decreasing patient anxiety about what to anticipate after surgery.

After surgery, maintenance of a patent airway is essential and a laryngectomy (tracheostomy) tube will be in place. The patient is placed in a semi-Fowler's position to decrease edema and tension on the suture lines. Vital signs should be monitored frequently because of the risk of hemorrhage and respiratory compromise. Immediately after surgery, the postlaryngectomy patient requires frequent suctioning by way of the laryngectomy tube.

- Patency of wound drainage tubes should be monitored every 4 hours for 24 hours to ensure that they are properly removing serous drainage. After the drainage tubes are removed, the area should be closely monitored to detect any swelling. If fluid continues to accumulate, aspiration may be necessary.
- Depression and changes in sexuality patterns because of altered body image are common in the patient who has had radical neck dissection. The nurse should expect to help the patient regain an acceptable self-concept.

- A speech therapist or speech pathologist should meet with the patient to discuss voice restoration. Options available include voice prosthesis, esophageal speech, and an electrolarynx.

▼ **Patient and Family Teaching**

- Instruct patient and family about the feeding and laryngectomy tubes and stoma care, allowing them to perform care repeatedly in the hospital to ensure correct performance of technique.
- Teach the patient to cover the stoma before performing activities such as shaving and the application of makeup to avoid inhalation of foreign materials.
- Encourage the patient to report changes, such as stoma narrowing, difficulty swallowing, and a lump in the throat. These changes may indicate tumor recurrence or tracheal stenosis.
- Measures to provide adequate humidity at home using a bedside humidifier or sitting in a steamy bathroom should be addressed.
- Changes following a total laryngectomy include loss of speech, loss of the ability to taste and smell, inability to produce audible sounds (including laughing and crying), and a permanent tracheal stoma. The patient should receive a referral for a home health care nurse to provide ongoing assistance and support.

HEADACHE

H

Description

Headache is probably the most common type of pain experienced by humans. The majority of people have functional headaches, such as migraine or tension type; the remainder have organic headaches caused by intracranial or extracranial disease.

- Primary classifications of headache include tension-type, migraine, and cluster headaches. Characteristics of these headaches are shown in Table 43. A patient may have more than one type of headache.

Tension-Type Headache

Tension-type headache is the most common type of headache and is characterized by its bilateral location and pressing/tightening quality. It is usually of mild or moderate intensity and is not aggravated by physical activity. It is likely that neurovascular factors similar to those involved in migraine headaches play a role in the development of tension-type headaches.

Clinical Manifestations. There is no prodrome (early manifestation of impending disease) in tension-type headache. The

Table 43 Comparison of Tension-Type, Migraine, and Cluster Headaches

Pattern	Tension-Type Headache	Migraine Headache	Cluster Headache
Site	Bilateral, bandlike pressure at base of skull, in face, or in both	Unilateral (in 60%), may switch sides, commonly anterior	Unilateral, radiating up or down from one eye
Quality	Constant, squeezing tightness	Throbbing, synchronous with pulse	Severe, bone-crushing
Frequency	Cycles for several years	Periodic; cycles of several months to years	May have months or years between attacks; attacks occur in clusters: 1-3 times/day over a period of 4-8 wk
Duration	Intermittent for months or years	Continuous for hours or days	30-90 min
Time and mode of onset	Not related to time	May be preceded by prodrome; onset after awakening; gets better with sleep	Nocturnal; commonly awakens patient from sleep
Associated symptoms	Palpable neck and shoulder muscles, stiff neck, tenderness	Nausea or vomiting, edema, irritability, sweating, photophobia, phonophobia, prodrome of sensory, motor, or psychic phenomena; family history (in 65%)	Vasomotor symptoms, such as facial flushing or pallor, unilateral lacrimation, ptosis, and rhinitis

headache does not involve nausea or vomiting but may involve sensitivity to light *(photophobia)* or sound *(phonophobia)*.

- Headaches may occur intermittently for weeks, months, or years. Many patients can have a combination of migraine and tension-type headaches with features of both headaches occurring simultaneously.

Diagnostic Studies. Careful history taking is the most important diagnostic tool. Electromyography (EMG) may or may not reveal sustained contraction of the neck, scalp, or facial muscles. If tension-type headache is present during physical examination, increased resistance to passive movement of the head and tenderness of head and neck may be present.

Migraine Headache

Migraine headache is a recurring headache characterized by unilateral or bilateral throbbing pain, a triggering event or factor, strong family history, and manifestations associated with neurologic and autonomic nervous system dysfunction. By the late teens, females are about twice as likely to suffer from migraine headaches as males. The incidence peaks for men and women between the ages of 25 to 55 years.

Pathophysiology. Three different theories attempt to explain the etiology of migraine headaches. The vascular theory suggests that vasoconstriction followed by vasodilation causes the throbbing pain. A second theory proposes that the pain is a result of muscular tension and thus is related to tension-type headache. The third theory proposes that changes in the serotonin pathway result in the headache pain.

Migraines can be preceded by prodrome and aura. The prodrome may precede the headache by several hours or several days.

- The aura (sensation of light and warmth) of migraine is associated with "spreading depression," a wave of oligemia (diminished cerebral blood flow) beginning in the occipital lobe and spreading forward in the brain.

In many cases, migraine headaches have no known precipitating events. However, for other patients, the headache may be triggered by foods, hormonal fluctuation, head trauma, physical exertion, fatigue, stress, and drugs.

Clinical Manifestations. *Migraine without aura* is the most common type of migraine headache. *Migraine with aura* occurs in only 10% of migraine headache episodes. The sharply defined aura may last 10 to 30 minutes before the start of the headache and may include sensory dysfunction (e.g., visual field defects, tingling or burning sensations, or paresthesias), motor dysfunction (e.g., weakness or paralysis), dizziness, confusion, and even loss of consciousness.

Clinical manifestations that can occur in migraine with and without aura are generalized edema, irritability, pallor, nausea and vomiting, and sweating. During the headache phase, patients with migraine tend to "hibernate"; that is, they seek shelter from noise, light, odors, people, and problems. The headache is described as a steady, throbbing pain that is synchronous with the pulse.

Diagnostic Studies. There are no specific laboratory or radiologic tests for migraine headache. The diagnosis is usually made from the history. Neurologic and other diagnostic examinations are often normal.

Cluster Headache

Cluster headaches are a rare form of headache that involve repeated headaches that can occur for weeks to months at a time, followed by periods of remission.

Pathophysiology. Neither the cause nor pathophysiology of cluster headache is fully known. The vasodilation that occurs in the affected part of the face is extracranial with the trigeminal nerve implicated in the production of pain. Cluster headaches involve dysfunction of intracranial blood vessels, the sympathetic nervous system, and pain modulation systems. Because of the circadian rhythmicity of the headaches, the hypothalamus is believed to play a role. These headaches can also be triggered by alcohol ingestion.

Clinical Manifestations. The pain of cluster headache is described as sharp and stabbing. It is one of the most severe forms of headache, with intense pain typically lasting about 1 hour. The headaches typically last for 4 to 8 weeks and then go into remission for months or years.

- It is not uncommon for this type of headache to start at night, awakening the patient after a few hours of sleep.
- The pain is generally located around the eye, radiating to the temple, forehead, cheek, nose, or gums.
- Other manifestations include swelling around the eye, lacrimation (tearing), facial flushing or pallor, rhinitis, and constriction of the pupil.
- Unlike the patient with migraine who seeks isolation and quiet, the patient with a cluster headache is often agitated and restless, unable to sit still or relax.

Diagnostic Studies. Diagnosis is primarily based on the history. However, a computed tomography (CT) scan, magnetic resonance imaging (MRI), or cerebral angiography may be performed to rule out an aneurysm, tumor, or infection.

Collaborative Care

If no systemic underlying disease is found, therapy is directed toward the functional type of headache. Table 59-3, Lewis and others, *Medical-Surgical Nursing,* edition 7, p. 1530 summarizes current therapies for prophylaxis and symptomatic relief of headaches. These therapies can include drugs, meditation, yoga, biofeedback, cognitive-behavioral therapy, and relaxation training.

Drug Therapy

Tension-Type Headache. Drug treatment usually involves a nonopioid analgesic (e.g., aspirin, acetaminophen) used alone or in combination with a sedative, muscle relaxant, tranquilizer, or codeine. Many of these drugs have potentially dangerous side effects.

Migraine Headache. Drug treatment is aimed at terminating or decreasing the symptoms of the attack. Many people with mild or moderate migraine can obtain relief with aspirin or acetaminophen. For moderate to severe headaches, the triptans have become the first line of therapy.

- Triptans affect selected serotonin receptors, reducing the neurogenic inflammation of the cerebral blood vessels and producing vasoconstriction. They include sumatriptan (Imitrex), naratriptan (Amerge), rizatriptan (Maxalt), almotriptan (Axert), frovatriptan (Frova), zolmitriptan (Zomig), and eletriptan (Relpax). Because these drugs cause constriction of coronary arteries, they are avoided in patients with heart disease. Triptan medications should be taken at the first symptom of migraine headache.
- Topiramate (Topamax), taken daily, has been shown to be an effective therapy for migraine prevention in adults. It must be used for 2 to 3 months to determine its effectiveness. Other preventive drugs for migraine headaches can include β-adrenergic blockers (e.g., propranolol [Inderal], atenolol [Tenormin]), tricyclic antidepressants (e.g., amitriptyline [Elavil]), selective serotonin reuptake inhibitors (e.g., fluoxetine [Prozac]), calcium channel blockers (e.g., verapamil [Isoptin]), divalproex (Depakote), clonidine (Catapres), and thiazides.
- Methysergide (Sansert) competitively blocks serotonin receptors to prevent migraines, but because of its side effects, it requires regular follow-up and drug holidays.
- Botox (BoNT-A) is being successfully used in the prophylactic treatment of chronic daily headaches and migraines with minimal side effects.

Cluster Headache. Because these headaches occur suddenly, often at night, and are not long lasting, drug therapy is not as useful as it is for other types of headache. Prophylactic medications may include verapamil (Isoptin), lithium, ergotamine, divalproex (Depakote), or nonsteroidal antiinflammatory drugs (NSAIDs). Acute treatment of cluster headache is inhalation of 100% oxygen (O_2) delivered at a rate of 7 to 9 L/min for 15 to 20 minutes, which may relieve headache by causing vasoconstriction. Sumatriptan is also effective in treating acute cluster headache.

Nursing Management
Goals
The patient with a headache will have reduced or no pain, experience increased comfort and decreased anxiety, demonstrate an understanding of triggering events and treatment strategies, use positive coping strategies to deal with chronic pain, and experience increased quality of life and decreased disability.

See NCP 59-1 for the patient with headache, Lewis and others, *Medical-Surgical Nursing,* edition 7, p. 1533.
Nursing Diagnoses
- Acute pain
- Anxiety
Nursing Interventions
Headaches may result from an inability to cope with daily stresses. The most effective therapy may be to help patients examine their lifestyle, recognize stressful situations, and learn to cope with them more appropriately. Precipitating factors can be identified, and ways of avoiding them can be developed. Daily exercise, relaxation periods, and socializing can be encouraged, since each can help decrease the recurrence of headache.
- The nurse can suggest alternative ways of handling the pain of headache through techniques such as relaxation, meditation, yoga, and self-hypnosis. Massage and moist hot packs to the neck and head can help a patient with tension-type headaches.
- The patient should learn about drugs prescribed for prophylactic and symptomatic treatment of headache and should be able to describe the purpose, action, dosage, and side effects.
- For the patient whose headaches are triggered by food, dietary counseling may be provided. The patient is encouraged to eliminate foods that may provoke headaches (e.g., chocolate, alcohol, excessive caffeine, cheese, fermented foods, monosodium glutamate).

▼ Patient and Family Teaching
A teaching guide for the patient with a headache is provided in Table 44.

Table 44	Patient and Family Teaching Guide: Headaches

1. Keep a diary or calendar of headaches and possible precipitating events
2. Avoid factors that can trigger a headache:
   Foods containing amines (cheese, chocolate), nitrites (meats such as hot dogs), vinegar, onions, monosodium glutamate
   Fermented or marinated foods
   Caffeine
   Oranges
   Tomatoes
   Aspartame
   Nicotine
   Ice cream
   Alcohol (particularly red wine)
   Emotional stress
   Fatigue
   Drugs such as ergot-containing and monoamine oxidase inhibitors
3. Describe the purpose, action, dosage, and side effects of drugs taken
4. Be able to self-administer sumatriptan (Imitrex) subcutaneously if prescribed
5. Use stress-reduction techniques, such as relaxation
6. Participate in regular exercise
7. Contact health care provider if the following occur:
   - Symptoms become more severe, last longer than usual, or are resistant to medication
   - Nausea and vomiting (if severe or not typical), change in vision, or fever occurs with the headache
   - Problems with drugs

H

HEART FAILURE

Description

Heart failure (HF) is an abnormal clinical condition involving impaired cardiac pumping that results in vasoconstriction and fluid retention. The term HF is preferred to the former term, congestive heart failure (CHF), because not all patients with HF have pulmonary congestion. HF is not a disease; it is associated with numerous types of heart disease, particularly with coronary artery disease (CAD) and long-standing hypertension. HF is characterized by ventricular dysfunction, reduced exercise tolerance, diminished quality of life, and shortened life expectancy. The incidence of HF is increasing due, in part, to increased survival after cardiovascular events and in part because of the increased aging population.

Risk factors for HF include CAD, advancing age, hypertension, diabetes mellitus, cigarette smoking, obesity, and high cholesterol levels.

Pathophysiology

HF may be caused by any interference with the normal mechanisms regulating cardiac output (CO). CO depends on (1) preload, (2) afterload, (3) myocardial contractility, (4) HR, and (5) metabolic state of the individual. Any alteration in these factors can lead to decreased ventricular function and subsequent HF.

- Major causes of HF may be divided into two subgroups: (1) primary causes, consisting of underlying cardiac diseases, such as CAD and cardiomyopathy, and (2) precipitating causes, such as anemia, pulmonary disease, and hypovolemia (see the complete listing of causes in Tables 35-1 and 35-2, Lewis and others, *Medical-Surgical Nursing,* edition 7, p. 822). Precipitating factors are generally more amenable to treatment than cardiac diseases.

Heart failure can be described as systolic or diastolic. *Systolic failure,* the most common cause of HF, is a defect in the ability of the ventricles to contract (pump). Systolic failure is caused by impaired contractile function (e.g., myocardial infarction [MI]), increased afterload (e.g., hypertension), cardiomyopathy, and mechanical abnormalities (e.g., valvular heart disease).

Diastolic failure is an impaired ability of the ventricles to relax and fill during diastole, resulting in high filling pressures and decreased ventricular filling. Decreased filling results in decreased stroke volume and CO and venous engorgement in both the pulmonary and systemic systems. The diagnosis of diastolic failure is based on the presence of pulmonary congestion, pulmonary hypertension, ventricular hypertrophy, and a normal ejection fraction. Diastolic failure is usually the result of left ventricular hypertophy from chronic hypertension, aortic stenosis, or hypertrophic cardiomyopathy.

Mixed systolic and diastolic failure is seen in disease states such as dilated cardiomyopathy, in which poor systolic function (weakened muscle function) is further compromised by dilated left ventricular walls that are unable to relax.

The patient with ventricular failure of any type has low systemic arterial blood pressure (BP), low CO, and poor renal perfusion. Whether a patient arrives at this point acutely (from an MI) or chronically (from worsening cardiomyopathy or hypertension), the body's response to this low CO is to mobilize compensatory mechanisms to maintain CO and BP. The main compensatory mechanisms include (1) sympathetic nervous system activation, (2) neurohormonal responses, (3) ventricular dilation, and (4) ventricular hypertrophy.

HF is usually manifested by biventricular failure, although one ventricle may precede the other in dysfunction.

- The most common form of initial heart failure is left-sided failure. Left-sided failure causes blood to back up through the left atrium and into the pulmonary veins. The increased pulmonary pressure causes fluid extravasation from the pulmonary capillary bed into the interstitium and then the alveoli, which is manifested as pulmonary congestion and edema.
- Right-sided failure causes backward blood flow to the right atrium and venous circulation. Venous congestion in the systemic circulation results in peripheral edema, hepatomegaly, and jugular venous distention. The primary cause of right-sided failure is left-sided failure. *Cor pulmonale* (right ventricular dilation and hypertrophy caused by pulmonary pathologic conditions) can also cause right-sided failure.

Manifestations of Acute Decompensated Heart Failure

Regardless of etiology, acute decompensated heart failure (ADHF) typically presents as *pulmonary edema,* an acute, life-threatening siutation in which the lung alveoli become filled with serosanguineous fluid. The most common cause of pulmonary edema is acute left ventricle (LV) failure secondary to CAD.

- Manifestations of pulmonary edema are unmistakable: the patient may be anxious, pale, and possibly cyanotic, with clammy and cold skin.
- The patient has severe dyspnea, as evidenced by obvious use of respiratory accessory muscles, respiratory rate >30 breaths/min, and orthopnea. Wheezing and coughing with production of frothy, blood-tinged sputum may also occur.
- Auscultation of the lungs may reveal bubbling crackles, wheezes, and rhonchi. The patient's HR is rapid, and BP may be elevated or decreased depending on the severity of edema.

Manifestations of Chronic Heart Failure

Manifestations of chronic HF depend on the patient's age, underlying type and extent of heart disease, and which ventricle is failing to pump effectively. Table 45 lists manifestations of left-sided and right-sided failure. The patient with chronic HF will probably have manifestations of biventricular failure.

- Fatigue after activities that normally are not tiring is one of the earliest symptoms.
- Dyspnea is a common sign. Shortness of breath occurs when the patient is in the recumbent position (orthopnea).

| Table 45 | Clinical Manifestations of Heart Failure |

Right-Sided Heart Failure	Left-Sided Heart Failure
Signs	
RV heaves	LV heaves
Murmurs	Pulsus alternans (alternating pulses: strong, weak)
Jugular venous distention	↑ HR
Edema (e.g., anterior tibias, medial malleoli, scrotum, sacrum)	PMI displaced inferiorly and posteriorly (LV hypertrophy)
Weight gain	↓ PaO_2, slight ↑ $PaCO_2$ (poor O_2 exchange)
↑ HR	Crackles (pulmonary edema)
Ascites	S_3 and S_4 heart sounds
Anasarca (massive generalized body edema)	Pleural effusion
	Changes in mental status
Hepatomegaly (liver enlargement)	Restlessness, confusion
Symptoms	
Fatigue	Weakness, fatigue
Anxiety, depression	Anxiety, depression
Dependent, bilateral edema	Dyspnea
Right upper quadrant pain	Shallow respirations up to 32-40/min
Anorexia and GI bloating	Paroxysmal nocturnal dyspnea
Nausea	Orthopnea (shortness of breath in recumbent position)
	Dry, hacking cough
	Nocturia
	Frothy pink-tinged sputum (advanced pulmonary edema)

GI, Gastrointestinal; *HR*, heart rate; *LV*, left ventricle; *PMI*, point of maximal impulse; *RV*, right ventricle.

- Paroxysmal nocturnal dyspnea (PND) occurs when the patient is asleep. The patient awakens in a panic, has feelings of suffocation, and has a strong desire to seek respiratory relief by sitting up.
- Other common signs include tachycardia; edema in the legs, liver, abdominal cavity, and lungs; nocturia; cool and dusky skin; restlessness and confusion; angina-type chest pain; and weight changes.

Complications

Pleural effusion results from increasing pressure in the pleural capillaries. Enlargement of the heart chambers in chronic HF can cause atrial fibrillation. Patients also have a high risk of fatal dysrhythmias.

Left ventricular thrombus may occur with ADHF or chronic HF in which the enlarged LV and poor CO combine to increase the chance of thrombus formation in the LV. Many health care providers administer anticoagulants in patients with HF and atrial fibrillation.

Hepatomegaly may result as liver lobules become congested with venous blood. Hepatic congestion leads to impaired liver function; eventually liver cells die, fibrosis occurs, and cirrhosis can develop.

Diagnostic Studies

- Laboratory data (cardiac enzymes, b-type natriuretic peptide [BNP] level, serum chemistries, arterial blood gases [ABGs], liver function tests, thyroid function studies, and complete blood count [CBC]) are studied.
- Chest x-ray to evaluate heart size and pulmonary congestion.
- Electrocardiogram (ECG) confirms cardiac changes. Exercise stress testing and nuclear imaging studies add additional information to ECG findings.
- Hemodynamic monitoring by means of a pulmonary artery catheter directly assesses cardiac function.
- Echocardiography measures CO and size of the cardiac chambers and assesses ventricular and valvular function.
- Cardiac catheterization helps detect underlying heart disease.

Nursing and Collaborative Management: Acute Decompensated Heart Failure and Pulmonary Edema

The goals of therapy for both ADHF and chronic HF are to decrease patient symptoms, reverse ventricular remodeling, improve quality of life, and decrease mortality and morbidity. The

Joint Commission on Accreditation of Healthcare Organizations (JCAHO) has established four core measures to promote the use of strategies that are associated with improved outcomes for patients with ADHF (see Table 35-8, Lewis and others, *Medical-Surgical Nursing,* edition 7, p. 828).

Treatment strategies should include improving LV function by decreasing intravascular volume, decreasing venous return (preload), decreasing afterload, controlling HR and rhythm, improving gas exchange and oxygenation, increasing CO, reducing anxiety, preserving target organ function (e.g., kidneys), and decreasing progression of the disease. Major components of management include:

- Decreasing intravascular volume:
  - Loop diuretics (e.g., furosemide [Lasix], bumetanide [Bumex]) are given following hemodynamic and renal function assessment.
  - Ultrafiltration or aquapheresis may remove up to 500 ml fluid /hr.
- Decreasing venous return (decreases preload):
  - Placing the patient in a high Fowler's position with feet horizontal in bed or dangling at bedside will pool blood in extremities.
  - Nitroglycerin intravenously (IV) causes systemic vasodilation, decreasing circulating volume and blood return to the heart; in high doses causes arterial dilation, decreasing afterload.
- Decreasing afterload (systemic resistance):
  - Nitroprusside (Nipride) IV is a potent arterial and venous dilator that reduces preload and afterload. Because of its rapid onset of action and potent effects, it is the drug of choice for the patient with ADHF and pulmonary edema.
  - Morphine sulfate also reduces preload and afterload. It dilates both the pulmonary and systemic blood vessels, thereby decreasing pulmonary pressures and improving gas exchange.
  - Nesiritide (Natrecor) is a recombinant form of BNP. Nesiritide reduces both preload and afterload by venous and arterial dilation, increases cardiac output, and increases diuresis and sodium excretion.
  - Nitroglycerin IV also causes arterial dilation in high doses, decreasing afterload.
- Improving gas exchange and oxygenation:
  - IV morphine sulfate improves gas exchange and decreases oxygen demands.

- Oxygen (O_2) administration increases the percentage of O_2 in inspired air (see Oxygen Therapy, p. 734). In severe pulmonary edema the patient may need to be intubated and placed on a mechanical ventilator.
- Improving cardiac function: inotropic therapy
  - Inotropic therapy is only recommended for use in the short-term management of patients with ADHF who have not responded to conventional pharmacotherapy and who have hemodynamic monitoring (see the section on hemodynamic monitoring, Lewis and others, *Medical-Surgical Nursing,* edition 7, pp. 827 to 829).
  - Digitalis is a positive inotrope that improves LV function but also increases myocardial oxygen consumption and has a slow onset of action.
  - β-Adrenergic agonists (e.g., dopamine [Intropin], dobutamine [Dobutrex], epinephrine, norepinephrine [Levophed]) increase cardiac contractility and heart rate: dopamine increases systemic vascular resistance (SVR) and is used for severe ADHF and cardiogenic shock; dobutamine does not increase SVR and may be preferred for short-term treatment of ADHF.
  - Phosphodiesterase inhibitors (e.g., inamrinone [Inocor], milrinone [Primacor]) increase myocardial contractility and promote peripheral vasodilation, resulting in increased CO and decreased afterload.
- Reducing anxiety:
  - Nursing interventions that promote effective coping, increased trust, and use of relaxation techniques are important measures.
  - Sedative medications (e.g., morphine sulfate, benzodiazepines) may be used.

Nursing care focuses on continual physical assessment, hemodynamic monitoring, and monitoring the patient's response to treatment.

Collaborative Care: Chronic Heart Failure

One of the most important goals in the treatment of chronic HF is to treat the underlying cause. The treatment of causes such as dysrhythmias, hypertension, valvular disorders, and CAD are discussed elsewhere in this book. Other goals and management are similar to those of ADHF.

Nonpharmacologic Therapy

- Administration of O_2 improves saturation and assists in meeting tissue oxygen needs, thereby decreasing dyspnea and fatigue.

- Physical and emotional rest conserves energy and decreases the need for additional O_2. A patient with severe HF may be on bed rest with limited activity. A patient with mild to moderate HF can be ambulatory with a restriction of strenuous activity.
- *Cardiac resynchronization therapy (CRT)*, unlike traditional pacing, coordinates right and left ventricular contractility through biventricular pacing. This therapy allows patients to increase their exercise capacity, as well as decrease their overall symptoms of failure.
- Cardiac transplantation is a desirable treatment for chronic HF. However, the lack of donor hearts makes it an option for only a small number of patients with HF.
- Mechanical options such as the intraaortic balloon pump (IABP) and ventricular assist devices (VADs) are available for patients with deteriorating conditions, especially those awaiting cardiac transplantation. The IABP is frequently used as a short-term bridge to cardiac surgery, including transplantation. VADs provide highly effective long-term support for up to 2 years.

Drug Therapy. Objectives include (1) identification of HF type, (2) correction of sodium and water retention and volume overload, (3) reduction of cardiac workload, (4) improvement of myocardial contractility, and (5) control of precipitating and complicating factors. Current approaches stress the role of diuretics, vasodilators, angiotensin-converting enzyme (ACE) inhibitors, and inotropic agents.

- Diuretics mobilize edematous fluid, reduce pulmonary venous pressure, and reduce preload.
  - Thiazide diuretics (e.g., hydrochlorothiazide [Hydrodiuril]) may be the first choice because of their convenience, safety, low cost, and effectiveness.
  - Loop diuretics such as furosemide (Lasix), bumetanide (Bumex), and torsemide (Demadex) are potent but can cause hypokalemia and ototoxicity.
  - Spironolactone (Aldactone), a potassium-sparing diuretic, also blocks the vasoconstrictor effect of aldosterone on the heart blood vessels and may be used in conjunction with other diuretics.
- Vasodilators are used to increase venous capacity, improve ejection fraction, slow the process of ventricular dysfunction, decrease heart size, block compensatory neurohormonal responses, and enhance neurohormonal blockade.
  - ACE inhibitors (e.g., captopril [Capoten], enalapril [Vasotec]) are useful in both systolic and diastolic heart failure and are the first-line therapy for chronic HF. A reduction in SVR seen with the use of ACE inhibitors

produces a significant increase in CO. Other hemodynamic changes include a reduction in (1) pulmonary artery pressure, (2) right arterial pressure, and (3) left ventricular filling pressure.
- Nitrates (e.g., nitroglycerin) increase venous capacitance by dilating the pulmonary vasculature and improving arterial compliance, decreasing preload.
- Combination isosorbide dinitrate/hydralazine (BiDil) can improve heart failure symptoms in blacks.
- Human BNP is being studied for its vasodilating effects in the treatment of patients with chronic HF.
- β-Adrenergic blockers, especially carvedilol (Coreg) and metoprolol (Toprol-XL), contribute to marked improvement in patient survival in chronic HF. These agents directly block the negative effects of the sympathetic nervous system on the failing heart.
- Positive inotropic agents are used to improve cardiac contractility.
  - Digitalis glycosides (e.g., digoxin [Lanoxin]) reduce symptoms of HF but have not been shown to prolong life. They are particularly useful in the treatment of HF accompanied by atrial flutter and/or fibrillation. Digitalis toxicity is not uncommon, especially in older adults.
  - Other inotropic agents include β-adrenergic agonists, phosphodiesterase inhibitors (milrinone [Primacor]), and calcium sensitizers (levosimendan [Simdax]).

Nutritional Therapy. Diet education and weight management are critical to the control of chronic HF.
- The edema of chronic HF is often treated by dietary restriction of sodium. A commonly prescribed diet for a patient with mild HF is a 2.5-g sodium diet. (For sample menu plans for sodium-restricted diets, see Table 35-11, Lewis and others, *Medical-Surgical Nursing,* edition 7, p. 834.) For more severe HF, sodium intake is restricted to 500 to 1000 mg, but compliance is poor with these diets because they are unpalatable. The patient should be taught what foods are low and high in sodium and ways to enhance food flavors without the use of salt (e.g., substituting lemon juice and various spices).
- Fluid restrictions are not commonly prescribed for mild to moderate HF. Diuretic therapy and digitalis preparations act as effective diuretics to promote fluid excretion. However, in moderate to severe HF, fluid restrictions are usually implemented.
- Patients should be instructed to weigh themselves at the same time each day, preferably before breakfast, while

wearing the same type of clothing. A weight gain of 3 lb (1.4 kg) over 2 days or a 5-lb (2.3-kg) gain over 1 week indicates fluid retention.

Nursing Management: Chronic Heart Failure

Goals

The patient with HF will have a decrease in symptoms (e.g., shortness of breath, fatigue), decreased peripheral edema, increased exercise tolerance, compliance with medical regimen, and no complications related to HF.

See NCP 35-1 for the patient with HF, Lewis and others, *Medical-Surgical Nursing,* edition 7, pp. 836 to 838.

Nursing Diagnoses

- Activity intolerance
- Excess fluid volume
- Disturbed sleep patterns
- Impaired gas exchange
- Anxiety
- Deficient knowledge

Nursing Interventions

Health Promotion. An important measure used to prevent HF is the treatment or control of underlying heart disease. For example, in rheumatic valvular disease, valve replacement should be planned before lung congestion develops.

- Early and continued treatment of hypertension is important. Hyperlipidemic states in persons with CAD should be managed with diet, exercise, and medication.
- The use of antidysrhythmic agents or pacemakers is indicated for people with serious dysrhythmias or conduction disturbances.
- When a patient is diagnosed with HF, preventive care should focus on slowing the progression of the disease. Knowing the importance of following the medication, diet, and exercise regimen is essential.

Acute Intervention. Many persons with HF will experience one or more episodes of ADHF. When they do, they are usually initially managed in a critical care unit and later transferred to a step-down general unit when their condition has stabilized. Nursing management presented here applies to the patient with stabilized ADHF or chronic HF.

Ambulatory and Home Care. HF is a chronic illness for most persons. Important nursing responsibilities are (1) teaching the patient about physiologic changes that have occurred, (2) assisting the patient to adapt to both physiologic and psychologic changes, and (3) integrating the patient and the patient's family or support system in the overall care plan. It must be emphasized to the patient that it is possible to live productively with this health problem.

- Home nursing care is a vital factor in preventing future hospitalization for this patient. Home care involves ongoing clinical assessments and monitoring of vital signs and response to therapies (Table 46).
- It must be stressed that the disease is chronic and that medication must be continued to keep the heart failure under control.

Table 46	Patient and Family Teaching Guide: Heart Failure

Health Promotion
1. Obtain annual flu vaccination.
2. Obtain pneumococcal vaccine (e.g., Pneumovax) and revaccination after 5 years (for people at high risk of infection or serious disease).
3. Consider smoking cessation and weight reduction, if appropriate.

Rest
1. Plan a regular daily rest and activity program.
2. After exertion, such as exercise and ADLs, plan a rest period.
3. Shorten working hours, or schedule rest periods during working hours.
4. Avoid emotional upsets. Verbalize any concerns, fears, feelings of depression, etc. to health care provider.

Drug Therapy
1. Take each drug as prescribed daily.
2. Develop a check-off system (e.g., daily chart) to ensure medications have been taken.
3. Take your pulse rate each day before taking medications (if appropriate). Know the parameters that your health care provider wants for your heart rate.
4. Learn to take your own BP at determined intervals (if appropriate). Know your target BP limits.
5. Know signs and symptoms of orthostatic hypotension and how to prevent them.
6. Know signs and symptoms of internal bleeding (bleeding gums, increased bruises, blood in stool or urine) and what to do if you take anticoagulants.
7. Know own INR if taking warfarin (Coumadin) and how often to have blood monitored.

ADLs, Activities of daily living; *BP,* blood pressure; *INR,* international normalized ratio.

Continued

Table 46	Patient and Family Teaching Guide: Heart Failure—cont'd

Dietary Therapy
1. Consult the written diet plan and list of permitted and restricted foods.
2. Examine labels to determine sodium content. Also examine the labels of over-the-counter drugs, such as laxatives, cough medicines, and antacids.
3. Avoid using salt when preparing foods or adding salt to foods.
4. Weigh yourself in the early morning after arising and emptying your bladder. Use the same scale and wear the same or similar clothes every day.
5. Report a weight gain of 3 lb (1.4 kg) in 2 days, or 3 to 5 lb (1.4 to 2.3 kg) in 1 week.
6. Eat smaller, more frequent meals.

Activity Program
1. Increase walking and other activities gradually, provided they do not cause fatigue and dyspnea.
2. Avoid extremes of heat and cold.
3. Keep regular appointments with health care provider.

Ongoing Monitoring
1. Know the signs and symptoms of recurring or progressing heart failure.
2. Recall the symptoms experienced when illness began; reappearance of previous symptoms may indicate a recurrence.
3. Report immediately to health care provider any of the following:
   - Difficulty breathing, especially with exertion or when lying flat
   - Waking up breathless at night
   - Frequent dry, hacking cough, especially when lying down
   - Fatigue, weakness
   - Swelling of ankles, feet, or abdomen; swelling of face or difficulty breathing (if taking ACE inhibitors)
   - Nausea with abdominal swelling, pain, and tenderness
   - Dizziness or fainting
   - Weight gain of 3 lb (1.4 kg) in 2 days, or 3 to 5 lb (1.4 to 2.3 kg) in 1 week
4. Follow-up with health care provider on regular basis.
5. Consider joining a local support group with your family members or support person or persons.

ACE, Angiotensin-converting enzyme.

- The patient should be taught the actions of prescribed drugs, manifestations of drug toxicity, and under what circumstances drugs should be withheld and a health care provider consulted.

HEMOPHILIA

Description
Hemophilia is a sex-linked recessive genetic disorder caused by defective or deficient coagulation factor. The two major forms of hemophilia that can occur in mild to severe forms are *hemophilia A* (classic hemophilia, factor VIII deficiency) and *hemophilia B* (Christmas disease, factor IX deficiency). *von Willebrand's disease* is a related disorder involving a deficiency of the von Willebrand's coagulation protein.

Hemophilia A is the most common form of hemophilia, accounting for about 80% of all cases. Von Willebrand's disease is considered the most common congenital bleeding disorder in humans, with estimates as high as 1 in 100 persons.

Deficiency and inheritance patterns of these three forms of inherited coagulopathies are compared in Table 47.

Clinical Manifestations and Complications
Clinical manifestations and complications related to hemophilia include (1) slow, persistent, prolonged bleeding from minor trauma and small cuts; (2) delayed bleeding after minor injuries (the delay may be several hours or days); (3) uncontrollable hemorrhage after dental extractions or irritation of the gingiva with a hard-bristle toothbrush; (4) epistaxis, especially after a blow to the face; (5) GI bleeding from ulcers and gastritis; (6) hematuria from genitourinary (GU) trauma and splenic rupture resulting from falls or abdominal trauma; (7) ecchymoses and subcutaneous (SC) hematomas; (8) neurologic signs, such as pain, anesthesia, and paralysis, that may develop from nerve compression caused by hematoma formation; and (9) hemarthrosis (bleeding into the joints), which may lead to joint deformity severe enough to cause crippling (commonly in knees, elbows, shoulders, hips, and ankles).

- All manifestations relate to bleeding. Any bleeding episode in persons with hemophilia may lead to life-threatening hemorrhage.
- The contamination of blood products with the human immunodeficiency virus (HIV) in the 1980s caused the majority of hemophilia deaths in the late 1980s. However,

Table 47 Comparison of Types of Hemophilia

Disorder	Deficiency	Laboratory Results*	Inheritance Pattern
Hemophilia A	Factor VIII	Bleeding time normal; prolonged partial thromboplastin time because of deficiency of coagulation factor	Recessive sex-linked (transmitted by female carriers, displayed almost exclusively in men)
Hemophilia B	Factor IX	Bleeding time normal; prolonged partial thromboplastin time because of deficiency of coagulation factor	Recessive sex-linked (transmitted by female carriers, displayed almost exclusively in men)
von Willebrand's disease	vWF and platelet dysfunction	Prolonged bleeding time because of defective platelets; prolonged partial thromboplastin time because of deficiency of coagulation factor	Autosomal dominant, seen in both genders; Recessive (in severe forms of the disease)

vWF, von Willebrand factor.
* Prothrombin time, thrombin time, and platelet count normal in hemophilia.

survival of up to 72 years old is now being observed because of improved preparation of replacement products, improved screening of blood donors, and use of recombinant replacement factors.

- Hepatitis C antibody screening is now routinely done on all donated blood and blood products to prevent hepatitis C transmission.

Diagnostic Studies

Laboratory studies affected by the deficient factor of hemophilia are presented in Table 47.

Collaborative Care

The goal of management is to prevent and treat bleeding. Care for persons with hemophilia or von Willebrand's disease requires the provision of preventive care, the use of replacement therapy during acute bleeding episodes and as prophylaxis, and treatment of complications of the disease and its therapy.

- Replacement of deficient clotting factors is the primary means of supporting patients with hemophilia. In addition to treating acute crises, replacement therapy may be given before surgery and dental care as a prophylactic measure.
- For mild hemophilia A or certain subtypes of von Willebrand's disease, desmopressin acetate (DDAVP), a synthetic analog of vasopressin, may be used to stimulate an increase in factor VIII and von Willebrand's factor (vWF).

Complications of treatment of hemophilia include development of inhibitors to factors VIII or IX, transfusion-transmitted infectious disorders, allergic reactions, and thrombotic complications with the use of factor IX because it contains activated coagulation factors.

The most common problem with acute management is starting factor replacement therapy too late and stopping it too soon. Generally, minor bleeding episodes should be treated for at least 72 hours. Surgery and traumatic injuries may need support for 10 to 14 days. In the long term, development of inhibitors to the factor products has occurred and requires individualized expert patient management.

Nursing Management

Because of the hereditary nature of hemophilia, referral for genetic counseling is essential when considering preventive measures. Counseling is especially important since persons with hemophilia are living into adulthood.

Interventions are related primarily to controlling the bleeding and include the following:

H

1. Stop the topical bleeding as quickly as possible by applying
    direct pressure or ice, packing the area with Gelfoam or
    fibrin foam, and applying topical hemostatic agents, such as
    thrombin.
2. Administer the specific coagulation factor concentrate as
    ordered.
3. When joint bleeding occurs, it is important to totally rest the
    involved joint to prevent crippling deformities from hemar-
    throsis. The joint may be packed in ice. Analgesics (e.g.,
    acetaminophen, codeine) are given to reduce severe pain;
    aspirin and aspirin-containing compounds should never be
    used. As soon as bleeding ceases, encourage mobilization of
    the affected area through range-of-motion (ROM) exercises
    and physical therapy. Weight bearing is avoided until all
    swelling has resolved and muscle strength has returned.
4. Manage life-threatening complications that may develop as
    a result of hemorrhage. Examples include prevention or
    treatment of airway obstruction from hemorrhage into the
    neck and pharynx, as well as early assessment and treatment
    of intracranial bleeding.

▼ **Patient and Family Teaching**

Quality and length of life may be significantly affected by the
patient's knowledge of the illness and how to live with it. The
nurse must provide ongoing assessment of the patient's adaptation
to the illness.

- The patient with hemophilia must be taught that immediate
  medical attention is required for severe pain or swelling of
  a muscle or joint that restricts movement or inhibits sleep
  and for a head injury, swelling in the neck or mouth, abdominal pain, hematuria, melena, and skin wounds in need of
  suturing.
- Daily oral hygiene must be performed without causing
  trauma.
- The patient should understand how to prevent injuries. The
  patient can learn to participate in noncontact sports (e.g.,
  golf) and wear gloves when doing household chores to
  prevent cuts or abrasions from knives, hammers, and other
  tools.
- The patient should wear a Medic-Alert tag to ensure that
  health care providers know about the hemophilia in case of
  an accident.
- The patient needs information about routine follow-up care,
  and compliance with scheduled visits must be assessed.
- A reliable person can be taught to self-administer some of
  the factor replacement therapies at home.

HEMORRHOIDS

Description
Hemorrhoids are dilated hemorrhoidal veins that may be internal (occurring above the internal sphincter) or external (occurring outside the external sphincter).

Pathophysiology
Hemorrhoids are thought to develop as a result of shearing forces during defecation. This force damages supporting muscles. When supporting tissues in the anal canal weaken, usually as a result of straining at defecation, the venules become dilated. In addition, blood flow through the veins of the hemorrhoidal plexus is impaired. Hemorrhoids may be precipitated by many factors, including pregnancy, prolonged constipation, straining in an effort to defecate, heavy lifting, prolonged standing and sitting, and portal hypertension (as found in cirrhosis).

Clinical Manifestations
Classic symptoms of hemorrhoids include bleeding, anal pruritus, prolapse, and pain.
- *Internal hemorrhoids* may be asymptomatic, but when they become constricted, pain occurs. Internal hemorrhoids can bleed, resulting in blood on toilet paper after defecation or blood on the outside of the stool. The patient may report a chronic, dull aching discomfort, particularly when hemorrhoids have prolapsed.
- *External hemorrhoids* are reddish blue and seldom bleed or cause pain unless a vein ruptures. Blood clots in external hemorrhoids cause pain and inflammation and are described as thrombosed. External hemorrhoids cause intermittent pain, pain on palpation, itching, and burning. Patients also report bleeding associated with defecation. Constipation or diarrhea can aggravate these symptoms.

Diagnostic Studies
Hemorrhoids are diagnosed by visual inspection, digital examination, anoscopy, or sigmoidoscopy.

Collaborative Care
Therapy is directed toward the causes of the condition and the patient's symptoms. A high-fiber diet and increased fluid intake prevent constipation and reduce straining. Ointments, creams, suppositories, and impregnated pads that contain antiinflamma-

tory agents (e.g., hydrocortisone) or astringents and anesthetics (e.g., witch hazel, benzocaine, pramoxine) may be used to shrink mucous membranes and relieve discomfort. The use of topical corticosteroids such as hydrocortisone agents should be limited to 1 week or less to prevent side effects such as contact dermatitis and mucosal atrophy. Stool softeners may be ordered to keep stools soft, and sitz baths may help relieve pain.

External hemorrhoids are usually managed by conservative therapy unless they become thrombosed. For internal hemorrhoids one of four nonsurgical approaches (band ligation, infrared coagulation, cryotherapy, laser treatment) can be used. A hemorrhoidectomy (surgical excision of hemorrhoids) is indicated when there is prolapse, excessive pain or bleeding, or large hemorrhoids. Surgical removal may be done by cautery, clamp, or excision.

- Hemorrhoids may recur. Occasionally anal strictures develop and dilation is necessary.

Nursing Management

Nursing care includes teaching measures to prevent constipation, avoidance of prolonged standing or sitting, proper use of over-the-counter medications available for hemorrhoidal symptoms, and instructions on when to seek medical care for symptoms (e.g., excessive pain and bleeding, prolapsed hemorrhoids).

- Pain is a common problem after a hemorrhoidectomy. Although the procedure is minor, the pain is severe, and opioids are usually given initially. Topical nitroglycerin preparations may be used to decrease pain and subsequent opioid use.
- Sitz baths (15 to 20 minutes) are started 1 or 2 days after surgery. A sponge ring in the sitz bath helps relieve pressure on the area. Initially the patient should not be left alone because of the possibility of weakness or fainting.
- Packing may be inserted into the rectum to absorb drainage. A T-binder may hold the dressing in place. If packing is inserted, it usually is removed the first or second postoperative day. The nurse should assess for rectal bleeding. The patient may be embarrassed when the dressing is changed, and privacy should be provided.
- A stool softener such as docusate sodium (Colace) is usually ordered the first few postoperative days. If the patient does not have a bowel movement within 2 or 3 days, an oil retention enema is given.
- The patient usually dreads the first bowel movement and often resists the urge to defecate. Pain medication may be given before the bowel movement to reduce discomfort.

▼ **Patient and Family Teaching**
- Patients should be taught the importance of diet, care of the anal area, symptoms of complications (especially bleeding), and avoidance of constipation and straining.
- Sitz baths are recommended for 1 to 2 weeks.
- The physician may order a stool softener to be taken for a time.
- Regular checkups are important in the prevention of any further problems.

HEPATITIS, VIRAL

Description
Hepatitis is an inflammation of the liver. Viral hepatitis is the most common cause of hepatitis. The types of infectious viral hepatitis are A, B, C, D, E, and G. Viral hepatitis is a major public health concern in the United States.
- Approximately 10 million cases of infection with hepatitis A virus (HAV) occur worldwide annually, and nearly 400 million people are infected with hepatitis B virus (HBV).
- Worldwide approximately 170 million people are infected with hepatitis C virus (HCV). HCV accounts for 45% of all cases of chronic viral hepatitis and is the most common liver disease in the United States. Approximately 20% of patients with chronic HCV progress to cirrhosis within 20 years.
- Co-infection of HCV and human immunodeficiency virus (HIV) is increasing. Approximately 40% of HIV-infected patients also have HCV. This high rate of co-infection is primarily related to intravenous (IV) drug use.

Etiology
Viral hepatitis can be caused by one of five viruses: A, B, C, D, and E. Hepatitis G virus has been recently recognized, and its exact role in liver disease has yet to be determined. Other viruses known to damage the liver include cytomegalovirus, Epstein-Barr virus, herpes virus, coxsackievirus, and rubella virus.
- The only definitive way to distinguish the various forms of viral hepatitis is by the presence of the antigens and the subsequent development of antibodies to them. HAV consistently causes outbreaks of hepatitis.
- Approximately 44% of viral hepatitis cases in adults in the United States are hepatitis B, 19% are hepatitis C, and 37% are hepatitis A. Table 48 lists characteristics of hepatitis viruses.

H

Table 48 Characteristics of Hepatitis Viruses

	Incubation Period	Mode of Transmission	Sources of Infection and Spread of Disease	Infectivity
Hepatitis A virus (HAV)	15-50 days (average 28 days)	Fecal-oral (fecal contamination and oral ingestion)	Crowded conditions; poor personal hygiene; poor sanitation; contaminated food, milk, water, and shellfish; persons with subclinical infections; infected food handlers; sexual contact	Most infectious during 2 wk before onset of symptoms; infectious until 1-2 wk after symptoms start
Hepatitis B virus (HBV)	45-180 days (average 56-96 days)	Percutaneous (parenteral)/permucosal exposure to blood or blood products; Sexual contact; Perinatal transmission	Contaminated needles, syringes, and blood products; sexual activity with infected partners; asymptomatic carriers; Tattoo/body piercing with contaminated needles; bites	Before and after symptoms appear; infectious for 4-6 mo; in carriers continues for patient's lifetime

Hepatitis C virus (HCV)	14-180 days (average 56 days)	Percutaneous (parenteral)/permucosal exposure to blood or blood products High-risk sexual contact Perinatal contact	Blood and blood products, needles and syringes, sexual activity with infected partners	1-2 wk before symptoms; continues during clinical course; 75%-85% develop chronic hepatitis
Hepatitis D virus (HDV)	2-26 wk HBV must precede HDV; chronic carriers of HBV always at risk	Can cause infection only when HBV is present; routes of transmission same as for HBV	Same as HBV	Blood infectious at all stages of HDV infection
Hepatitis E virus (HEV)	15-64 days (average 26-42 days in different epidemics)	Fecal-oral Outbreaks associated with contaminated water supply in developing countries	Contaminated water; poor sanitation; found in Asia, Africa, and Mexico; not common in the United States and Canada	Not known; may be similar to HAV

H

- Infection with HAV or HBV provides immunity to that virus (homologous immunity). However, the patient can still develop another type of viral hepatitis, and patients with hepatitis C can be reinfected with another strain of hepatitis C. For a more complete description of each hepatitis virus, see Lewis and others, *Medical-Surgical Nursing,* edition 7, pp. 1088 to 1091.

Pathophysiology

The pathophysiologic changes in the various types of viral hepatitis are similar. Hepatitis involves widespread inflammation of liver tissue.

- During acute infection, liver damage is mediated by cytotoxic cytokines and natural killer cells that cause lysis of infected hepatocytes. Liver cell damage results in hepatic cell necrosis. There are proliferation and enlargement of Kupffer cells. Inflammation of the periportal areas may interrupt bile flow. Cholestasis may occur.
- Liver cells regenerate in an orderly manner, and if no complications occur, they should resume their normal appearance and function.
- The antigen-antibody complexes between the virus and its corresponding antibody form a circulating immune complex in the early phases of hepatitis. The circulating immune complexes activate the complement system. Manifestations of this activation are rash, angioedema, arthritis, fever, and malaise. Cryoglobulinema (abnormal proteins found in the blood), glomerulonephritis, and vasculitis have also been found secondary to immune complex disease.

Clinical Manifestations

A large number of patients have no symptoms. Manifestations of viral hepatitis may be classified into acute and chronic phases.

- The acute phase usually lasts 1 to 4 months. During the incubation period, symptoms may include malaise, anorexia, fatigue, nausea, occasional vomiting, and right upper quadrant abdominal discomfort. The anorexia can be severe, and other symptoms may include headache, low-grade fever, arthralgias, and skin rashes. Physical examination may reveal hepatomegaly, lymphadenopathy, and sometimes splenomegaly. This is the period of maximal infectivity for hepatitis A.
- The acute phase may be *icteric* (symptomatic, including jaundice) or anicteric. Jaundice results when bilirubin diffuses into the tissues. The urine may darken because of excess bilirubin being excreted by the kidneys. If conju-

gated bilirubin cannot flow out of the liver because of bile duct obstruction, stools will be light or clay colored. Pruritus, caused by bile salts beneath the skin, may result if cholestasis is present.

- When jaundice occurs, the fever usually subsides, but the gastrointestinal (GI) symptoms usually remain and fatigue may continue.
- The convalescence following the acute phase begins as jaundice is disappearing and lasts weeks to months, with an average of 2 to 4 months. During this period the patient's major complaints are malaise and easy fatigability. Hepatomegaly remains for several weeks. Relapses may occur, and the disappearance of jaundice does not mean the patient has totally recovered.

Additional considerations include:

- Many HBV infections and the majority of HCV infections result in chronic (lifelong) viral infection. Some patients may be asymptomatic, but others may have intermittent or ongoing malaise, fatigue, myalgias, arthralgias, and hepatomegaly.
- Not all patients with viral hepatitis have jaundice. This is referred to as *anicteric hepatitis*. A high percentage of persons with HAV are anicteric and do not have symptoms.
- There is slight variation in manifestations between the types of hepatitis. In hepatitis A the onset is more acute and the symptoms are usually mild, flulike manifestations. In hepatitis B the onset is more insidious and the symptoms are usually more severe. In hepatitis C the majority of cases are mild or asymptomatic, but HCV has a high rate of persistence and often leads to chronic liver disease.

Complications

Most patients with acute viral hepatitis recover completely with no complications. The overall mortality rate is 1%.

Complications include fulminant hepatic failure, chronic hepatitis, cirrhosis of the liver (see Cirrhosis, p. 131), and hepatocellular carcinoma (see Liver Cancer, p. 386).

It is not known what factors contribute to the persistence of the virus in some patients, causing chronic disease. HAV does not cause chronic hepatitis. Chronic HBV is identified by the persistence of hepatitis B surface antigen (HBsAg) for longer than 6 months. Chronic HBV and HCV are risk factors for the development of cirrhosis and hepatocellular carcinoma.

- *Fulminant viral hepatitis* is a clinical syndrome that results in severe impairment or necrosis of liver cells and potential liver failure.

- Fulminant viral hepatitis develops in a small percentage of patients. The disorder may occur as a complication of hepatitis B or C, particularly hepatitis B accompanied by infection with hepatitis D virus (HDV). Toxic reactions to drugs and congenital metabolic disorders may also cause fulminant hepatitis and liver failure. Hepatocellular failure with death usually occurs.

Diagnostic Studies

- Many of the liver function tests show significant abnormalities.
- Physical assessment reveals hepatic tenderness, hepatomegaly, and splenomegaly.
- Liver biopsy allows for histologic examination of liver cells in chronic hepatitis.
- Table 49 presents the serologic tests for the different types of viral hepatitis.

Collaborative Care

There is no specific treatment for acute viral hepatitis. Most patients can be managed at home. Emphasis is on measures to rest the body and assist the liver in regenerating. Adequate nutrients and rest seem to be most beneficial for healing and liver cell regeneration. Dietary emphasis is on a well-balanced diet that the patient can tolerate.

- Rest reduces liver metabolic demands and promotes cell regeneration. The degree of rest ordered depends on symptom severity; usually alternating periods of activity with rest is adequate.

Drug Therapy

There are no specific drug therapies for the treatment of acute viral hepatitis. Supportive drug therapy may include antiemetics, such as dimenhydrinate (Dramamine) or trimethobenzamide (Tigan).

Drug therapy for chronic HBV is focused on decreasing the viral load, serum levels of aspartate aminotransferase (AST) and alanine aminotransferase (ALT), the rate of disease progression, and the rate of drug-resistant HBV. Two categories of drugs available for suppressing viral activity and decreasing viral load in patients with HBV include α-interferon and nucleoside analogs.

- α-Interferon interferes with viral replication and is available in long-acting preparations (Pegasys, PEG-Intron). The long-acting preparations are administered subcutaneously once per week and are preferred to conventional α-interferon that must be injected. One third of the patients receiving α-interferon will have a significant reduction of

Table 49	Hepatitis Serology

Virus	Tests	Significance
A	Anti-HAV IgM	Acute infection
	Anti-HAV IgG	Previous infection and long-term immunity or immunization
B	HBsAg (hepatitis B surface antigen)	Current infection (but not necessarily acute)*; positive in chronic carriers
	Anti-HBs (antibody to surface antigen)	Indicates previous infection with hepatitis B or immunization; marker of response to vaccine
	HBeAg (hepatitis B e antigen)	Indicates high infectivity; present in acute, active infection
	Anti-HBe (antibody to e antigen)	Indicates previous infection
	HBcAg (hepatitis B core antigen)	Ongoing infection with hepatitis B
	Anti-HBc IgM	Acute infection*
	Anti-HBc IgG (antibody to HB core antigen)	Indicates previous infection or ongoing infection with hepatitis B; does not appear after vaccination
	HBV DNA	Indicates active ongoing viral replication; best indicator of viral replication
	HBV genotyping	Indicates the genotype of HBV
C	Anti-HCV (antibody to hepatitis C)	Marker for acute or chronic infection with HCV
	Enzyme immunoassay (EIA)	Used in initial screening for HCV
	Recombinant immunoblot assay (RIBA)	More sensitive antibody test
	HCV RNA (RNA polymerase chain reaction [PCR] assay)	Indicates active ongoing viral replication
	HCV genotyping	Indicates the genotype of HCV
D	Anti-HDV	Present in past or current infection with hepatitis D
	HDV Ag	Present within a few days after infection

H

A, Hepatitis A virus (HAV); Ag, antigen; B, hepatitis B virus (HBV); C, hepatitis C virus (HCV); D, hepatitis D virus (HDV); DNA, deoxyribonucleic acid; IgG, immunoglobulin G; IgM, immunoglobulin M; RNA, ribonucleic acid.
* If positive HBsAg and anti-HBc IgM, it indicates the presence of acute infection.

serum HBV DNA levels, normalization of ALT levels, and
loss of HBV e antigen (HBeAg).
- Nucleoside analogs suppress HBV replication by inhibiting
  viral DNA synthesis. The preparations used in the treatment
  of chronic HVB when there is evidence of active viral replication include lamivudine (Epivir), adefovir (Hepsera),
  entecavir (Baraclude), and telbivudine (Tyzeka). The
  drugs are taken orally and can reduce viral load and liver
  damage. However, seroconversion (loss of HBeAg) is low,
  and the majority of patients return to pretreatment levels
  of HBV DNA and liver inflammation when treatment is
  stopped.

Drug therapy for hepatitis C is directed at reducing the viral
load, decreasing progression of the disease, and promoting seroconversion. Treatment for HCV includes a combination of ribavi-
rin (Rebetol, Copegus) and long-acting α-interferon (PEG-Intron,
Pegasys).

Drug therapy is also used for prevention of HAV and HBV
infection.

Both hepatitis A vaccine and immune globulin (IG) are used
for prevention of hepatitis A. The vaccine is used for preexposure
prophylaxis, and IG can be used either before or after exposure.
- IG provides temporary (6 to 8 weeks) passive immunity and
  is effective for preventing hepatitis A if given within 1 to
  2 weeks after exposure.
- IG is recommended for persons who do not have anti-HAV
  antibodies and are exposed because of close contact with
  persons who have HAV.
- Although IG may not prevent infection in all persons, it may
  modify the illness to a subclinical infection.
- Twinrix, a combined HAV and HBV vaccine, is available
  for persons over the age of 18 years.

Immunization with hepatitis B vaccine is the most effective
method of preventing HBV infection.
- For postexposure prophylaxis, the vaccine and hepatitis B
  immune globulin (HBIG) are used. HBIG contains antibodies to HBV and confers temporary passive immunity. HBIG
  is recommended for postexposure prophylaxis in cases of
  needle stick, mucous membrane contact, or sexual exposure
  and for infants born to mothers who are positive for HBsAg.

Nutritional Therapy
An important measure in assisting hepatocytes to regenerate is
adequate nutrition. No special diet is required. However, a diet
high in carbohydrates and proteins with a low fat content is usually
recommended.

Nursing Management

Goals

The patient with viral hepatitis will have relief of discomfort, be able to resume normal activities, and return to normal liver function without complications.

See NCP 44-1 for the patient with viral hepatitis, Lewis and others, *Medical-Surgical Nursing,* edition 7, pp. 1097 to 1098.

Nursing Diagnoses

- Imbalanced nutrition: less than body requirements
- Activity intolerance
- Ineffective therapeutic regimen management

Nursing Interventions

Viral hepatitis is a community health problem. The nurse must assume a significant role in the control and prevention of this disease.

Hepatitis A. Vaccination is the best protection against HAV. Preventive measures include personal and environmental hygiene and health education to promote good sanitation.

Hand washing is essential and is probably the most important precaution. Health teaching should include careful hand washing after bowel movements and before eating.

Hepatitis B. Vaccination is the best protection against HBV. Control and prevention of hepatitis B also focus on the identification of possible exposure through percutaneous and sexual transmission.

- Good hygienic practices, including hand washing and the use of gloves when expecting contact with blood, are important. A condom is advised for sexual intercourse, and the partner should be vaccinated. Razors, toothbrushes, and other personal items should not be shared. Close contacts of the patient with hepatitis B who are HBsAg negative and antibody negative should be vaccinated.

Hepatitis C. There currently is no vaccine available. Primary measures to prevent HCV transmission are similar to those of HBV, including the screening of blood, organ, and tissue donors; use of infection control measures; and modification of high-risk sexual behavior.

During acute intervention, promoting good nutrition and promoting rest are major goals.

- The patient's response to rest and activity should be assessed. Diversional activities may help. Psychologic and emotional rest is as essential as physical rest.
- The nurse should try to determine whether there is something that appeals to the patient with anorexia. Small, frequent meals may be preferable to three large ones and may also help prevent nausea.

- The patient should be assessed for patterns of jaundice and manifestations indicative of complications, including bleeding tendencies with increasing prothrombin time values, symptoms of encephalopathy, or markedly abnormal liver function tests.

▼ **Patient and Family Teaching**

- Teach the patient and family about preventive measures and how to prevent transmission to other family members. The patient should know what symptoms need to be reported to the physician.
- Stress the importance of regular follow-up visits for at least 1 year after the diagnosis of hepatitis. Because relapses are fairly common with hepatitis B and C, the patient should be instructed about the symptoms of recurrence. Alcohol should be avoided in patients with chronic hepatitis B and C.
- A patient who remains positive for HBsAg is a chronic carrier and should never be a blood donor.
- The patient who is receiving α-interferon for the treatment of hepatitis B or C requires education regarding the medication. α-Interferon is administered intramuscularly or subcutaneously; thus the patient or a family member needs to be taught how to administer the drug.

HERNIA

Description

A hernia is a protrusion of a viscus through an abnormal opening or a weakened area in the wall of the cavity in which it is normally contained. A hernia may occur in any part of the body, but it usually occurs within the abdominal cavity.

- Hernias that easily return to the abdominal cavity are called *reducible*. The hernia can be reduced manually or may reduce spontaneously when the person lies down.
- If the hernia cannot be placed back into the abdominal cavity, it is known as *irreducible* or *incarcerated*. In this situation intestinal flow may be obstructed. When the hernia is irreducible and intestinal flow and blood supply are obstructed, the hernia is *strangulated*. The result is an acute intestinal obstruction.

Types

The types of hernias include inguinal, femoral, umbilical, and ventral (incisional).

- *Inguinal hernia* is the most common type of hernia and occurs at the point of weakness in the abdominal wall where the spermatic cord in men and the round ligament in women emerge. When the protrusion escapes through the inguinal ring and follows the spermatic cord or round ligament, it is termed an indirect hernia. When it escapes through the posterior inguinal wall, it is a direct hernia. An inguinal hernia is more common in men.
- *Femoral hernia* occurs when there is a protrusion through the femoral ring into the femoral canal. It becomes strangulated easily and occurs more frequently in women.
- *Umbilical hernia* occurs when the rectus muscle is weak (as with obesity) or the umbilical opening fails to close after birth.
- *Ventral,* or *incisional, hernia* is due to a weakness of the abdominal wall at the site of a previous incision. It occurs most commonly in patients who are obese, who have had multiple surgical procedures in the same area, or who have had inadequate wound healing because of poor nutrition or infection.

Clinical Manifestations

A hernia may be readily visible, especially when the person tenses the abdominal muscles. Discomfort may result from tension. If the hernia becomes strangulated, the patient will experience severe pain and symptoms of a bowel obstruction, such as vomiting, cramping abdominal pain, and distention.

Collaborative Care

Surgery is the treatment of choice for hernias and prevents strangulation. Surgical repair of a hernia is known as a *herniorrhaphy.* Repairs are by laparoscopic surgery and are usually an outpatient procedure. The reinforcement of the weakened area with wire, fascia, or mesh is known as a *hernioplasty.* Strangulated hernias are treated immediately with resection of the involved area or a temporary colostomy so that necrosis and gangrene do not occur.

Nursing Management

Some patients with hernias may wear a truss, which is a pad placed over the hernia and held in place with a belt. The truss is worn to keep the hernia from protruding. If a patient wears a truss, the nurse should check for skin irritation caused by continual rubbing of the truss.

After a hernia repair, the patient may have difficulty voiding. Therefore the nurse should observe for a distended bladder.

- Scrotal edema is a painful complication after inguinal hernia repair. A scrotal support with application of an ice bag may help relieve pain and edema.
- Coughing is not encouraged, but deep breathing and turning should be done. If the patient needs to cough or sneeze, the incision should be splinted during coughing, and sneezing should be done with mouth open.
- After discharge the patient may be restricted from heavy lifting or physical activities for 6 to 8 weeks.

HERPES, GENITAL

Description

Two different strains of herpes simplex virus (HSV) cause infection.

- HSV type 1 (HSV-1) generally causes infection above the waist, involving the gingivae, dermis, upper respiratory tract, and central nervous system (CNS).
- HSV type 2 (HSV-2) most frequently involves the genital tract and perineum (i.e., locations below the waist).

However, either strain can cause disease on the mouth or genitals. When a person is infected with HSV, the virus usually persists within the individual for life. It is estimated that more than 50 million people are infected with genital herpes.

- Most people (80%) infected with HSV are asymptomatic or unaware of their infection.

Pathophysiology

The HSV enters through the mucous membranes or breaks in the skin during contact with an infected person. HSV then reproduces inside the cell and spreads to surrounding cells. It next enters the peripheral or autonomic nerve endings and ascends to the sensory or autonomic nerve ganglion, where it often becomes dormant. Viral reactivation may occur when the virus travels down to the initial site of infection. Additional sexual contact is not necessary for a recurrence of HSV infection. The recurrent infection produces a syndrome similar to, but less intense than, the primary infection.

Because HSV is readily inactivated at room temperature and by drying, airborne spread and fomite spread have not been documented as significant means of transmission. There does not appear to be any period of time when viral transmission is not possible once primary HSV-2 infection has occurred. Women with recurrent symptomatic genital herpes shed the virus up to 1% of the time even when no visible lesions are present.

Clinical Manifestations

A patient with a primary (initial) HSV-2 infection initially experiences burning or tingling at the site of inoculation. Vesicular lesions, which may occur on the penis, scrotum, vulva, perineum, perianal region, vagina, or cervix, contain large quantities of infectious viral particles. The lesions rupture and form shallow, moist ulcerations. Finally, crusting and epithelialization of the erosions occur.

- Primary infections tend to be associated with local inflammation and pain accompanied by systemic manifestations of fever, headache, malaise, myalgia, and regional lymphadenopathy.
- Urination may be painful from urine touching active lesions. Urinary retention may occur as a result of HSV urethritis or cystitis. A purulent vaginal discharge may develop with HSV cervicitis.
- Primary lesions are generally present for 17 to 20 days.
- The duration of symptoms is longer, with a greater frequency of complications in women.

After the first infection, HSV-2 establishes latency in the sacral ganglia and may be reactivated periodically. Recurrent attacks occur in about 50% to 80% of all persons during the year after the primary episode. Stress, fatigue, menses, and sunburn tend to trigger recurrence. Many patients can predict a recurrence by noticing early symptoms of tingling, burning, and itching at the site where lesions eventually arise. Symptoms of recurrent episodes are less severe, and the unilateral lesions heal within 8 to 12 days. With time, recurrent lesions generally occur less frequently.

Complications

Although most infections are relatively benign, complications of genital herpes may involve the CNS, causing aseptic meningitis and lower motor neuron damage.

- Neuron damage may result in atonic bladder, impotence, and constipation. The most common complication is autoinoculation of the virus to extragenital sites such as fingers (whitlow), lips, and breasts.

Diagnostic Studies

- Diagnosis is usually based on the patient's symptoms and history.
- Isolation of the virus by tissue culture from active lesions confirms diagnosis. Cultures are more positive in primary infection versus recurrent infection.

- Type-specific immunoassays for HSV infection test for the presence of antibodies to HSV and determine the presence of a chronic HSV infection.

Collaborative Care
Symptomatic Care. Symptomatic treatment, such as good genital hygiene and wearing of loose-fitting cotton undergarments, should be encouraged. The lesions should be kept clean and dry. To ensure complete drying of the perineal area women may use a hair dryer set on a cool setting. Drying agents such as colloidal oatmeal (Aveeno) and aluminum salts (Burow's solution) may provide relief from the burning and itching.

- Frequent sitz baths may soothe the area and reduce inflammation. Pain may require a local anesthetic, such as lidocaine (Xylocaine), or systemic analgesics, such as codeine and aspirin.
- Barrier forms of contraception, especially condoms, used during asymptomatic periods, decrease the transmission of the disease. When lesions are present, the patient should avoid sexual activity altogether because even barrier protection is not satisfactory in eliminating disease transmission.

Drug Therapy. Three antiviral agents are available for the treatment of HSV: acyclovir (Zovirax), valacyclovir (Valtrex), and famciclovir (Famvir). These drugs inhibit herpetic viral replication and are prescribed for primary and recurrent infections. They also are used to suppress frequent recurrences (more than six episodes per year). Although not a cure, these drugs shorten the duration of viral shedding and healing time of genital lesions and reduce outbreaks by 75%. Continued use of oral acyclovir for up to 5 years is safe and effective. Acyclovir ointment appears to have no clinical benefit in the treatment of recurrent lesions, either in speed of healing or in resolution of pain. Intravenous (IV) acyclovir is reserved for severe or life-threatening infections.

Nursing Management: Genital Herpes
See Sexually Transmitted Diseases, p. 562.

HIATAL HERNIA

Description
Hiatal hernia is herniation of a portion of the stomach into the esophagus through an opening (or hiatus) in the diaphragm. It is

also referred to as diaphragmatic hernia or esophageal hernia. Hiatal hernias are common in older adults and occur more frequently in women than in men.

Hiatal hernias are classified into two types (Fig. 5).

- A *sliding hernia* occurs at the junction of the stomach and esophagus and is located above the hiatus of the diaphragm. It "slides" into the thoracic cavity when the patient is supine and usually goes back into the abdominal cavity when the patient is standing upright. This is the most common type of hiatal hernia.
- A *paraesophageal* or *rolling hernia* occurs at the esophagogastric junction where the fundus and greater curvature of the stomach roll up through the diaphragm to form a pocket alongside the esophagus.

Pathophysiology
The actual cause of hiatal hernia is unknown. Many factors contribute to the development of hiatal hernia, including structural changes, such as weakening of the muscles in the diaphragm around the esophagogastric opening. Factors that increase intraabdominal pressure, including obesity, pregnancy, ascites, intense physical exertion, and heavy lifting on a continual basis, may also contribute to the development of a hiatal hernia. In some cases, congenital weakness is a contributing factor.

Clinical Manifestations
When present, signs and symptoms of hiatal hernia are similar to those described for gastroesophageal reflux disease (GERD). Frequently the symptoms mimic gallbladder disease, peptic ulcer disease, and angina.

- Heartburn, especially after a meal or after lying supine, is a common symptom. Bending over may cause a severe burning pain, which is usually relieved by sitting or standing. Large meals, alcohol, and smoking may precipitate pain.
- Nocturnal attacks are common, especially if the person has eaten before lying down.

Complications may include GERD, esophagitis, hemorrhage from erosion, stenosis, ulcerations of the herniated portion of the stomach, strangulation of the hernia, and regurgitation with tracheal aspiration.

Diagnostic Studies
- Barium swallow may show gastric mucosa protrusion through the esophageal hiatus.

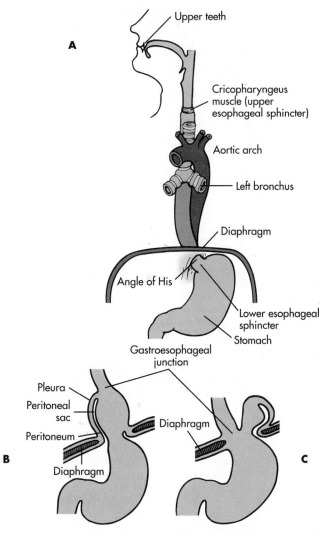

Fig. 5. A, Normal esophagus. **B,** Sliding hiatal hernia. **C,** Rolling or paraesophageal hernia.

- Upper gastrointestinal (GI) endoscopy with biopsy and cytologic analysis determines if lower esophageal sphincter (LES)
  is incompetent and whether gastric reflux is present
- pH of gastric and esophageal secretions may be monitored.
- Esophageal motility (manometry) studies determine pressure
  gradients.

Nursing and Collaborative Management

Conservative management is similar to that described under Gastroesophageal Reflux Disease, including lifestyle modifications
(elimination of constricting garments, avoidance of lifting and
straining, and elimination of alcohol and smoking) and the administration of antacids and antisecretory agents (see Gastroesophageal Reflux Disease, p. 242). Elevation of the bed on 4- to 6-inch
blocks assists gravity in maintaining the stomach in the abdominal
cavity and also helps prevent reflux and tracheal aspiration. If
overweight, the patient is encouraged to lose weight.

The objectives of surgical therapy are to reduce the hernia,
provide an acceptable LES pressure, and prevent movement of the
gastroesophageal junction.

- Surgical approches include reduction of the herniated
  stomach into the abdomen, *herniotomy* (excision of the
  hernia sac), *herniorraphy* (closure of the hiatal defect), an

H

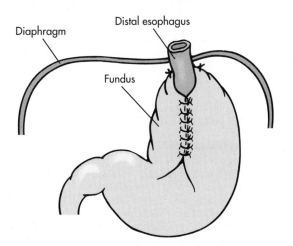

Fig. 6. Nissen fundoplication for repair of hiatal hernia.
Fundus of stomach is wrapped around distal esophagus and sutured
to itself.

antireflux procedure, and *gastropexy* (attachment of the stomach subdiaphragmatically to prevent reherniation).
- Laparoscopically performed Nissen and Toupet fundoplication techniques are the standard antireflux surgeries for hiatal hernia (Fig. 6).

HODGKIN'S LYMPHOMA

Description

Hodgkin's lymphoma, formerly called Hodgkin's disease, is a malignant condition characterized by proliferation of abnormal, giant, multinucleated cells called *Reed-Sternberg cells,* which are located in the lymph nodes. The disease makes up 12% of all lymphomas and has a bimodal age-specific incidence, occurring most frequently in persons from 15 to 35 years old and over 50 years old. In adults, it is twice as prevalent in men as in women, and its prevalence is increased among patients with human immunodeficiency virus infection.

Pathophysiology

Although the cause of Hodgkin's lymphoma remains unknown, several key factors are thought to play a role in its development. The main interacting factors include infection with the Epstein-Barr virus, genetic predisposition, and exposure to occupational toxins.

In Hodgkin's lymphoma the normal structure of the lymph nodes is destroyed by hyperplasia of monocytes and macrophages. The disease is believed to arise in a single location (it originates in the lymph nodes in 90% of patients) and then spread along adjacent lymphatics. It eventually infiltrates other organs, especially the lungs, spleen, and liver. In about two thirds of patients the cervical lymph nodes are the first to be affected.

Clinical Manifestations

The initial sign is most often an enlargement of the cervical, axillary, or inguinal lymph nodes. The enlarged nodes are not painful unless pressure is exerted on adjacent nerves.
- The patient may note weight loss, fatigue, weakness, fever, chills, tachycardia, or night sweats. A group of initial findings, including fever, night sweats, and weight loss (referred to as *B symptoms*), correlates with a worse prognosis.
- Generalized pruritus without skin lesions may develop. Cough, dyspnea, stridor, and dysphagia may all reflect mediastinal node involvement.

- In more advanced disease there is hepatomegaly and splenomegaly. Anemia results from increased destruction as
  well as decreased production of erythrocytes. Intrathoracic
  involvement may lead to superior vena cava syndrome.
  Enlarged retroperitoneal nodes may cause palpable abdominal masses or interfere with renal function.
- Jaundice may result from liver involvement.
- Spinal cord compression leading to paraplegia may occur
  with extradural involvement.

Diagnostic Studies

- Peripheral blood analysis often reveals microcytic hypochro-
  mic anemia; neutrophilic leukocytosis (15,000 to 28,000/µl
  [15 to 28×10^9/L]), which may be associated with lymphopenia; and an increased platelet count.
- Other blood studies may show hypoferremia caused by excessive iron uptake by the liver and spleen, elevated alkaline
  phosphatase from liver and bone involvement, hypercalcemia
  from bone involvement, and hypoalbuminemia.
- Excisional lymph node biopsy offers a definitive diagnosis. If
  removed, the node is examined histologically for the presence
  of Reed-Sternberg cells.
- Bone marrow biopsy is performed as an important aspect of
  staging.
- Computed tomography (CT) or magnetic resonance imaging
  (MRI) scans are used as initial staging tools. Positron emission
  tomography (PET) scans may show increased uptake of carbohydrate by cancer cells, and concurrent CT scans may identify
  masses such as mediastinal lymphadenopathy, renal displacement caused by retroperitoneal node enlargement, abdominal
  lymph node enlargement, and liver, spleen, bone, and brain
  infiltration.

Collaborative Care

Treatment decisions are made based on the clinical stage of the
disease. The standard of chemotherapy is the ABVD regimen:
doxorubicin (Adriamycin), bleomycin, vinblastine, and dacarbazine given for two to eight cycles of treatment depending on
disease stage and prognosis. The role of radiation as a supplement
to chemotherapy varies depending on site of disease and the presence of resistant disease after chemotherapy.

   Intensive chemotherapy with or without the use of autologous
or allogeneic hematopoietic stem cell transplantation (HSCT)
and hematopoietic growth factors is the treatment of choice for
advanced, refractory, or relapsed Hodgkin's lymphoma.

Nursing Management

Nursing care for Hodgkin's lymphoma is largely based on managing problems related to the disease, such as pain, and side effects of therapy, such as pancytopenia.

- Because the survival of patients with Hodgkin's lymphoma depends on their response to treatment, supporting the patient through the immunosuppressive state is extremely important.
- Psychosocial considerations are just as important as they are with leukemia (see Leukemia, p. 380). Although the prognosis for Hodgkin's lymphoma is better than that for many forms of cancer or leukemia, patients must still be helped to deal with the physical, psychologic, social, and spiritual consequences of their disease.
- Evaluation of patients for long-term effects of therapy is important because delayed consequences of the disease and treatment, such as secondary malignancies and long-term endocrine, cardiac, and pulmonary toxicities, may not be apparent for many years.

HUMAN IMMUNODEFICIENCY VIRUS INFECTION

Description

In 1985 the human immunodeficiency virus (HIV) was identified as the causative agent of a chronic, progressive immune function disorder, the final stage of which is known as acquired immunodeficiency syndrome (AIDS). Today more than 39 million people worldwide are infected with HIV. Although advances in diagnosis and treatment of AIDS have been made over the years, the epidemic continues to grow in marginalized individuals.

Pathophysiology

HIV is a fragile virus. It can be transmitted under specific conditions through infected body fluids, including blood, semen, vaginal secretions, and breast milk. Sexual contact with an infected partner is the most common method of transmission. An HIV-infected individual can transmit HIV to others within a few days of becoming infected. The ability to transmit HIV is lifelong.

HIV is a ribonucleic acid (RNA) virus. RNA viruses are called retroviruses because they replicate in a "backward" manner, going from RNA to deoxyribonucleic acid (DNA). Like all viruses, HIV cannot replicate unless it is in a living cell. HIV infects human cells that have CD4 receptors on their surfaces. These include lymphocytes, monocytes/macrophages, astrocytes, and oligodendrocytes. Immune dysfunction in HIV disease is caused predominantly by destruction of CD4$^+$ T cells (also known as T-helper cells or CD4$^+$ lymphocytes). The major concern related to immune suppression is the development of opportunistic diseases (infections and cancers that occur in immunosuppressed patients that can lead to disability, disease, and death).

Clinical Manifestations

The typical course of untreated HIV infection follows the pattern shown in Fig. 7. It is important to remember that disease progression is highly individualized and that treatment can significantly alter the pattern.

Acute Infection. During acute HIV infection, HIV-specific antibodies are produced (seroconversion) and a flulike syndrome of fever, lymphadenopathy, pharyngitis, headache, malaise, nausea, and/or a diffuse rash may occur.

- Symptoms generally occur 1 to 3 weeks after initial infection and last for 1 to 2 weeks.

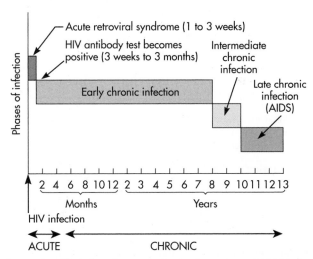

Fig. 7. Timeline for the spectrum of untreated HIV infection. The timeline represents the course of the illness from the time of infection to clinical manifestations of disease.

- During this time a high viral load is noted and CD4$^+$ T-cell counts fall temporarily but quickly return to baseline. In most people these symptoms are mild and may be mistaken for a cold or flu.

Early Chronic Infection. The median interval between untreated HIV infection and a diagnosis of AIDS is about 11 years. During this time CD4$^+$ lymphocyte counts remain above 500 cells/μl (normal or slightly decreased) and the viral load in the blood is low. This phase has been referred to as asymptomatic disease, but fatigue, headache, low-grade fever, night sweats, persistent generalized lymphadenopathy (PGL), and other symptoms often occur.

Intermediate Chronic Infection. When the CD4$^+$ T-cell count drops below 200 to 500 cells/μl, the viral load increases and HIV advances to a more active stage.

- Symptoms include persistent fever, frequent drenching night sweats, chronic diarrhea, headaches, and fatigue. Other problems that may occur include localized infections (oropharyngeal candidiasis, shingles, oral hairy leukoplakia, oral or genital herpes, Kaposi sarcoma), lymphadenopathy, and neurologic manifestations (myopathy and aseptic meningitis).

Late Chronic Infection. A diagnosis of AIDS cannot be made until the HIV-infected patient meets the criteria established by the Centers for Disease Control and Prevention (CDC), which include the development of at least one of these conditions:

1. CD4$^+$ lymphocyte count below 200/μl
2. Development of an opportunistic infection (see Table 15-11, Lewis and others, *Medical-Surgical Nursing*, edition 7, pp. 254 to 255)
3. Development of an opportunistic cancer (e.g., Kaposi sarcoma)
4. Wasting syndrome (defined as a loss of 10% or more of ideal body mass)
5. Development of AIDS dementia complex (ADC)

Diagnostic Studies

The most useful screening tests are those that detect HIV-specific antibodies. The major problem is that there is a median delay of 2 months after infection before antibodies can be detected. This creates a period during which an infected individual will not test positive for HIV antibody. HIV antibody testing can now be done on oral fluids and urine.

Diagnosis of HIV Infection

- Highly sensitive enzyme immunoassay (EIA) detects serum antibodies that bind to HIV antigens.

- Western blot or immunofluorescence assay (IFA) more specifically confirms HIV if a repeat EIA indicates the blood is HIV antibody positive.
- New "rapid" HIV-antibody testing provides highly accurate results within 20 minutes and is strongly recommended by the CDC.

Progression of HIV Infection
- CD4$^+$ T-cell count monitors the progression of the infection.
- Measurements of viral loads provide an assessment of disease progression.
- White blood cell (WBC) count, red blood cell (RBC) count, and platelets decrease with progression of HIV.

Collaborative Care

Management of the patient with HIV infection focuses on monitoring the disease progression and immune function, initiating and monitoring antiretroviral therapy (ART), preventing the development of opportunistic diseases, detecting and treating opportunistic diseases, managing symptoms, preventing or decreasing the complications of treatment, and preventing further transmission of HIV.

Drug Therapy. The goals of drug therapy in HIV infection are to decrease the viral load, maintain or raise CD4$^+$ T-cell counts, and delay the development of HIV-related symptoms and opportunistic diseases.

Drugs currently approved to treat HIV infection include three drug classifications that inhibit the ability of HIV to make a DNA copy early in replication, one drug classification that inhibits the ability of the virus to reproduce in the late stages of replication, and one classification that prevents entry of HIV into the cell (Table 50). Indications for initiation of antiretroviral therapy and adverse effects of the drugs are described in Tables 15-14 and 15-15, Lewis and others, *Medical-Surgical Nursing,* edition 7, pp. 262 to 263.

- Resistance to antiretroviral drugs develops rapidly when they are used alone or taken in inadequate doses. For that reason combinations of three or more antiretroviral drugs prescribed at full strength should be used.
- Many antiretroviral agents cause serious and potentially fatal interactions when used in combination with other commonly used drugs, including over-the-counter drugs and herbal therapies.

Opportunistic diseases associated with HIV can be delayed or prevented through prophylactic interventions, including pneumococcal, influenza, and hepatitis B vaccines, isoniazid (INH) for tuberculosis (TB) if a positive tuberculin skin test is present, trimethoprim-sulfamethoxazole (TMP-SMX) inhalation for

Table 50	Antiretroviral Agents Used to Treat HIV

Mechanism of Action	Drugs
Nucleoside Reverse Transcriptase Inhibitors (NRTIs)	
Insert a piece of DNA into the developing HIV DNA chain, blocking further development of the chain and leaving the new strand of HIV DNA incomplete	zidovudine (AZT, ZDV, Retrovir) didanosine (ddI, Videx, Videx EC [time-released]) stavudine (d4T, Zerit) lamivudine (3TC, Epivir) abacavir (Ziagen) emtricitabine (FTC, Emtriva) Combivir (lamivudine and zidovudine combination) Epzicom (lamivudine and abacavir combination)
Nonnucleoside Reverse Transcriptase Inhibitors (NNRTIs)	
Combine with reverse transcriptase enzyme to block the process needed to convert HIV RNA into HIV DNA	nevirapine (Viramune) delavirdine (Rescriptor) efavirenz (Sustiva)
Nucleotide Reverse Transcriptase Inhibitors (NtRTIs)	
Inhibit the action of reverse transcriptase	tenofovir DF (Viread) Truvada (tenofovir and emtricitabine combination)
Protease Inhibitors (PIs)	
Prevent the protease enzyme from cutting HIV proteins into the proper lengths needed to allow viable virions to assemble and bud out from the cell membrane	saquinavir (Fortovase, Invirase) indinavir (Crixivan) ritonavir (Norvir) nelfinavir (Viracept) amprenavir (Agenerase) Kaletra (lopinavir and ritonavir combination) atazanavir (Reyataz) fosamprenavir (Lexiva) tipranavir (Aptivus) darunavir (Prezista)
Entry Inhibitors	
Prevent binding of HIV to cells, thus preventing entry of HIV into cells where replication would occur	enfuvirtide (Fuzeon)
Combination Therapy	
Combined NtRTI, NRTI, and NNRTI mechanisms	Atripla (tenofovir, emcitrabine, efavirenz combination)

DNA, Deoxyribonucleic acid; *HIV*, human immunodeficiency virus; *RNA*, ribonucleic acid.

Pneumocystis jiroveci and toxoplasma, and rifabutin (Mycobutin) for *Mycobacterium avium* complex. See Table 15-9, Lewis and others, *Medical-Surgical Nursing,* edition 7, p. 249 for a complete description.

Nursing Management

Goals

The patient with HIV infection will adhere to drug regimens; promote a healthy lifestyle that includes avoiding exposure to additional sexual and blood-borne diseases; protect others from HIV; maintain or develop healthy and supportive relationships; maintain activities and productivity; explore spiritual issues; come to terms with issues related to disease, disability, and death; and cope with the frequent symptoms caused by HIV and its treatments. Goals are individualized and change as new treatment protocols develop and/or as HIV disease progresses.

Nursing Diagnoses

- Acute pain
- Anxiety
- Fear
- Imbalanced nutrition: less than body requirements
- Disturbed thought processes
- Ineffective coping
- Diarrhea

Nursing Interventions

The initial nursing focus is to prevent HIV infection. Currently, education and behavioral changes are the only effective prevention tools. The goal is for the person to develop safer, healthier, and less risky behaviors than are currently being used, especially decreasing risks related to sexual intercourse and drug use.

- Any individual who is at risk for HIV should be encouraged to be tested. HIV testing should be accompanied by pretest and posttest counseling.
- Early intervention after detection of HIV infection can promote health and delay or limit disability. It should focus on early detection of symptoms, opportunistic diseases, and psychosocial problems.

Useful interventions for HIV-infected patients include nutritional support; moderation or elimination of alcohol, tobacco, and drug use; keeping recommended vaccines up to date; adequate rest, exercise, and stress reduction; avoiding exposure to new infectious agents; mental health counseling; and getting involved in support groups and community activities.

- Facilitating empowerment is particularly important because the individual with HIV infection often experiences multiple losses, including an overwhelming feeling of loss of control.

- During acute exacerbations of opportunistic diseases or adverse effects of treatment, symptomatic care may include education and treatment for diarrhea, pneumonia, fatigue, wasting syndrome, and AIDS-dementia complex.
- The focus of terminal care is patient comfort, facilitation of emotional and spiritual issues, and helping significant others deal with grief and loss.

▼ **Patient and Family Teaching**

HIV education emphasizes prevention and risk-reducing activities. Teaching that outlines the proper use of male and female condoms and the proper use of drug-using equipment promotes risk reduction (see Tables 15-19, 15-20, and 15-21, Lewis and others, *Medical-Surgical Nursing,* edition 7, pp. 262 to 263). For an infected patient, teaching is directed toward health promotion, managing the problems caused by HIV infection, and maximizing the patient's quality of life.

- Teach the patient and family about symptoms to report to ensure early recognition and treatment (see Table 15-23, Lewis and others, *Medical-Surgical Nursing,* edition 7, p. 265 for a patient teaching guide).
- Teach advantages and disadvantages of new treatments, including drug therapy, dangers of nonadherence to therapeutic regimens, how and when to take each medication, drug interactions to avoid, and side effects that need to be reported to the primary care provider. Tables 15-21 and 15-23, Lewis and others, *Medical-Surgical Nursing,* edition 7, pp. 263 and 265 provide guidance for patient teaching in these areas.
- Teach energy conservation measures and the use of assistive devices to increase safety and decrease fatigue.
- Discuss infection control measures with the patient, family, and visitors.
- Provide information about support groups and community resources.

HUNTINGTON'S DISEASE

Description

Huntington's disease (HD) is a genetically transmitted, autosomal dominant disorder that affects both men and women of all races. The offspring of a person with this disease have a 50% risk of inheriting it. The onset is usually between 30 and 50 years. Like Parkinson's disease, the pathology of HD involves the basal ganglia and the extrapyramidal system. Instead of a deficiency of dopamine (DA), however, HD involves a deficiency of the neurotransmitters acetylcholine (ACh) and γ-aminobutyric acid (GABA). The net effect is an excess of DA, which leads to symptoms opposite those of Parkinson's disease.

Clinical manifestations are characterized by abnormal and excessive involuntary movements (chorea). These are writhing, twisting movements of the face, limbs, and body that get worse as the disease progresses.

- Facial movements involving speech, chewing, and swallowing are affected; this may cause aspiration and malnutrition. The gait deteriorates, and ambulation eventually becomes impossible. Perhaps the most devastating deterioration is in mental functioning, including symptoms of intellectual decline, emotional lability, and psychotic behavior.
- Death usually occurs 10 to 20 years after the onset of symptoms.

Diagnosis in the past was based on family history and clinical symptoms. However, since the gene for HD has been discovered, one can now be tested for the presence of the gene.

Because there is no cure, collaborative care is palliative. Antipsychotic, antidepressant, and antichorea medications are prescribed and have some benefit. However, they do not alter the course of the disease. This disease presents a great challenge to health care professionals.

The goal of nursing care is to provide the most comfortable environment possible for the patient and family by maintaining physical safety, treating physical symptoms, and providing emotional and psychologic support.

- Because of the choreic movements, caloric requirements are high. Patients may require as many as 4000 to 5000 kcal/day to maintain body weight. As the disease progresses, meeting caloric needs becomes a greater challenge when the patient has difficulty swallowing and holding the head still. Depression and mental deterioration can also compromise nutritional intake.

HYPERPARATHYROIDISM

Description

Hyperparathyroidism is a condition involving increased secretion of parathyroid hormone (PTH). PTH helps regulate calcium and phosphate levels by stimulating bone resorption, renal tubular reabsorption of calcium, and activation of vitamin D. Thus over-secretion of PTH is associated with increased serum calcium levels.

Hyperparathyroidism is classified as primary, secondary, or tertiary.

- *Primary hyperparathyroidism* is due to an increased secretion of PTH leading to disorders of calcium, phosphate, and bone metabolism. The most common cause is a benign adenoma in the parathyroid gland. Previous head and neck radiation may be a predisposing factor for a parathyroid adenoma.
- *Secondary hyperparathyroidism* is a compensatory response to conditions that induce or cause hypocalcemia, the main stimulus of PTH secretion. These conditions include vitamin D deficiencies, malabsorption, chronic renal failure, and hyperphosphatemia.
- *Tertiary hyperparathyroidism* occurs when there is hyperplasia of the parathyroid glands and a loss of negative feedback from circulating calcium levels. This causes autonomous secretion of PTH even with normal calcium levels. It is observed in the patient who has had a kidney transplant after a long period of dialysis treatment for chronic kidney disease.

Pathophysiology

Excessive levels of circulating PTH usually lead to hypercalcemia and hypophosphatemia, creating a multisystem effect (see Table 50-11, Lewis and others, *Medical-Surgical Nursing,* edition 7, p. 1310).

- In the bones, decreased bone density, cyst formation, and general weakness can occur as a result of the effect of PTH on osteoclastic (bone resorption) and osteoblastic (bone formation) activity.
- In the kidneys, excess calcium cannot be reabsorbed, which leads to hypercalciuria. This urinary calcium, along with a large amount of urinary phosphate, can lead to calculi formation. In addition, PTH stimulates the synthesis of a form of vitamin D, which increases gastrointestinal (GI) absorption of calcium and leads to high serum calcium levels.

Clinical Manifestations

Hyperparathyroidism has varying symptoms, including weakness, loss of appetite, emotional disorders, constipation, increased need for sleep, and shortened attention span.

- Major signs include loss of calcium from the bones (osteoporosis), fractures, and kidney stones (nephrolithiasis).
  Neuromuscular abnormalities are characterized by muscle
  weakness, particularly in proximal muscles of the lower
  extremities.

Complications include renal failure; pancreatitis; cardiac
changes; and long bone, rib, and vertebral fractures.

Diagnostic Studies
- Radioimmunoassay measurement of PTH, which is elevated
- Serum calcium levels elevated with decreased phosphorous
  levels
- Urine calcium, serum chloride, serum uric acid, and serum
  creatinine elevated
- Serum amylase (if pancreatitis present) and alkaline phospha-
  tase (if bone disease present) both elevated
- Bone density tests to detect bone loss
- Magnetic resonance imaging (MRI), computed tomography
  (CT) scan, and ultrasound to localize adenoma

Collaborative Care
Treatment objectives are to relieve the symptoms and prevent
complications caused by excess PTH. The choice of therapy
depends on the urgency of the clinical situation, the degree of
hypercalcemia, the underlying disorder, and the status of renal and
hepatic function.

- The most effective treatment of primary and secondary
  hyperparathyroidism is partial or complete surgical removal
  of the parathyroid glands. The procedure most commonly
  used involves the use of an endoscope on an outpatient
  basis. Autotransplantation of normal parathyroid tissue
  in the forearm or near the sternocleidomastoid muscle is
  usually done, allowing PTH secretion to continue with normalization of calcium levels.
- If the patient does not meet surgical criteria or if the patient
  is elderly or at increased surgical risk from other health
  problems, a conservative management approach is used.
  This includes an annual examination with tests for serum
  PTH, calcium, phosphorous, and alkaline phosphatase
  levels and renal function; x-rays to assess for metabolic bone
  disease; and measurement of urinary calcium excretion.

Additional measures include maintenance of a high fluid intake,
a moderate calcium intake, and phosphorous supplementation,
unless contraindicated by an increased risk for urinary calculi
formation.

- Estrogen or progestin therapy can reduce serum and urinary calcium levels in postmenopausal women and may retard demineralization of the skeleton.
- Bisphosphonates (e.g., alendronate [Fosamax]) inhibit osteoclastic bone resorption and rapidly normalize serum calcium levels. Oral phosphate may be used to inhibit the calcium-absorbing effects of vitamin D in the intestine.
- Calcimimetic agents (e.g., cinacalcet [Sensipar]) are a class of drugs that increase the sensitivity of the calcium receptor on the parathyroid gland, resulting in decreased PTH secretions and calcium blood levels, thus sparing calcium stores in the bone.
- Diuretics may be given to increase urinary excretion of calcium.

Nursing Management

Nursing care after surgery is similar to that for the patient after thyroidectomy (see Hyperthyroidism, p. 333). The major postoperative complications are hemorrhage and fluid and electrolyte disturbances. Tetany is usually apparent early in the postoperative period but may develop over several days. Mild tetany, characterized by an unpleasant tingling of the hands and around the mouth, may be present but should resolve without problems. Intravenous calcium should be readily available for use if tetany becomes more severe (e.g., muscular spasms or laryngospasms develop).

- Strict monitoring of intake and output is necessary to evaluate fluid status.
- Calcium, potassium, phosphate, and magnesium levels are assessed frequently.
- Mobility is encouraged to promote bone calcification.
- If surgery is not performed, treatment to relieve symptoms and prevent complications is initiated.

▼ **Patient and Family Teaching**
- The nurse can assist the patient with hyperparathyroidism to adapt the meal plan to his or her lifestyle. A referral to a dietitian may be useful.
- Because immobility can aggravate bone loss, the nurse needs to stress the importance of an exercise program.
- The patient should be encouraged to keep annual appointments. All tests being performed should be explained. The patient should also be instructed in the symptoms of hypocalcemia or hypercalcemia and when to report these should they occur.

HYPERTENSION

Description

- Hypertension is a persistent systolic blood pressure (SBP) greater than or equal to 140 mm Hg, diastolic blood pressure (DBP) greater than or equal to 90 mm Hg, or current use of antihypertensive medication. In the United States, at least 65 million people (32%) have high blood pressure. Hypertension makes the heart work harder than normal and increases the risk of myocardial infarction, heart failure, stroke, and renal disease.

- Prehypertension (SBP of 120 to 139 or DBP of 80 to 89) increases the risk of developing hypertension and affects another 59 million Americans.

- Prevalence of hypertension increases with age; and African Americans, as compared with other ethnic groups, have the highest prevalence of hypertension in the world.

- Hypertension is more prevalent in men than in women until the age of 55 years; after age 55 years it is more prevalent in women than men.

The status of hypertension control has improved considerably over the last 20 years. Large-scale education programs provided by various organizations have increased hypertension control over the last 20 years. However, even though the percentage of patients with hypertension on medication who have their BP contolled has improved from 10% to 34%, two thirds of hypertensive patients do not have their BP controlled.

Classification of hypertension according to stages is described in Table 51.

Two subtypes of hypertension include *isolated systolic hypertension (ISH)* and *pseudohypertension*. ISH is an average SBP ≥ 140 mm Hg coupled with an average DBP <90 mm Hg and is associated with loss of elasticity in larger arteries from atherosclerosis in older adults. Pseudohypertension, or false hypertension, can occur with rigid, calcified arteries resulting from advanced atherosclerosis.

The etiology of hypertension can be classified as primary (essential) or secondary. *Primary (essential) hypertension* accounts for up to 90% of all cases of hypertension. Although the exact cause of essential hypertension is unknown, several contributing factors, including greater than ideal body weight, diabetes mellitus (DM), increased sympathetic nervous system (SNS) activity, increased sodium intake, and excessive alcohol intake, have been identified.

H

| Table 51 | Classification of Hypertension | | |

Blood Pressure (mm Hg)

Category	Systolic		Diastolic
Normal	<120	and	<80
Prehypertension	120-139	or	80-89
Hypertension, stage 1	140-159	or	90-99
Hypertension, stage 2	≥160	or	≥100

From the U.S. Department of Health and Human Services: *Seventh Report of the Joint National Committee on Prevention, Detection, Evaluation, and Treatment of High Blood Pressure (JNC-7)*, Washington, DC, 2003, National Institutes of Health.

Secondary hypertension is elevated BP with a specific cause that often can be identified and corrected. This type of hypertension accounts for 5% to 10% of hypertension in adults and more than 80% of hypertension in children. Causes of secondary hypertension include coarctation or congenital narrowing of the aorta, renal artery stenosis, endocrine disorders such as Cushing syndrome, neurologic disorders such as brain tumors and head injury, sleep apnea, and pregnancy-induced hypertension. Treatment of secondary hypertension is directed at eliminating the underlying cause.

Pathophysiology of Primary Hypertension

The hemodynamic hallmark of hypertension is persistently increased systemic vascular resistance (SVR). Factors that are known to be related to the development of primary hypertension or contribute to the disease are presented in Table 52.

Clinical Manifestations

Hypertension is often called the "silent killer" because it is frequently asymptomatic until it becomes severe and target organ disease has occurred. A patient with severe hypertension may experience a variety of symptoms secondary to effects on blood vessels in the various organs and tissues or to the increased workload of the heart. These secondary symptoms include fatigue, reduced activity tolerance, dizziness, palpitations, angina, and dyspnea.

The most common complications of hypertension are target organ diseases, including the heart (hypertensive heart disease), brain (cerebrovascular disease), peripheral vasculature (peripheral

Table 52	Risk Factors for Primary Hypertension
Age	SBP rises progressively with increasing age. After age 50 years a SBP >140 mm Hg is a more important cardiovascular risk factor than DBP.
Alcohol	Excessive alcohol intake is strongly associated with hypertension. Patients with hypertension should limit their daily intake to 1 oz of alcohol.
Cigarettes	Smoking greatly increases the risk of cardiovascular disease. People with hypertension who smoke are at even greater risk for cardiovascular disease.
Diabetes mellitus	Hypertension is more common in people with diabetes. When hypertension and diabetes coexist, complications (e.g., target organ disease) are more severe.
Elevated serum lipids	Elevated levels of cholesterol and triglycerides are primary risk factors in atherosclerosis. Hyperlipidemia is more common in people with hypertension.
Excess dietary sodium	High sodium intake can contribute to sodium hypertension in some patients and can decrease the effectiveness of certain antihypertensive medications.
Gender	Hypertension is more prevalent in men in young adulthood and early middle age. After age 55 years, hypertension is more prevalent in women.
Family history	History of a close blood relative (e.g., parents, sibling) with hypertension is associated with an increased risk for developing hypertension.
Obesity	Weight gain is associated with increased frequency of hypertension. The risk is greatest with central abdominal obesity.
Ethnicity	Incidence of hypertension is twice as high in African Americans as in whites.
Sedentary lifestyle	Regular physical activity can help control lifestyle weight and reduce cardiovascular risk. Physical activity may decrease BP.

H

BP, Blood pressure; *DBP,* diastolic blood pressure; *SBP,* systolic blood pressure.

Continued

Table 52	Risk Factors for Primary Hypertension—cont'd
Socioeconomic status	Hypertension is more prevalent in lower-status socioeconomic groups and among less educated people.
Stress	People exposed to repeated stress may develop hypertension more frequently than others. People who develop hypertension may respond differently to stress than those who do not develop hypertension.

vascular disease), kidney (nephrosclerosis), and eyes (retinal damage).

Hypertensive Heart Disease. Hypertension is a major risk factor for coronary artery disease (CAD). The mechanisms by which hypertension contributes to the development of atherosclerosis are not fully known. Injury to the coronary artery endothelium causes arteriolar changes that result in the high incidence of CAD. Sustained high BP also increases the cardiac workload and produces left ventricular hypertrophy (LVH). Progressive LVH, especially in association with CAD, is associated with the development of heart failure.

Heart failure occurs when the heart's compensatory adaptations are overwhelmed and the heart can no longer pump enough blood to meet the metabolic needs of the body.

- The patient may complain of shortness of breath on exertion, paroxysmal nocturnal dyspnea, and fatigue. Signs of an enlarged heart may be present on x-ray, and an electrocardiogram (ECG) may show electrical changes indicative of LVH.

Cerebrovascular Disease. Hypertension is a major risk factor for stroke and cerebral atherosclerosis. Atherosclerotic plaques are commonly distributed at the bifurcation of the common carotid artery. Portions of the atherosclerotic plaque, or the blood clot that forms on the plaque, may break off and travel to intracerebral vessels, producing a thromboembolism. The patient may experience transient ischemic attacks or a stroke.

Peripheral Vascular Disease. As it does with other vessels, hypertension speeds up the process of atherosclerosis in peripheral blood vessels, leading to the development of aortic aneurysm, aortic dissection, and peripheral vascular disease. *Intermittent claudication* (ischemic muscle pain precipitated by activity and relieved with rest) is a classic symptom of peripheral arterial disease.

Nephrosclerosis. Hypertension is one of the leading risk factors for end-stage renal disease, especially among African Americans. Some degree of renal dysfunction is usually present in the hypertensive patient, even one with a minimally elevated BP. This disorder is the result of ischemia caused by the narrowed lumen of intrarenal blood vessels. Gradual narrowing of arteries and arterioles leads to the destruction of glomeruli, atrophy of tubules, and eventual death of nephrons. These changes may eventually lead to renal failure. The earliest symptom of renal dysfunction is usually nocturia.

Retinal Damage. The appearance of the retina provides important information about the severity of the hypertensive process. The retina is the only place in the body where the blood vessels can be directly visualized. Therefore retinal damage provides an indication of vessel damage in the heart, brain, and kidneys. Manifestations of severe retinal damage include blurring of vision, retinal hemorrhage, and loss of vision.

Diagnostic Studies

Initially, the BP is taken at least twice in each arm, at least 1 minute apart, with the arm with the higher average pressure used for all subsequent BP measurements. If the first two readings differ by more than 5 mm Hg, additional readings should be obtained. Basic laboratory studies are performed to evaluate target organ disease, determine overall cardiovascular risk, or establish baseline levels before initiating therapy.

- Routine urinalysis, blood urea nitrogen (BUN), and serum creatinine levels to screen for renal involvement
- Serum electrolytes, especially potassium (K^+) levels, to detect hyperaldosteronism
- Blood glucose (fasting, if possible) level to assess for diabetes mellitus
- Lipid profile (serum cholesterol and triglyceride levels) to assess for atherosclerosis risk factors
- ECG for baseline cardiac status

Collaborative Care

- The goal in treating a hypertensive patient is to reduce overall cardiovascular risk and to control BP. Lifestyle modifications are indicated for all patients with prehypertension and hypertension. These modification measures include weight reduction, Dietary Approaches to Stop Hypertension (DASH) eating plan, dietary sodium reduction, regular aerobic physical activity, moderation of alcohol intake, and avoidance of tobacco use.
- Dietary therapy consists of restricting sodium intake to less than 2.4 g/day and following the DASH eating plan, which is

H

rich in vegetables, fruit, and nonfat dairy products. (See Table 33-7, Lewis and others, *Medical-Surgical Nursing,* edition 7, p. 770 for a description of the DASH diet.) Men should limit their intake of alcohol to no more than two drinks per day and women to no more than one drink per day (one drink = $\frac{1}{2}$ oz alcohol [e.g., 12 oz beer, 5 oz wine, 1.5 oz 80-proof whiskey]).

- Moderate aerobic physical activity, such as brisk walking, jogging, or swimming, can help control BP, promote relaxation, and decrease or control body weight. It is recommended that all adults have regular physical activity at least 30 min/day most days of the week. The patient with heart disease or other serious health problems needs a thorough examination, possibly including a stress test, before beginning an exercise program.
- The nicotine contained in tobacco causes vasoconstriction and increases BP in hypertensive people. Everyone, especially a hypertensive patient, should be strongly advised to avoid tobacco use.

Drug Therapy

Drug therapy may be indicated for some patients with hypertension that is not controlled by lifestyle changes. The general goals of drug therapy are to achieve a BP of <140/90 mm Hg (<130/80 mm Hg for patients with diabetes or chronic kidney disease). The drugs currently available for treating hypertension have two main actions: reducing SVR and decreasing the volume of circulating blood.

- Drugs used in treatment of hypertension include diuretics, adrenergic (SNS) inhibitors, direct vasodilators, angiotensin inhibitors, and calcium channel blockers. (See Table 33-8, Lewis and others, *Medical-Surgical Nursing,* edition 7, pp. 773 to 776 for a description of antihypertensive drug therapy.)
- Periodic monitoring of BP is important during drug therapy. After the BP has stabilized, it should be monitored every 3 to 6 months to ensure control.

Nursing Management

Goals

The patient with hypertension will achieve and maintain desired BP; understand, accept, and implement the therapeutic plan; experience minimal or no unpleasant side effects of therapy; and be confident of ability to manage and cope with this condition.

Nursing Diagnoses/Collaborative Problems

- Ineffective health maintenance
- Anxiety

- Ineffective therapeutic regimen management
- Potential complication: stroke
- Potential complication: hypertensive crisis

Nursing Interventions

The nurse in routine screening settings is in an ideal position to assess for the presence of hypertension, identify risk factors for hypertension and CAD, and teach the patient about these conditions.

  - Effort and resources should be focused on controlling BP in persons already identified as having hypertension; identifying and controlling BP in high-risk groups such as African Americans, obese persons, and relatives of people with hypertension; and screening those with limited access to the health care system.

The primary nursing responsibilities for long-term management of hypertension are to assist the patient in reducing BP and complying with the treatment plan. Nursing actions include patient and family teaching, detection and reporting of adverse treatment effects, compliance assessment and enhancement, and evaluation of therapeutic effectiveness.

▼ **Patient and Family Teaching**

Patient and family education includes nutritional therapy, drug therapy, physical activity, and, if appropriate, home BP monitoring and tobacco cessation (Table 53).

Nutritional Therapy. The patient and family, especially the member who prepares the meals, should be educated about sodium-restricted diets. Instruction should include reading the labels of over-the-counter drugs as well as packaged foods and health products to identify hidden sources of sodium. It is helpful to review the patient's normal diet and to identify foods high in sodium.

Drug Therapy. Side effects of antihypertensive drug therapy are common. The number or severity of side effects may be related to dosage, and it may be necessary to change the drug or decrease the dosage. Side effects may decrease with long-term use of the drug.

Physical Activity. Generally, physical activity is more likely to be sustained if it is safe and enjoyable, fits easily into the daily schedule, and does not generate financial or social costs. Nurses can assist patients to increase their physical activity by identifying and communicating the need for increased activity, explaining the difference between physical activity and exercise, assisting in initiating activity, and following up appropriately.

Home BP Monitoring. Some patients benefit from regularly monitoring their BP at home. A log of BP measurements should be maintained by the patient and brought to office visits. Home BP

| Table 53 | Patient and Family Teaching Guide: Hypertension |

When presenting information to the patient and/or family, the nurse should do the following:

General Instructions
1. Provide the numeric value of the patient's BP and explain what it means (e.g., high, low, normal, borderline). Encourage patient to monitor BP at home.
2. Inform patient that hypertension is usually asymptomatic and symptoms do not reliably indicate BP levels.
3. Explain that hypertension means high blood pressure and does not relate to a "hyper" personality.
4. Explain that long-term follow-up care and therapy are necessary to treat hypertension. Therapy involves lifestyle changes (e.g., weight management, sodium reduction, smoking cessation) and, in most cases, medications.
5. Explain that therapy will not cure but should control hypertension.
6. Tell patient that controlled hypertension is usually compatible with an excellent prognosis and a normal lifestyle.
7. Explain the potential dangers of uncontrolled hypertension.

Instructions Related to Medications
1. Be specific about the names, actions, dosages, and side effects of prescribed medications.
2. Tell patient to plan regular and convenient times for taking medications and measuring BP.
3. Tell patient not to discontinue drugs abruptly because withdrawal may cause a severe hypertensive reaction.
4. Tell patient not to double up on doses when a dose is missed.
5. Inform patient that if BP increases, the patient should not take an increased medication dosage before consulting the health care provider.
6. Tell patient not to take a medication belonging to someone else.
7. Tell patient to supplement diet with foods high in potassium (e.g., citrus fruits and green leafy vegetables) if taking potassium-losing diuretics.
8. Tell patient to avoid hot baths, excessive amounts of alcohol, and strenuous exercise within 3 hours of taking medications that promote vasodilation.

BP, Blood pressure.

Table 53	Patient and Family Teaching Guide: Hypertension—cont'd

9. Many medications cause orthostatic hypotension. Explain that the effects of orthostatic hypotension can be reduced by instructing the patient to arise slowly from bed, sit on the side of the bed for a few minutes, stand slowly, not stand still for prolonged periods of time, do leg exercises to increase venous return, sleep with head of bed raised or on pillows, and lie or sit down when dizziness occurs.

10. Many medications cause sexual problems (e.g., erectile dysfunction, decreased libido). Encourage the patient to consult with the health care provider about changing drugs or dosages if sexual problems develop.

11. Inform the patient that side effects of medications often diminish with time.

12. Caution about potentially high-risk over-the-counter medications, such as high-sodium antacids, appetite suppressants, and cold and sinus medications. Advise patient to read warning labels and to consult with pharmacist.

measurement may give a more valid indication of BP because the patient is more relaxed.

Patient Compliance. Active patient participation increases the likelihood of adherence to the treatment plan. Measures such as involving the patient in scheduling medications convenient to a daily routine, helping the patient link pill taking with another daily activity, and involving family members (if necessary) help increase patient compliance.

H

HYPERTHYROIDISM

Description

Hyperthyroidism is hyperactivity of the thyroid gland with a sustained increase in synthesis and release of thyroid hormones. The most common form of hyperthyroidism is Graves' disease. Other causes include toxic nodular goiter, thyroiditis, pituitary tumors, and thyroid cancer. *Thyrotoxicosis* is hypermetabolism that results from excess circulating levels of thyroxine (T_4), triiodothyronine (T_3), or both. Hyperthyroidism and thyrotoxicosis usually occur together as in Graves' disease, but in some cases, thyrotoxicosis may occur without hyperthyroidism.

- The incidence of hyperthyroidism is greater in women, with the highest frequency in persons 20 to 40 years old.

Pathophysiology

Graves' disease is an autoimmune disease of unknown etiology marked by diffuse thyroid enlargement and excessive thyroid hormone secretion. The patient develops antibodies to the thyroid-stimulating hormone (TSH) receptor. These antibodies attach to receptors and stimulate the thyroid gland to release T_3, T_4, or both. The excessive release of thyroid hormones leads to the clinical manifestations associated with thyrotoxicosis.

- The disease is characterized by remissions and exacerbations, with or without treatment. It may progress to destruction of thyroid tissue, causing hypothyroidism.
- Precipitating factors, such as insufficient iodine supply, infections, and emotions, may interact with genetic factors to cause Graves' disease.

Nodular goiters are characterized by nodules that secrete thyroid hormone independent of TSH stimulation. If associated with hyperthyroidism, a nodule is termed *toxic.* There may be multiple nodules or a single nodule. The frequency of toxic multinodular goiter is highest in people over 40 years of age.

Clinical Manifestations

The manifestations of hyperthyroidism are related to the effects of excess thyroid hormones. Manifestations are numerous and include hypertension, palpitations, dysrhythmias, angina, fatigue, nervousness, insomnia, weight loss, increased appetite, diarrhea, diaphoresis, intolerance to heat, menstrual irregularities in women, and impotence in men.

- When the thyroid gland is excessively large, a goiter may be palpated and noted on inspection.
- *Exophthalmos,* a protrusion of the eyeballs from the orbits, is due to impaired venous drainage from the orbit leading to increased deposits of fat and fluid (edema) in the retro-orbital tissues. This sign is seen in 20% to 40% of patients with Graves' disease. When the eyelids do not close completely, exposed corneal surfaces become dry and irritated. Serious consequences, such as corneal ulcers and eventual loss of vision, can occur.
- A patient with advanced disease may exhibit many symptoms, whereas a patient in the early stages of hyperthyroidism may only exhibit weight loss and increased nervousness. Table 50-6, Lewis and others, *Medical-Surgical Nursing,*

edition 7, p. 1301 compares features of hyperthyroidism in younger and older adult patients.

Complications

Thyrotoxic crisis (thyroid storm) is an acute, rare condition in which all hyperthyroid manifestations are heightened. The cause is presumed to be stressors such as infection, trauma, or surgery in a patient with preexisting hyperthyroidism.

- Manifestations include severe tachycardia, heart failure, shock, hyperthermia (up to 105.3° F [40.7° C]), restlessness, agitation, abdominal pain, nausea, vomiting, diarrhea, delirium, and coma.
- Aggressive measures must be taken to prevent death. Treatment is aimed at reducing circulating thyroid hormone levels by appropriate drug therapy, fever reduction, fluid replacement, and elimination or management of the initiating stressor or stressors.

Diagnostic Studies

- Diagnosis is confirmed with findings of decreased serum TSH levels and elevated free T_4 levels.
- Total T_3 and T_4 may be assessed.
- Radioactive iodine uptake (RAIU) differentiates Graves' disease from other forms of thyroiditis.
- Ophthalmic examination is done.

Collaborative Care

The therapeutic goals are to block the adverse effects of thyroid hormones and stop their oversecretion. Three primary treatment options are antithyroid medications, radioactive iodine therapy, and subtotal thyroidectomy. Generally the treatment of choice in nonpregnant adults is radioactive iodine therapy. If surgery is to be performed, the patient is usually given antithyroid drugs and iodine to produce a euthyroid state. Drugs used in the treatment of hyperthyroidism are useful in controlling symptoms in thyrotoxic states, but they are not curative.

Drug Therapy

Antithyroid Drugs. The first-line antithyroid drugs commonly used are propylthiouracil (PTU) and methimazole (Tapazole). These drugs inhibit the synthesis of thyroid hormones; PTU also blocks the peripheral conversion of T_4 to T_3. Indications for their use include Graves' disease in the young patient, hyperthyroidism during pregnancy, and the need to achieve a euthyroid state before surgery or radiation therapy.

Iodine. In large doses, iodine (e.g., Lugol's solution, saturated solution of potassium iodide [SSKI]) inhibits the synthesis of T_3 and T_4 and blocks the release of these hormones into circulation. Iodine decreases thyroid vascularity, making surgery safer and easier. The maximal effect is usually seen within 1 to 2 weeks.

β-Adrenergic Blockers. Propranolol (Inderal) is the most frequently used β-adrenergic blocker. It relieves the symptoms of thyrotoxicosis that result from increased β-adrenergic receptor stimulation caused by excess thyroid hormones.

Radioactive Iodine. Radioactive iodine limits thyroid hormone secretion by damaging or destroying thyroid tissue. Because of a delayed response, the maximum effect may not be seen for 2 to 3 months, and other drug therapy may be used until the effects of irradiation become apparent. This treatment is effective but often results in hypothyroidism.

Surgical Therapy

Thyroidectomy is indicated for individuals who have been unresponsive to antithyroid therapy, for individuals with very large goiters causing tracheal compression, and for individuals with a possible malignancy.

For subtotal thyroidectomy to be effective, approximately 90% of the thyroid tissue must be removed. If too much tissue is taken, the gland will not regenerate after surgery and hypothyroidism will develop. Postoperative complications include hypothyroidism, damage or inadvertent removal of the parathyroid glands, hemorrhage, injury to the recurrent or superior laryngeal nerve, thyrotoxic crisis, and infection.

Nutritional Therapy

The potential for nutritional deficits is high when an increased metabolic rate is present. A high-calorie diet (4000 to 5000 kcal/day) may be ordered to satisfy hunger and prevent tissue breakdown. This is accomplished with six full meals each day and snacks high in protein, carbohydrates, minerals, and vitamins, particularly vitamin A, thiamine, vitamin B_6, and vitamin C. Highly seasoned and high-fiber foods should be avoided because they stimulate the already hypermotile gastrointestinal (GI) tract.

Nursing Management

Goals

The patient with hyperthyroidism will experience relief of symptoms, have no serious complications related to the disease or treatment, maintain nutritional balance, and cooperate with the therapeutic plan.

See NCP 50-1 for the patient with hyperthyroidism, Lewis and others, *Medical-Surgical Nursing,* edition 7, p. 1303.

Nursing Diagnoses
- Activity intolerance
- Risk for injury (corneal ulceration)
- Risk for injury
- Imbalanced nutrition: less than body requirements
- Anxiety
- Insomnia

Nursing Interventions

A restful, calm, quiet room should be provided because increased metabolism causes sleep disturbances. Provision of adequate rest may be a challenge because of the patient's irritability and restlessness.

- Interventions may include placing the patient in a cool room away from very ill patients and noisy, high-traffic areas; using light bed coverings and changing the linen frequently if the patient is diaphoretic; encouraging and assisting with exercise involving large muscle groups (tremors can interfere with small-muscle coordination) to allow the release of nervous tension and restlessness; and establishing a supportive, trusting relationship to help the patient cope with aggravating events and lessen anxiety.

If exophthalmos is present, there is a potential for corneal injury. The patient may also have orbital pain. Interventions to relieve eye discomfort and prevent corneal ulceration include applying artificial tears to soothe and moisten conjunctival membranes, restricting salt, elevating the patient's head to reduce periorbital edema, and providing dark glasses to reduce glare and prevent irritation from smoke, air currents, dust, and dirt. If the eyelids cannot be closed, they should be lightly taped shut for sleep.

- To maintain flexibility, the patient should be taught to exercise intraocular muscles several times each day by turning the eyes in the complete range of motion.

Nursing Management: Patient Receiving Radioactive Iodine Therapy

Radioactive iodine therapy (ablation) is administered on an outpatient basis. Because the usual therapeutic dose of iodine is low, no radiation safety precautions are necessary.

- The patient should be instructed that radiation thyroiditis and parotiditis are possible and may cause dryness and irritation of the mouth and throat. Relief may be obtained with frequent sips of water, ice chips, or the use of a salt and soda gargle three or four times per day. Discomfort should subside in 3 to 4 days.
- Because of the high frequency of hypothyroidism after radioactive iodine therapy, the patient and significant others

should be taught the symptoms of hypothyroidism and instructed to seek medical help if these symptoms occur.

Nursing Management: Patient Having Thyroid Surgery

When subtotal thyroidectomy is the treatment of choice, the patient must be adequately prepared to avoid postoperative complications.

- Preoperative teaching should include comfort and safety measures in which the patient can participate and practice the importance of deep breathing and leg exercises. The patient should also be taught how to support the head manually while turning in bed to minimize stress on the surgery suture line. Range-of-motion (ROM) exercises of the neck should be practiced, and the patient should be told that talking is likely to be difficult for a short time after surgery.
- The hospital room must be prepared before the patient's return from surgery. Oxygen, suction equipment, and a tracheostomy tray should be readily available.
- Recurrent laryngeal nerve damage leads to vocal cord paralysis. If there is paralysis of both cords, spastic airway obstruction will occur, requiring an immediate tracheostomy.
- Respiration may become difficult because of excess swelling of the neck tissue, hemorrhage, and hematoma formation.
- Laryngeal stridor (harsh, vibratory sound) may occur during respiration as a result of edema of the laryngeal nerve or because of tetany, which occurs if the parathyroid glands are removed or damaged during surgery. To treat tetany, calcium salts such as calcium gluconate should be readily available for intravenous (IV) administration.

After a thyroidectomy the nurse should do the following:

- Assess the patient every 2 hours for 24 hours for signs of hemorrhage or tracheal compression, such as irregular breathing, neck swelling, frequent swallowing, sensations of fullness at the incision site, choking, and blood on anterior or posterior dressings.
- Place the patient in a semi-Fowler's position, and support the head with pillows, avoiding flexion of the neck and any tension on the suture lines.
- Monitor vital signs. Check for signs of tetany secondary to hypoparathyroidism (e.g., tingling of toes, fingers, or around the mouth; muscular twitching; apprehension) and by evaluating any difficulty in speaking and hoarseness.
- Control postoperative pain by giving medication.
- The appearance of the incision may be quite distressing; the patient can be reassured that the scar will fade in color and eventually look like a normal neck wrinkle.

▼ **Patient and Family Teaching**

Follow-up care is important for the patient who has undergone thyroid surgery.

- Hormone balance should be monitored periodically to ensure normal function has returned.
- Caloric intake must be reduced substantially below the amount that was required before surgery to prevent weight gain.
- Adequate iodine is necessary to promote thyroid function, but excesses inhibit the thyroid. Seafood once or twice per week or the normal use of iodized salt should provide sufficient intake.
- Regular exercise helps stimulate the thyroid and should be encouraged.
- High environmental temperatures should be avoided because they inhibit thyroid regeneration.
- If a complete thyroidectomy has been performed, the patient needs instruction in lifelong thyroid replacement therapy.

HYPOPARATHYROIDISM

Description

Hypoparathyroidism is an uncommon condition characterized by inadequate circulating parathyroid hormone (PTH) that results in hypocalcemia. PTH resistance at the cellular level may also occur. This is caused by a genetic defect resulting in hypocalcemia in spite of normal or high PTH levels and is often associated with hypothyroidism and hypogonadism.

Pathophysiology

The most common cause of hypoparathyroidism is the accidental removal of parathyroids or damage to the vascular supply of the glands during neck surgery (e.g., thyroidectomy, radical neck surgery).

- Idiopathic hypoparathyroidism resulting from absence, fatty replacement, or atrophy of the glands is a rare disease that usually occurs early in life and may be associated with other endocrine disorders. Affected patients may have antiparathyroid antibodies.
- Severe hypomagnesemia also leads to suppression of PTH secretion.

Clinical Manifestations

Clinical features of acute hypoparathyroidism are due to hypocalcemia (see Table 50-11, Lewis and others, *Medical-Surgical Nursing,* edition 7, p. 1310).

Sudden decreases in calcium concentration give rise to a syndrome called *tetany.*

- This state is characterized by tingling of the lips, fingertips, and occasionally feet, as well as increased muscle tension leading to paresthesias and stiffness.
- Dysphagia, painful tonic spasms of smooth and skeletal muscles (particularly of the extremities and face), and laryngospasms are also present. *Chvostek sign* (a facial muscle spasm when the face is tapped below the temple) and *Trousseau sign* (a carpopedal spasm when arterial circulation is interrupted by applying a blood pressure [BP] cuff for 3 minutes) are usually positive.

Respiratory function may be severely compromised by accessory muscle spasm and laryngeal spasm–induced airway obstruction. Patients are usually anxious and apprehensive.

Diagnostic studies include decreased serum calcium and PTH levels and increased serum phosphate levels.

Collaborative Care

The main objective is to treat tetany when present and to prevent long-term complications by maintaining normal calcium levels.

- Emergency treatment of tetany requires administration of IV calcium. Calcium can cause hypotension and cardiac arrest; thus a slow IV push is required. For long-term management, oral calcium supplements may be prescribed.
- Specific hormone replacement of PTH is not used to treat hypoparathyroidism because of the expense and the need for parenteral administration.
- Vitamin D is used in chronic and resistant hypocalcemia to enhance intestinal calcium absorption and bone resorption. Preferred preparations are dihydrotachysterol (Hytakerol) and calcitriol (Rocaltrol). These drugs are more potent, raise calcium levels rapidly, and are quickly metabolized.

Nursing Management

- If tetany or generalized muscle cramps develop, rebreathing may partially alleviate the symptoms. The patient who can cooperate should be instructed to breathe in and out of a paper bag or breathing mask. This reduces carbon dioxide excretion from the lungs and lowers body pH. Because an acidic environment enhances both solubility and the degree of ionization of calcium, ionized calcium is increased, temporarily relieving the hypocalcemia.

▼ **Patient and Family Teaching**

The patient with hypoparathyroidism needs instruction in the management of long-term nutrition and drug therapy.

- A high-calcium meal plan includes foods such as dark green vegetables, soybeans, and tofu. The patient should be told that foods containing oxalic acid (e.g., spinach, rhubarb), phytic acid (e.g., bran, whole grains), and phosphorus reduce calcium absorption.
- The patient should be instructed about the signs and symptoms of hypocalcemia and hypercalcemia and to contact the health care provider if they occur.
- Patient calcium levels should be monitored three or four times per year. Treatment modification is often necessary because hypercalcemia can develop.
- The need for lifelong treatment and health supervision should be stressed.

HYPOTHYROIDISM

Description

Hypothyroidism results from insufficient circulating thyroid hormone as a result of a variety of abnormalities. Hypothyroidism can be *primary* (related to destruction of thyroid tissue or defective hormone synthesis) or *secondary* (related to pituitary disease with decreased thyroid-stimulating hormone [TSH] secretion or hypothalamic dysfunction with decreased thyrotropin-releasing hormone [TRH] secretion). It may also be transient related to a thyroiditis or discontinuance of thyroid hormone therapy.

- The most common cause of primary hypothyroidism in adults is atrophy of the thyroid gland as the result of Hashimoto's thyroiditis and Graves' disease. These autoimmune diseases destroy the thyroid gland.
- Hypothyroidism that develops in infancy *(cretinism)* is caused by thyroid hormone deficiencies during fetal or early neonatal life.

Clinical Manifestations

All hypothyroid states have certain features in common, regardless of the cause. Manifestations vary depending on severity and duration of thyroid deficiency, as well as the patient's age at onset of the deficiency.

Hypothyroidism has systemic effects characterized by an insidious and nonspecific slowing of body processes. Clinical presentation can range from a patient with no symptoms to a patient with classic symptoms and physical changes easily detected on examination.

- The adult with hypothyroidism often is fatigued and lethargic and experiences personality and mental changes including impaired memory, slowed speech, decreased initiative, and somnolence.
- Hypothyroidism is associated with decreased cardiac output and decreased cardiac contractility. Anemia is a common feature. Increased serum cholesterol and triglyceride levels and the accumulation of mucopolysaccharides in the intima of small blood vessels can result in coronary atherosclerosis.
- Gastrointestinal (GI) motility is decreased in hypothyroidism, and *achlorhydria* (absence or decreased secretion of hydrochloric acid) is common. Constipation, which is a common complaint, may progress to obstipation and, rarely, to intestinal obstruction.
- Other physical changes include cold intolerance, hair loss, dry and coarse skin, brittle nails, hoarseness, muscle weakness and swelling, and weight gain.

Those with severe long-standing hypothyroidism may display *myxedema*, the accumulation of hydrophilic mucopolysaccharides in the dermis and other tissues. This mucinous edema causes the characteristic facies of hypothyroidism (i.e., puffiness, periorbital edema, and masklike affect).

Complications

The mental sluggishness, drowsiness, and lethargy of hypothyroidism may progress gradually or suddenly to a notable impairment of consciousness or coma. This situation, termed *myxedema coma,* constitutes a medical emergency.

- Myxedema coma can be precipitated by infection, drugs (especially opioids, tranquilizers, and barbiturates), exposure to cold, and trauma. It is characterized by subnormal temperature, hypotension, and hypoventilation.
- For the patient to live, vital functions must be supported, and IV thyroid hormone replacement must be administered.

Diagnostic Studies

- Serum TSH and free thyroxine (FT_4) are the most reliable indicators of thyroid function.
- Serum TSH levels help determine the cause of hypothyroidism. If high, the defect is in the thyroid; if low, it is in the pituitary.

- TRH stimulation test shows an increase in TSH if the problem is hypothalamic dysfunction; no change in TSH suggests anterior pituitary dysfunction.
- Serum cholesterol and triglycerides are increased.

Collaborative Care

The therapeutic objective in hypothyroidism is the restoration of the euthyroid state as safely and rapidly as possible with hormone replacement therapy. Levothyroxine (Synthroid, Levothroid) is the drug of choice to treat hypothyroidism. In the young, otherwise healthy patient, the maintenance replacement dose can be started at once. In the older adult patient and the person with compromised cardiac status, a small or initial dose is recommended because the usual dose may increase myocardial oxygen (O_2) consumption. Any chest pain experienced by a patient starting thyroid replacement should be reported immediately, and electrocardiogram (ECG) and serum cardiac enzyme tests must be performed. The dose is increased at 4- to 6-week intervals. It is important that the patient take replacement medication regularly.

- With treatment, striking transformations occur in both appearance and mental function. Most adults return to a normal state. Cardiovascular conditions and (occasionally) psychosis may persist despite corrections of the hormonal imbalance. Relapses occur if treatment is interrupted.

Nursing Management

Goals

The patient with hypothyroidism will experience relief of symptoms, maintain an euthyroid state, maintain a positive self-image, and comply with lifelong thyroid replacement therapy.

See NCP 50-2 for the patient with hypothyroidism, Lewis and others, *Medical-Surgical Nursing,* edition 7, pp. 1307 to 1308.

Nursing Diagnoses

- Imbalanced nutrition: more than body requirements
- Constipation
- Activity intolerance
- Disturbed thought processes

Nursing Interventions

Most individuals with hypothyroidism are managed on an outpatient basis. However, the patient who develops myxedema coma requires acute nursing care, often in an intensive care setting. Mechanical respiratory support is frequently necessary, and the patient will require cardiac monitoring. The nurse should monitor core temperature, because the patient with myxedema coma is often hypothermic.

- For assessment of the patient's progress, vital signs, body weight, fluid intake and output, and visible edema should be monitored. Cardiac assessment is especially important because the cardiovascular response to the hormone determines the medication regimen.
- Energy level and mental alertness should be noted. These should increase within 2 to 14 days and continue to rise steadily to normal levels.

▼ **Patient and Family Teaching**

Repeated patient education is imperative. Initially the hypothyroid patient needs more time than usual to comprehend all the necessary information.

- The need for lifelong drug therapy must be stressed. Signs and symptoms of hypothyroidism or hyperthyroidism that indicate hormone imbalance should be included in the teaching plan. Toxic symptoms should be clearly defined.
- The patient must be taught to contact a health care provider immediately if signs of overdose, such as orthopnea, dyspnea, rapid pulse, palpitations, nervousness, or insomnia, appear.
- The patient with diabetes mellitus (DM) should test his or her capillary blood glucose at least daily because a return to the euthyroid state frequently increases insulin requirements.
- In addition, thyroid preparations potentiate the effects of other common drugs, such as anticoagulants, antidepressants, and digitalis compounds. The patient should be taught the toxic signs and symptoms of these medications and remain under close medical observation until stable.

INCREASED INTRACRANIAL PRESSURE

Description

Increased intracranial pressure (ICP) is a life-threatening situation that results from an increase in any or all of the three components of the skull: brain tissue, blood, and cerebrospinal fluid (CSF). Cerebral edema is an important factor contributing to increased ICP. Regardless of the cause (Table 54), cerebral edema results in an increase in tissue volume that has the potential for increased ICP. The extent and severity of the original insult are factors that determine the degree of cerebral edema.

Three types of cerebral edema—vasogenic, cytotoxic, and interstitial—have been identified. More than one type may be present from a single insult in the same patient.

Table 54	Causes of Cerebral Edema

Mass Lesions
Brain abscess
Brain tumor (primary or metastatic)
Hematoma (intracerebral, subdural, epidural)
Hemorrhage (intracerebral, cerebellar, brainstem)

Head Injuries
Contusion
Hemorrhage
Posttraumatic brain swelling

Brain Surgery

Cerebral Infections
Meningitis
Encephalitis

Vascular Insult
Anoxic and ischemic episodes
Cerebral infarction (thrombolic or embolic)

Toxic or Metabolic Encephalopathic Conditions
Lead or arsenic intoxication
Hepatic encephalopathy
Uremia

- *Vasogenic cerebral edema* is the most common type of edema. It occurs mainly in the white matter and is attributed to changes in the endothelial lining of the cerebral capillaries. These changes result in the flow of fluid from the intravascular to the extravascular space.
- *Cytotoxic cerebral edema* results from local disruption of the functional or morphologic integrity of the cell membranes and occurs most often in the gray matter. This type of edema develops from destructive lesions or trauma to brain tissue.
- *Interstitial cerebral edema* is the result of periventricular diffusion of ventricular CSF in a patient with uncontrolled hydrocephalus. It can also be caused by enlargement of the extracellular space as a result of systemic water excess (hyponatremia).

Pathophysiology

Increased ICP can be caused by many factors, including a mass lesion (e.g., hematoma), cerebral edema associated with brain tumors, head injury, or brain inflammation, or by metabolic insult. These insults may result in hypercapnia, cerebral acidosis, impaired autoregulation, and systemic hypertension, which promote the formation and spread of cerebral edema. This edema distorts brain tissue, further increasing ICP, which leads to more tissue hypoxia and acidosis. Figure 8 illustrates the progression of increased ICP.

Sustained increases in ICP result in brainstem compression and herniation of the brain from one compartment to another. With brain displacement and herniation, ischemia and edema are further increased. Fig. 57-4, Lewis and others, *Medical-Surgical Nursing,* edition 7, p. 1471 illustrates herniation.

- Herniations force the cerebellum and brainstem downward through the foramen magnum. If compression of the brainstem is unrelieved, respiratory arrest may occur.

Clinical Manifestations

Manifestations of increased ICP can take many forms, depending on the cause, location, and rate at which the pressure increase occurs. The earlier the condition is recognized and treated, the better the prognosis.

- *Change in the level of consciousness (LOC).* LOC is a sensitive and important indicator of the patient's neurologic status. The change in consciousness may be dramatic, as in coma, or subtle, such as a change in orientation or a decrease in the level of attention.
- *Changes in vital signs.* Manifestations such as Cushing triad consisting of increasing systolic pressure (widening pulse pressure), bradycardia with a full and bounding pulse, and irregular respiratory pattern may be present but often do not appear until ICP has been increased for some time or markedly increased suddenly (e.g., head trauma). The effect of increased ICP on the hypothalamus can cause a change in body temperature.
- *Ocular signs.* Compression of the oculomotor nerve (CN III) results in dilation of the pupil ipsilateral to the mass, sluggish or no response to light, an inability to move the eye upward, and ptosis of the eyelid. A fixed, unilaterally dilated pupil is a neurologic emergency that indicates brain herniation. Other cranial nerves may also be affected, with signs of blurred vision, diplopia, and changes in extraocular eye movements. Papilledema, a nonspecific sign that is associated with persistent increases in ICP, is also seen.
- *Decrease in motor function.* As ICP continues to rise, the patient manifests changes in motor ability. A contralateral

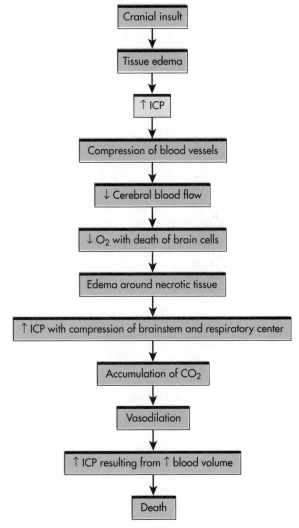

Fig. 8. Progression of increased intracranial pressure.

hemiparesis or hemiplegia may be seen. If painful stimuli are used to elicit a motor response, the patient may exhibit a localization to the stimuli or a withdrawal from it. Decorticate (flexor) and decerebrate (extensor) posturing may also be elicited by noxious stimuli (see Fig. 57-6, Lewis and others, *Medical-Surgical Nursing,* edition 7, p. 1472).

- *Headache.* Although the brain itself is insensitive to pain, compression of other intracranial structures, such as the walls of arteries and veins and the cranial nerves, can produce headache. The headache is often continuous but is worse in the morning. Straining or movement may accentuate the pain.
- *Vomiting.* Vomiting, usually not preceded by nausea, is often a nonspecific sign of increased ICP.

Diagnostic Studies

- Magnetic resonance imaging (MRI) and computed tomography (CT) scan
- Vital signs, neurologic checks, ICP measurements
- Skull, chest, and spinal x-ray studies
- Electroencephalogram (EEG), angiography
- Cerebral blood flow and velocity studies, positron emission tomography (PET)
- Laboratory studies, including complete blood count (CBC), coagulation profile, electrolytes, creatinine, arterial blood gases (ABGs), ammonia level, general drug and toxicology screen, and CSF protein

Collaborative Care

The goals of management are to identify and treat the underlying cause of increased ICP and to support brain function. A careful history is an important diagnostic aid that can direct the search for the underlying cause.

Ensuring adequate oxygenation to support brain function is the first step. ABG analysis guides the oxygen therapy. To meet the goal of maintaining the partial pressure of oxygen in arterial blood (PaO_2) at 100 mm Hg or greater, an endotracheal tube or tracheostomy and mechanical ventilation may be necessary.

- If the condition is caused by a mass lesion, such as a tumor or hematoma, surgical removal of the mass is the best management (see Brain Tumors, p. 78).
- Nonsurgical intervention for the reduction of tissue volume related to cerebral tissue swelling and edema includes the use of diuretics and corticosteroids.

Drug Therapy

Drug therapy plays an important part in the management of increased ICP. Osmotic diuretics are used to reduce the volume of brain water, and corticosteroids are used to control the cerebral edema.

- IV mannitol (Osmitrol) is an osmotic diuretic that decreases ICP in two ways: plasma expansion and osmotic effect. The plasma expansion effect reduces the hematocrit and blood viscosity, thereby increasing cerebral blood flow and cerebral oxygenation. The osmotic effect causes fluid to move from the tissue into the blood vessels, resulting in a decrease in total brain fluid content.

- Corticosteroids (e.g., dexamethasone [Decadron]) are thought to control the vasogenic edema surrounding tumors and abscesses but are not recommended in the management of head-injured patients. They are also thought to improve cerebral blood flow and restore autoregulation.

- High-dose barbiturates (e.g., pentobarbital [Nembutal] and thiopental [Pentothal]) are used in patients with an increased ICP refractory to treatment. These drugs produce a decrease in cerebral metabolism and a subsequent decrease in increased ICP.

Hyperventilation Therapy

Although the use of aggressive hyperventilation (a partial pressure of carbon dioxide in arterial blood [$PaCO_2$] < 25 mm Hg) to constrict cerebral blood vessels is performed less than in the past to treat increased ICP, brief periods of less aggressive hyperventilation (target $PaCO_2$ 30 to 35 mm Hg) may be useful for refractory intracranial hypertension.

Nutritional Therapy

The patient with increased ICP is in a hypermetabolic and hypercatabolic state that increases the need for glucose to provide the necessary fuel for metabolism of the injured brain. Because malnutrition promotes continued cerebral edema, maintenance of optimal nutrition is imperative. If the patient cannot maintain an adequate oral intake, other means of meeting the nutritional requirements, such as enteral or parenteral nutrition, should be started. Current fluid therapy is directed at keeping patients normovolemic.

Nursing Management

Goals

The overall goals are that the patient with increased ICP will have ICP within normal limits, maintain a patent airway, demonstrate

normal fluid and electrolyte balance, and have no complications
secondary to immobility and decreased LOC.

See NCP 57-1 for the patient with increased intracranial pressure, Lewis and others, *Medical-Surgical Nursing,* edition 7,
pp. 1479 to 1480.

Nursing Diagnoses

- Ineffective tissue perfusion (cerebral)
- Decreased intracranial adaptive capacity
- Risk for disuse syndrome
- Interrupted family processes

Nursing Interventions

Maintenance of Respiratory Function. Maintenance of a patent
airway is critical with increased ICP and is a primary nursing
responsibility. As the LOC decreases, the patient is at increased
risk of airway obstruction. Altered breathing patterns may become
evident.

- Airway patency can be aided by keeping the patient lying
  on one side, with frequent position changes. Snoring sounds,
  which may indicate obstruction, should be noted. Accumulated secretions should be removed by suctioning. An oral
  airway facilitates breathing and provides an easier suctioning route in the comatose patient.

The nurse must use measures to prevent hypoxia and hypercapnia. Proper positioning of the head is important.

- Elevation of the head of the bed by 30 degrees enhances
  respiratory exchange and aids in decreasing cerebral edema.
- Suctioning and coughing can cause transient increases in
  ICP and decreases in PaO_2. Suctioning should be kept to a
  minimum.
- Abdominal distention can interfere with respiratory function and should be prevented. Insertion of a nasogastric tube
  to aspirate the stomach contents can prevent distention,
  vomiting, and possible aspiration. In patients with facial and
  skull fractures, a nasogastric tube is contraindicated, and
  oral insertion of a gastric tube is preferred.
- ABGs should be measured and evaluated regularly. The
  appropriate ventilatory support can be ordered on the basis
  of the PaO_2 and $PaCO_2$ values.

Fluid and Electrolyte Balance. Fluid and electrolyte disturbances
can have an adverse effect on ICP. IV fluids should be closely
monitored. Intake and output, with insensible losses and daily
weights taken into account, are important parameters in the assessment of fluid balance.

- Electrolyte determinations should be made daily. It is especially important to monitor serum glucose, sodium (Na^+),

potassium (K^+), and osmolality. Urinary output is monitored for problems related to diabetes insipidus (DI) and syndrome of inappropriate antidiuretic hormone (SIADH) (see Diabetes Insipidus, p. 162, and Syndrome of Inappropriate Antidiuretic Hormone, p. 612).

Monitoring of Intracranial Pressure. Measurement of ICP is valuable in detecting the early rise of ICP and the patient's response to treatment. Methods are discussed in detail in Chapter 57, Lewis and others, *Medical-Surgical Nursing,* edition 7.

Body Position. Patients should be maintained in the head-up position. The nurse must take care to prevent extreme neck flexion, which can cause venous obstruction and increased ICP. The bed should be positioned so that it lowers the ICP while maintaining cerebral perfusion pressure (CPP).

- Care should be taken to turn the patient with slow, gentle movements because rapid changes in position may increase ICP. Caution should be used to prevent discomfort in turning and positioning of the patient because pain or agitation also increases pressure. Increased intrathoracic pressure contributes to increased ICP; thus coughing, straining, and the Valsalva maneuver should be avoided. Extreme hip flexion should also be avoided to decrease the risk of raising the intraabdominal pressure, which increases ICP.

Protection From Injury. The patient with increased ICP and a decreased LOC needs protection from self-injury. Confusion, agitation, and the possibility of seizures can put the patient at risk of injury. Restraints should be used judiciously in the agitated patient. The patient can benefit from a quiet, nonstimulating environment and the presence of a family member. Touching and talking to the patient, even one who is in coma, are always an appropriate approach. The nurse must create a balance between sensory deprivation and overload.

Psychologic Considerations. Anxiety over the diagnosis and prognosis for the patient with neurologic problems can be distressing to the patient, family, and nursing staff. Short, simple explanations are appropriate and allow the patient and family to acquire the amount of information they desire. There is a need for support, information, and education of both patients and families.

The nurse should assess the family members' desire and need to assist in providing care for the patient and allow for their participation as appropriate.

INFLAMMATORY BOWEL DISEASE

Description

Crohn's disease and *ulcerative colitis* are autoimmune disorders that are referred to as *inflammatory bowel disease* (IBD). Both diseases are characterized by chronic inflammation of the intestine with periods of remission interspersed with periods of exacerbation. The cause is unknown, and there is no cure.

Both genetic and environmental factors seem to play a role in IBD. An antigen probably initiates the inflammation, but the actual tissue damage is due to an overactive, inappropriate, and sustained inflammatory response. The prevalent theory is that an unidentified organism that is usually innocuous stimulates a poorly regulated immune response in genetically susceptible people. Although the antigen that initiates IBD is unknown, there is strong support for the existence of at least five susceptibility genes. Not only are family members of patients with Crohn's disease at increased risk for Crohn's disease, but also they have an increased risk of ulcerative colitis and vice versa.

Both ulcerative colitis and Crohn's disease commonly occur during adolescence and early adulthood and have a second peak in the sixth decade. Both are more prevalent in whites and in industrialized regions of the world.

Certain criteria are used to differentiate ulcerative colitis from Crohn's disease, but a clear differentiation between the two cannot be made in about one third of the cases. Crohn's disease and ulcerative colitis are compared in Table 55.

Pathophysiology

Although symptoms of the diseases are often the same, the pattern of inflammation is different for the two diseases.

Crohn's Disease

- The inflammation in Crohn's disease involves all layers of the bowel wall and can occur anywhere in the gastrointestinal (GI) tract from the mouth to the anus. It most commonly occurs in the terminal ileum and colon.
- Areas of involvement are usually discontinuous skip lesions, with segments of normal bowel occurring between diseased portions. Typically, ulcerations are deep and longitudinal and penetrate between islands of inflamed edematous mucosa, causing a classic cobblestone appearance.
- Strictures at the areas of inflammation may cause bowel obstruction.

Table 55	Comparison of Ulcerative Colitis and Crohn's Disease	

Characteristic	Ulcerative Colitis	Crohn's Disease
Clinical		
Age at onset	Young to middle age	Young
Diarrhea	Common	Common
Abdominal crampy pain	Possible	Common
Fever (intermittent)	During acute attacks	Common
Weight loss	Common	Severe
Rectal bleeding	Common	Infrequent
Tenesmus	Severe	Rare
Malabsorption and nutritional deficiencies	Minimal incidence	Common
Pathologic		
Location	Starts distally and spreads in a continuous pattern up the colon	Occurs anywhere along GI tract in characteristic skip lesions; most frequent site is terminal ileum
Distribution	Continuous	Segmental
Depth of involvement	Mucosa and submucosa	Entire thickness of bowel wall (transmural)
Granulomas	Absent	Common
Cobblestoning of mucosa	Rare	Common
Pseudopolyps	Common	Rare
Small bowel involvement	Minimal	Common
Complications		
Fistulas	Rare	Common
Strictures	Rare	Common
Anal abscesses	Rare	Common
Perforation	Common	Common
Toxic megacolon	Common	Rare
Carcinoma	Increased incidence after 10 yr of disease	Slightly greater than general population
Recurrence after surgery	Cure with colectomy	40%-60% or more recurrence after segmental resections of small or large intestine

GI, Gastrointestinal.

- Because the inflammation goes through the entire bowel wall, peritonitis, abscesses, or fistula tracts that communicate with adjacent areas of bowel, bladder, vagina, or skin can develop.

Ulcerative Colitis

- The inflammation of ulcerative colitis usually starts in the rectum and moves in a continuous pattern toward the cecum.
- Inflammation and ulcerations occur in the mucosal layer, the innermost layer of bowel. Fistulas and abscesses are rare because it does not extend through the bowel wall.
- Areas of inflamed mucosa form pseudopolyps, tongue-like projections into the bowel lumen.

Clinical Manifestations

Manifestations depend largely on the anatomic site of involvement, extent of the disease process, and presence or absence of complications.

Crohn's Disease

- Diarrhea and colicky abdominal pain are common symptoms of Crohn's disease.
- If the small intestine is involved, weight loss occurs because of malabsorption and a mass is sometimes felt in the right iliac fossa.
- Rectal bleeding sometimes occurs with Crohn's disease although not as often as with ulcerative colitis.
- Systemic symptoms such as fever may occur.

Ulcerative Colitis

- The primary symptoms of ulcerative colitis are bloody diarrhea and abdominal pain. Pain may vary from the mild, lower abdominal cramping associated with diarrhea to the severe, constant abdominal pain associated with acute perforation.
- With mild disease, diarrhea may consist of one or two semi-formed stools daily that contain small amounts of blood. The patient may have no other systemic manifestations.
- In moderate disease there is increased stool output (four or five stools/day), increased bleeding, and systemic symptoms including fever, malaise, and anorexia.
- In severe disease, diarrhea is bloody, contains mucus, and occurs 10 to 20 times a day. In addition, fever, weight loss (10% of total body weight), anemia, tachycardia, and dehydration are present.

Complications

Patients with IBD experience both gastrointestinal (GI) and systemic complications.

- GI tract complications include hemorrhage, strictures, perforation, fistulas, and colonic dilation. *Toxic megacolon* is

colonic dilation greater than 5 cm and may require an emergency colectomy to prevent perforation.
- Toxic megacolon is more common with ulcerative colitis, whereas strictures and fistulas occur more often with Crohn's disease.
- Hemorrhage, malabsorption, and cellular breakdown lead to anemia, fluid and electrolyte imbalances, and nutritional deficiencies.
- Ulcerative colitis increases the risk for colorectal cancer, whereas Crohn's disease increases the risk for small bowel cancer.
- Systemic complications of IBD include fever, anorexia, and malaise.
- Arthritis, ankylosing spondylitis, eye inflammation, and skin lesions such as erythema nodosum and pyoderma gangrenosum are other extraintestinal manifestations.
- Primary sclerosing cholangitis, gallstones, and kidney stones are additional complications of IBD.

Diagnostic Studies
Diagnosis of IBD includes ruling out other diseases with similar symptoms and then determining whether the patient has Crohn's disease or ulcerative colitis.
- Stool is examined for blood, pus, and mucus and cultured to rule out infectious diarrhea.
- Laboratory studies may indicate electrolyte disturbances, anemia, leukocytosis, hypoalbuminemia, and an elevated erythrocyte sedimentation rate.
- Sigmoidoscopy and colonoscopy directly examine large intestine mucosa for inflammation, ulcerations, pseudopolyps, and strictures.
- Biopsies may be taken by means of a sigmoidoscope or colonoscope.
- Double-contrast barium enema may show areas of granular inflammation with ulcerations.

Collaborative Care
The goals of treatment are to rest the bowel, control inflammation and infection, correct malnutrition, alleviate stress, provide symptomatic relief, and improve quality of life.

A variety of medications are available to treat IBD and are the preferred treatment in Crohn's disease because there is a high recurrence rate following surgical treatment. Hospitalization is indicated if the patient does not respond to drug therapy or if complications occur.

Drug Therapy
Drugs are used to induce and maintain a remission of IBD in order to improve quality of life. Five major classes of medications are used to treat IBD. All five classes are used to treat Crohn's disease; aminosalicylates and corticosteroids are mainstays of treatment for ulcerative colitis.

- *Aminosalicylates* are combination drugs that contain 5-aminosalicylic acid (5-ASA) and an agent that delivers 5-ASA to the colon when it is taken orally. 5-ASA suppresses proinflammatory cytokines and other inflammatory mediators when applied to the intestinal mucosa. Sulfasalazine (Azulfidine) contains 5-ASA and sulfapyridine, but newer agents that are better tolerated include olsalazine (Dipentum), mesalamine (Pentasa), and balsalazide (Colazal). Preparations with 5-ASA can be administerd orally or rectally as suppositories, enemas, and foams. They are first-line therapies for Crohn's disease, especially when the colon is involved, but are more effective for ulcerative colitis.
- *Antimicrobials* are used to treat IBD although no specific infectious agent has been discovered. Metronidazole (Flagyl), ciprofloxacin (Cipro), and clarithromycin (Biaxin) have been effective for Crohn's disease but not as effective for ulcerative colitis.
- *Corticosteroids* such as prednisone are used to achieve remission from acute flare-ups in IBD but are not effective for maintaining the remission. When the disease affects the left colon, sigmoid, and rectum, corticosteroid suppositories, enemas, and foams can be used to deliver the drug directly to inflamed tissue with minimal systemic effects. Oral prednisone is given to patients who do not respond to either 5-ASA or topical corticosteroids. IV corticosteroids are reserved for those with severe inflammation.
- *Immunosuppressants* (azathioprine [Imuran] and 6-mercaptopurine [Purinethol]) are given orally and take 3 to 6 months to be fully effective. They are most useful for patients with Crohn's disease who do not respond to other medications.
- *Biologic drug therapy* includes the use of infliximab (Remicade), a monoclonal antibody to the cytokine tumor necrosis factor. It is given IV to induce and maintain remission in patients with active Crohn's disease and in patients with draining fistulas who do not respond to conventional drug therapy.

Surgical Therapy

In the patient with Crohn's disease, surgery is usually reserved for emergency situations, such as excessive bleeding, obstruction, or peritonitis, or when medical treatment has failed. Unlike ulcerative colitis, which can be cured by total proctocolectomy, Crohn's disease is not cured by surgery.

- The principal surgical treatment for Crohn's disease is strictureplasty to widen areas of narrowed bowel.
- If diseased bowel is resected with an anastomosis of bowel ends, the disease commonly recurs at the area of anastomosis.

In the patient with ulcerative colitis, surgery is indicated if the patient fails to respond to treatment; if exacerbations are frequent and debilitating; or if massive bleeding, perforation, strictures, obstruction, dysplasia, or carcinoma develops. Since ulcerative colitis affects only the colon, a total proctocolectomy is curative.

- Surgical procedures include total colectomy with rectal mucosal stripping and ileoanal reservoir, total proctocolectomy with permanent ileostomy, and total proctocolectomy with continent ileostomy.

For descriptions of these procedures, see Lewis and others, *Medical-Surgical Nursing,* edition 7, pp. 1055 to 1056, 1069 to 1070, and NCP 43-3 for the patient with a colostomy or ileostomy, pp. 1073 to 1075.

Nutritional Therapy

Diet is an important component in the treatment of IBD. The dietitian is a vital member of the team and should be consulted regarding dietary recommendations.

- The goals of diet management are to provide adequate nutrition without exacerbating symptoms, to correct and prevent malnutrition, to replace fluid and electrolyte losses, and to prevent weight loss. Parenteral nutrition may be necessary to provide positive nitrogen balance while resting the bowel. Promoting good nutrition is essential for patients with IBD, and the diet for each patient must be individualized to correct nutritional deficiencies and meet needs for nutrients.

Nursing Management

Goals

The patient with IBD will experience a decrease in the number and severity of acute exacerbations, maintain normal fluid and electrolyte balance, be free from pain or discomfort, comply with medical regimens, maintain nutritional balance, and have improved quality of life.

See NCP 43-2 for the patient with inflammatory bowel disease, Lewis and others, *Medical-Surgical Nursing,* edition 7, pp. 1058 to 1059.

Nursing Diagnoses

- Diarrhea
- Impaired skin integrity
- Anxiety
- Imbalanced nutrition: less than body requirements
- Ineffective coping
- Ineffective therapeutic regimen management

Nursing Interventions

During the acute phase, attention is focused on hemodynamic stability, pain control, fluid and electrolyte balance, and nutritional support. Accurate intake and output records must be maintained, with the number and appearance of stools also noted. Nursing care is directed toward an intensive therapeutic and supportive program.

- Honesty, patience, and understanding are essential in the relationships with the patient. An explanation of all procedures and treatments will build trust and may reduce some anxiety.
- Psychotherapy may be indicated if the patient has emotional problems, but any person who has 10 to 20 bowel movements each day, rectal discomfort, and an unpredictable disease may be anxious, frustrated, discouraged, and depressed. Nurses and other team members can assist patients to learn strategies to cope with the chronicity of IBD.
- Severe fatigue limits the patient's energy for physical activity. Nutritional deficiencies and anemia may leave the patient feeling weak and listless. Rest is important because patients may lose sleep because of frequent episodes of diarrhea and abdominal pain. Activities should be scheduled around rest periods.
- Until diarrhea is controlled, the patient must be kept clean, dry, and free of odor. A deodorizer should be placed in the room, and patients must have ready access to a toilet. Meticulous perianal skin care using plain water (no harsh soap) is necessary to treat and prevent skin breakdown. Sitz baths, dibucaine (Nupercainal), witch hazel, or other soothing compresses or prescribed ointments may reduce irritation and relieve anal discomfort.

▼ **Patient and Family Teaching**

In the majority of patients the disease course is chronic and intermittent, regardless of the site of involvement. The patient and family may need help in setting realistic short- and long-term goals.

- Specific teaching should address (1) the importance of rest and diet management, (2) perianal care, (3) action and side effects of medications, (4) symptoms of disease recurrence, (5) when to seek medical care, and (6) the use of diversional activities to reduce stress.
- Excellent teaching resources written in easily comprehensible language are available from the Crohn's and Colitis Foundation of America.

INTERSTITIAL CYSTITIS/PAINFUL BLADDER SYNDROME

Description

Interstitial cystitis (IC) is a chronic, painful inflammatory disease of the bladder characterized by symptoms of urgency/frequency and pain in the bladder and/or pelvis. *Painful bladder syndrome* (PBS) is suprapubic pain related to bladder filling, accompanied by other symptoms such as frequency, in the absence of urinary tract infection (UTI) or other obvious pathologic condition. The average age at onset is 40 years, and the ratio of women to men with IC/PBS is 10:1 to 12:1.

Although the etiology of IC remains unknown, probable contributing factors include chronic inflammation with mast cell invasion of the bladder wall (possibly resulting from an infection or autoimmune disorder), defects of the glycosaminoglycan layer that protects bladder mucosa from the irritating effects of urine exposure, abnormal constituents in the urine, dysfunction of the sympathetic innervation of the lower urinary tract, and reflex sympathetic dystrophy.

Clinical Manifestations

Two primary clinical manifestations of IC include pain and bothersome lower urinary tract symptoms (e.g., frequency, urgency).

- The pain is usually located in the suprapubic area but may involve the vagina, labia, or entire perineal region. It varies from moderate to severe in intensity and is exacerbated by bladder filling, postponing urination, physical exertion, pressure against the suprapubic area, dietary intake of certain foods, or emotional distress. The pain is transiently relieved by urination.
- Bothersome lower urinary tract symptoms are very similar to a UTI, and the condition is frequently misdiagnosed as a recurring or chronic UTI or, in men, chronic prostatitis.

The pain and bothersome voiding symptoms produced by IC remit and exacerbate over time.

Diagnostic Studies

IC is a diagnosis of exclusion. The condition is suspected whenever a patient experiences symptoms of a UTI despite the absence of bacteriuria, pyuria, or a positive urine culture.

- History and physical examination are necessary to exclude other disorders that produce somewhat similar symptoms, such as UTI or endometriosis.
- Cystoscopic examination may reveal a small bladder capacity and superficial ulceration with bladder filling.

Collaborative Care

Because the etiology of IC is unknown, no single treatment has been identified that consistently reverses or relieves symptoms.

Dietary and lifestyle alterations are used to relieve pain and diminish voiding frequency and nocturia. Dietary alterations include elimination of foods and beverages likely to exacerbate the symptoms. A diet low in acidic foods and avoiding beverages such as coffee, tea, and carbonated or alcoholic drinks may be helpful.

- Patients may be advised that an over-the-counter (OTC) dietary supplement, calcium glycerophosphate (Prelief), alkalinizes the urine and can provide relief from the irritating effects of certain foods.
- Because stress can exacerbate IC/PBS, basic relaxation techniques (e.g., sitz baths, application of heat or cold to perineum or bladder, stress reduction tapes) may be helpful.

Two tricyclic antidepressants, amitriptyline (Elavil) and nortriptyline (Aventyl), are used to reduce the burning pain and urinary frequency. Pentosan (Elmiron) is used to enhance the protective effects of the glycosaminoglycan layer of the bladder.

- Although these drugs are effective over time (weeks to months), they do not provide the immediate relief that may be needed with an acute exacerbation of symptoms. In this case, a short course of opioid analgesics may be given.

Several agents may be instilled directly into the bladder through a small catheter.

- Dimethyl sulfoxide (DMSO) probably acts by desensitizing pain receptors in the bladder wall.
- Heparin and hyaluronic acid also may be instilled into the bladder to enhance the protective properties of the glycosaminoglycan layer of the bladder and relieve symptoms.
- Bacille Calmette-Guérin (BCG), an attenuated form of the *Myocbacterium bovis,* administered intravesically is a

common treatment for IC. Its mechanism of action is unclear, but it may alleviate inflammation induced by a possible autoimmune disorder.

Distention of the bladder during endoscopic examination relieves IC-related pain and voiding frequency, probably by temporarily disrupting sensory nerve endings in the bladder wall. Several surgical procedures, such as urinary diversion, can be used in an attempt to relieve severe, debilitating pain.

Nursing Management

Reassurance that IC is a real condition experienced by others and that it can be effectively treated may relieve the anxiety, anger, guilt, and frustration related to experiences of chronic pain and voiding dysfunction in the absence of a definitive diagnosis and treatment strategy.

The patient also needs to be given instruction about the need to maintain good nutrition, particularly in light of the dietary restrictions often necessary to control IC-related pain.

- Elimination of a variety of foods and beverages from the diet likely to irritate the bladder typically provides modest to profound relief from symptoms. The patient should be taught to self-use Prelief.
- The patient is also advised to avoid clothing that creates suprapubic pressure, including pants with tight belts or restrictive waistlines.
- Written educational materials concerning diet, coping with the need for frequent urination, and strategies for coping with the emotional burden of IC are available from the Interstitial Cystitis Association (*http://www.ichelp.com*).

INTERVERTEBRAL LUMBAR DISK DAMAGE

Pathophysiology

An intervertebral disk is interposed between the vertebrae from the cervical axis to the sacrum. Structural degeneration of the lumbar disk is often caused by *degenerative disk disease* (DDD). This progressive degeneration is a normal process of aging and results in the intervertebral disks losing their elasticity, flexibility, and shock-absorbing capabilities. Most persons by age 60 years have some degree of DDD, and compression of the nerve roots and cord may then occur.

An acute *herniated intervertebral disk* (slipped disk) can be the result of natural degeneration with age or repeated stress and

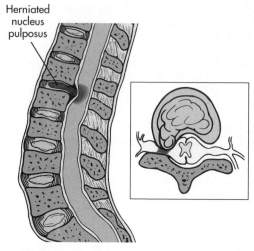

Herniated
nucleus
pulposus

Fig. 9. Compression of spinal cord caused by herniation of nucleus pulposus into spinal cord. *Inset,* Pressure on nerves as they leave the spinal canal.

trauma to the spine. The nucleus pulposus (gelatinous center of the disk) may first bulge and then it can herniate, placing pressure on nearby nerves (Fig. 9). The most common sites of rupture are the lumbosacral disks, specifically L4-5 and L5-S1.

Clinical Manifestations

The most common feature of lumbar disk damage is low back pain. Radicular pain that radiates down the buttock and below the knee along the distribution of the sciatic nerve generally indicates disk herniation. The straight-leg raise test may be positive indicating nerve root irritation. Back or leg pain may be reproduced by raising the leg and flexing the foot at 90 degrees.

Reflexes may be depressed or absent, depending on the spinal nerve root involved. The patient may report paresthesia or muscle weakness in the legs, feet, or toes. Multiple nerve root (cauda equina) compression may be manifested as bowel or bladder incontinence, or impotence.

Diagnostic Studies

- X-rays are done to note structural defects.
- A myelogram, magnetic resonance imaging (MRI), or computed tomography (CT) scan is helpful in localizing the herniation site.

- An epidural venogram or diskogram may be necessary if other methods of diagnosis are unsuccessful.
- An electromyogram (EMG) of the extremities can be performed to determine severity of nerve irritation caused by herniation or to rule out other pathologic conditions, such as peripheral neuropathy.

Collaborative Care
Conservative Therapy
The patient with suspected disk damage is usually managed first with conservative therapy. This includes limitation of extremes of spinal movement (brace/corset/belt), local heat or ice, ultrasound and massage, traction, and transcutaneous electrical nerve stimulation (TENS). Drug therapy includes nonsteroidal antiinflammatory drugs (NSAIDs), short-term opioids, and muscle relaxants. Epidural corticosteroid injections may be effective in reducing inflammation and relieving acute pain. Conservative treatment can result in a healing over of the damaged area with a concomitant decrease in pain.

Once symptoms subside, back-strengthening exercises are begun twice per day and are encouraged for a lifetime. The patient should be taught the principles of good body mechanics. Extremes of flexion and torsion are strongly discouraged.

Most patients initially recover with a conservative treatment plan. If the radiculopathy *(nerve root pain)* becomes progressively worse or there is a loss of bowel or bladder control, surgery may be indicated.

Surgical Therapy
Surgery should be carefully considered because some patients, for unknown reasons, do not improve and symptoms may actually worsen after surgery.

- The traditional and most common procedure for lumbar disk disease is a *laminectomy*. It involves the surgical excision of part of the posterior arch of the vertebra (referred to as the lamina) to gain access to part or all of the entire protruding disk to remove it. A minimal hospital stay is usually required.
- A *diskectomy* is another common type of surgical procedure that may be performed to decompress the nerve root. Microsurgical diskectomy is a version of the standard diskectomy in which the surgeon uses a microscope to allow better visualization of the disk to aid in the removal of the damaged portion.
- A *percutaneous laser diskectomy* is an outpatient surgical procedure that is done by using fluoroscopy and passing a

tube through retroperitoneal soft tissues to the lateral border of the disk. A laser is then used to remove the herniated portion of the disk.

■ An *intradiskal electrothermoplasty* is a minimally invasive outpatient procedure that involves x-ray–guided insertion of a needle into the affected disk. A wire is then threaded into the disk through the needle. The wire is then heated to denervate the small nerve fibers that have grown into the cracks and have invaded the degenerating disk.

■ A similar outpatient technique is *radiofrequency diskal nucleoplasty,* in which a special radiofrequency probe is inserted into the disk and generates energy that breaks up the molecular bonds of the gel in the nucleus.

■ Another procedure uses an *interspinous process decompression system* (X stop) that fits onto a mount that is placed on vertebrae in the lower back. The device works by pushing open the spinal cord by pressing against parts of either side of the vertebrae. The effect is similar to and less invasive than a laminectomy.

A *spinal fusion* may be performed if an unstable bony mechanism is present. The spine is stabilized by creating an ankylosis (fusion) of contiguous vertebrae with a bone graft from the patient's fibula or iliac crest or from donated cadaver bone. Metal fixation with rods, plates, or screws may be implanted. A posterior lumbar interbody fusion may be performed to provide extra support for bone grafting or a prosthetic device. A newer device, the Infuse Bone Graft/LT-CAGE, contains genetically engineered protein that stimulates the body to grow new bone at the spinal fusion site.

Nursing Management: Spinal Surgery

Postoperative care focuses on maintaining proper spine alignment at all times until healing has occurred. Flat bed rest may be maintained for 1 to 2 days depending on the surgery. Logrolling patients when turning is essential to maintain proper body alignment. Pillows can be used under the thighs of each leg when supine and between the legs when in the side-lying position to provide comfort and ensure alignment.

The patient often fears turning or any movement that increases pain. The nurse must offer reassurance to the patient that the proper technique is being used to maintain body alignment.

Most patients require the postoperative use of opioids, such as morphine, intravenously for 24 to 48 hours. Patient-controlled analgesia (PCA) allows for optimal analgesic levels and is the preferred method of continued pain management during this time.

- After fluids are being taken, the patient may be switched to oral drugs such as acetaminophen with codeine, hydrocodone (Vicodin), or oxycodone (Percocet). Diazepam (Valium) may be prescribed for muscle relaxation.

- Because the spinal canal may be entered during the surgical procedure, there is potential for cerebrospinal fluid (CSF) leakage. Severe headache or leakage of CSF on the dressing should be reported immediately.

- Frequent monitoring of peripheral neurologic signs of the extremities is a nursing responsibility after spinal surgery. Movement of arms and legs and assessment of sensation should be unchanged when compared with preoperative status. Paresthesias, such as numbness and tingling, may not be relieved immediately after surgery. Any new muscle weakness or paresthesias should be documented and reported immediately.

- Paralytic ileus and interference with bowel function may occur for several days and may manifest as nausea, abdominal distention, and constipation. The nurse should assess whether the patient is passing flatus, has bowel sounds in all quadrants, and has a flat, soft abdomen. Stool softeners (e.g., docusate sodium [Colace]) may aid in relieving and preventing constipation.

- Adequate bladder emptying may be altered because of activity restrictions, opioids, or anesthesia. Patients should use the commode or ambulate to the bathroom when allowed to promote adequate emptying of the bladder. Intermittent catheterization or an indwelling catheter may be necessary for patients who have difficulty urinating.

- Activity prescriptions vary with surgeons, but the patient who has had spinal surgery usually ambulates early in the postoperative period. It is a nursing responsibility to know the specific orders related to activity for any patient.

Additional nursing responsibilities are required if the patient has also had a spinal fusion. Because a bone graft is usually involved, the postoperative healing time is prolonged compared with that for a laminectomy. Immobilization over an extended time may be necessary. A rigid orthosis (thoracic-lumbar-sacral orthosis or chair-back brace) is often used during the period of immobilization.

In addition to the primary surgical site, the donor site for the bone graft must be regularly assessed. The donor site usually causes greater postoperative pain than the fused area. A pressure dressing is applied to the donor site to prevent excessive bleeding. If the donor site is the fibula, neurovascular extremity assessments are a postoperative nursing responsibility.

The patient should be instructed to avoid sitting or standing for prolonged periods. Activities that should be encouraged include walking, lying down, and shifting weight from one foot to the other when standing.

- The patient should learn to think through an activity before starting any potentially injurious task, such as bending, lifting, or stooping. Any twisting movement of the spine is contraindicated. The thighs and knees, rather than the back, should be used to absorb the shock of activity and movement.
- A firm mattress or bed board is essential to provide vertebral support.

INTESTINAL OBSTRUCTION

Description

Intestinal obstruction occurs when intestinal contents cannot pass through the gastrointestinal (GI) tract. The obstruction may occur in the small intestine or colon and can be partial or complete. Causes of intestinal obstruction can be classified as mechanical or nonmechanical.

- *Mechanical obstruction* is a detectable occlusion of the intestinal lumen. Most intestinal obstructions occur in the small intestine. Surgical adhesion is the most common cause of small bowel obstructions and can occur within days of surgery or several years later. Hernias and tumors are the next most common causes. Carcinoma is the most common cause of large bowel obstruction, followed by volvulus and diverticular disease.
- *Nonmechanical obstruction* may result from a neuromuscular or vascular disorder. *Paralytic (adynamic) ileus* is the most common form of nonmechanical obstruction. It occurs to some degree after any abdominal surgery. Other causes of paralytic ileus include inflammatory reactions (e.g., acute pancreatitis, acute appendicitis), electrolyte abnormalities, and thoracic or lumbar spinal fractures. Vascular obstructions are rare and are due to an interference with the blood supply to a portion of the bowel. The most common causes of vascular bowel obstructions are emboli and atherosclerosis of the mesenteric arteries.

Pathophysiology

When fluid, gas, and intestinal contents accumulate proximal to the intestinal obstruction, distention occurs, and the distal bowel may collapse. As the fluid increases, so does the pressure in the lumen of the bowel. The increased pressure leads to an increase in capillary permeability and extravasation of fluids and electrolytes into the peritoneal cavity. Retention of fluid in the intestine and peritoneal cavity can lead to a severe reduction in circulating blood volume and result in hypotension and hypovolemic shock.

- The most dangerous obstruction is when the bowel becomes twisted, cutting off the blood supply. If not corrected quickly, the bowel will become necrotic and rupture, leading to massive infection and death.
- The location of the obstruction determines the extent of fluid, electrolyte, and acid-base imbalances. With a high obstruction, metabolic alkalosis may result from the loss of gastric hydrochloric (HCl) acid through vomiting or nasogastric (NG) intubation. When the obstruction is in the small bowel, dehydration occurs rapidly. If the obstruction is below the proximal colon, solid fecal material accumulates until symptoms of discomfort appear.

Clinical Manifestations

Manifestations vary, depending on the location of the intestinal obstruction, and include nausea, vomiting, abdominal pain, distention, inability to pass flatus, and obstipation.

- An obstruction located high in the small intestine produces rapid-onset, sometimes projectile vomiting with bile-containing vomitus. Vomiting from more distal obstructions of the small intestine is more gradual in onset. Vomitus may be orange-brown and fecal smelling because of bacterial overgrowth.
- Vomiting usually relieves abdominal pain in high intestinal obstructions. Persistent, colicky abdominal pain is seen with lower intestinal obstruction. A characteristic sign of mechanical obstruction is pain that comes and goes in waves. This is due to intestinal peristalsis trying to move bowel contents past the obstructed area. In contrast, paralytic ileus produces a more constant generalized discomfort. Strangulation causes severe, constant pain that is rapid in onset.
- Abdominal distention is a common manifestation of intestinal obstructions. It is usually absent or minimally noticeable in high obstructions of the small intestine and greatly

increased in lower intestinal obstructions. Abdominal tenderness and rigidity are usually absent unless strangulation or peritonitis has occurred.

- Auscultation of bowel sounds reveals high-pitched sounds above the area of obstruction. Bowel sounds may also be absent. Borborygmi (audible abdominal sounds caused by hyperactive intestinal motility) are often noted by the patient. The patient's temperature rarely rises above 100° F (37.8° C) unless strangulation or peritonitis has occurred.

Diagnostic Studies

- Upright and lateral abdominal x-rays show the presence of gas and fluid in the intestines. The presence of intraperitoneal air indicates perforation.
- Barium enemas are helpful in locating large intestinal obstructions but are not used if perforation is suspected.
- Sigmoidoscopy or colonoscopy may provide direct visualization of an obstruction in the colon.
- Computed tomography (CT) scans may also be used in diagnosis.
- An elevated white blood cell (WBC) count may indicate strangulation or perforation; elevated hematocrit (Hct) values may reflect hemoconcentration; decreased hemoglobin and Hct values may indicate bleeding from a neoplasm or strangulation with necrosis.
- Serum sodium (Na^+), potassium (K^+), and chloride (Cl^-) concentrations are decreased in small bowel obstruction.
- Blood urea nitrogen (BUN) and serum creatinine should be monitored to determine if fluid resuscitation is adequate.
- Stool should be checked for occult blood.

Collaborative Care

Emergency surgery is indicated if the bowel is strangulated, but many obstructions resolve with conservative treatment. Treatment is directed toward relief of the obstruction and correction and maintenance of fluid and electrolyte balance.

- Initial treatment of bowel obstruction caused by adhesions includes maintaining nothing-by-mouth (NPO) status of the patient, insertion of an NG tube to decompress the bowel, intravenous (IV) fluid resuscitation, and analgesics for pain control.
- Long intestinal tubes (10 feet [300 cm]) such as Cantor or Miller-Abbott tubes may be used instead of NG tubes to decompress the bowel. Their use is controversial and limited because they are more difficult and time consuming to insert, and they may not be any more effective than NG tubes.

- IV infusions of normal saline or Ringer's lactate that contain K^+ should be given to maintain the fluid and electrolyte balance. Parenteral nutrition may be necessary in some cases to correct nutritional deficiencies, improve the patient's nutritional status before surgery, and promote postoperative healing.

If the situation does not improve within 24 to 48 hours or if the patient's condition deteriorates, surgery is performed to relieve the obstruction.

- Surgery may involve simply resecting the obstructed segment of bowel and anastomosing the remaining healthy bowel back together. Partial or total colectomy, colostomy, or ileostomy may be required when extensive obstruction or necrosis is present.
- Occasionally obstructions can be removed nonsurgically. A colonoscope can be used to remove polyps, dilate strictures, and remove and destroy tumors with a laser.

Nursing Management
Goals
The patient with an intestinal obstruction will have relief from the obstruction and a return to normal bowel function, minimal to no discomfort, and normal fluid and electrolyte status.
Nursing Diagnoses
- Acute pain
- Deficient fluid volume
- Imbalanced nutrition: less than body requirements
Nursing Interventions
The patient should be monitored closely for signs of dehydration and electrolyte imbalance.

- A strict intake and output record should be maintained that includes all emesis and tube drainage. IV fluids should be administered as ordered.
- Serum electrolyte levels should be monitored closely. A patient with a high obstruction is more likely to have metabolic alkalosis; a patient with a low obstruction is at greater risk of metabolic acidosis.
- The patient is often restless and constantly changes position to relieve the pain.
- The nurse should provide comfort measures, promote a restful environment, and keep distractions and visitors to a minimum.
- Nursing care of the patient after surgery for an intestinal obstruction is similar to the care of the patient after a laparotomy (see Abdominal Pain, Acute, p. 3).

IRRITABLE BOWEL SYNDROME

Description

Irritable bowel syndrome (IBS) is a symptom complex characterized by intermittent and recurrent abdominal pain and stool
pattern irregularities. It is classified as IBS with diarrhea, IBS with
constipation, and IBS with alternating diarrhea and constipation.
Other common symptoms include abdominal distention, bloating,
excessive flatulence, a continual defecation urge, urgency, and a
sensation of incomplete evacuation.

IBS affects approximately 10% to 15% of the Western population, of whom two or three times as many women as men seek
care for IBS. Stress, psychologic factors, and specific food intoler-
ances are factors that precipitate IBS symptoms.

- In IBS the presence of stool or gas in the gastrointestinal
  (GI) tract stimulates visceral afferent fibers that results
  in the perception of discomfort or pain. Several neuro-
  chemicals including serotonin are likely involved in
  bowel symptoms of diarrhea, constipation, and pain
  sensitivity.
- Because a diagnosis of IBS is made when the patient displays the characteristic symptoms and other conditions are
  ruled out, the key to accurate diagnosis is a thorough health
  history and physical examination. Emphasis should be on
  symptoms, past health history (e.g., psychosocial aspects
  including physical or sexual abuse), family history, and
  drug and dietary history.
- Standardized, symptom-based criteria for IBS are referred
  to as the Rome criteria and include abdominal discomfort
  or pain for at least 12 weeks (not necessarily consecutive)
  within 12 months that has at least two of the following
  characteristics:
- Relieved with defecation
- Onset associated with a change in stool frequency
- Onset associated with a change in stool appearance

Because treatment is often focused on symptoms, patients are
encouraged to keep a diary of symptoms, diet, and episodes of
stress to help identify factors that seem to trigger IBS symptoms.

- A diet containing dietary fiber, at least 20 g/day, or a
  bulking agent such as Metamucil has been traditionally
  prescribed, but fermentation of large amounts of fiber can
  increase bloating and gas pain, two symptoms that are
  already problematic for many patients with IBS.

- The patient whose primary symptoms are abdominal distention and increased flatulence should be advised to eliminate common gas-producing foods such as broccoli and cabbage and to substitute yogurt for milk products if there is lactose intolerance.
- Antispasmodic agents, such as dicyclomine (Bentyl), may be tried before meals to alleviate the pain associated with ingestion of food, but their effectiveness has been questioned.
- Loperamide (Imodium), a synthetic opioid that decreases intestinal transit and enhances intestinal water absorption and sphincter tone, has been found effective for IBS patients with diarrhea.
- Two serotonergic agents used for IBS include tegaserod (Zelnorm) for women whose primary bowel symptom is constipation and alosetron (Lotronex) for women with severe IBS and diarrhea. Because of serious, sometimes fatal complications from constipation, alosetron is available only in a restricted access program for women who have not responded to other IBS therapies.
- Other therapies may include relaxation and stress management techniques, acupuncture, hypnosis, and Chinese herbs, although no single therapy has been found to be effective for all patients with IBS.

KIDNEY CANCER

Kidney cancers arise from the cortex or pelvis. Adenocarcinoma (renal cell carcinoma) is the most common type of malignant kidney tumor. Kidney cancer is twice as frequent in men as in women and is typically discovered when the person is 50 to 70 years old. The most significant risk factor is cigarette smoking. Other risk factors include obesity, hypertension, and exposure to cadmium, asbestos, and gasoline.

There are no characteristic early symptoms. The most common manifestations are hematuria, flank pain, and a palpable mass in the flank or abdomen. Other symptoms include weight loss, fever, hypertension, and anemia. Local extension of kidney cancer into the renal vein and vena cava is common. The most common sites of metastases include the lungs, liver, and long bones and are present in about 30% of patients at the time of diagnosis.

Diagnostic Studies

- Intravenous pyelogram (IVP) with nephrotomography is primary method of detection and evaluation of masses.
- Ultrasound helps differentiate between a tumor and a cyst.
- Angiography, percutaneous needle aspiration, computed tomography (CT) scan, and magnetic resonance imaging (MRI) are also used for diagnosis.

The treatment of choice for patients with stage I or II tumors is a radical nephrectomy, which is removal of the kidney, adrenal gland, surrounding fascia, part of the ureter, and draining lymph nodes. Radiation therapy is used palliatively in inoperable cases and when there are metastases to the bone or lungs. Although renal cell carcinoma is refractory to most chemotherapy drugs, 5-FU, floxuridine (FUDR), and gemcitabine (Gemzar) may be used to treat metastatic disease. Biologic therapies, including α-interferon and interleukin-2, are also used in metastatic disease. Targeted therapy for metastatic disease includes the use of sunitinib malate (Sutent) and sorafenib (Nexavar).

KIDNEY DISEASE, CHRONIC

Description

Chronic kidney disease (CKD) is defined as the presence of kidney damage for at least 3 months with functional or structural abnormalities of the kidneys, with or without decreased glomerular filtration rate (GFR). The damage can be evident through either pathologic abnormalities or markers of kidney damage, such as abnormalities in blood or urine specimens, or imaging studies. CKD is also defined as a GFR of less than 60 ml/min/1.73 m^2 for at least 3 months, with or without kidney damage. Five stages of chronic kidney disease have been identified based on the level of kidney function as determined by the GFR (Table 56). The last stage of kidney failure (end-stage renal disease [ESRD]) occurs when the GFR is less than 15 ml/min.

Although there are many different causes of CKD, the end result is a systemic disease involving every body organ. In the United States the leading causes of ESRD are diabetes mellitus (DM) and hypertension.

Pathophysiology

In the majority of cases the individual passes through the early stages of CKD without recognizing the disease state because the remaining nephrons hypertrophy to compensate. The prognosis

Table 56	Stages and Descriptions of Chronic Kidney Disease	
	Description	**GFR (ml/min/1.73 m²)**
	At increased risk for CKD	≥90 (with CKD risk factors)
Stage 1	Kidney damage with normal or ↑ GFR	≥90
Stage 2	Kidney damage with mild ↓ GFR	60-89
Stage 3	Moderate ↓ GFR	30-59
Stage 4	Severe ↓ GFR	15-29
Stage 5	Kidney failure (end-stage renal disease)	<15 (or dialysis)

From National Kidney Foundation: *The K/DOQI clinical practice guidelines for chronic kidney disease: evaluation, classification and stratification*, 2002. Available at *www.kidney.org/professionals/kdoqi/guidelines_ckd/Gif_File/kck_t3.gif* (accessed July 23, 2006).
CKD, Chronic kidney disease, *GFR,* glomerular filtration rate.

and course of CKD are highly variable depending on the etiology, patient's condition and age, and adequacy of medical follow-up care. Some individuals live normal, active lives with compensated renal failure, whereas others may rapidly progress to ESRD.

When the GFR falls below 15 ml/min (from normal range of 85 to 135 ml/min for the average adult), some form of dialysis or transplantation is required for survival.

Clinical Manifestations

As renal function progressively deteriorates, every body system becomes affected. Many of the early clinical manifestations are similar to those of acute renal failure (see Renal Failure, Acute, p. 529). Manifestations are a result of retained substances including urea, creatinine, phenols, hormones, water, electrolytes, and many other substances. *Uremia* is a syndrome that incorporates all the signs and symptoms seen in the various systems throughout the body in CKD (see Fig. 47-5 in Lewis and others, *Medical-Surgical Nursing,* edition 7, p. 1206). Manifestations of uremia vary among patients according to the etiology of kidney disease, comorbid conditions, age, and the degree of compliance with the prescribed medical regimen.

Specific manifestations include:

▪ *Urinary system.* Persistent proteinuria; polyuria, nocturia, and a fixed specific gravity at 1.010 because of decreased

K

renal concentrating ability, followed by oliguria and anuria as renal disease progresses. Possible casts, pyuria, and hematuria depending on cause of kidney disease.

- *Metabolic disturbances.* Blood urea nitrogen (BUN) and creatinine levels increase, leading to nausea, vomiting, lethargy, and impaired thought processes; a cellular insensitivity to insulin of an unknown cause results in defective carbohydrate metabolism with moderate hyperglycemia, hyperinsulinemia, and abnormal glucose tolerance tests; hyperinsulinemia stimulates hepatic production of triglycerides, and hyperlipidemia results from decreased levels of the enzyme lipoprotein lipase that is important in the breakdown of lipoproteins.

- *Electrolyte and acid-base imbalances.* Hyperkalemia results from decreased renal excretion, breakdown of cellular protein, metabolic acidosis, and dietary intake; sodium (Na^+) may also be retained, resulting in water retention, edema, hypertension, and heart failure; calcium, phosphate, and magnesium imbalances occur.

- *Hematologic system.* Anemia results from a lack of erythropoietin, bleeding tendencies occur because of a defect in platelet function, and an altered chemotactic response by both neutrophils and monocytes increases the risk for infection.

- *Alterations of calcium and phosphate metabolism.* Impaired calcium absorption occurs because the kidneys cannot activate vitamin D and resulting low serum calcium levels stimulate the release of parathyroid hormone (PTH). PTH stimulates the resorption of calcium and phosphate from bone. The excess phosphate binds with calcium, forming insoluble metastatic calcifications that are deposited throughout the body.

Additional systemic signs include pulmonary edema, diarrhea, peripheral neuropathy, osteomalacia, yellow-gray discoloration of skin, deposition of calcium phosphate and urea in the skin, mucosal ulcerations in the gastrointestinal (GI) tract, hypothyroidism, infertility, and personality and behavior changes.

Diagnostic Studies

- Urinalysis detects protein, red blood cells (RBCs), white blood cells (WBCs), casts, and glucose.
- Urine culture may identify microorganisms in the urine.
- BUN and serum creatinine are elevated.
- GFR, obtained from 24-hour urine creatinine clearance measures, is decreased.

- Reversible renal disease is identified by renal scan, computed tomography (CT) scan, renal ultrasound, and renal biopsy.
- Hematocrit (Hct) and hemoglobin (Hb) levels are decreased.

Collaborative Care

When a patient is diagnosed as having chronic renal insufficiency, conservative therapy is attempted before maintenance dialysis begins. Every effort is made to detect and treat potentially reversible causes of renal failure (e.g., cardiac failure, dehydration, pyelonephritis, nephrotoxins, lower urinary tract obstruction). Conservative therapy is directed toward preserving existing renal function, treating symptoms, preventing complications, and providing for patient comfort. This therapy consists primarily of drug and nutritional therapy and supportive care.

Drug Therapy

Drug therapy includes administration of erythropoietin, calcium supplements, phosphate binders, antihypertensive medication, and measures to lower potassium (K^+). Drug dosages and frequency of administration are adjusted for decreased renal function.

- Acute hyperkalemia may require treatment with intravenous (IV) glucose and insulin to move potassium into the cells, or IV 10% calcium gluconate. Sodium polystyrene sulfonate (Kayexalate), a cation-exchange resin, is used to lower potassium levels in stage 4 CKD. Dialysis may be required to decrease potassium if dysrhythmias are present.
- In addition to diet, weight loss, and lifestyle changes, treatment of hypertension includes the use of antihypertensive drugs. Drugs most commonly used include diuretics, β-adrenergic blockers, calcium channel blockers, angiotensin-converting enzyme (ACE) inhibitors, and angiotensin receptor blockers (ARBs).
- Calcium-based phosphate binders such as calcium carbonate (e.g., Tums) and calcium acetate (e.g., PhosLo) are used to bind phosphate in the GI tract, which is then excreted in the stool. Newer phosphate binders that do not contain calcium include sevelamer (Renagel) and lanthanum (Fosrenol).
- Human erythropoietin (epoetin alfa [Epogen, Procrit]) produced with recombinant DNA technology is available to treat the anemia of CKD.

Nutritional Therapy

Nutritional therapy includes the restriction of protein, potassium, sodium, phosphate, and water (see specific recommended restric-

K

tions in Lewis and others, *Medical-Surgical Nursing,* edition 7, pp. 1202 to 1203). In the attempt to restrict specific nutrients that are affected by CKD, deficiencies of vitamins, calcium, and protein are likely to occur.

Nursing Management
Goals
The patient with chronic kidney disease will demonstrate the knowledge and ability to comply with the therapeutic regimen, participate in decision making for the plan of care and future treatment modality, demonstrate effective coping strategies, and continue with activities of daily living (ADLs) within physiologic limitations.

See NCP 47-1 for the patient with chronic kidney disease, Lewis and others, *Medical-Surgical Nursing,* edition 7, pp. 1214 to 1215.

Nursing Diagnoses
- Excess fluid volume
- Imbalanced nutrition: less than body requirements
- Grieving
- Risk for injury (fracture)
- Activity intolerance
- Impaired skin integrity

Nursing Interventions
If a patient has a personal or family history of renal disease, hypertension, or DM, regular checkups, including serum creatinine, BUN, and urinalysis, are essential.

- Individuals at risk can take measures to prevent or delay the progression of CKD by maintaining glycemic control if diabetic, controlling blood pressure (BP), and obtaining early and definitive treatment of urinary tract infections.
- When potentially nephrotoxic drugs are prescribed, it is important to monitor the patient's renal function with serum creatinine and BUN.
- Any changes in urine appearance (color, odor), frequency, or volume must be reported to the health care provider.
- While the patient with CKD is being maintained on conservative therapy, the decision regarding future therapies should be made. This should be done before complications such as mental status changes, bleeding, progressive neuropathies, and fluid overload occur.
- The patient and family need a clear explanation of what is involved in dialysis and transplantation. The patient should be informed that if dialysis is chosen, the option of transplantation still remains, and if a transplanted organ fails, the patient can return to dialysis.

| Table 57 | Patient and Family Teaching Guide: Chronic Kidney Disease |

1. Explain dietary (protein, sodium, potassium, phosphate) and fluid restrictions.
2. Encourage discussion of difficulties in modifying diet and fluid intake.
3. Explain signs and symptoms of electrolyte imbalance, especially high potassium.
4. Teach alternative ways of reducing thirst, such as sucking on ice cubes, lemon, or hard candy.
5. Explain the rationale for prescribed medications and common side effects. Examples:
   Phosphate binders should be taken with meals.
   Iron supplements should be taken between meals.
6. Explain the importance of reporting any of the following:
   Weight gain greater than 4 lb (2 kg)
   Increasing blood pressure
   Shortness of breath
   Edema
   Increasing fatigue or weakness
   Confusion or lethargy
7. Encourage patient and family to share concerns about lifestyle changes, living with a chronic illness, and decisions about type of dialysis or transplantation.

▼ Patient and Family Teaching

It is important to teach the patient and family because the patient is responsible for diet, medications, and follow-up care (Table 57).

- The patient should weigh daily, learn to take a daily BP, and be able to identify the signs and symptoms of fluid overload, hyperkalemia, and other electrolyte imbalances.
- The patient and family must understand the importance of strict dietary adherence. The dietitian should meet with the patient and family on a regular basis for nutritional planning. A diet history and a consideration of cultural variations will facilitate diet planning and adherence.
- The patient needs a complete understanding of the drugs, dosages, and common side effects. It may be helpful to make a list of medications and the times of administration that can be posted in the home. The patient must be instructed to avoid certain over-the-counter drugs, such as nonsteroidal antiinflammatory drugs (NSAIDs) and magnesium-based laxatives and antacids.

K

LACTASE DEFICIENCY

Description
Lactase deficiency is a condition in which the lactase enzyme that breaks down lactose into two simple sugars (glucose and galactose) is deficient or absent.

Primary lactase insufficiency is most commonly due to genetic factors. Certain ethnic or racial groups, especially those with Asian or African ancestry, develop low lactase levels at about age 5 years. Other causes of lactose malabsorption include conditions that lead to bacterial overgrowth with lactose fermentation in the small bowel and intestinal mucosal damage that interferes with absorption. Gastrointestinal (GI) diseases that damage the mucosa include inflammatory bowel disease (ulcerative colitis, Crohn's disease), gastroenteritis, and celiac disease.

Clinical Manifestations
Symptoms of lactose intolerance include bloating, flatulence, crampy abdominal pain, and diarrhea. They may occur within one-half hour to several hours after drinking a glass of milk or ingesting a milk product. Undigested lactose creates an osmotic action, pulling fluid into the small intestines, resulting in diarrhea.

Diagnostic Studies
Many lactose-intolerant persons are aware of their milk intolerance and simply avoid milk and milk products. Lactose intolerance can be diagnosed by a lactose tolerance test or a lactose hydrogen breath test. The hydrogen breath test detects lung excretion of hydrogen produced by bacterial metabolism of undigested lactose in the colon.

Nursing and Collaborative Management
Treatment consists of eliminating lactose from the diet by avoiding milk and milk products and/or replacing lactase with commercially available preparations. The objective of care is to teach the importance of adherence to the diet.

- A lactose-free diet is given initially and is gradually advanced to a low-lactose diet as tolerated by the patient.
- Many lactose-intolerant persons may not exhibit symptoms if lactose is taken in small amounts.
- Cheese is better tolerated than milk and ice cream.
- If the milk has been fermented (e.g., cultured buttermilk, yogurt, sour cream), the patient with low lactase levels may tolerate it better.

- Lactase enzyme (Lactaid) is available as an over-the-counter product. It is mixed with milk and breaks down lactose before the milk is ingested.

LEIOMYOMAS

Leiomyomas (fibroids) are benign smooth muscle tumors within the uterus. They are the most common benign tumors of the female genital tract. By 30 years of age, 10% of white women and 30% of African American women will have uterine leiomyomas.

The cause of leiomyomas is unknown. They appear to depend on ovarian hormones because they grow slowly during the woman's reproductive years and undergo atrophy after menopause.

The majority of women with leiomyomas do not have any symptoms. Of the women who develop symptoms, the most common include abnormal uterine bleeding, pain, and symptoms associated with pelvic pressure. Pain is thought to be associated with an infection or twisting of the pedicle from which the tumor is growing.

Pressure on surrounding organs may result in rectal, bladder, and lower abdominal discomfort. Large tumors may cause a general enlargement of the lower abdomen. These tumors are sometimes associated with miscarriage and infertility.

Diagnosis is based on the characteristic pelvic findings of an enlarged uterus distorted by nodular masses.

Treatment depends on the symptoms, age of the patient, her desire to bear children, and the location and size of the tumor or tumors. If the symptoms are minor, the health care provider may elect to monitor the patient closely for a time.

- Persistent heavy menstrual bleeding causing anemia and large or rapidly growing tumors are indications for surgery. When so indicated, leiomyomas are removed by hysterectomy or myomectomy. A myomectomy is performed for women who wish to have children. In this case, only the fibroids are removed to preserve the uterus. Small fibroids may be removed using a hysteroscope and laser resection instruments.
- Cryosurgery and magnetic resonance imaging (MRI)–guided focused ultrasound may also be used to destroy smaller tumors.

LEUKEMIA

Description

Leukemia is a general term used to describe a group of malignant disorders affecting the blood and blood-forming tissues of the bone marrow, lymph system, and spleen. It results in an accumulation of dysfunctional cells because of a loss of regulation in cell division. Although leukemia is often thought of as a disease of children, the number of adults affected is 10 times that of children.

Regardless of the specific type, there is generally no single causative agent in the development of leukemia. Most leukemias result from a combination of factors including genetic and environmental influences.

Classification

Leukemia can be classified as acute versus chronic and as of myelogenous origin or of lymphocytic origin. By combining the acute and chronic categories with the cell type involved, four major types of leukemia can be identified. Table 58 summarizes the relative incidence and features of the four types of leukemia.

Acute myelogenous leukemia (AML) represents only one fourth of all leukemias, but it makes up approximately 85% of the acute leukemias in adults. Its onset is often abrupt and dramatic. A patient may have serious infections and abnormal bleeding from the onset of the disease.

Acute lymphocytic leukemia (ALL) is the most common type of leukemia in children and accounts for 15% of acute leukemias in adults. The 5-year survival rate is nearly 80% for children and about 40% for adults. In ALL, immature lymphocytes proliferate in the bone marrow; most are of B-cell origin. Fever is present in the majority of patients at time of diagnosis. Signs and symptoms may appear abruptly with bleeding or fever, or they may be insidious with progressive weakness, fatigue, and bleeding tendencies.

Chronic myelogenous leukemia (CML) is caused by excessive development of mature neoplastic granulocytes in the bone marrow. These cells contain a distinctive cytogenetic abnormality, the Philadelphia chromosome. CML usually has a chronic stable phase that lasts for several years, followed by the development of an acute aggressive phase (blastic phase) that is often refractory to therapy.

Chronic lymphocytic leukemia (CLL) is characterized by the production and accumulation of functionally inactive but long-lived, small, mature-appearing lymphocytes. The lymphocyte

Table 58 Types of Leukemia

Type	Age of Onset	Clinical Manifestations	Diagnostic Findings
Acute myelogenous leukemia (AML)	Increase in incidence with advancing age, peak incidence between 60-70 yr of age	Fatigue and weakness, headache, mouth sores, minimal hepatosplenomegaly and lymphadenopathy, anemia, bleeding, fever, infection, sternal tenderness	Low RBC count, Hb, Hct; low platelet count; low to high WBC count with myeloblasts; high LDH; greatly hypercellular bone marrow with myeloblasts
Acute lymphocytic leukemia (ALL)	Before 14 yr of age, peak incidence between 2-9 yr of age and in older adults	Fever; pallor; bleeding; anorexia; fatigue and weakness; bone, joint, and abdominal pain; generalized lymphadenopathy; infections; weight loss; hepatosplenomegaly; headache; mouth sores; neurologic manifestations, including CNS involvement, increased intracranial pressure (nausea, vomiting, lethargy, cranial nerve dysfunction), secondary to meningeal infiltration	Low RBC count, Hb, Hct; low platelet count; low, normal, or high WBC count; high LDH; transverse lines of rarefaction at ends of metaphysis of long bones on x-ray; hypercellular bone marrow with lymphoblasts; lymphoblasts also possible in cerebrospinal fluid; presence of Philadelphia chromosome (20%-25% of patients)

Continued

CNS, Central nervous system; Hb, hemoglobin; Hct, hematocrit; LDH, lactic dehydrogenase; RBC, red blood cell; WBC, white blood cell.

L

Table 58 Types of Leukemia—cont'd

Type	Age of Onset	Clinical Manifestations	Diagnostic Findings
Chronic myelogenous leukemia (CML)	25-60 yr of age, peak incidence around 45 yr of age	No symptoms early in disease; and weakness, fever, sternal tenderness, weight loss, joint pain, bone pain, massive splenomegaly, increase in sweating	Low RBC count, Hb, Hct; high platelet count early, lower count later; increase in polymorphonuclear neutrophils, normal number of lymphocytes, and normal or low number of monocytes; low leukocyte alkaline phosphatase; presence of Philadelphia chromosome in 90% of patients
Chronic lymphocytic leukemia (CLL)	50-70 yr of age, rare below 30 yr of age, predominance in men	No symptoms frequently; detection of disease often during examination for unrelated condition; chronic fatigue, anorexia, splenomegaly and lymphadenopathy, hepatomegaly	Mild anemia and thrombocytopenia with disease progression; total WBC count >100,000/μl, increase in peripheral lymphocytes; increase in presence of lymphocytes in bone marrow; hypogammaglobulinemia; may have autoimmune hemolytic anemia (4%-11%), idiopathic thrombocytopenia purpura (2%-4%)

involved is usually the B cell. Lymph node enlargement (lymph-adenopathy) throughout the body is present, and there is an increased incidence of infection because of T-cell deficiencies or hypogammaglobulinemia. Because CLL is usually a disease of older adults, treatment decisions must be made by considering disease progression and treatment of side effects. Fifty percent of patients with early-stage CLL experience rapid progressive disease and will require some therapy.

Hairy cell leukemia accounts for 2% of all adult leukemias and is a chronic disease of lymphoproliferation. This leukemia type predominantly involves B lymphocytes that infiltrate the bone marrow and spleen. The disease is often indolent, and some patients may not need therapy for up to 10 years.

Clinical Manifestations

Manifestations of leukemia vary (see Table 58). Essentially they relate to problems caused by bone marrow failure and the formation of leukemic infiltrates. The patient is predisposed to anemia, thrombocytopenia, and decreased function of white blood cells (WBCs).

- WBC infiltration into the patient's organs leads to problems such as splenomegaly, hepatomegaly, lymphadenopathy, bone pain, meningeal irritation, and oral lesions.

Diagnostic Studies

- Peripheral blood evaluation and bone marrow examination are the primary methods of diagnosing and classifying the sub-types of leukemia.
- Morphologic, histochemical, immunologic, and cytogenetic methods are all used to identify cell subtypes and the stage of development of leukemic cell populations.
- Studies such as lumbar puncture and computed tomography (CT) scan can determine the presence of leukemic cells outside the blood and bone marrow.

Collaborative Care

Collaborative care first focuses on the initial goal of attaining remission. Although a patient may not be cured, attaining remission or disease control is a realistic option for the majority of patients. In some cases, cure is a realistic goal.

- Because cytotoxic chemotherapy is the mainstay of treatment, the nurse must understand the principles of cancer chemotherapy, including cellular kinetics, the use of multiple drugs rather than single agents, and the cell cycle (see Chemotherapy, p. 712).

- Corticosteroids and radiation therapy may have a role in therapy for the patient with leukemia. Total body radiation may be used to prepare a patient for bone marrow transplantation, or radiation may be restricted to certain areas (fields), such as the liver, spleen, or other organs affected by infiltrates.
- In ALL, prophylactic intrathecal methotrexate is given to decrease central nervous system (CNS) involvement, which is common in this type of leukemia. When CNS leukemia does occur, cranial radiation may be given. The use of biologic therapy may be indicated for specific leukemias (see Lewis and others, *Medical-Surgical Nursing,* edition 7, pp. 719 to 723).

Chemotherapeutic agents used to treat leukemia vary. Combination chemotherapy is the mainstay of treatment for leukemia. The three purposes for using multiple drugs are to (1) decrease drug resistance, (2) minimize drug toxicity to the patient by using multiple drugs with varying toxicities, and (3) interrupt cell growth at multiple points in the cell cycle.

Hematopoietic stem cell transplantation (HSCT) is another type of therapy used for patients with different forms of leukemia. The goal of HSCT is to totally eliminate leukemia cells from the body using combinations of chemotherapy with or without total body radiation. This treatment also eradicates the patient's hematopoietic stem cells, which are then replaced with those of a human leukocyte antigen (HLA)–matched sibling, a volunteer donor (allogeneic), or an identical twin (syngeneic) or with the patient's own (autologous) stem cells that were removed (harvested) before the intensive therapy. (See the sections on HSCT in Lewis and others, *Medical-Surgical Nursing,* edition 7, p. 721.)

The primary complications of patients with allogeneic HSCT are graft-versus-host disease (GVHD), relapse of leukemia (especially ALL), and infection (especially interstitial pneumonia). Because transplantation has serious associated risks, the patient must weigh the significant risks of treatment-related death or treatment failure (relapse) with the hope of cure.

Nursing Management
Goals
The patient with leukemia will understand and cooperate with the treatment plan, experience minimal side effects and complications associated with both the disease and its treatment, and feel hopeful and supported during the periods of treatment, relapse, or remission.

See NCPs 31-1, pp. 688 to 689; 31-2, p. 706; and 31-3, p. 716, Lewis and others, *Medical-Surgical Nursing,* edition 7.

Nursing Diagnoses

Nursing diagnoses related to leukemia include those appropriate for anemia (see Anemia, p. 28), thrombocytopenia (see Thrombocytopenic Purpura, p. 635), and neutropenia (see the section on neutropenia in Lewis and others, *Medical-Surgical Nursing,* edition 7, pp. 713 to 716).

Nursing Interventions

The nursing role during acute phases of leukemia is extremely challenging because the patient has many physical and psychosocial needs. As with other forms of cancer, the diagnosis of leukemia can evoke great fear and be equated with death.

- The nurse must help the patient realize that although the future may be uncertain, one can have a meaningful quality of life while in remission or with disease control.
- Families need help in adjusting to the stress of the abrupt onset of serious illness (e.g., dependence, withdrawal, changes in role responsibilities, alterations in body image) and the losses imposed by the sick role. The diagnosis of leukemia often brings with it the need to make difficult decisions at a time of profound stress for the patient and family.

The nurse is an important advocate in helping the patient and family understand the complexities of treatment decisions and manage the side effects and toxicities. A patient may require isolation or may need to temporarily relocate to an appropriate treatment center. These situations can lead patients to feel deserted and isolated at a time when support is most needed.

- From a physical care perspective, the nurse is challenged to make assessments and plan care to help the patient deal with the severe side effects of chemotherapy. The life-threatening problems of bone marrow suppression (anemia, thrombocytopenia, neutropenia) require aggressive nursing interventions.
- The nurse must be knowledgeable about all drugs being administered. In addition, the nurse must know how to assess laboratory data reflecting the effects of the drugs. Patient survival and comfort during aggressive chemotherapy are significantly affected by the quality of nursing care.

▼ Patient and Family Teaching

The patient and family must be educated to understand the importance of their continued diligence in disease management and the need for follow-up care.

- Assistance may be needed to reestablish various relationships that are a part of the patient's life. Friends and family may not know how to interact with the patient.
- Involving the patient in survivor networks, support groups, or services, such as CanSurmount and Make Today Count, may help the patient adapt to living with a life-threatening illness. Exploring community resources (e.g., American Cancer Society, Leukemia Society, Meals-on-Wheels) may reduce the financial burden and feelings of dependence. Spiritual support may give the patient inner strength and peace.

LIVER CANCER

Description
Primary carcinoma of the liver is the fourth most common cancer in the world, with the majority of cases occurring in males. Hepatocellular carcinoma is the most common primary malignant tumor of the liver. About 80% of people with primary liver cancer have cirrhosis of the liver. Hepatitis C infection is responsible for 50% to 60% of all liver cancers, whereas hepatitis B is responsible for about 20%.

The liver is a common site of metastatic cancer growth because of its high rate of blood flow and extensive capillary network. Cancer cells in other parts of the body are commonly carried to the liver by way of the portal circulation. Primary liver tumors commonly metastasize to the lung.

- The prognosis for patients with liver cancer is poor. The cancer grows rapidly, and death may occur within 4 to 7 months as a result of hepatic encephalopathy or massive blood loss from gastrointestinal (GI) bleeding.

Clinical Manifestations
It is difficult to diagnose and differentiate liver cancer from cirrhosis in its early stages because of similar clinical manifestations (e.g., hepatomegaly, splenomegaly, jaundice, weight loss, peripheral edema, ascites, portal hypertension).

- Other common manifestations include dull abdominal pain in the epigastric or right upper quadrant region, anorexia, nausea and vomiting, and increased abdominal girth.

Diagnostic Studies
- Liver scan, computed tomography (CT), magnetic resonance imaging (MRI), magnetic resonance angiography, hepatic

angiography, endoscopic retrograde cholangiopancreatography (ERCP), and a liver biopsy assist in diagnosis.

■ α-Fetoprotein (AFP) may be positive in hepatocellular carcinoma. AFP is elevated in as many as 75% of patients with hepatocellular carcinoma and helps distinguish primary cancer from metastatic cancer.

Nursing and Collaborative Management

Treatment depends on the size and number of tumors, presence of metastasis, and overall health of the patient. Overall the management is similar to that for liver cirrhosis (see Cirrhosis, p. 131). Surgical excision (lobectomy) or liver transplant is sometimes performed if the tumor is localized to one portion of the liver. Only about 15% of patients have surgically resectable disease, but surgical interventions offer the best chance for cure. Other treatment options are radiofrequency ablation (RFA), cryosurgery, percutaneous ethanol injection, alcohol injection, and chemotherapy. Chemotherapy is used for patients with hepatocellular cancer who are not likely to benefit from other procedures.

Nursing interventions focus on keeping the patient as comfortable as possible. Because the patient with liver cancer manifests the same problems as the patient with advanced liver disease, the nursing interventions discussed for cirrhosis of the liver apply (see Cirrhosis, p. 131).

LOW BACK PAIN, ACUTE

Description

Low back pain is common and probably affects 80% of adults in the United States at least once during their lifetime. Risk factors associated with low back pain include smoking, stress, poor posture, lack of muscle tone, and excess weight. Jobs that require repetitive heavy lifting, vibration (e.g., jackhammer operator), and extended periods of driving are also associated with low back pain.

Pathophysiology

Pain in the lumbar region is a common problem because this area (1) bears most of the weight of the body, (2) is the most flexible region of the spinal column, (3) has nerve roots that are vulnerable to injury or disease, and (4) has an inherently poor biomechanical structure.

Low back pain is most often due to a musculoskeletal problem.

- The causes of low back pain of musculoskeletal origin include acute lumbosacral strain, instability of lumbosacral bony mechanism, osteoarthritis of the lumbosacral vertebrae, intervertebral disk degeneration, and herniation of the intervertebral disks.

Acute low back pain is defined as lasting 4 weeks or less. It is usually associated with some type of activity that causes undue stress (often hyperflexion) on tissues of the lower back. Often symptoms do not appear at the time of injury but develop later because of a gradual increase in paravertebral muscle spasms.

Few definitive diagnostic abnormalities are present with paravertebral muscle strain. The straight-leg raise test is positive for disk herniation when radicular pain occurs. Magnetic resonance imaging (MRI) and computed tomography (CT) scans are generally not done unless trauma or systemic disease (e.g., cancer, spinal infection) is suspected.

Collaborative Care

If the acute muscle spasms and accompanying pain are not severe, the patient may be treated on an outpatient basis with a combination of the following: analgesics such as nonsteroidal antiinflammatory drugs (NSAIDs), muscle relaxants, massage and back manipulation, and alternating use of heat and cold compresses. Severe pain may require a brief course of opioid analgesics.

A brief period of rest (1 to 2 days) at home may be necessary for some persons, whereas most persons do better with a continuation of regular activities.

- All patients during this time should avoid activities that aggravate the pain, including lifting, bending, twisting, and prolonged sitting. Most cases spontaneously improve within 2 weeks.
- Invasive treatments, such as epidural corticosteroid injections and implanted devices that deliver pain medication, are reserved for patients with chronic back pain who are refractory to the usual therapeutic options.

Nursing Management
Goals

The patient with low back pain will have satisfactory pain relief, avoid constipation secondary to medication and immobility, learn back-sparing practices, and return to previous level of activity within prescribed restrictions.

See NCP 64-2 for the patient with low back pain, Lewis and others, *Medical-Surgical Nursing,* edition 7, pp. 1678 to 1680.

Nursing Diagnoses
Acute Management
- Acute pain
- Impaired physical mobility

Chronic Management
- Chronic pain
- Ineffective coping
- Ineffective therapeutic regimen management

Nursing Interventions
Primary nursing responsibilities are to assist the patient to maintain activity limitations, promote comfort, and teach the patient about the health problem and appropriate exercises.

- Although actual muscle-strengthening and stretching exercises are often taught by the physical therapist, it is the nurse's responsibility to ensure that the patient understands the type and frequency of exercise prescribed, as well as the rationale for the program. Specific exercises are presented in Table 64-7, Lewis and others, *Medical Surgical Nursing,* edition 7, p. 1677.
- The frustration, pain, and disability imposed on the patient with low back pain problems require emotional support and understanding care by the nurse.
- The nurse is a significant role model and teacher for patients with low back problems. The nurse should use proper body mechanics at all times. This should be a primary consideration when teaching transfer and turning techniques to patients and care providers.

▼ **Patient and Family Teaching**
The nurse should assess the patient's use of body mechanics and offer instruction regarding activities that could produce back strain (Table 59).

- Patients are advised to maintain an appropriate weight. Excess body weight places extra stress on the lower back and weakens abdominal muscles that support the lower back.
- The position assumed while sleeping is also important in preventing low back pain. Sleeping in a prone position should be avoided because it produces excessive lumbar lordosis, placing excessive stress on the lower back. A firm mattress is recommended. The patient should sleep in either a supine or side-lying position, with the knees and hips flexed to prevent unnecessary pressure on support muscles, ligamentous structures, and lumbosacral joints.
- Patients should be advised to avoid or cease smoking. Nicotine has been shown to decrease circulation to the vertebral disks and has a causal link to some types of low back pain.

Table 59	Patient and Family Teaching Guide: Low Back Problems

Do Not
- Lean forward without bending knees
- Lift anything above level of the elbows
- Stand in one position for a prolonged time
- Sleep on abdomen or on back or side with legs out straight
- Exercise without consulting health care provider if having severe pain
- Exceed prescribed amount and type of exercises without consulting health care provider

Do
- Prevent lower back from straining forward by placing a foot on a step or stool during prolonged standing
- Sleep in a side-lying position with knees and hips bent
- Sleep on back with a lift under knees and legs or on back with a 10-inch–high pillow under knees to flex hips and knees
- Exercise 15 minutes in the morning and in the evening regularly; begin exercises with a 2- or 3-minute warm-up period by moving arms and legs, by alternately relaxing and tightening muscles; exercise slowly with smooth movements
- Maintain appropriate body weight
- Use local heat and cold application
- Use a lumbar roll or pillow for sitting

LOW BACK PAIN, CHRONIC

Description

Chronic low back pain lasts more than 3 months or is a repeated incapacitating episode. Causes of chronic low back pain include degenerative disk disease, lack of physical exercise, prior injury, obesity, structural and postural abnormalities, and systemic disease. Osteoarthritis (OA) may cause chronic pain in the lumbar area in patients over age 50 years or in the thoracic or lumbar area of younger patients with OA.

Spinal stenosis is a narrowing of the vertebral canal or nerve root canals caused by encroachment of bone on the space, and when it occurs in the lumbar area, it is a common cause of chronic or recurrent low back pain. Compression of the nerve roots can result with subsequent disk herniation. The pain associated with lumbar spinal stenosis often starts in the low back and then radiates to the buttock and leg. It worsens with walking and standing without walking.

Treatment regimens are much the same as for acute low back pain: a reduction in the pain associated with daily activities, a formal back pain program, and ongoing medical care. Cold, damp weather aggravates the back pain but can be relieved with rest and local heat application.

- Relief of pain and stiffness using mild analgesics, such as nonsteroidal antiinflammatory drugs (NSAIDs), is integral to the daily comfort of the patient with chronic low back pain.
- Weight reduction, sufficient rest periods, local heat/cold application, and exercise and activity throughout the day help keep the muscles and joints mobilized.
- Tricyclic antidepressants (e.g., amitriptyline [Elavil]) and selective serotonin reuptake inhibitors (e.g., sertraline [Zoloft]) have been shown to improve the chronic symptoms of low back pain through their actions on spinal neurotransmitters.
- Surgery may be indicated in patients with severe chronic low back pain who do not respond to conservative care and/or have continued neurologic deficits. (See Surgical Therapy, Intravertebral Lumbar Disk Damage, Lewis and others, *Medical Surgical Nursing*, edition 7, pp. 1681 to 1683.)

LUNG CANCER

Description

Lung cancer is the leading cause of cancer-related deaths in men and women in the United States and accounts for 28% of all cancer deaths. The overall 5-year survival rate is 15%. The disease is found most frequently in persons 40 to 75 years old.

- Cigarette smoking as a chronic respiratory irritant is the greatest risk factor for lung cancer. Smoking is responsible for approximately 80% to 90% of all lung cancers. Tobacco smoke contains 60 carcinogens in addition to substances that interfere with normal cell development. Cigarette smoke causes a change in the bronchial epithelium, which usually returns to normal when smoking is discontinued.
- Sidestream smoke (smoke from burning cigarettes, cigars) contains the same carcinogens found in mainstream smoke

(smoke inhaled and exhaled from the smoker). This environmental tobacco smoke inhaled by nonsmokers poses a 35% increased risk of the development of lung cancer in nonsmokers.
- Those who smoke pipes and cigars also have an increased risk of developing lung cancer, which is slightly higher than that of nonsmokers.
- Inhaled occupational carcinogens are another major risk factor and include asbestos, radon, nickel, iron and iron oxides, uranium, polycyclic aromatic hydrocarbons, and arsenic.

Pathophysiology

The pathogenesis of lung cancer is not well understood. More than 90% of cancers originate from the epithelium of the bronchus (bronchogenic). They grow slowly, and it takes 8 to 10 years for a tumor to reach 1 cm, which is the smallest lesion detectable on x-ray. Lung cancers occur primarily in the segmental bronchi or beyond and have a preference for the upper lobes of the lungs.

Pathologic changes in the bronchial system show nonspecific inflammatory changes with hypersecretion of mucus, desquamation of cells, reactive hyperplasia of basal cells, and metaplasia of normal respiratory epithelium to stratified squamous cells. Primary lung cancers are often categorized into two broad types: *non–small cell lung cancer* (NSCLC) and *small cell lung cancer* (SCLC). Lung cancer metastasizes primarily by direct extension and by way of the blood and lymph system. Common sites for metastasis are the liver, brain, bones, lymph nodes, and adrenal glands.

Clinical Manifestations

Manifestations are usually nonspecific, appear late in the disease process, and depend on the type of primary lung cancer, its location, and metastatic spread.
- Persistent pneumonitis as a result of obstructed bronchi may be one of the earliest manifestations, causing fever, chills, and cough.
- A significant symptom often reported first is a persistent cough that may be productive of sputum. Hemoptysis is not a common early symptom.
- Chest pain may be localized or unilateral and range from mild to severe.
- Dyspnea and an auscultatory wheeze may be present with bronchial obstruction.

Later manifestations may include nonspecific symptoms such as anorexia, fatigue, weight loss, and nausea and vomiting. Hoarseness may be present as a result of involvement of the recurrent laryngeal nerve. Unilateral paralysis of the diaphragm, dysphagia, and superior vena cava obstruction may occur because of intrathoracic spread of malignancy. There may be palpable lymph nodes in the neck or axilla. Mediastinal involvement may lead to pericardial effusion, cardiac tamponade, and dysrhythmias.

Paraneoplastic syndrome is caused by certain lung cancers, especially SCLCs. The syndrome is characterized by various manifestations resulting from certain substances (e.g., hormones, antigens, and enzymes) produced by the tumor itself or in response to the tumor. Systemic manifestations may include hormonal syndromes (Cushing syndrome, syndrome of inappropriate antidiuretic hormone [SIADH]), neuromuscular signs (peripheral neuropathy), dermatologic signs (dermatomyositis), vascular and hematologic signs (anemia, thrombophlebitis), and connective tissue disease (arthralgias, digital clubbing).

Diagnostic Studies

- Chest x-ray is used for diagnosis, evidence of metastasis, and presence of pleural effusion.
- Computed tomography (CT) scanning is the single most effective noninvasive technique for evaluating lung cancer; scans of brain and bones evaluate metastatic disease.
- Magnetic resonance imaging (MRI) may be used in combination with or instead of CT for diagnosis, lymph node enlargement, and mediastinal involvement.
- Positron emission tomography (PET) scan is used for early clinical staging.
- Additional diagnostic studies include sputum specimens, biopsy, bronchoscopy, pulmonary angiography, lung scans, and mediastinoscopy.

Collaborative Care

Surgical resection is the treatment of choice in NSCLC stages I and II because the disease is potentially curable with resection. However, 50% of all NSCLCs are not resectable at the time of diagnosis. In SCLC stage I disease (which is rare), surgical resection, chemotherapy, and radiation therapy may be recommended. Small cell carcinomas usually have widespread metastasis at the time of diagnosis. Surgical procedures that may be performed include pneumonectomy (removal of one entire lung), lobectomy (removal of one or more lung lobes), or lung-conserving resection or segmental or wedge resection procedures.

Radiation therapy used with the intent to cure may be used in the individual who is unable to tolerate sugical resection because of comorbidities.

- Radiation is also done for symptom relief of dyspnea and hemoptysis from bronchial obstruction tumors and to treat superior vena cava syndrome.
- Radiation can be used to treat the pain of metastatic bone lesions or cerebral metastasis, to reduce tumor mass preoperatively, or as an adjuvant measure postoperatively.

Chemotherapy may be used for nonresectable tumors or as an adjuvant therapy to surgery in NSCLC. Chemotherapy has improved survival in patients with advanced NSCLC and is now considered standard treatment (see Chemotherapy, p. 712).

One type of biologic therapy, or targeted therapy, approved for patients with locally advanced and metastatic NSCLC is erlotinib (Tarceva). Erlotinib was developed to block the stimulatory signals in the cancer cells and is used to treat patients whose cancer has progressed despite other treatments.

Nursing Management
Goals
The patient with lung cancer will have effective breathing patterns, adequate airway clearance, adequate oxygenation of tissues, minimal to no pain, and a realistic attitude toward treatment and prognosis.

Nursing Diagnoses
- Ineffective airway clearance
- Anxiety
- Acute pain
- Imbalanced nutrition: less than body requirements
- Ineffective health maintenance
- Ineffective breathing pattern

Nursing Interventions
When obtaining a health history, it is important to obtain information related to respiratory carcinogens. The patient should be asked about occupational exposure to carcinogens and excessive exposure to air pollution.

- A detailed history of cigarette smoking should also be obtained. This information should be used to evaluate the patient's risk for lung cancer and also to teach about early recognition of symptoms.

It is important to determine the understanding of the patient and the family concerning the diagnostic tests, the diagnosis or potential diagnosis, the treatment options, and the prognosis. Initially the patient will require support and reassurance during the diagnostic evaluation. When a diagnosis is established, the nurse should help patients and their families deal with the diagnosis of lung cancer. Patients may feel guilty about their cigarette smoking having caused the cancer and need to discuss this feeling with someone who has a nonjudgmental attitude. Questions regarding each patient's condition should be answered honestly. Additional counseling from a social worker, psychologist, or member of the clergy may be needed.

Specific care of the patient depends on the treatment plan.

See NCP 28-2 for the patient after thoracotomy, Lewis and others, *Medical-Surgical Nursing,* edition 7, p. 594 for postoperative care of the patient with chest surgery.

- Postoperative care for the patient having surgery is discussed in Chapter 20, Lewis and others, *Medical-Surgical Nursing,* edition 7.
- Care of the patient with cancer undergoing radiation therapy and chemotherapy is discussed in Chapter 16.

The nurse has a major role in providing patient comfort, teaching methods to reduce pain, and assessing indications for hospitalization.

▼ **Patient and Family Teaching**
- The best way to halt the epidemic of lung cancer is for people to stop smoking. Important nursing activities to assist in the progress toward this goal include promoting smoking cessation programs and actively supporting education and policy changes related to smoking.
- For the individual who does have a smoking habit, efforts should be made to assist the smoker to stop smoking. Nicotine's addictive properties make quitting a difficult task that requires much support. Agents and strategies to assist patients to stop smoking are discussed in Chapter 12 and in Tables 12-4, 12-5, and 12-6 (pp. 171 to 173) in Lewis and others, *Medical-Surgical Nursing,* edition 7.
- Discharge instructions for the patient who has had a surgical resection with an intent to cure should include manifestations of metastasis. The patient and family should be told to contact the physician if symptoms such as hemoptysis, dysphagia, chest pain, and hoarseness develop.

L

LYME DISEASE

Description
Lyme disease is a spirochetal infection caused by *Borrelia burgdorferi* and is transmitted by the bite of an infected deer tick. It is the most common vector-borne disease in the United States. The

peak season for human infection is during the summer months. Most cases occur in three U.S. endemic areas: (1) along the northeastern coast from Maryland to Massachusetts, (2) in Wisconsin and Minnesota, and (3) along the northwestern coast of northern California and Oregon.

Clinical Manifestations

The most characteristic sign is *erythema migrans* (EM), a skin lesion that occurs at the site of the tick bite within 2 to 30 days after exposure. This lesion begins as a red macule or papule that slowly expands to form a large round lesion with a bright red border and central clearing. The EM lesion is often accompanied by other acute symptoms, such as fever, headache, fatigue, stiff neck, swollen lymph nodes, and migratory joint and muscle pain.

- If not treated, Lyme disease can progress in several weeks or months to neurologic abnormalities, including severe headaches, temporal facial paralysis, and poor motor coordination.
- In late disease, which can occur from months to years after the initial infection, arthritis pain and swelling can occur in large joints.
- Neurologic disorders, such as neuroborreliosis, can also occur in the late stage, causing confusion and forgetfulness.

Diagnostic Studies

Diagnosis is based on the clinical manifestations and history of exposure in an endemic area.

- Routine laboratory tests play only a minor role in diagnosis. Complete blood count (CBC) and erythrocyte sedimentation rate (ESR) results are usually normal.
- Lyme serology tests for antibodies are not usually positive initially because it takes many weeks to get clinically detectable levels of circulating antibodies.
- Cerebrospinal fluid should be examined in individuals with neurologic involvement.

Nursing and Collaborative Management

Active lesions can be treated with antibiotic therapy. Oral doxycycline (Vibramycin), cefuroxime (Ceftin), and amoxicillin are often effective in early-stage infection and in prevention of later stages of the disease. Doxycycline has also been shown to be effective in preventing Lyme disease when given within 3 days after the bite of a deer tick. Long-standing infection may require extended intravenous (IV) antibiotic therapy. IV ceftriaxone (Rocephin) is used for cardiac or neurologic abnormalities.

- Patient and family teaching for the prevention of Lyme disease in endemic areas is outlined in Table 65-11, Lewis and others, *Medical-Surgical Nursing*, edition 7, p. 1714.

MACULAR DEGENERATION, AGE-RELATED

Description

Age-related macular degeneration (AMD) is a degeneration of the retina involving the macula that results in varying degrees of central vision loss. AMD is divided into two classic forms, dry (atrophic), which is more common, and wet (exudative), which is more severe. It is the most common cause of irreversible central vision loss in persons over 60 years old.

Pathophysiology

AMD is related to retinal aging. Family history is a major risk factor, and a gene responsible for some cases of AMD has been identified. In addition, long-term exposure to ultraviolet light, hyperopia, cigarette smoking, and light-colored eyes may be additional risk factors. Nutritional factors suh as vitamins C, E, beta-carotene, and zinc may play a role in the progression of AMD.

- In dry AMD, people notice that reading and other close-vision tasks become more difficult. This form starts with the abnormal accumulation of yellowish colored extracellular deposits called *drusen* in the retinal pigment epthelium. Atrophy and degeneration of macular cells then result, leading to a slowly progressive and painless vision loss.
- Wet AMD is characterized by the growth of new blood vessels from their normal location in the choroids to an abnormal location in the retinal epithelium. As the new blood vessels leak, scar tissue gradually forms. Acute vision loss may occur in some cases from bleeding.

Clinical Manifestations

The patient may experience blurred and darkened vision, the presence of scotomas (blind spots in the visual fields), or metamorphopsia (distortion of vision).

Diagnostic Studies

- Visual acuity measurement
- Ophthalmoscopic examination to look for drusen and other changes in the fundus

M

- Amsler grid test to define the involved area and provide a baseline for future comparison
- Fundus photography and IV fluorescein angiography to help to further define the extent and type of AMD

Nursing and Collaborative Management

Laser photocoagulation of abnormal blood vessels when visual acuity is compromised has been the therapy of choice. However, the laser beam also destroys the retinal pigment epithelium and photoreceptor cells, leaving a blind spot from the scarred area.

- A newer therapy for patients with wet AMD is called photodynamic therapy. This procedure destroys the abnormal blood vessels without permanent damage to the retinal pigment epithelium and photoreceptor cells. Current criteria for its use are very specific, and not all patients with wet AMD may be eligible.
- Pegaptanib (Macugen), an intravitreous injectable drug, is a selective inhibitor of endothelial growth factor that helps to slow vision loss in wet AMD.
- Patients at risk for AMD (in consultation with their health care provider) should consider supplements of vitamins and minerals.
- When no treatment is possible, or when treatment fails, the patient with AMD can benefit from low-vision aids, such as magnifying lenses and amplification lamps.

The permanent loss of central vision associated with AMD has significant psychosocial implications for nursing care. Nursing management of the patient with uncorrectable visual impairment is discussed in Lewis and others, *Medical-Surgical Nursing,* edition 7, pp. 419 to 421 and is appropriate for the patient with AMD. It is especially important when caring for patients to avoid giving them the impression that "nothing can be done" about their problem. Although it is true that therapy will not recover lost vision, much can be done to augment the remaining vision.

MALABSORPTION SYNDROME

Malabsorption results from impaired absorption of fats, carbohydrates, proteins, minerals, and vitamins. Lactose intolerance is the most common malabsorption disorder, followed by inflammatory bowel disease, celiac disease, tropical sprue, and cystic fibrosis.

- The stomach, small intestine, liver, and pancreas regulate normal digestion and absorption. Nutrients are broken down so that absorption can take place through the intestinal mucosa and nutrients can enter the bloodstream. If there is an interruption in this process, malabsorption may occur.
- Malabsorption can be caused by (1) biochemical or enzyme deficiencies, (2) bacterial proliferation, (3) disruption of small intestine mucosa, (4) disturbed lymphatic and vascular circulation, or (5) surface area loss.

The most common clinical manifestation of malabsorption is steatorrhea (bulky, foul-smelling, yellow-gray, greasy stools with puttylike consistency).

Diagnostic studies include qualitative examination of stool for fat (Sudan stain), a 72-hour stool collection for quantitative measurement of fecal fat, and the D-xylose absorption-excretion test to evaluate carbohydrate absorption. Additional studies may include (1) bile acid breath test to evaluate bile-salt malabsorption or malabsorption from bacterial overgrowth; (2) triolein breath test, which measures carbon dioxide excretion after ingestion of a radioactive triglyceride; and (3) excretion of breath hydrogen after ingestion of lactose, which is a sensitive, specific, and noninvasive test for detection of lactase deficiency.

- A pancreatic secretin test may be performed to rule out pancreatic insufficiency.
- Endoscopy may be used to obtain a small bowel biopsy specimen for diagnosis.
- Small bowel barium enema is used to identify abnormal mucosal patterns.
- Capsule endoscopy can be used to assess the small intestine for absorption problems.
- Laboratory studies to evaluate nutritional status (complete blood count [CBC], prothrombin, serum vitamin A and carotene levels, serum electrolytes, calcium, and cholesterol) are frequently ordered.

See the specific disorders of Celiac Disease (Sprue), p. 105; Cystic Fibrosis, p. 159; Inflammatory Bowel Disease, p. 352; Lactase Deficiency, p. 378.

MALIGNANT MELANOMA

M

Description

Malignant melanoma is a tumor arising in cells producing melanin; these are usually the melanocytes of the skin. Melanoma has the ability to metastasize to any organ, including the brain and heart. This is the deadliest form of skin cancer, and its incidence is increasing at a faster rate than any other cancer.

The precise cause of melanoma is unknown, but risk factors include long-term ultraviolet (UV) exposure or overexposure to artificial light, such as a tanning bed. Persons with fair skin and eyes and those with a prior diagnosis of melanoma or having a first-degree relative diagnosed with melanoma have an increased risk. Immunosuppression, dysplastic nevi, and exposure to environmental hazards, including herbicides, also increase a person's risk.

Clinical Manifestations

About one third of melanomas occur in existing nevi or moles. Melanoma frequently occurs on the lower legs in women and on the trunk, head, and neck in men. Because most melanoma cells continue to produce melanin, melanoma tumors are often brown or black. Individuals should consult their health care provider immediately if their moles or lesions show any of the clinical signs (ABCDs) of melanoma (see Fig. 24-3, Lewis and others, *Medical-Surgical Nursing,* edition 7, p. 466). The ABCDs of melanoma include **A**symmetry, **B**order irregularity, **C**olor varied from one area of the lesion to another, and **D**iameter >6 mm. Any sudden or progressive increase in the size, color, or shape of a mole should be checked. When melanoma begins in the skin it is called *cutaneous melanoma.* Melanoma can also occur in the eyes, meninges, lymph nodes, digestive tract, and anywhere else in the body where melanocytes are found.

Collaborative Care

Biopsies should be done of all suspicious lesions using an excisional biopsy technique. Shave-biopsy, shave-excision, or electrocautery should never be done of lesions suspected to be melanoma.

Treatment depends on the site of the original tumor, stage of the cancer, and patient's age and general health. The initial treatment of malignant melanoma is surgery. Melanoma that has spread to the lymph nodes or nearby sites usually requires additional therapy, such as chemotherapy, biologic therapy (e.g., α-interferon, interleukin-2), and/or radiation therapy. Examples of chemotherapeutic agents that are used include dacarbazine (DTIC), temozolomide (TMZ), procarbazine (Matulane), carmustine (BCNU), and lomustine (CCNU). Gene and vaccine therapies are currently being examined as additional treatment options.

Cutaneous melanoma is nearly 100% curable by excision if diagnosed early when the malignant cells are restricted to the epidermis. The most important prognostic factor is tumor thickness at the time of presentation. If spread to regional lymph nodes occurs, the patient has a 50% 5-year survival. If metastasis occurs, treatment is largely palliative.

▼ **Patient and Family Teaching**

Emphasize the importance of protection from the damaging effects of the sun, such as wearing a large-brimmed hat, sunglasses, and a long-sleeved shirt of a lightly woven fabric.

- Inform patients that the rays of the sun are most dangerous between 10 AM and 2 PM standard time and 11 AM and 3 PM daylight savings time. Recommend that patients use a sunscreen with a minimum SPF of 15 on a daily basis.
- Patients should be taught to self-examine their skin at least monthly to detect persistent skin lesions.

MALNUTRITION

Description

Malnutrition is an excess, deficit, or imbalance of the essential components of a balanced diet. Malnutrition is also described as undernutrition or overnutrition. *Undernutrition* describes a state of poor nourishment as a result of inadequate diet or diseases that interfere with normal appetite and assimilation of ingested foods. *Overnutrition* refers to the ingestion of more food than is required for body needs, as in obesity.

- The incidence of malnutrition in hospitalized patients is 30% to 55%. The prevalence of malnutrition in older long-term care residents ranges from 23% to 85%.

Pathophysiology

Protein-calorie malnutrition (PCM) is the most common form of undernutrition and can result from primary (poor eating habits) or secondary (alteration or defect in ingestion, digestion, absorption, or metabolism) factors. Secondary malnutrition may occur as a result of gastrointestinal (GI) obstruction, surgical procedures, cancer, malabsorption syndromes, drugs, or infectious diseases.

- In the initial process of starvation, the body's selective use of carbohydrates (glycogen) rather than fat and protein to meet metabolic needs will deplete glycogen stores within 18 hours.
- When carbohydrate stores are depleted, protein begins to be converted to glucose for energy, resulting in a negative nitrogen balance.

M

- Within 5 to 9 days, body fat is mobilized to supply needed energy.
- In prolonged starvation up to 97% of calories are provided by fat, and protein is conserved. Depletion of fat stores depends on the amount available, but fat stores are generally used up in 4 to 6 weeks. Once fat stores are used, body proteins, including those in internal organs and plasma, can no longer be spared and rapidly decrease because they are the only remaining body source of available energy.
- When the diet is extremely deficient in calories and essential proteins, the sodium-potassium exchange pump fails, leaving sodium inside the cell (along with water causing cell expansion), and potassium levels in extracellular fluid rise.
- The liver is the body organ that loses the most mass during protein deprivation. It gradually becomes infiltrated with fat secondary to decreased synthesis of lipoproteins. Immediate restoration to a diet of protein and other necessary constituents must be instituted or death rapidly ensues.

Clinical Manifestations

Malnutrition signs are particularly evident in the skin, eyes, mouth, muscles, and central nervous system (CNS).

- These signs include conjunctival and corneal dryness; dental caries, loose teeth, and discolored enamel; constant hunger, diarrhea, and flatulence; hepatomegaly; decreased blood pressure (BP); increased number of infections; and depression, confusion, and motor weakness.
- Major complications of PCM are delayed wound healing and increased susceptibility to infection.

Diagnostic Studies

- Serum albumin, prealbumin, and transferrin levels are decreased.
- Serum potassium (K^+) may be elevated.
- Red blood cell (RBC) count and hemoglobin (Hb) levels are decreased and may indicate anemia.
- White blood cell (WBC) count and total lymphocyte count are decreased.
- Liver enzyme studies may be elevated.
- Serum levels of fat-soluble and water-soluble vitamins are often decreased.
- Anthropometric measurements help evaluate response to therapy.

Collaborative Care

Early management of uncomplicated PCM is usually achieved without hospitalization by means of a diet high in calories and protein and by close supervision. In severe PCM the patient may be hospitalized for correction of fluid and electrolyte imbalances and for infections secondary to a compromised immune system. Enteral feedings, both oral and tube, can be used to supplement the diet. In cases of severe PCM, parenteral nutrition (PN) may be initiated (see Tube Feeding, p. 751, and Parenteral Nutrition, p. 743).

Nursing Management

Goals

The patient with malnutrition will achieve weight gain, consume a specified number of calories per day (with a diet individualized for the patient), and have no adverse consequences related to malnutrition or nutrition therapies.

Nursing Diagnoses

- Imbalanced nutrition: less than body requirements
- Feeding self-care deficit
- Constipation or diarrhea
- Deficient fluid volume
- Risk for impaired skin integrity
- Noncompliance
- Activity intolerance

Nursing Interventions

The nurse must assess the patient's nutritional status, as well as focus on the other physical problems of the patient. It is important for the nurse to identify patients who are at risk, why they are at risk, and how to intervene appropriately.

- Daily weight can give an ongoing record of body weight gain or loss. The body weight, in conjunction with accurate recording of food and fluid intake, provides a clear picture of the patient's fluid and nutritional state.
- The nurse and the dietitian working with the patient and family can assist in the selection of high-calorie and high-protein foods.
- Between-meal supplements should be provided for the undernourished patient. If the patient is unable to consume enough nutrition with a high-calorie, high-protein diet, oral liquid nutrition supplements can be added.
- Some patients may benefit from appetite stimulants, such as megestrol acetate (Megace) or dronabinol (Marinol), to improve nutritional intake.

M

▼ **Patient and Family Teaching**
- Discuss with the patient and family the importance of high-caloric, high-protein foods. The family can be encouraged to bring the patient's favorite food while the patient is still hospitalized.
- Discharge preparation for both patient and family is important. They must be carefully instructed on the cause of the under-nourished state and ways to avoid the problem in the future.
- Diet instruction is usually done by the dietitian, but it is important for the nurse to assess patient understanding and reinforce the information whenever possible.

MÉNIÈRE'S DISEASE

Description
Ménière's disease is an inner ear disease characterized by episodic vertigo, tinnitus, aural fullness, and fluctuating sensorineural hearing loss. Symptoms are incapacitating as a result of sudden, severe attacks of vertigo with nausea and vomiting. Symptoms usually begin between ages 30 and 60 years.

Pathophysiology
The cause of the disease is unknown, but it results in an excessive accumulation of endolymph in the membranous labyrinth. The volume of endolymph increases until the membranous labyrinth ruptures, mixing high-potassium endolymph with low-potassium perilymph.

Clinical Manifestations
- Attacks may occur without warning or be preceded by an aura consisting of a sense of fullness in the ear, increasing tinnitus, and a decrease in hearing.
- The patient reports a whirling sensation and may experience the feeling of being pulled to the ground ("drop attack").
- Autonomic symptoms include pallor, sweating, nausea, and vomiting.
- The duration of the attacks may be hours or days, and attacks may occur several times per year. The clinical course is highly variable.
- Low-pitched tinnitus may be present continuously in the affected ear or may be intensified during an attack.
- Hearing loss fluctuates, decreasing with each vertigo attack and eventually leading to permanent hearing loss.

Diagnostic Studies
- Audiometric studies demonstrate mild, low-frequency hearing loss.
- Vestibular tests indicate decreased function.
- Glycerol test supports the diagnosis if hearing improvement occurs.
- Neurologic testing is done to rule out central nervous system (CNS) disease.

Nursing and Collaborative Management
During an acute attack, antihistamines, anticholinergics, and benzodiazepines can be used to decrease the abnormal sensation and lessen symptoms such as nausea and vomiting. Acute vertigo is treated symptomatically with bed rest, sedation, and antiemetics or antivertigo drugs for motion sickness. Diazepam (Valium), meclizine (Antivert), and fentanyl with droperidol (Innovar) may be used to reduce the vertigo. Most patients respond to the prescribed medications but must learn to live with the unpredictability of the attacks.

- During an acute attack a patient needs reassurance that the condition is not life threatening. The nurse should focus on providing only essential care, because movement aggravates vertigo.
- Side rails should be up and the bed in low position if the patient is in bed. Avoid the use of lights and TV, which exacerbate symptoms. Have an emesis basin available because vomiting is common. Assist with ambulation because unsteadiness remains after an attack.
- Inform the patient that severe tinnitus and vertigo may exist for days to weeks after the attack.

Management between attacks may include vasodilators, diuretics, antihistamines, and a low-sodium diet.

With frequent incapacitating attacks and reduced quality of life, surgical therapy is indicated. Surgical options include endolymphatic shunt, vestibular nerve resection, and labyrinth ablation. Careful management can decrease the possibility of progressive sensorineural loss in many patients.

MENINGITIS

M

Description
Meningitis is an acute inflammation of the meningeal tissues surrounding the brain and spinal cord. Meningitis specifically

refers to infection of the arachnoid mater and the cerebrospinal fluid (CSF). Bacterial meningitis is considered a medical emergency; if it is left untreated, the mortality rate approaches 100%. See Table 39, pp. 208 to 209, for a comparison of meningitis and encephalitis.

Pathophysiology

Meningitis usually occurs in the fall, winter, or early spring and is often secondary to viral respiratory disease. *Streptococcus pneumoniae* and *Neisseria meningitidis* are the leading causes of bacterial meningitis. Organisms usually gain entry to the central nervous system (CNS) through the upper respiratory tract or bloodstream, but they may enter by direct extension from penetrating wounds of the skull or through fractured sinuses in basal skull fractures.

The inflammatory response to the infection tends to increase CSF production with a moderate increase in intracranial pressure (ICP). The purulent secretion produced by bacteria quickly spreads to other areas of the brain through the CSF.

- Because most patients develop increased ICP and altered mental status, all patients must be observed closely for manifestations of ICP (see Increased Intracranial Pressure, p. 344).

Clinical Manifestations

Fever, severe headache, nausea, vomiting, and nuchal rigidity (resistance to flexion of the neck) are key signs.

- A positive Kernig's sign, a positive Brudzinski's sign, photophobia, a decreased level of consciousness (LOC), and signs of increased ICP may also be present.
- If the infecting organism is a meningococcus, a skin rash is common and petechiae may be seen.
- Seizures occur in one third of all cases of meningitis.
- Coma is associated with a poor prognosis and occurs in 5% to 10% of patients with bacterial meningitis.

Complications

In bacterial meningitis, cranial nerve dysfunction, which usually disappears within a few weeks, often occurs with cranial nerves III, IV, VI, VII, or VIII.

- Cranial nerve irritation can have serious sequelae; the optic nerve (CN II) is compressed by increased ICP. Papilledema is often present, and blindness may occur.
- When the oculomotor (CN III), trochlear (CN IV), and abducens (CN VI) nerves are irritated, ocular movements

are affected. Ptosis, unequal pupils, and diplopia are common.

- Irritation of the trigeminal nerve (CN V) is evidenced by sensory losses and loss of the corneal reflex, with irritation of the facial nerve (CN VII) resulting in facial paresis. Irritation of the vestibulocochlear nerve (CN VIII) causes tinnitus, vertigo, and deafness.
- Hemiparesis, dysphasia, and hemianopsia may also occur, with these signs resolving over time.
- Acute cerebral edema may occur with bacterial meningitis, causing seizures, optic nerve palsy, bradycardia, hypertensive coma, and death.
- Hearing loss may be permanent after bacterial meningitis, but it is not a complication of viral meningitis.
- A complication of meningococcal meningitis is the Waterhouse-Friderichsen syndrome. The syndrome is manifested by petechiae, disseminated intravascular coagulation (DIC), and adrenal hemorrhage.

Diagnostic Studies

When bacterial meningitis is suspected, specimens of blood, CSF, sputum, and nasopharyngeal secretions are taken for culture to identify the causative organism. Diagnosis is verified by doing a lumbar puncture with analysis of the CSF.

- Analysis of CSF includes (1) cultures to identify the causative organism, (2) protein levels (often elevated; are even higher in bacterial meningitis), (3) glucose concentration (decreased in bacterial meningitis), and (4) gross examination (purulent and turbid in bacterial meningitis).
- Skull x-rays may detect infected sinuses.
- Computed tomography (CT) scans may reveal increased ICP or hydrocephalus.

Collaborative Care

A rapid diagnosis based on a history and physical examination is crucial because the patient is usually in a critical state when health care is sought. When meningitis is suspected, antibiotic therapy is instituted after the collection of specimens for cultures, even before the diagnosis is confirmed. Penicillin, ampicillin, vancomycin, and a third-generation cephalosporin (e.g., ceftriaxone [Rocephin] or cefotaxime [Claforan]) are common drugs of choice to treat bacterial meningitis. Dexamethasone may be prescribed before or with the first dose of antibiotics to decrease mortality rate and reduce incidence of hearing loss in patients with bacterial meningitis.

Nursing Management

Goals

The patient with meningitis will have a return to maximal neurologic functioning, resolution of infection, and control of pain and discomfort.

See NCP 57-2 for the patient with bacterial meningitis, Lewis and others, *Medical-Surgical Nursing,* edition 7, pp. 1496 to 1497.

Nursing Diagnoses/Collaborative Problems

- Ineffective tissue perfusion (cerebral)
- Decreased intracranial adaptive capacity
- Disturbed sensory perception
- Acute pain
- Hyperthermia
- Potential complication: seizure activity

Nursing Interventions

Prevention of respiratory infections through vaccination programs for pneumococcal pneumonia and influenza should be supported by the nurse. A vaccine is available for protection against *Neisseria meningitidis* and is recommended for children ages 11 or 12 years. In addition, early and vigorous treatment of respiratory and ear infections is important. Persons who have close contact with anyone who has meningitis should be given prophylactic antibiotics.

The patient with meningitis is acutely ill. The fever is high, and head pain is severe. Irritation of the cerebral cortex may result in seizures with changes in mental status and LOC dependent on the level of ICP.

- Assessment of vital signs, neurologic evaluation, fluid intake and output, and evaluation of lung fields and skin should be performed at regular intervals based on the patient's condition.
- Head and neck pain secondary to movement requires attention. Codeine provides some pain relief without undue sedation for most patients. A darkened room and cool cloth over the eyes relieve the discomfort of photophobia. For the delirious patient, additional low lighting may be necessary to decrease hallucinations.
- All patients suffer some degree of mental distortion and hypersensitivity and may be frightened and misinterpret the environment. Every attempt should be made to minimize environmental stimuli and the resulting exaggerated perception.

If seizures occur, protective measures should be taken. Antiseizure medications are administered as ordered. Problems associated with increased ICP need to be managed (see Increased Intracranial Pressure, p. 344). Restraints should be avoided. The presence of a familiar person at the bedside has a calming effect.

Fever must be vigorously managed because it increases cerebral edema and the frequency of seizures. Aspirin or acetaminophen may be used to reduce fever. If the fever is resistant to aspirin or acetaminophen, however, more vigorous means are necessary, such as an automatic cooling blanket. If a cooling blanket is not available, tepid sponge baths with water may be effective. Because high fever greatly increases the metabolic rate, the patient should be assessed for dehydration and adequacy of intake. Supplemental feedings to maintain adequate nutritional intake by means of tube or oral feedings may be necessary.

- Meningitis generally requires respiratory isolation until the cultures are negative. Meningococcal meningitis is highly contagious, whereas other causes of meningitis may pose a minimal to no infection risk with patient contact.

After the acute period has passed, good nutrition should be stressed with an emphasis on a high-protein, high-caloric diet in small, frequent feedings.

- Muscle rigidity may persist in the neck and backs of the legs. Progressive range-of-motion (ROM) exercises and warm baths are useful. Activity should be gradually increased as tolerated, but adequate bed rest and sleep should be encouraged.

- Residual effects can result in sequelae such as dementia, seizures, deafness, hemiplegia, and hydrocephalus. Vision, hearing, cognitive skills, and motor and sensory abilities should be assessed after recovery with appropriate referrals as indicated.

- Throughout the acute and convalescent periods, the nurse should be aware of the anxiety and stress experienced by individuals close to the patient.

METABOLIC SYNDROME

M

Description

Metabolic syndrome, also known as *syndrome X, insulin resistance syndrome, and dysmetabolic syndrome,* is a collection of risk factors that increase an individual's chance of developing cardiovascular disease and diabetes mellitus. It is estimated that one in five Americans has metabolic syndrome. Metabolic syndrome is diagnosed if an individual has three or more of the following conditions:

- Waist circumference of ≥40 inches (≥102 cm) in men or ≥35 inches (≥88 cm) in women
- Triglycerides of >105 mg/dl (>1.7 mmol/L) or drug treatment for elevated triglycerides
- High-density lipoprotein (HDL) cholesterol of <40 mg/dl (<1.0 mmol/L) in men or <50 mg/dl (<1.3 mmol/L) in women or drug treatment for reduced HDL cholesterol
- Blood pressure of ≥130 mm Hg systolic or ≥85 mm Hg diastolic or drug treatment for hypertension
- Fasting glucose of ≥100 mg/dl (5.6 mmol/L) or drug treatment for elevated glucose

Pathophysiology

The main underlying risk factors for metabolic syndrome are abdominal obesity and insulin resistance, although physical inactivity, presence of inflammatory markers, prothrombotic tendencies, hormonal imbalance, aging, and genetic predispositions are also associated with the condition. At risk are African Americans, Hispanics, American Indians, and Asians. Patients who have been diagnosed with metabolic syndrome typically are individuals who have diabetes who cannot maintain a proper level of glucose, have hypertension, and secrete a large amount of insulin, or who have survived a heart attack and have hyperinsulinemia.

Nursing and Collaborative Management

First-line interventions to reduce the risk factors for metabolic syndrome are lifestyle therapies that reduce the major risk factors of cardiovascular disease: reducing low-density lipoprotein (LDL) cholesterol, stopping smoking, lowering blood pressure, and reducing glucose levels. Weight should be reduced to a desirable level, physical activity should be increased, and healthy dietary habits should be established.

Nurses should assist patients by providing information on positive lifestyle changes. Patients who are unable to lower risk factors with lifestyle therapies alone or those at high risk for a coronary event may be considered for drug therapy. Although no medication is available for metabolic syndrome specifically, medication can be prescribed to lower individual risk factors, such as metformin (Glucophage) to reduce glucose levels or antihypertensive drugs to control blood pressure.

MULTIPLE MYELOMA

Description

Multiple myeloma, or plasma cell myeloma, is a condition in which neoplastic plasma cells infiltrate the bone marrow and destroy bone. The disease is twice as common in men as in women and usually develops after age 40 years.

Pathophysiology

The cause of multiple myeloma is unknown. Exposure to radiation, organic chemicals (e.g., benzene), herbicides, and insecticides may play a role. Genetic factors and viral infection may also influence the risk of developing multiple myeloma.

- The disease process involves the excessive production of plasma cells that infiltrate the bone marrow and produce abnormal and excessive amounts of immunoglobulins (usually IgG, IgA, IgD, and IgE). The abnormal immunoglobulin is known as myeloma protein.
- Production of excessive and abnormal amounts of interleukins (IL-4, IL-5, IL-6) also contributes to the pathologic process of bone destruction.
- The body's normal immune response is compromised by the reduction of normal plasma cells and immunoglobulins.
- Ultimately, the malignant plasma cells destroy bone and invade the lymph nodes, liver, spleen, and kidneys.

Clinical Manifestations

Multiple myeloma develops slowly and insidiously.

- The patient often does not manifest symptoms until the disease is advanced, at which time skeletal pain is the major symptom. Pain in the pelvis, spine, and ribs is common.
- Diffuse osteoporosis develops as the myeloma protein destroys more bone. Osteolytic lesions are seen in the skull, vertebrae, and ribs. Vertebral destruction can lead to vertebral collapse with compression of the spinal cord.
- Loss of bone integrity can lead to the development of pathologic fractures. Bony degeneration causes calcium loss from bones, resulting in hypercalcemia. Hypercalcemia may cause renal, gastrointestinal (GI), or neurologic changes, such as polyuria, anorexia, confusion, and ultimately seizures, coma, and cardiac problems.
- High protein levels caused by the myeloma protein can result in renal failure from renal tubular obstruction and interstitial nephritis from uric acid precipitates.

M

- The patient may display symptoms of anemia, thrombocytopenia, and granulocytopenia, all of which are related to the replacement of normal bone marrow with plasma cells.

Diagnostic Studies

- Pancytopenia, hyperuricemia, hypercalcemia, and elevated creatinine may be found.
- Monoclonal (M) antibody protein is found in blood and urine.
- An abnormal globulin known as Bence Jones protein is often found in urine.
- Bone marrow analysis shows significantly increased numbers of plasma cells.
- X-rays show distinct areas of bone erosions, generalized thinning of the bones, and/or fractures, especially in the vertebrae, ribs, pelvis, and bones of the thigh and upper arms.
- The simplest measure of prognosis in multiple myeloma is based on blood levels of two markers: β_2-microglobulin and albumin. In general, higher levels of β_2-microglobulin and lower levels of albumin are associated with a poorer prognosis.

Collaborative Care

The therapeutic approach involves managing both the disease and its symptoms. Multiple myeloma is seldom cured, but treatment can relieve symptoms, produce remission, and prolong life. Current treatment options include "watchful waiting" (for early multiple myeloma), chemotherapy, biologic therapy, and hematopoietic stem cell transplantation (HSCT).

Ambulation and adequate hydration are used to treat hypercalcemia, hyperuricemia, and dehydration. Weight bearing helps the bones reabsorb some calcium, and fluids dilute calcium and prevent protein precipitates from causing renal tubular obstruction.

Control of pain and prevention of pathologic fractures are other goals of collaborative care. Analgesics, orthopedic supports, and localized radiation help reduce skeletal pain.

Chemotherapy is usually the first treatment recommended and is used to reduce the number of plasma cells (see Chemotherapy, p. 712). Corticosteroids may be added because they exert an antitumor effect in some patients. High-dose chemotherapy, such as melphalan, followed by autologous HSCT has evolved as the standard of care in eligible patients. α-Interferon has been used after chemotherapy. Radiation therapy is used for its palliative effect on localized lesions.

Bisphosphonates, such as pamidronate (Aredia), zoledronic acid (Zometa), and etidronate (Didronel), inhibit bone breakdown and are used for skeletal pain and hypercalcemia. Thalidomide (Thalomid) is an immune-modulating and antiangiogenic drug that may slow the growth of plasma cells and reduce their number.

- Drugs may be used to treat the complications of multiple myeloma. For example, allopurinol (Zyloprim) may be given to reduce hyperuricemia, and intravenous (IV) furosemide (Lasix) promotes renal excretion of calcium. Calcitonin can be used to decrease the risk of fractures and reduce bone pain.

Nursing Management

Maintaining adequate hydration is a primary nursing consideration to minimize problems from hypercalcemia. Fluids are administered to attain a urinary output of 1.5 to 2 L/day. This may require an intake of 3 to 4 L. In addition, weight bearing helps bones to reabsorb some of the calcium, and corticosteroids may augment the excretion of calcium.

Once chemotherapy is initiated, uric acid levels increase because of the increased cell destruction. Hyperuricemia must be resolved by ensuring adequate hydration and using allopurinol.

- Because of the potential for pathologic fractures, the nurse must be careful when moving and ambulating the patient. A slight twist or strain in the wrong area (e.g., weak area in patient's bones) may be sufficient to cause a fracture.

Pain management requires innovative and knowledgeable nursing interventions. Analgesics, such as nonsteroidal antiinflammatory drugs (NSAIDs), acetaminophen, or acetaminophen with codeine, may be more effective than opioids alone in diminishing bone pain. Braces, especially for the spine, may also help control pain.

- Assessment and prompt treatment of infection are important. Fifty to seventy percent of patients with multiple myeloma will die as a result of bacterial infections. Hematologic function is impaired as a result of the disease and effects of treatment. Nursing care presented in NCP 31-1, pp. 688 to 689; NCP 31-2, p. 706; and NCP 31-3, p. 716, Lewis and others, *Medical-Surgical Nursing,* edition 7 applies to the patient with multiple myeloma.
- The patient's psychosocial needs require sensitive, skilled management. As with leukemia (see Leukemia, p. 380), it is important to help the patient and significant others adapt to changes fostered by chronic illness and to adjust to the losses related to the disease process.

M

- The way in which patients and families deal with confronting death may be affected by the manner in which they have learned to accept and live with the chronic nature of the disease.

MULTIPLE SCLEROSIS

Description

Multiple sclerosis (MS) is a chronic, progressive, degenerative disorder of the central nervous system (CNS) characterized by demyelination of the nerve fibers of the brain and spinal cord. It is an autoimmune disease of young to middle-age adults, with the onset usually between ages 15 and 50 years. Women are affected more often than men.

- Incidence of MS is highest in temperate climates (between 45 and 65 degrees of latitude), such as those found in Europe, Canada, and the northern United States, as compared with tropical regions.
- It is not known exactly how many people have MS. The average life expectancy after the onset of symptoms is more than 25 years.

Pathophysiology

The cause of MS is unknown, although research findings suggest MS is related to infectious (viral), immunologic, and genetic factors and perpetuated as a result of intrinsic factors (e.g., faulty immunoregulation). Susceptibility to MS appears to have an inherited tendency; first-, second-, and third-degree relatives of patients with MS are at a slightly increased risk. Possible precipitating factors include infection, physical injury, emotional stress, excessive fatigue, and pregnancy.

MS is characterized by chronic inflammation, demyelination, and gliosis (scarring) in the CNS (Fig. 10). The primary neuropathologic condition is an autoimmune disease caused by autoreactive T cells (lymphocytes). A virus in genetically susceptible individuals may initially trigger this process. The activated T cells migrate to the CNS. This is likely the initial event in the development of MS. Subsequent antigen-antibody reaction within the CNS results in an inflammatory response and leads to axon demyelination.

- The disease process consists of loss of myelin, disappearance of oligodendrocytes, and proliferation of astrocytes.

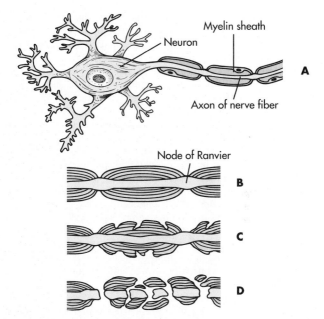

Fig. 10. Pathogenesis of multiple sclerosis. A, Normal nerve cell with myelin sheath. **B,** Normal axon. **C,** Myelin breakdown. **D,** Myelin totally disrupted; axon not functioning.

- Early in the disease the damaged myelin can regenerate, the symptoms will disappear, and the patient experiences a remission.
- Eventually the characteristic plaque formation, or sclerosis, occurs with plaques scattered throughout multiple regions of the CNS.
- As the disease progresses, the myelin is totally disrupted and is replaced by glial scar tissue. Without myelin, nerve impulses slow down, and with the destruction of nerve axons, impulses are totally blocked, resulting in a permanent loss of function.

Clinical Manifestations

Because the onset is often insidious and gradual, with vague symptoms that occur intermittently over months or years, the disease may not be diagnosed until long after the onset of the first symptom.

M

- Because the disease process has a spotty distribution in the CNS, signs and symptoms vary over time. The disease is characterized by chronic progressive deterioration in some persons and by remissions and exacerbations in others. Clinical manifestations vary according to areas of the CNS involved. A classification scheme that identifies various courses of MS is shown in Table 59-13, Lewis and others, *Medical-Surgical Nursing,* edition 7, p. 1543.

Common signs and symptoms include motor, sensory, cerebellar, and emotional problems.

- Motor symptoms include weakness or paralysis of the limbs, trunk, or head; diplopia; and spasticity of muscles.
- Sensory symptoms include numbness and tingling, patchy blindness (scotomas), blurred vision, vertigo, tinnitus, decreased hearing, and chronic neuropathic pain.
- Cerebellar signs include nystagmus, ataxia, dysarthria, and dysphagia.
- Bowel and bladder function can be affected if the sclerotic plaque is located in the areas of the CNS that control elimination. Problems usually involve constipation and a spastic (uninhibited) bladder.
- Sexual dysfunction occurs in many persons. Physiologic erectile dysfunction may result from spinal cord involvement in men. Women may experience decreased libido, difficulty with orgasmic response, painful intercourse, and decreased vaginal lubrication.
- Although intellectual functioning generally remains intact, emotional stability may be affected. Persons may experience anger, depression, or euphoria. Signs and symptoms are aggravated or triggered by physical and emotional trauma, fatigue, and infection.

Death usually occurs because of the infectious complications (e.g., pneumonia) of immobility or because of unrelated disease.

Diagnostic Studies

Because there is no definitive diagnostic test for MS, the diagnosis is based primarily on the history, clinical manifestations, and presence of multiple sclerotic plaques identified by magnetic resonance imaging (MRI). Laboratory tests are adjuncts to the clinical examination.

- Cerebrospinal fluid (CSF) analysis may show an increase in immunoglobulin G (IgG) or a high number of lymphocytes and monocytes.

- Evoked potential response testing results are often delayed as a result of decreased nerve conduction from the eye and ear to the brain.

Collaborative Care

Because there is currently no cure for MS, collaborative care is aimed at treating the disease process and providing symptomatic relief. The disease process is treated with drugs, and the symptoms are controlled with a variety of medications and other therapy.

Drug Therapy

- Adrenocorticotropic hormone (ACTH), methylprednisolone (Medrol), and prednisone are helpful in treating acute exacerbations.
- Immunosuppressive drugs, such as azathioprine (Imuran), methotrexate, and cyclophosphamide (Cytoxan), have been shown to produce some beneficial effects in patients with progressive-relapsing, secondary-progressive, and primary-progressive MS.
- Immunomodulator drugs modify the disease process. These drugs include interferon β-1b (Betaseron), interferon β-1a (Avonex, Rebif), and glatiramer acetate (Copaxone).
- Mitoxantrone (Novantrone), a newer immunosuppressant drug, reduces both B and T lymphocytes and impairs antigen presentation.

Many other drugs are used to treat the symptoms of MS. Antispasmodics are used for spasticity. Amantadine (Symmetrel), CNS stimulants (pemoline [Cylert], methylphenidate [Ritalin], and modafinil [Provigil]) are used for fatigue. Anticholinergics used to treat bladder symptoms. Tricyclic antidepressants and antiseizure medications are used for chronic pain. Table 59-15, Lewis and others, *Medical-Surgical Nursing,* edition 7, pp. 1544 to 1545 lists drugs used for symptomatic treatment of MS.

Other Therapy

- Surgery (e.g., neurectomy, rhizotomy, cordotomy) or dorsal-column electrical stimulation may be required if spasticity is not controlled with antispasmodics.
- Tremors that become unmanageable with medication are sometimes treated by thalamotomy or deep brain stimulation.
- Neurologic dysfunction sometimes improves with physical therapy and speech therapy.

Nutritional Therapy

A nutritious, well-balanced diet is essential. Although there is no standard prescribed diet, a high-protein diet with supplementary

M

vitamins is often advocated. A diet high in roughage may help relieve constipation.

Nursing Management

Goals

The patient with MS will maximize neuromuscular function, maintain independence in activities of daily living for as long as possible, manage disabling fatigue, optimize psychosocial well-being, adjust to the illness, and reduce factors that precipitate exacerbations.

See NCP 59-3 for the patient with multiple sclerosis, Lewis and others, *Medical-Surgical Nursing,* edition 7, pp. 1547 to 1548.

Nursing Diagnoses

- Impaired physical mobility
- Impaired urinary elimination
- Sexual dysfunction
- Interrupted family processes
- Dressing/grooming self-care deficit
- Risk for impaired skin integrity

Nursing Interventions

The patient with MS should be aware of triggers that may cause exacerbations or worsening of the disease. Exacerbations of MS are triggered by infection (especially upper respiratory infections), trauma, childbirth, stress, fatigue, and climatic changes. The nurse should help the patient identify particular triggers and develop ways to avoid them or minimize their effects.

The most common reasons for hospitalization are for a diagnostic workup and for treatment of an acute exacerbation.

- During the diagnostic phase the patient needs reassurance that even though there is a tentative diagnosis of MS, certain diagnostic studies must be made to rule out other neurologic disorders. The patient with recently diagnosed MS may need assistance with the grieving process.
- During an acute exacerbation the patient may be immobile and confined to bed. The focus of nursing intervention at this phase is to prevent the hazards of immobility, such as respiratory and urinary tract infections and pressure ulcers.

▼ Patient and Family Teaching

- Patient teaching should focus on building a general resistance to illness. This includes avoiding fatigue, extremes of heat and cold, and exposure to infection.
- It is important to teach the patient to achieve a good balance of exercise and rest, eat nutritious and well-balanced meals, and avoid the hazards of immobility (contractures and pressure sores).

- Patients should know their treatment regimens, the side effects of drugs, and drug interactions with over-the-counter medications.
- Some patients may need to be taught self-catheterization to control bladder problems.
- Increasing dietary fiber may help some patients achieve regularity in bowel habits.
- Inform patients about the National Multiple Sclerosis Society, which offers a variety of services to meet the needs of MS patients and their families.

MUSCULAR DYSTROPHY

Description

Muscular dystrophy (MD) is a group of genetically transmitted diseases characterized by progressive symmetric wasting of skeletal muscle without evidence of neurologic involvement. In all forms of MD an insidious loss of strength occurs with increasing disability and deformity. The types of MD differ in the groups of muscles affected, age of onset, rate of progression, and mode of genetic inheritance. The age of onset of symptoms varies from before age 5 years to early adulthood. Types of MD are presented in Table 64-4, Lewis and others, *Medical-Surgical Nursing*, edition 7, p. 1645.

Duchenne's MD and *Becker's MD* are sex-lined recessive disorders usually seen in males. In these disorders there is a genetic mutation of the dystrophin gene. Abnormalities in dystrophin can lead to defects in the plasma membrane of muscle fiber with subsequent muscle fiber degeneration.

Diagnostic studies include muscle serum enzymes (especially creatinine kinase [CK]), electromyogram (EMG) testing, muscle fiber biopsy, electrocardiogram (ECG) abnormalities reflective of cardiomyopathy, and genetic pedigree.

- Muscle biopsy confirms the diagnosis, with classic findings of fat and connective tissue deposits, degeneration and necrosis of muscle fibers, and a deficiency of dystrophin.

Presently, there is no definitive therapy available to stop the progressive wasting. Corticosteroid therapy may significantly halt the disease progression for up to 3 years. The goal of treatment is to preserve mobility and independence through exercise, physical therapy, and orthopedic appliances.

- The nurse should encourage communication among family members to cope with the emotional and physical strains of

M

MD. Emphasis should be placed on teaching the patient and family range-of-motion (ROM) exercises, nutrition, and signs of progression.

- Genetic testing and counseling may be recommended for individuals with a family history of MD.
- Nursing care should focus on keeping the patient active as long as possible. Prolonged bed rest should be avoided, because immobility can lead to further muscle wasting.
- As the disease progresses, the focus shifts to teaching the patient to limit sedentary periods during which skin integrity or respiratory complications could develop.

MYASTHENIA GRAVIS

Description
Myasthenia gravis (MG) is an autoimmune disease of the neuromuscular junction characterized by fluctuating weakness of certain skeletal muscle groups. Women are affected slightly more often than men. Peak age at onset in women is 20 to 30 years.

Pathophysiology
MG is caused by an autoimmune process in which antibodies are produced that attack acetylcholine (ACh) receptors. A reduction in the number of ACh receptor sites at the neuromuscular junction prevents ACh molecules from attaching to the receptors and stimulating muscle contraction. Anti-ACh receptor antibodies are detectable in the serum of most patients with MG. Thymic tumors are found in about 15% of all patients with MG, and abnormal thymus tissue is found in most others.

Clinical Manifestations
The primary feature is fluctuating weakness of skeletal muscle. Strength is usually restored after a period of rest. The muscles most often involved are those used for moving the eyes and eyelids, chewing, swallowing, speaking, and breathing. The muscles are generally the strongest in the morning and become exhausted with continued activity. By the end of the day, muscle weakness is prominent.

- In 90% of cases, the eyelid muscles or extraocular muscles are involved. Facial mobility and expression can be impaired. There may be difficulty in chewing and swallowing food.

Speech is affected, and the voice often fades during long conversations.

- No other signs of neural disorder accompany MG; there is no sensory loss, reflexes are normal, and muscle atrophy is rare.

The course of the disease is highly variable. Some patients may have short-term remissions, others may stabilize, and still others may have severe progressive involvement. Restricted ocular myasthenia, usually seen only in men, has a good prognosis.

- Exacerbations of MG can be precipitated by emotional stress, pregnancy, menses, secondary illness, trauma, temperature extremes, and hypokalemia. A wide variety of drugs, including β-adrenergic blockers and psychotropic drugs, have been associated with worsening of MG.

The major complications of MG result from muscle weakness in areas that affect swallowing and breathing. An acute exacerbation of MG that results in aspiration and respiratory insufficiency is known as a *myasthenic crisis*.

Diagnostic Studies

The diagnosis of MG can be made on the basis of history and physical examination.

- Muscle weakness is present on examination.
- Fatigibility and progressive drooping of eyelids with upward gaze for 2 to 3 minutes occur. After a brief rest, the eyes can open again.
- Acetylcholine receptor antibodies are found in serum of 85% to 90% of patients with generalized MG.
- Electromyogram (EMG) may show a decremental response to repeated stimulation of the hand muscles, indicative of muscle fatigue.
- The Tensilon test reveals improved muscle contractility after an intravenous (IV) injection of the anticholinesterase agent edrophonium chloride (Tensilon chloride).

Collaborative Care

Drug Therapy

Drug therapy for MG includes anticholinesterase drugs, alternate-day corticosteroids, and immunosuppressants.

- Acetylcholinesterase is the enzyme responsible for the breakdown of ACh in the synaptic cleft. Acetylcholinesterase inhibitors prolong the action of ACh and facilitate transmission of impulses at the neuromuscular junction. Neostigmine (Prostigmin) and pyridostigmine (Mestinon) are the most successful drugs of this group.

M

- Because of the autoimmune nature of MG, corticosteroids (specifically prednisone) are used to suppress the immune response. Cytotoxic drugs such as azathioprine (Imuran) and cyclophosphamide (Cytoxan) may also be used for immunosuppression.

Other Therapies

- Because the thymus gland appears to enhance the production of ACh receptor antibodies, removal of the thymus gland results in improvement in a majority of patients.
- Removal of anti-ACh receptor antibodies with plasmapheresis can provide short-term improvement and is indicated for patients in crisis or in preparation for surgery when corticosteroids must be avoided.
- IV immunoglobulin G has been used with some success and may be better than plasmapheresis for treating exacerbations or moderately severe MG.

Nursing Management

Goals

The patient with MG will have a return of normal muscle endurance, manage fatigue, avoid complications, and maintain a quality of life appropriate to disease course.

Nursing Diagnoses

- Ineffective breathing pattern
- Ineffective airway clearance
- Impaired verbal communication
- Imbalanced nutrition: less than body requirements
- Disturbed sensory perception
- Activity intolerance
- Disturbed body image

Nursing Interventions

The patient who is admitted to the hospital usually has a respiratory tract infection or is in acute myasthenic crisis. Nursing care is aimed at maintaining adequate ventilation, continuing drug therapy, and watching for side effects of therapy. The nurse must be able to distinguish cholinergic from myasthenic crisis because the causes and treatment of the two differ greatly (Table 60).

- As with other chronic illnesses, care focuses on the neurologic deficits and their impact on daily living.
- A balanced diet that can be chewed and swallowed easily should be prescribed. Semisolid foods may be easier to eat than solids or liquids. Scheduling doses of medication so that peak action is reached at mealtime may make eating less difficult.

Table 60 Comparison of Myasthenic Crisis and Cholinergic Crisis

	Myasthenic Crisis	Cholinergic Crisis
Causes	Exacerbation of myasthenia following precipitating factors or failure to take drug as prescribed or drug dose too low	Overdose of anticholinesterase drugs resulting in increased ACh at the receptor sites, remission (spontaneous or after thymectomy)
Differential diagnosis	Improved strength after IV administration of anticholinesterase drugs; increased weakness of skeletal muscles manifesting as ptosis, bulbar signs (e.g., difficulty in swallowing, difficulty in signs articulating words), or dyspnea	Weakness within 1 hr after ingestion of anticholinesterase; increased weakness of skeletal muscles manifesting as ptosis, bulbar signs, dyspnea; effects on smooth muscle include pupillary miosis, salivation, diarrhea, nausea or vomiting, abdominal cramps, increased bronchial secretions, sweating, or lacrimination

ACh, Acetylcholine; IV, intravenous.

M

- Diversional activities that require little physical effort and match the interests of the patient should be arranged.
▼ **Patient and Family Teaching**
Teaching should focus on the importance of following the medical regimen, potential adverse reactions to specific drugs, planning activities of daily living to avoid fatigue, availability of community resources, and complications of the disease and therapy (crisis conditions) and what to do about them.

- Contact with the Myasthenia Gravis Society or an MG support group may be helpful and should be explored.

MYOCARDITIS

Description

Myocarditis is a focal or diffuse inflammation of the myocardium that has been associated with viruses, bacteria, fungi, radiation therapy, pharmacologic and chemical factors, and autoimmune disorders. Viruses, particularly coxsackievirus type A and B, are the most common etiologic agent in the United States and Canada.

- Myocarditis is frequently associated with acute pericarditis, particularly when it is caused by coxsackievirus B strains.

Pathophysiology

When the myocardium becomes infected, the causative agent invades the myocytes and causes cellular damage and necrosis. The immune response is activated, cytokines and oxygen-free radicals are released, and an autoimmune response occurs, resulting in further destruction of myocytes. The myocarditis results in cardiac dysfunction and possibly dilated cardiomyopathy (see Cardiomyopathy, p. 96).

Clinical Manifestations

Clinical features of myocarditis are variable, ranging from a benign course without overt manifestations to severe heart involvement or sudden cardiac death. Fever, fatigue, malaise, myalgias, pharyngitis, dyspnea, lymphadenopathy, and nausea and vomiting are early systemic manifestations of the viral illness.

- Early cardiac manifestations appear 7 to 10 days after viral infection and include pericardial chest pain with a pericardial friction rub and effusion.

- Late cardiac signs relate to the development of heart failure and may include S_3, crackles, jugular venous distention, syncope, peripheral edema, and angina.
- Most patients with myocarditis recover spontaneously although some may develop dilated cardiomyopathy.

Diagnostic Studies

- Electrocardiogram (ECG) changes are often nonspecific and reflect associated pericardial involvement, including diffuse ST segment abnormalities. Dysrhythmias and conduction disturbances may be present.
- Laboratory findings are also often inconclusive, with mild to moderate leukocytosis and atypical lymphocytes, increased erythrocyte sedimentation rate (ESR) and C-reactive protein (CRP) levels, elevated levels of myocardial markers such as troponin, and elevated viral titers (virus is generally only present in tissue and fluid samples during the initial 8 to 10 days of illness).
- Histologic confirmation is possible through endomyocardial biopsy. A biopsy done during the initial 6 weeks of acute illness is most diagnostic because this is the period in which lymphocytic infiltration and myocyte damage indicative of myocarditis are present.
- Other studies include the use of echocardiography, nuclear scans, and magnetic resonance imaging (MRI) to evaluate cardiac function.

Collaborative Care

A specific therapy for myocarditis has yet to be established and usually consists of managing associated cardiac decompensation.

- Digoxin is often used to treat ventricular failure because it improves myocardial contractility and reduces ventricular rate. Digoxin should be used cautiously in patients with myocarditis because of increased heart sensitivity to the adverse effects of this drug.
- Diuretics may be used to reduce fluid volume and decrease preload; nitroprusside (Nitropress), inamrinone (Inocor), and milrinone (Primacor) may be used to reduce afterload and improve cardiac output by decreasing arterial resistance.
- Oxygen (O_2) therapy, bed rest, restricted activity, and maintenance of standby emergency equipment are general supportive measures.

Immunosuppression therapy with agents such as prednisone, azathioprine (Imuran), and cyclosporine has been used on a limited basis to reduce myocardial inflammation and to prevent irreversible myocardial damage. The use of this therapy remains controversial because of the associated serious side effects and lack of clear documentation for its efficacy.

Nursing Management

Interventions focus on an assessment for the signs and symptoms of heart failure and instituting measures to decrease cardiac workload (e.g., use of semi-Fowler's position, spaced activity and rest periods, provisions for a quiet environment). Medications that increase the heart's contractility and decrease the preload, afterload, or both require careful monitoring.

The patient may be anxious about the diagnosis of myocarditis, recovery from myocarditis, and therapy. Nursing measures include assessing the level of anxiety, instituting measures to decrease anxiety, and keeping the patient and family informed about therapeutic measures.

The patient who receives immunosuppressive therapy may have additional problems of alterations in immune response with the potential for infection and complications related to the therapy. Guidelines for care include monitoring for complications and providing the patient with a clean, safe environment according to proper infection control standards.

NAUSEA AND VOMITING

Description

Nausea and vomiting are the most common manifestations of gastrointestinal (GI) diseases. Although each symptom can occur independently, they are closely related and usually treated as one problem. They are also found in a wide variety of conditions unrelated to GI disease. These include pregnancy, infectious diseases, central nervous system (CNS) disorders (e.g., meningitis), cardiovascular problems (e.g., myocardial infarction [MI], heart failure [HF]), metabolic disorders (e.g., uremia), side effects of drugs (e.g., digitalis, antibiotics), and psychologic factors (e.g., stress, fear).

Nausea is a feeling of discomfort in the epigastrium with a conscious desire to vomit. Anorexia usually accompanies nausea and is brought on by unpleasant stimulation involving any of the five senses. Generally, nausea occurs before vomiting and is characterized by contraction of the duodenum and by the slowing of gastric motility and emptying.

Vomiting is a complex act that results in the forceful ejection of partially digested food and secretions from the upper GI tract. It occurs when the gut becomes overly irritated, excited, or distended. Vomiting can be a protective mechanism to rid the body of spoiled or irritating foods and liquids.

Pathophysiology

The vomiting center in the brainstem coordinates the multiple components involved in vomiting. Neural impulses reach the vomiting center by way of afferent pathways through branches of the autonomic nervous system. Visceral receptors for these afferent fibers are located in the GI tract, kidneys, heart, and uterus. When stimulated, these receptors relay information to the vomiting center, which initiates the vomiting reflex. The simultaneous closure of the glottis, deep inspiration with contraction of the diaphragm in the inspiratory position, closure of the pylorus, relaxation of the stomach and lower esophageal sphincter, and contraction of the abdominal muscles with increasing intra-abdominal pressure force stomach contents up and out of the mouth.

In addition, the chemoreceptor trigger zone (CTZ) located in the brain responds to chemical stimuli of drugs and toxins. Once stimulated (e.g., motion sickness), the CTZ transmits impulses to the vomiting center.

Clinical Manifestations

Signs of severe or prolonged nausea and vomiting include rapid dehydration with loss of essential electrolytes (e.g., potassium [K^+], hydrogen [H^+]). As vomiting persists, there may be severe electrolyte imbalances, loss of extracellular fluid (ECF) volume, decreased plasma volume, and eventual circulatory failure. Metabolic alkalosis may result from loss of hydrochloric acid from the stomach, but more frequently metabolic acidosis occurs as a result of loss of the contents of the small intestine. Weight loss may occur in a short time when vomiting is severe.

Collaborative Care

The goals of management are to determine and treat the underlying cause of nausea and vomiting and to provide symptomatic relief. Determining the cause is often difficult because nausea and vomiting are manifestations of many conditions of the GI tract and of disorders of other body systems. Evaluation of the amount, frequency, character (e.g., projectile), content (e.g., feces, bile, blood), and color (e.g., red, "coffee ground") of vomitus helps to determine the cause.

N

Many different drugs are used to treat nausea and vomiting, but they are used with caution until the cause of the vomiting is determined. Drugs may include anticholinergics (e.g., scopolamine), antihistamines (e.g., promethazine [Phenergan]), phenothiazines (e.g., prochlorperazine [Compazine]), and butyrophenones (e.g., droperidol [Inapsine]). Other drugs with antiemetic effects include benzamides (metoclopramide [Reglan]) and 5-HT3 (serotonin) receptor antagonists (e.g., ondansetron [Zofran]). A comprehensive list of drugs used for nausea and vomiting is included in Table 42-1, Lewis and others, *Medical-Surgical Nursing,* edition 7, p. 992.

Alternative therapies such as acupressure or acupuncture have been effective in reducing postoperative nausea and vomiting, and botanicals such as ginger and peppermint oil may be used by patients.

The patient with severe vomiting requires intravenous (IV) fluid therapy with electrolyte replacement until able to tolerate oral intake. In some cases a nasogastric (NG) tube and suction are used to decompress the stomach. Once symptoms have subsided, oral nourishment beginning with clear liquids is started. Water is the initial fluid of choice for rehydration. As the condition improves, a diet high in carbohydrates and low in fatty foods is preferred.

Nursing Management

Goals

The patient with nausea and vomiting will experience minimal or no nausea and vomiting, have normal electrolyte levels and hydration status, and return to a normal pattern of fluid balance and nutrient intake.

See NCP 42-1 for the patient with nausea and vomiting, Lewis and others, *Medical-Surgical Nursing,* edition 7, p. 994.

Nursing Diagnoses

- Nausea
- Deficient fluid volume
- Imbalanced nutrition: less than body requirements
- Impaired oral mucous membranes

Nursing Interventions

Until a diagnosis is confirmed, the patient is kept on nothing by mouth (NPO) status and given IV fluids. An NG tube connected to suction may be necessary for persistent vomiting. Keeping the stomach empty reduces the stimulus to vomit.

- The environment should be quiet, free of noxious odors, and well ventilated.
- Use of relaxation techniques and diversional tactics may help prevent or relieve nausea and vomiting.

- Cleansing the face and hands with a cool washcloth and providing mouth care between episodes increase the person's comfort level. When symptoms occur, all foods and medications should be stopped until the acute phase is past.

With prolonged vomiting, interventions include accurate intake and output with vital signs, assessment for dehydration, proper positioning to prevent aspiration, and observation for changes in comfort and mentation.

▼ **Patient and Family Teaching**
- Provide explanations for diagnostic tests and procedures.
- The patient and family may need instructions on how to deal successfully with the unpleasant sensations of nausea, discussion of methods for preventing nausea and vomiting, and strategies to maintain fluid and nutritional intake during periods of nausea.
- When food is identified as the precipitating cause of nausea and vomiting, help the patient identify the specific food and associated circumstances.

NEPHROTIC SYNDROME

Description
Nephrotic syndrome results when the glomerulus of the kidney is excessively permeable to plasma protein, causing proteinuria leading to low plasma albumin and tissue edema. Common causes include primary glomerular disease (e.g., focal glomerulonephritis), infections (e.g., hepatitis, streptococcal), neoplasms (e.g., Hodgkin's lymphoma), allergens (e.g., bee sting), drugs (e.g., nonsteroidal antiinflammatory agents [NSAIDs]), and multisystem diseases (e.g., diabetes mellitus [DM]).

Pathophysiology and Clinical Manifestations
The increased glomerular membrane permeability found in nephrotic syndrome is responsible for massive excretion of protein in the urine. This results in decreased serum protein and subsequent edema formation, including ascites and anasarca.

- Diminished plasma oncotic pressure from the decrease in serum proteins stimulates hepatic lipoprotein synthesis, which results in hyperlipidemia. Fat bodies (fatty casts) commonly apear in the urine.
- Immune responses, both humoral and cellular, are altered in nephrotic syndrome. As a result, infection is a major cause of morbidity and mortality.

N

- Calcium and skeletal abnormalities may occur, including hypocalcemia, blunted calcemic response to parathyroid hormone, hyperparathyroidism, and osteomalacia.
- Hypercoagulability with thromboembolism is potentially the most serious complication of nephrotic syndrome. The renal vein is the most commonly involved site for thrombus formation. Pulmonary emboli occur in about 40% of nephrotic patients with thrombosis.

Characteristic manifestations include peripheral edema, massive proteinuria, hyperlipidemia, and hypoalbuminemia. Characteristic blood chemistries include decreased serum albumin, decreased total serum protein, and elevated serum cholesterol.

Collaborative Care

The goals of treatment are to relieve edema and cure or control the primary disease. Management of edema includes the cautious use of angiotensin-converting enzyme (ACE) inhibitors, NSAIDs, low-sodium intake (2 to 3 g/day), and a low to moderate protein diet (0.5 to 0.6 g/kg/day).

- Dietary salt restrictions are key to managing edema. In some patients, thiazide or loop diuretics may be needed.
- If protein loss exceeds 10 g/24 hr, additional dietary protein may be needed.
- Treatment with lipid-lowering agents, such as colestipol (Colestid) and lovastatin (Mevacor), may result in moderate decreases in serum cholesterol levels. Treatment of hyperlipidemia is frequently unsuccessful.
- Corticosteroids and cyclophosphamide (Cytoxan) may be used for the treatment of severe cases. Prednisone has been effective in some persons with early-stage nephrosis, membranous glomerulonephritis, proliferative glomerulonephritis, and lupus nephritis.
- Management of DM and treatment of edema are the only measures used for nephrotic syndrome related to DM.

Nursing Management

The major focus of care is related to edema. It is important to assess edema by weighing the patient daily, accurately recording intake and output, and measuring abdominal girth or extremity size. Comparing this information daily provides the nurse with a tool for assessing the effectiveness of treatment. Edematous skin needs careful cleaning. Trauma should be avoided, and the effectiveness of diuretic therapy must be monitored. The person is often ashamed of the edematous appearance and may need support in dealing with an altered body image.

The patient has the potential to become malnourished from the excessive loss of protein in the urine. Maintaining a low to moderate protein diet that is also low in sodium is not always easy. The patient is usually anorexic; serving small, frequent meals in a pleasant setting may encourage better dietary intake.

- Because the patient is susceptible to infection, measures should be taken to avoid exposure to persons with known infections.

NON-HODGKIN'S LYMPHOMAS

Description
Non-Hodgkin's lymphomas (NHLs) are a heterogeneous group of malignant neoplasms of primarily B- or T-cell origin that affect all ages. B-cell lymphomas constitute about 90% of all NHLs. They are classified according to different cellular and lymph node characteristics. Common names for different types of NHL include Burkitt's lymphoma, reticulum cell sarcoma, and lymphosarcoma. NHL is the most commonly occurring hematologic cancer and the fifth leading cause of cancer death.

Pathophysiology
The cause of NHLs is usually unknown, but an increased incidence is associated with advanced age, use of immunosuppressive medications, chemotherapy or radiation therapy, and occupational exposure to carcinogens. Epstein-Barr virus is associated with Burkitt's lymphoma. Although there is no hallmark feature in NHL, all NHLs involve lymphocytes arrested in various stages of development.

Clinical Manifestations
NHLs can originate outside the lymph nodes, and the method of spread can be unpredictable. The majority of patients have widely disseminated disease at the time of diagnosis. The primary clinical manifestation is painless lymph node enlargement (*adenopathy*). Because the disease is usually disseminated when diagnosed, other symptoms are present depending on where the disease has spread (e.g., hepatomegaly with liver involvement, neurologic symptoms with central nervous system disease). NHL can also present nonspecifically with airway obstruction, renal failure, pericardial tamponade, and gastrointestinal complaints.

- Patients with high-grade (very aggressive) lymphomas may have lymphadenopathy and constitutional ("B") symptoms,

N

such as fever, night sweats, and weight loss. The peripheral blood is usually normal, but some lymphomas may occur in a "leukemic" phase.

Diagnostic Studies
Diagnostic studies for NHL resemble those used for Hodgkin's lymphoma. Lymph node biopsy establishes the cell type and pattern. Staging, as described for Hodgkin's lymphoma, is used to guide therapy. The prognosis for NHL is generally not as good as that for Hodgkin's lymphoma.

Nursing and Collaborative Management
Treatment for NHL involves chemotherapy and sometimes radiation therapy (see Chemotherapy, p. 712). Ironically, aggressive lymphomas are more responsive to treatment and more likely to be cured. Indolent lymphomas have a naturally long course but are more difficult to treat effectively.

- Initial therapy for patients with low-grade (indolent) lymphoma who are asymptomatic may include rituximab (Rituxan), a genetically engineered monoclonal antibody against the CD20 antigen on the surface of normal and malignant B lymphocytes, to reduce time to progression of disease.
- Once the disease is symptomatic, rituximab with chemotherapy, such as cyclophosphamide (Cytoxan) with or without prednisone or the CHOP regimen (cyclophosphamide, doxorubicin [Adriamycin], vincristine [Oncovin], prednisone, and rituximab) may be used.
- Complete remissions are uncommon, but the majority of patients respond with improvement in adenopathy and symptoms.
- Aggressive lymphomas may be treated similarly, depending on the extent of the disease and the patient's prognosis. High-dose chemotherapy with autologous hematopoietic stem cell transplant has show a better outcome than conventional chemotherapy in the treatment of patients with relapsed, aggressive NHL.
- Because NHL represents a large variety of neoplasms, some subtypes may be treated differently from the general standards described above. A variety of immunosuppressive agents, biologic agents, and monoclonal antibodies may be used.

Nursing care for patients with NHL is similar to those with Hodgkin's lymphoma, but NHL is often more extensive and involves specific organs.

- Care is based on managing problems related to the disease (pain, spinal cord compression, tumor lysis syndrome), pancytopenia, and other effects of therapy.
- Because most of these patients receive therapy that is potentially myelosuppressive, nursing care presented in NCPs 31-1, pp. 688 to 689; 31-2, p. 706; and 31-3, p. 716, Lewis and others, *Medical-Surgical Nursing,* edition 7, applies.
- Psychosocial considerations are very important. Helping the patient and family understand the disease, treatment, and expected and potential untoward side effects is paramount in enlisting their help in the patient's well-being and safety.

OBESITY

Description
Obesity is an abnormal increase in the proportion of fat cells. An imbalance between energy expenditure and energy intake from a long-term sedentary lifestyle and/or excessive calorie intake causes an individual to become overweight or obese. Obesity has reached epidemic proportions in the United States, where 65% of people over the age of 20 years are either overweight or obese. Obesity is a major health problem because of adverse health conditions. It is the second leading cause of preventable deaths after smoking and the third leading reason for liver transplantation. Health risks associated with obesity include higher rates of hypertension, dyslipidemia, obesity hypoventilation syndrome, sleep apnea, type 2 diabetes mellitus, osteoarthritis, gout, gastroesophageal reflux disease, gallstones, nonalcoholic steatohepatitis, and cancers of the breast, endometrium, ovary, cervix, colon, and prostate.

Pathophysiology
The cause of obesity involves complex genetic/biologic susceptibility factors influenced by environmental and psychosocial factors.

- Strong evidence of a genetic predisposition to obesity is suggested in studies of twin and adoptive children.
- Biologic components related to obesity include hormones and peptides such as leptin, insulin, ghrelin, and peptide YY that interact at the level of the hypothalamus to influence eating behavior, energy metabolism, and body fat metabolism.

- Adipocytes (fat cells) themselves secrete a number of hormones and cytokines known as adipokines that are altered by visceral fat accumulation.
- Environmental factors include greater access to prepackaged and fast foods, larger portion sizes, lack of physical activity and sedentary recreation, and high-calorie foods that are more accessible to those of low socioeconomic status.
- The association of food with comfort, reward, pleasure, and fun is a powerful incentive for overeating and must be included when considering the etiology and treatment of obesity.

Diagnostic Studies

- History and physical examination to reveal extent and duration of obesity and differentiate *primary* (excess calories for metabolic demand) from *secondary* (biologic disorders) obesity
- Laboratory tests of liver function, fasting glucose level, triglyceride level, and low- and high-density lipoprotein cholesterol levels to assist in evaluating the cause and effects of obesity
- Classifications of body weight and obesity defined by body mass index (BMI), standardized height-weight charts, anthropometric measurements, or hip/waist ratio (Table 61)

Collaborative Care

When no organic cause can be found for obesity, it should be considered a chronic, complex illness. A supervised plan of care should focus on:

- Successful weight loss, requiring a short-term energy deficit
- Successful weight control, requiring long-term behavioral changes

A multipronged approach should be taken with attention to dietary intake, physical activity, behavioral modification, and perhaps drug therapy. Restricting dietary intake so that it is below energy requirements is an effective way to reduce body weight (see Table 41-6, Nutritional Therapy in Lewis and others, *Medical-Surgical Nursing,* edition 7, p. 978). Weight reduction diets found in popular media that advocate the elimination of any one category of foods should be discouraged. A well-balanced, low-calorie diet is essential to weight loss and weight control.

- The loss of 1 to 2 pounds per week is a realistic and healthy goal to set with the patient.
- During normal plateau periods, when no weight is lost for several days to several weeks, patients need encouragement and support to prevent giving up on the weight loss plan.

Table 61 Classification of Overweight and Obesity by BMI, Waist Circumference, and Associated Disease Risk*

	BMI (kg/m²)	Obesity Class	Disease Risk Based on Waist Circumference*	
			Men ≤40 in (102 cm) Women ≤35 in (88 cm)	Men >40 in (102 cm) Women >35 in (88 cm)
Underweight	<18.5		—	—
Normal†	18.5-24.9		—	—
Overweight	25.9-29.9		Increased	High
Obese	30.0-34.9	Class I	High	Very high
	35.0-39.9	Class II	Very high	Very high
Morbid obesity	≥40.0	Class III	Extremely high	Extremely high

From National Heart, Lung, and Blood Institute North American Association for the Study of Obesity: *The practical guide: identification, evaluation, and treatment of overweight and obesity in adults*, pub no 00-4084, Washington, DC, 2000, U.S. Department of Health and Human Services. *BMI*, Body mass index.

* Disease risk for type 2 diabetes, hypertension, and cardiovascular disease relative to person of normal weight.
† Increased waist circumference can also be a marker for increased risk in persons of normal weight.

Daily exercise for at least 30 to 60 minutes per day is an essential part of a weight control program. Walking, swimming, and cycling are good forms of exercise.

- The patient should be encouraged to wear a pedometer to document the recommendation of 10,000 steps per day.
- Psychologic benefits of exercise include reduced tension and stress, better-quality sleep and rest, and increased stamina and energy, factors that improve the patient's overall health.
- Behavior therapy to deemphasize the diet and change eating behaviors uses the basic techniques of self-monitoring, stimulus control, and rewards. Persons who have undergone behavior therapy are more successful in maintaining their losses over an extended time than those who do not participate in such training.
- The person who is on any type of weight control program may be encouraged to join a support or self-help group if the support of others having the same problems and experiences is helpful.

Drug Therapy

Medications have been used in the treatment of obesity as adjuncts to a good diet and exercise program. Drugs approved for weight loss can be classified into two categories: those that decrease food intake by reducing appetite or increasing satiety (sense of feeling full after eating) and those that decrease nutrient absorption. Drugs that increase energy expenditure (e.g., ephedrine) are not approved by the Food and Drug Administration for weight loss in the United States at this time.

- Appetite-suppressant drugs reduce food intake through noradrenergic (drugs that mimic norepinephrine) or serotonergic mechanisms in the central nervous system (CNS). Noradrenergic agents include phentermine (Adipex-P, Fastin, Ionamin), diethylpropion (Tenuate, Tepanil), phendimetrazine (Bontril, Plegine), and benzphetamine (Didrex). Phendimetrazine and benzphetamine are Schedule III drugs that are only to be used for short-term treatment.
- Serotonergic drugs that increase the effect of serotonin (e.g., fenfluramine [Pondimin], dexfenfluramine [Redux]) have serious side effects and have been withdrawn from the market.
- Nutrient absorption–blocking drugs such as orlistat (Xenical) work by blocking fat breakdown and absorption in the intestine.

Because drugs do not cure obesity without substantial changes in food intake and increased physical activity, weight gain occurs when short-term drug therapy is stopped. As with any pharmacologic treatment, patients should be taught about administration and side effects.

Surgical Therapy

Bariatric surgery is a surgical procedure that is used to treat morbid obesity. To be considered for bariatric surgery, an individual has to meet a number of criteria, including severe or morbid obesity with one or more severe obesity-related medical complications, such as hypertension or heart failure.

- Bariatric surgeries are categorized as restrictive, malabsorptive, or a combination of restrictive and malabsorptive.
- Gastric restrictive surgeries include vertical banded gastroplasty and adjustable gastric banding; gastric malabsorptive surgeries include biliopancreatic diversion and biliopancreatic diversion with duodenal switch; a combination procedure is a Roux-en-Y gastric bypass. These surgeries are discussed further on pp. 982 to 984 in Lewis and others, *Medical-Surgical Nursing,* edition 7.

Cosmetic surgeries may be used to reduce fatty tissue and skinfolds. These procedures include a *lipectomy* (adipectomy) to remove unsightly adipose folds and *liposuction* for cosmetic purposes.

Nursing Management

Goals

The overall goals are that the patient with obesity will modify eating patterns, participate in a regular physical activity program, achieve weight loss to a specified level, maintain weight loss at a specified level, and minimize or prevent health problems related to obesity.

Nursing Diagnoses

- Imbalanced nutrition: more than body requirements
- Impaired skin integrity
- Ineffective breathing pattern
- Chronic low self-esteem
- Health-seeking behaviors

Nursing Interventions

When assessing obese patients, the nurse should consider several different types of questions, such as the following:

- What is the individual's history with weight gain and weight loss?
- Is the patient interested in losing weight or managing his or her weight differently?
- What do patients think contributes to their weight?

- What sort of barriers do they feel impede their weight loss efforts?
- What does food mean to them? Or how do they use food (e.g., to relieve stress, provide comfort)?
- Do members of the patient's family have a tendency to be overweight?
- Are there environmental or genetic factors influencing the weight gain?

The nurse, working closely with other members of the health care team, plays a major role in the planning for and management of the obese patient. Nurses are in a pivotal position to help overweight and obese people deal with negative experiences and to educate other health care professionals to prevent bias against overweight patients.

Preoperative care for gastric surgery includes planning for special needs of an obese patient, such as the availability of an oversized blood pressure (BP) cuff, oversized bed and chair; and a reinforced trapeze bar. Consideration should be given to questions such as how the patient will be weighed, how the patient will be transported through the hospital, and how simple physical assessment strategies may have to be adjusted.

- The patient must be instructed in the proper coughing technique, deep breathing, use of an incentive spirometer, and methods of turning and positioning to prevent pulmonary complications after surgery.

Postoperative care and teaching emphasize facilitating patient respiratory efforts (elevating the head of the bed, turning, coughing, deep breathing), monitoring the abdominal wound for healing, early ambulation, and monitoring nasogastric (NG) tube patency. Extra nurses and other personnel may be necessary to turn and ambulate the patient.

- The patient has considerable abdominal pain after surgery, and pain medications should be given as frequently as necessary during the immediate postoperative period.
- Anticipate and recognize several potential psychologic problems after surgery. Some patients express guilt feelings concerning the fact that the only way they could lose weight was by surgical means rather than by the "sheer willpower" of reduced dietary intake. The nurse should be ready to provide support so that this patient does not dwell on negative feelings.
- Discharge teaching includes the importance of strict adherence to a diet high in protein and low in carbohydrates, fat, and roughage, with six small feedings daily, and prompt recognition of complications such as anemia, diarrhea,

vitamin deficiencies, and psychiatric problems, especially episodes of depression.
- The nurse needs to reinforce physical activity programs and cognitive training such as self-help support groups or professional counseling to facilitate the patient's adjustment to a new body image and social reintegration.

ORAL CANCER

Description
Oral cancer may occur on the lips or anywhere within the mouth (e.g., tongue, floor of mouth, buccal mucosa, hard palate, soft palate, pharyngeal walls, or tonsils). Head and neck squamous cell carcinoma (HNSCC) is an umbrella term for cancers of the oral cavity, pharynx, and larynx and accounts for 90% of malignant oral tumors. Carcinoma of the lips has the most favorable prognosis of any of the oral tumors, because lip lesions are more apparent to the patient than other oral lesions and are usually diagnosed earlier.
- Oral cancer is more common after age 40 years, with age 60 years being the average age of onset. The 5-year survival rate for all stages of cancer of the oral cavity and pharynx is 53%.

Pathophysiology
Although the cause of oral cancers is not definitive, there are a number of predisposing factors, including constant overexposure to ultraviolet (UV) radiation from the sun, tobacco use (cigar, cigarette, pipe, snuff), excessive alcohol intake, and chronic irritation, such as from a jagged tooth or poor dental care.

Clinical Manifestations
Common manifestations include leukoplakia, erythroplakia, ulcerations, a sore that bleeds easily and does not heal, and a rough area felt with the tongue.
- *Leukoplakia,* called "white patch" or "smoker's patch," is a whitish precancerous lesion on the mucosa of the mouth or tongue that results from chronic irritation, especially from smoking. The patch becomes keratinized (hard and leathery) and is sometimes described as hyperkeratosis.
- *Erythroplakia,* which is seen as a red velvety patch on the mouth or tongue, is also considered a precancerous lesion.

Fifty percent of cases of erythroplakia progress to squamous cell carcinoma.
- Cancer of the lip appears as an indurated, painless lip ulcer.
- The first sign of tongue cancer is an ulcer or area of thickening. Soreness or pain of the tongue may occur, especially on eating hot or highly seasoned foods. Some patients experience limitation of movement of the tongue. Later symptoms of tongue cancer include increased salivation, slurred speech, dysphagia, toothache, and earache.
- Approximately 30% of patients with oral cancer present with an asymptomatic neck mass.

Diagnostic Studies
- Biopsy of suspected lesion with cytologic examination
- Oral exfoliative cytology and toluidine blue test to screen for oral cancer

Collaborative Care
Management usually consists of surgery, radiation, chemotherapy, or a combination of these. Surgery remains the most effective treatment. Many of the operations are radical procedures involving extensive resections. Various surgical procedures may be performed, including hemiglossectomy (removal of one half of the tongue), glossectomy (removal of the entire tongue), and radial neck dissection. A tracheostomy (see Tracheostomy, p. 746) is commonly done with radical neck dissection.

Chemotherapy and radiation are used together when the lesions are more advanced or involve several structures of the oral cavity. Chemotherapy may also be used when surgery and radiation fail or as the initial therapy for smaller tumors (see Chemotherapy, p. 712).

Palliative treatment may be indicated when the prognosis is poor, the cancer is inoperable, or the patient decides against surgery. If it becomes difficult for the patient to swallow, a gastrostomy may be performed to provide adequate nutritional intake and frequent suctioning will be necessary. Analgesic medication should be given freely.

Nursing Management
Goals
The patient with oral cancer will have a patent airway, be able to communicate, have adequate nutritional intake to promote wound healing, and have relief of pain and discomfort.

Nursing Diagnoses
- Imbalanced nutrition: less than body requirements
- Chronic pain
- Anxiety
- Ineffective coping
- Ineffective health maintenance

Nursing Interventions

The nurse has a significant role in the early detection and treatment of oral cancer. Inspection of a patient's oral cavity to detect suspicious lesions should be included in a routine physical examination. A patient who smokes should be encouraged to stop smoking.

Preoperative care for the patient who is having radical neck dissection involves consideration of the patient's physical and psychosocial needs with a special emphasis on oral hygiene. Because the risk of oral cancer is high with the use of alcohol, a thorough assessment of alcohol intake should be done, and measures to assess and treat withdrawal if it is a problem should be implemented early (see Chapter 12, Lewis and others, *Medical-Surgical Nursing,* edition 7).

Postoperative care focuses on the maintenance of a patent airway, including tracheostomy care and observing for signs of respiratory distress (see NCP 27-1 and NCP 27-2 for the patient with a tracheostomy and the patient with a radical neck surgery, Lewis and others, *Medical-Surgical Nursing,* edition 7, pp. 548 to 549 and 554 to 555).

- Oral hygiene decreases the probability of infection, with the patient needing proper positioning to prevent aspiration (lying on the side or supine with the head turned to one side). The dressing should be observed for signs of hemorrhage or infection.
- Malnourishment delays wound healing; tube feedings may be started following surgery.
- The patient with a tracheostomy will need alternate forms of communication, such as chalkboard or pad and pencil.
- Allow for personal verbalization of feelings regarding surgery. Obtain a psychiatric referral for prolonged or severe depression.
- Facial disfigurement and other mutilating aspects of radical head and neck surgery may have a major long-term impact on the patient's body image and lifestyle, which may include learning to swallow again, altered physical appearance, taste and sensation changes, speech therapy, and reconstruction.

▼ **Patient and Family Teaching**
- Teach correct oral hygiene and dental care and encourage the patient to seek preventive dental care.
- Instruct the patient to examine the mouth and to recognize the danger signals of oral cancer. If any of these signals are present, the patient should be instructed to visit a health care provider. Danger signals are unexplained pain or soreness in the mouth, unusual bleeding from the oral cavity, dysphagia, swelling or a lump in the neck, and any ulcerative lesion that does not heal within 2 to 3 weeks.
- Answer questions about the patient's body image honestly and assure the patient of his or her self-worth.

The patient is often discharged with a tracheostomy and gastrostomy tube. The patient and family need to be taught how to manage these tubes and who to call if there are problems. Initially, home health care may be needed to evaluate the family or the patient's ability to perform self-care activities.

OSTEOARTHRITIS

Description

Osteoarthritis (OA), the most common form of joint (articular) disease in North America, is a slowly progressive noninflammatory disorder of the diarthrodial (synovial) joints. Previously identified as degenerative joint disease (DJD), it is now known to involve the formation of new joint tissue in response to cartilage destruction.

Although OA is not considered to be a normal part of the aging process, growing older continues to be a consistently identified risk factor. Cartilage destruction can actually begin between ages 20 and 30 years, and the majority of adults are affected by age 40 years. Few patients experience symptoms until after age 50 or 60 years, but more than half of those older than 65 years of age have x-ray evidence of the disease in at least one joint. The incidence of OA after age 50 years is higher in women than in men. This increased incidence is believed to be due to estrogen reduction at menopause.

- Genetic factors appear to play a significant role in the occurrence of OA. Modifiable risk factors include obesity, which contributes to hip and knee OA. Regular moderate exercise decreases the likelihood of disease development and progression, but overuse of knees by strenuous exercise is linked to an increased risk of knee OA.

OA may occur as a primary idiopathic or secondary disorder. The cause of idiopathic OA is unknown. Secondary OA has an identifiable precipitating event, such as previous trauma, infection, or a skeletal deformity, that is believed to predispose the person to later degenerative changes.

Pathophysiology

OA results from cartilage damage that triggers a metabolic response at the level of the chondrocytes. Progression of OA causes cartilage to gradually become softer, less elastic, and less able to resist wear with heavy use. Continued changes in the cartilage collagen lead to fissuring, fibrillation, and erosion of the articular surfaces. Incongruity in joint surfaces creates an uneven distribution of stress across the joint and contributes to a reduction in motion.

Although inflammation is not characteristic of OA, a secondary synovitis may result when phagocytic cells try to rid the joint of small pieces of cartilage torn from the joint surface. These inflammatory changes contribute to the early pain and stiffness of OA. Contact between exposed bony joint surfaces after cartilage has completely deteriorated can occur in later stages of OA.

Clinical Manifestations

Systemic manifestations such as fatigue or fever are not present in OA. Organ involvement is absent as well, which is an important differentiation between OA and inflammatory joint disorders, such as rheumatoid arthritis (Table 62).

Joints. Manifestations of OA range from mild discomfort to significant disability. Joint pain is the predominant symptom of OA. Pain generally worsens with joint use. In the early stages of OA, joint pain is relieved by rest. In advanced disease, however, the patient may complain of pain with rest or experience sleep disruptions resulting from increasing joint discomfort. The pain of OA may be referred to the groin, buttock, or medial side of the thigh or knee. Sitting down becomes difficult, as does rising from a chair when the hips are lower than the knees. As OA develops in intervertebral (apophyseal) joints of the spine, localized pain and stiffness are common.

Unlike pain, which is typically provoked by activity, joint stiffness occurs after periods of rest or static position. Early-morning stiffness is common but generally resolves within 30 minutes, a factor distinguishing OA from inflammatory arthritic disorders.

- Overactivity temporarily increases stiffness. *Crepitation,* a grating sensation caused by loose particles of cartilage in the joint cavity, can also contribute to stiffness.

Table 62 Comparison of Rheumatoid Arthritis and Osteoarthritis

Parameter	Rheumatoid Arthritis	Osteoarthritis
Age at onset	Young to middle age	Usually >40 yr old
Gender	Female 2:1 or 3:1, less marked gender difference after age 60 yr	Before age 50 yr more men than women After age 50 yr more women than men
Weight	Lost or maintained weight	Often overweight
Disease	Systemic disease with exacerbations and remissions	Localized disease with variable, progressive course
Affected joints	Small joints first (PIPs, MCPs, MTPs), wrists, elbows, shoulders, knees; usually bilateral, symmetric	Weight-bearing joints (knees, hips), MCPs, DIPs, PIPs, cervical and lumbar spine; often asymmetric
Pain characteristics	Stiffness lasts 1 hr to all day and may decrease with use; pain is variable, may disrupt sleep	Stiffness occurs on arising but usually subsides after 30 min; pain gradually worsens with joint use and time, lessens with rest
Effusions	Common	Uncommon
Nodules	Present, especially on extensor surfaces	Heberden's (DIPs) and Bouchard's (PIPs) nodes
Synovial fluid	WBC count >2000/μl with mostly neutrophils	WBC count <2000/μl (mild leukocytosis)
X-rays	Joint space narrowing, erosion, subluxation with advanced disease; osteoporosis related to corticosteroid use	Joint space narrowing, osteophytes, subchondral cysts, sclerosis
Laboratory findings	RF positive in 80% of patients Elevated ESR, CRP indicate active inflammation	RF negative Transient elevation in ESR related to synovitis

CRP, C-reactive protein; DIP, distal interphalangeal; ESR, erythrocyte sedimentation rate; MCP, metacarpophalangeal; MTP, metatarsophalangeal;

- OA usually affects joints asymmetrically. The most commonly involved joints are shown in Fig. 11.

Deformity. Deformity or instability associated with OA is specific to the involved joint. For example, *Heberden's nodes* occur on the distal interphalangeal joints as an indication of osteophyte formation and loss of joint space. *Bouchard's nodes* on the proximal interphalangeal joints indicate similar disease involvement. Heberden's and Bouchard's nodes are often red, swollen, and tender. These bony enlargements do not usually cause significant loss of function.

Knee OA often leads to joint malalignment as a result of cartilage loss in the medial compartment. The patient has a character-

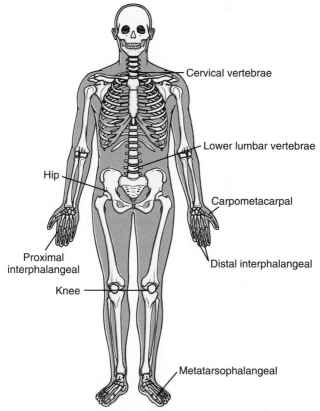

Fig. 11. Joints most frequently involved in osteoarthritis.

istic bow-legged appearance and may develop an altered gait. In advanced hip OA, one of the patient's legs may become shorter because of loss of joint space.

Diagnostic Studies

- A bone scan, computed tomography (CT) scan, or magnetic resonance imaging (MRI) may be useful in early OA to monitor joint changes. X-rays also confirm disease and monitor treatment effectiveness. As OA progresses, x-rays typically show joint space narrowing, bony sclerosis, and osteophyte formation.
- No laboratory abnormalities are a specific diagnostic indicator. The erythrocyte sedimentation rate (ESR) is normal except in instances of acute synovitis, when minimal elevations may be noted.
- Synovial fluid analysis allows differentiation between OA and other forms of inflammatory arthritis. In OA, fluid remains clear yellow with few or no signs of inflammation.

Collaborative Care

Therapy focuses on managing pain and inflammation, preventing disability, and maintaining and improving joint function. Non-pharmacologic interventions are the foundation of management. Drug therapy serves as an adjunct to nonpharmacologic treatments. Symptoms are often managed conservatively for many years, but the patient's loss of joint function, unrelieved pain, and diminished ability to independently perform self-care may require surgery. Arthroscopic surgery to repair cartilage or ligament tears or remove bone bits or cartilage may be effective in OA.

Rest and Joint Protection

The affected joint should be rested during any periods of acute inflammation and maintained in a functional position with splints or braces if necessary. Immobilization should not exceed 1 week because joint stiffness increases with inactivity. The patient may need to modify usual activities or use an assistive device to decrease stress on affected joints.

Heat and Cold Applications

Applications of heat and cold may help reduce complaints of pain and stiffness. Heat therapy is helpful for stiffness, including hot packs, whirlpool, ultrasound, and paraffin wax baths.

Nutritional Therapy and Exercise

If the patient is overweight, a weight reduction program is a critical part of the treatment plan. The nurse should help the patient evaluate the current diet to make appropriate changes. Aerobic conditioning and specific programs for muscle strengthening can lead to a reduction in pain and disability for some patients.

Complementary and Alternative Therapies

Complementary and alternative therapies for symptom management of arthritis have become increasingly popular with patients
who have failed to find relief through traditional medical care.
Therapies include yoga, acupuncture, massage, guided imagery,
and therapeutic touch. In particular, the use of nutritional supplements such as glucosamine and chondroitin sulfate for relieving
moderate to severe arthritis pain in the knees and improving joint
mobility has shown promising results.

Drug Therapy

Drug therapy is based on the severity of the patient's symptoms
(see Table 65-3, Lewis and others, *Medical-Surgical Nursing,*
edition 7, pp. 1698 to 1700). The patient with mild to moderate
joint pain may receive relief from acetaminophen (Tylenol). The
patient may receive up to 1000 mg every 6 hours, with a daily dose
not to exceed 4 g. A topical agent such as capsaicin cream (Zostrix)
may also be beneficial. It blocks pain by locally interfering with
substance P, which is responsible for pain impulse transmission.
Other topical over-the-counter products that contain salicylates,
camphor, eucalyptus oil, and menthol may also provide temporary
pain relief.

For the patient who cannot obtain adequate pain management
with acetaminophen, or for the patient with moderate to severe OA
pain, a nonsteroidal antiinflammatory drug (NSAID) may provide
greater relief. NSAID therapy is typically initiated in low-dose,
over-the-counter strengths (e.g., ibuprofen [Motrin], 200 mg up
to 4 times per day), with the dose increased as the patient's symptoms indicate. If the patient is at risk for or experiences gastrointestinal (GI) side effects with NSAID use, supplemental treatment
with a protective agent such as misoprostol (Cytotec) may be
indicated.

As an alternative to traditional NSAIDs, treatment with the
COX-2 inhibitor celecoxib (Celebrex) may be considered in
selected patients. Other COX-2 inhibitors have been withdrawn
from the market until further evaluation of the cardiovascular risks
of these drugs can be completed.

- Intraarticular injections of corticosteroids may be appropriate for the older patient with local inflammation and
  effusion.
- Intraarticular hyaluronic acid (HA) injections have been
  shown to be safe and effective in treating the pain and
  functional impairment of mild to moderate knee OA. These
  compounds appear to have antiinflammatory benefits and a
  short-term lubricant effect.

Nursing Management

Goals

The patient with OA will maintain or improve joint function through a balance of rest and activity, use joint protection measures to improve activity tolerance, achieve independence in self-care and maintain optimal role function, and use pharmacologic and nonpharmacologic pain management techniques to manage pain satisfactorily.

Nursing Diagnoses

- Acute and chronic pain
- Insomnia
- Impaired physical mobility
- Self-care deficits
- Imbalanced nutrition: more than body requirements
- Chronic low self-esteem

Nursing Interventions

Community education should focus on decreasing modifiable risk factors for OA through weight loss and the reduction of occupational and recreational hazards. Athletic instruction and physical fitness programs should include safety measures that protect and reduce trauma to the joint structures.

The patient with OA is usually treated on an outpatient basis, often by an interdisciplinary team of health care providers that includes a rheumatologist, a nurse, an occupational therapist, and a physical therapist.

- The hospital or home health nurse should assist the patient with activities of daily living (ADLs) as necessary and help the patient plan rest periods during the day. The patient needs sufficient time to move stiff, painful joints, especially when arising in the morning or after any period of sustained inactivity. Proper body alignment should be maintained at all times.

- Safety measures in the home and work environment are important. Measures include removing scatter rugs, providing rails at the stairs and bathtub, using night-lights, and wearing well-fitting supportive shoes. Assistive devices such as canes, walkers, elevated toilet seats, and grab bars reduce joint load and promote safety.

- Sexual counseling may help the patient and significant other to enjoy physical closeness by introducing the idea of alternate positions and timing for intercourse.

- Drugs are administered for the relief of pain and inflammation. Nonpharmacologic techniques such as massage, application of heat and cold, relaxation, and guided imagery may be helpful in relieving pain. The nurse should be open to

helping the patient and family to develop creative new
approaches to symptom management.

▼ **Patient and Family Teaching**

Education is an important nursing responsibility that should be
carried out regardless of patient setting.

- Teaching should include information about the nature and
  treatment of the disease, pain management, correct posture
  and body mechanics, correct use of assistive devices such
  as a cane or walker, principles of joint protection and energy
  conservation, and a therapeutic exercise program.
- The nurse needs to assist the patient in developing long-
  term strategies to manage OA.
- Home care goals must be individualized to meet the patient's
  needs. Family and social support systems should be included
  in goal setting and education.
- Support and understanding of the disease process can be
  gained through community resources such as the Arthritis
  Foundation's Self-Help Course *(www.arthritis.org)*.

OSTEOMALACIA

Osteomalacia is a rare condition of adult bone associated with
vitamin D deficiency, resulting in bone decalcification and softening. This disease is the same as rickets in children except that the
epiphyseal growth plates are closed in the adult.

- Vitamin D is required for absorption of calcium from the
  intestine. Insufficient vitamin D intake can interfere with
  the normal bone mineralization, causing failure or insufficient calcification of bone, which results in bone
  softening.

Vitamin D deficiency results from a lack of exposure to ultraviolet (UV) rays, gastrointestinal (GI) malabsorption, chronic
diarrhea, pregnancy, and kidney disease.

The most common clinical features are localized bone pain,
difficulty rising from a chair, and difficulty walking. Other
manifestations include low back pain, progressive muscular weakness, weight loss, and progressive deformities of the spine (kyphosis) or extremities. Fractures are common and demonstrate delayed
healing.

Laboratory findings include decreased serum calcium or phosphorous levels, decreased serum 25-hydroxyvitamin D, and elevated serum alkaline phosphatase. X-rays may demonstrate the

effects of generalized bone demineralization, especially a loss of calcium in the bones of the pelvis, and the presence of associated bone deformity.

- *Looser's transformation zones* (ribbons of decalcification in bone found on x-ray) are diagnostic of osteomalacia. Significant osteomalacia may exist without demonstrable x-ray changes.

Collaborative care is directed toward the correction of the vitamin D deficiency. Vitamin D_3 (cholecalciferol) and vitamin D_2 (ergocalciferol) can be supplemented, and the patient often shows a dramatic response. Calcium or phosphorous supplements may also be prescribed. A diet high in calcium and vitamin D and exposure to sunlight are also valuable.

OSTEOMYELITIS

Description
Osteomyelitis is a severe infection of the bone, bone marrow, and surrounding soft tissue. The most common infecting micro-organism is *Staphylococcus aureus.* A variety of microorganisms can cause osteomyelitis, and aerobic gram-negative bacteria alone or mixed with gram-positive organisms are often found (Table 63).

- Use of antibiotics in conjunction with surgical treatment has significantly reduced the mortality rate and complications associated with osteomyelitis.

Pathophysiology
Infecting microorganisms can invade by indirect or direct entry. The *indirect entry (hematogenous)* of microorganisms in osteo-myelitis most frequently affects growing bone in boys less than 12 years old and is associated with their higher incidence of blunt trauma. Adults with vascular insufficiency disorders (e.g., diabetes mellitus) and genitourinary and respiratory infections are at higher risk for a primary infection to spread by way of the blood to the bone. The pelvis, tibia, and vertebrae are the most common sites of infection.

Direct-entry osteomyelitis can occur at any age when there is an open wound (e.g., penetrating wounds, fractures) and microor-ganisms gain entry to the body. Osteomyelitis may also occur in the presence of a foreign body, such as an implant or an orthopedic prosthetic device (e.g., plate, total joint prosthesis).

Table 63	Causative Organisms in Osteomyelitis

Organism	Possible Predisposing Problem
Staphylococcus aureus	Pressure ulcer, penetrating wound, open fracture, orthopedic surgery, abscessed tooth, vascular insufficiency disorders (e.g., diabetes, atherosclerosis)
Staphylococcus epidermidis	Indwelling prosthetic devices (e.g., joint replacements, fractured fixation devices)
Escherichia coli	Urinary tract infection (UTI)
Mycobacterium tuberculosis	Tuberculosis (TB)
Neisseria gonorrhoeae	Gonorrhea
Pseudomonas	Puncture wounds, intravenous (IV) drug use
Salmonella	Sickle cell disease
Fungi, mycobacteria	Immunocompromised host

After gaining entrance to the bone by way of the blood, the microorganisms then lodge in an area of bone in which circulation slows, usually the metaphysis.

- The microorganisms grow, resulting in increased pressure because of the nonexpanding nature of most bone. This leads to ischemia and vascular compromise of the periosteum.
- Eventually the infection passes through the bone cortex and marrow cavity, ultimately resulting in cortical devascularization and necrosis. Once ischemia occurs, the bone dies.

The devitalized bone eventually separates from surrounding living bone, forming *sequestra*. Once formed, a sequestrum continues to be an infected island of bone, surrounded by pus and difficult to reach by blood-borne antibiotics or white blood cells (WBCs). Sequestrum may enlarge and serve as a site for microorganisms that spread to other sites, including the lungs and brain. Sequestrum also can move out of the bone and into the soft tissue. If necrotic sequestrum is not resolved naturally or surgically, it may develop a sinus tract, resulting in a chronic, purulent cutaneous drainage.

Chronic osteomyelitis is either a continuous, persistent problem or a process of exacerbations and remission. Granulation tissue turns to scar tissue, and this avascular tissue provides an ideal site for continued microorganism growth and is impenetrable to antibiotics.

Clinical Manifestations

Acute osteomyelitis refers to the initial infection or an infection of less than 1 month in duration.

- Systemic manifestations include fever, night sweats, restlessness, nausea, and malaise.
- Local manifestations include constant bone pain that is unrelieved by rest and worsens with activity; swelling, tenderness, and warmth at the infection site; and restricted movement of the affected part.
- Later signs include drainage from the sinus tracts to the skin and fracture site.

Chronic osteomyelitis refers to a bone infection that persists for longer than 1 month or an infection that has failed to respond to the initial course of antibiotic therapy.

- Systemic signs may be diminished, with local signs of infection more common, including constant bone pain and swelling, tenderness, and warmth at the infection site.

Diagnostic Studies

- Bone or soft tissue biopsy is the definitive way to determine the causative microorganism.
- Blood and/or wound cultures are frequently positive for microorganisms.
- Elevated WBC and erythrocyte sedimentation rate (ESR) may be found.
- Radiologic signs suggestive of osteomyelitis usually do not appear until 10 days to weeks after the appearance of clinical symptoms, by which time the disease will have progressed.
- Radionuclide bone scans (gallium and indium) are helpful in diagnosis and usually positive in the area of infection.
- Magnetic resonance imaging (MRI) and computed tomography (CT) scans may be used to help identify the extent of the infection including soft tissue involvement.

Collaborative Care

Vigorous and prolonged intravenous (IV) antibiotic therapy is the treatment of choice if ischemia has not occurred. If antibiotic therapy is delayed, surgical debridement and decompression are often necessary.

Patients are often discharged to home care with IV antibiotics delivered through a central venous catheter or peripherally inserted central catheter (PICC). IV antibiotic therapy may initially be started in the hospital and continued in the home for 4 to 6 weeks or as long as 3 to 6 months. A variety of antibiotics may be prescribed depending on the microorganism. These drugs include penicillin, nafcillin (Nafcil), neomycin, vancomycin, and cephalexin (Keflex).

- In adults with chronic osteomyelitis, oral therapy with a fluoroquinolone (ciprofloxacin [Cipro]) for 6 to 8 weeks may be prescribed instead of IV antibiotics.
- Oral antibiotic therapy may also be given after IV therapy is complete to ensure resolution of the infection.
- Patient response to drug therapy is monitored through bone scans and ESR tests.
- Surgical treatment for chronic osteomyelitis includes removal of the poorly vascularized tissue and dead bone and extended use of antibiotics. Antibiotic-impregnated polymethylmethacrylate bead chains may also be implanted during surgery.
- Intermittent or constant irrigation of the affected bone with antibiotics may also be initiated.
- Hyperbaric oxygen therapy using 100% oxygen may be administered as an adjunct therapy in refractory cases of chronic osteomyelitis.

Orthopedic prosthetic devices may need to be removed. Muscle flaps or skin and bone grafting may be necessary if destruction is extensive. Amputation of the extremity may be indicated to preserve life or improve quality of life (see Amputation, p. 691).

- Rare complications of osteomyelitis include septicemia, septic arthritis, pathologic fractures, squamous cell carcinoma, and amyloidosis.

Nursing Management

Goals
The patient with osteomyelitis will have satisfactory pain and fever control, will not experience any complications associated with osteomyelitis, will cooperate with the treatment plan, and will maintain a positive outlook on the disease outcome.

See NCP 64-1 for the patient with osteomyelitis, Lewis and others, *Medical-Surgical Nursing,* edition 7, pp. 1671 to 1672.

Nursing Diagnoses
- Acute pain
- Impaired physical mobility
- Ineffective therapeutic regimen management

Nursing Interventions
Control of infections already in the body (e.g., urinary and respiratory tract) is important in preventing osteomyelitis. Adults who are immunocompromised, have orthopedic devices, and/or have vascular insufficiencies such as diabetes mellitus are especially susceptible. These patients and their families should be

instructed regarding the local and systemic manifestations of osteomyelitis.

- Symptoms of bone pain, fever, swelling, and restricted limb movement should be reported.

Some immobilization of the affected limb (e.g., splint, traction) is usually indicated to decrease pain. The involved limb should be handled carefully to avoid excessive manipulation, which increases pain and may cause a pathologic fracture.

- An important nursing responsibility is to assess the patient's pain. Minor to severe pain may be experienced with muscle spasms. Nonsteroidal antiinflammatory drugs (NSAIDs), opioid analgesics, and muscle relaxants may be prescribed.
- Dressings are used to absorb the exudate from draining wounds and to debride devitalized tissue from the wound site when removed. When the dressing is changed, sterile technique is essential.

The patient is frequently on bed rest in the early stages of acute infection. Good body alignment and frequent position changes prevent complications associated with immobility and promote comfort.

- The patient should be instructed to avoid any activities such as exercise or heat application that increase circulation and serve as stimuli to the spread of infection.
- Peak and trough blood levels of most antibiotics need to be carefully monitored throughout the course of therapy to avoid adverse drug effects.

▼ **Patient and Family Teaching**

- The patient should be taught the potential adverse and toxic reactions associated with prolonged and high-dose antibiotic therapy. These reactions include hearing deficit, fluid retention, and neurotoxicity, which can occur with the aminoglycosides. Jaundice, colitis, and photosensitivity have been noted with extended use of the cephalosporins.
- Long-term antibiotic therapy can result in an overgrowth of *Candida albicans* in the genitourinary and oral cavities. The nurse should instruct the patient to report any whitish yellow, curdlike lesions to the health care provider.
- If at home, the patient and family must be instructed on the management of the venous access device. They must also be taught how to administer the antibiotic when scheduled and the need for follow-up laboratory testing.
- Patient and family are often frightened and discouraged because of the serious nature of the disease, uncertainty of the outcome, and the lengthy cost and course of treatment. Con-

tinued psychologic and emotional support is an integral part of
nursing management.

OSTEOPOROSIS

Description

Osteoporosis, or porous bone (fragile bone disease), is a chronic,
progressive metabolic bone disease characterized by low bone
mass and structural deterioration of bone tissue, leading to
increased bone fragility. At least 10 million persons in the United
States have osteoporosis, and with the projected increase in life
expectancy, this number is expected to grow. *Osteopenia* is defined
as bone loss that is more than normal, but not yet at the level for
a diagnosis of osteoporosis. More than 14 million women over age
50 have osteopenia. One in two women and one in eight men older
than the age of 50 years will sustain an osteoporosis-related fracture during their lifetime.

Osteoporosis is eight times more common in women than in men
for several reasons: (1) women tend to have lower calcium intake
than men throughout their lives (men between 15 and 50 years old
consume twice as much calcium as women); (2) women have less
bone mass because of their generally smaller frame; and (3) pregnancy and breast-feeding can deplete a woman's skeletal system.

Risk factors for osteoporosis are female gender, increasing age,
white or Asian race, oophorectomy, family history, small stature,
anorexia, early menopause, sedentary lifestyle, and insufficient
dietary calcium. Increased risk is also associated with cigarette
smoking and alcoholism. Decreased risk is associated with regular
weight-bearing exercise and fluoride and vitamin D ingestion.

Pathophysiology

Peak bone mass (maximum bone tissue) is mainly achieved before
age 20 years. It is determined by a combination of four major
factors: heredity, nutrition, exercise, and hormone function. Heredity may be responsible for up to 70% of peak bone mass.

- Bone loss from midlife (age 35 to 40 years) onward is
  inevitable, but the rate of loss varies. At menopause, women
  experience rapid bone loss when the decline in estrogen
  production is the sharpest. This rate of loss then slows and
  eventually matches the rate of bone lost by men 65 to 70
  years old.

Bone is continually being deposited by osteoblasts and resorbed
by osteoclasts, a process called *remodeling.* Normally the rates of

bone deposition and resorption are equal to each other so that the total bone mass remains constant. In osteoporosis, bone resorption exceeds bone deposition.

- Although resorption affects the entire skeletal system, osteoporosis occurs most commonly in the bones of the spine, hips, and wrists. Over time, wedging and fractures of the vertebrae produce a gradual loss of height and a humped back known as *dowager's hump* or *kyphosis.*
- The usual first signs of osteoporosis are back pain or spontaneous fractures. The loss of bone substance causes the bone to become mechanically weakened and prone to either spontaneous fractures or fractures from minimal trauma.
- Specific diseases associated with osteoporosis include intestinal malabsorption, kidney disease, rheumatoid arthritis, hyperthyroidism, chronic alcoholism, cirrhosis of the liver, and diabetes mellitus (DM).
- Many medications can interfere with bone metabolism, including corticosteroids, antiseizure drugs (phenytoin [Dilantin]), heparin, aluminum-containing antacids, certain cancer treatments, and excessive thyroid hormones.

Clinical Manifestations

Osteoporosis is often called the "silent disease" because bone loss occurs without symptoms. People may not know they have osteoporosis until their bones become so weak that a sudden strain, bump, or fall causes a hip or vertebral fracture.

- Collapsed vertebrae may initially be manifested as back pain, loss of height, or spinal deformities, such as kyphosis or severely stooped posture.

Diagnostic Studies

Osteoporosis often goes unnoticed because it cannot be detected by conventional x-ray until more than 25% to 40% of the calcium in the bone is lost.

- Serum calcium, phosphorous, and alkaline phosphatase levels remain normal, although alkaline phosphatase may be elevated after a fracture.
- Bone mineral density (BMD) measurements are used to measure bone density.
- Quantitative ultrasound (QUS) measures bone density in the hip, kneecap, or shin with sound waves.
- One of the most common BMD studies is the *dual-energy x-ray absorptiometry (DEXA),* which measures bone density in the spine, hips, and forearm (the most common sites of fractures resulting from osteoporosis). DEXA scores are frequently reported as T-scores: osteoporosis is quantita-

tively defined as a BMD of at least 2.5 standard deviations below the mean BMD of young adults; osteopenia is defined as a BMD of a T-score less than or equal to a range of 1.0 to 2.5, not yet at the level for a diagnosis of osteoporosis.

Nursing and Collaborative Management

Care of the patient with osteoporosis focuses on proper nutrition, calcium and vitamin D supplementation, exercise, prevention of fractures, and medication. Treatment is recommended for post-menopausal women who have a T-score of less than or equal to −2.0, a T-score less than or equal to −1.5 with additional risk factors, or a prior history of a hip or vertebral fracture. Prevention and treatment of osteoporosis focus on adequate calcium intake (1000 mg/day in premenopausal women and postmenopausal women taking estrogen and 1500 mg/day in postmenopausal women who are not receiving supplemental estrogen).

- If dietary intake of calcium is inadequate, supplemental calcium should be taken. The amount of elemental calcium varies in different calcium preparations (see Table 64-16, Lewis and others, *Medical-Surgical Nursing,* edition 7, p. 1689). Calcium supplementation inhibits age-related bone loss; however, no new bone is formed.
- Moderate amounts of exercise are important to build up and maintain bone mass. The best exercises are those that are weight bearing and force an individual to work against gravity, such as walking, hiking, weight training, stair climbing, tennis, and dancing. Walking is preferred to high-impact aerobics or running, both of which may put too much stress on the bones of patients with osteoporosis.
- Patients should be instructed to quit smoking and limit alcohol intake.

Drug Therapy

Estrogen replacement therapy after menopause may be used to prevent osteoporosis. Although the exact mechanism for the protective function of estrogen is not known, it is believed that estrogen inhibits osteoclast activity, leading to decreased bone resorption and preventing both cortical and trabecular bone loss.

- Estrogen replacement therapy is most effective when combined with calcium. The greatest benefit of estrogen is probably in the first 10 years after menopause. Transdermal estrogen treatment has been shown to be effective in the treatment of postmenopausal women with established osteoporosis.
- Calcitonin is secreted by the thyroid gland and inhibits osteoclastic bone resorption by directly interacting with

active osteoclasts. It is available in intramuscular (IM), subcutaneous (SC), and intranasal forms. When calcitonin is used, calcium supplementation is necessary to prevent secondary hyperparathyroidism.

- Bisphosphonates inhibit osteoclast-mediated bone resorption, thereby increasing BMD and total bone mass. This group of drugs includes etidronate (Didronel), alendronate (Fosamax), pamidronate (Aredia), risedronate (Actonel), clodronate (Bonefos), tiludronate (Skelid), and ibandronate (Boniva). Alendronate is available as a weekly oral tablet, and ibandronate is available as a monthly oral tablet. An injectable version of ibandronate that would last 3 months is under development.

Patients should be instructed on the proper administration of a bisphosphonate to aid in its absorption. It should be taken on rising in the morning with a full glass of water. The patient should not eat or drink anything for 30 minutes after taking it. The patient should also be instructed not to lie down after taking this medication. These precautions have been proven to decrease gastrointestinal (GI) side effects (especially esophageal irritation) and increase drug absorption.

- Other drugs include selective estrogen receptor modulators, such as raloxifene (Evista). These drugs mimic the effect of estrogen on bone by reducing bone resorption without stimulating breast or uterine tissues. Raloxifene in postmenopausal women significantly increases BMD.
- Teriparatide (Forteo) is a portion of human parathyroid hormone that is used for the treatment of osteoporosis by increasing the action of osteoblasts. It is the first drug for osteoporosis that stimulates new bone formation rather than just preventing further bone loss. Limitations of its use include subcutaneous injection administration, cost, and possible increased risk for osteosarcoma with long-term use.

OVARIAN CANCER

Description

Ovarian cancer is a malignant neoplasm of the ovaries. Because most patients with ovarian cancer have advanced disease at diagnosis, it causes more deaths than any other cancer of the female reproductive system. White women of North American or European descent are at greater risk for ovarian cancer than are African American women.

Table 64	Risk Factors for Ovarian Cancer

Increased Risk	Decreased Risk
Family history of ovarian cancer	Oral contraceptive use
Family history of breast or colon cancer	(>5 yr)
Personal history of breast or colorectal cancer	Breast-feeding
Personal history of hereditary nonpolyposis colorectal cancer	Multiple pregnancies
	Early age at first birth
Mutant *BRCA* gene	
Increasing age	
Nulliparity	
Early menarche and late menopause	
Hormone replacement therapy	
High-fat diet	

The cause of ovarian cancer is unknown, but multiple factors affect its occurrence (Table 64).

Pathophysiology

About 90% of ovarian cancers are epithelial carcinomas. Germ cell tumors account for another 10%. Histologic grading is an important prognostic determinant.

Ovarian cancer can metastasize directly by shedding malignant cells that frequently implant on the uterus, bladder, bowel, and omentum. Metastasis also occurs by lymphatic drainage through the retroperitoneal nodes and the iliac and inguinal lymphatics.

Clinical Manifestations

In its early stages, symptoms are vague and may include general abdominal discomfort (gas, indigestion, bloating, cramps), sense of pelvic heaviness, loss of appetite, feeling of fullness, and change in bowel habits. Pain is not an early symptom.

- As the malignancy grows, a variety of symptoms, such as an increase in abdominal girth, bowel and bladder dysfunction, persistent pelvic or abdominal pain, menstrual irregularities, and ascites, can occur.

Diagnostic Studies

- No screening test exists for ovarian cancer. Yearly bimanual pelvic examinations should be performed to identify the presence of an ovarian mass. Abdominal or vaginal ultrasound can be used to detect ovarian masses.

- For women with a high risk of ovarian cancer, a combination of serum CA-125 (a tumor marker) and ultrasound is recommended in addition to a yearly pelvic examination. CA-125 is positive in 80% of women with epithelial ovarian cancer and is used to monitor the disease course.
- If the mass is malignant, staging is critical for guiding treatment decisions. Because of the numerous metastatic pathways for ovarian cancer, accurate staging usually involves multiple biopsies.

Collaborative Care

The usual treatment for stage I disease (limited to the ovaries) is a total abdominal hysterectomy and bilateral salpingo-oophorectomy with the removal of as much of the tumor as possible (i.e., tumor debulking). Ascitic fluid is submitted for cytologic study, and appropriate biopsies are performed to determine the stage of the disease. The addition of chemotherapy or the instillation of intraperitoneal radioisotopes is usually done for stage I disease (see Chemotherapy, p. 712).

The patient with stage II disease (limited to the true pelvis) may receive external abdominal and pelvic radiation, intraperitoneal radiation, or systemic combined chemotherapy after tumor-reducing surgery. After the completion of systemic chemotherapy in patients who are clinically free of symptoms, a "second-look" surgical procedure is often performed to determine whether there is any evidence of disease. This option does not necessarily improve the outcome. If no disease is found, the patient is monitored for recurrent disease.

Chemotherapy (e.g., cisplatin [Platinol], carboplatin [Paraplatin]) is used for the treatment of stage III (limited to the abdominal cavity) and stage IV (distant metastases) diseases. Altretamine (Hexalen) is used for the palliative treatment of persistent, recurrent ovarian cancer. Paclitaxel (Taxol) and topotecan (Hycamtin) are used to treat metastatic ovarian cancer. Surgical debulking is often done in conjunction with chemotherapy for advanced disease. Intraperitoneal chemotherapy may be used for patients who have minimum residual disease after surgery.

- Radiation and chemotherapy may be used to shrink the size of metastatic tumors, which relieves both pressure and pain.

Nursing Management: Cancers of the Female Reproductive Tract

See Cervical Cancer, p. 108.

PAGET'S DISEASE

P

Description
Paget's disease (osteitis deformans) is a skeletal bone disorder in which there is excessive bone resorption followed by replacement of normal marrow by vascular, fibrous connective tissue and new bone that is larger, more disorganized, and weaker. It occurs most often after the fourth decade of life and most commonly in men. Up to 40% of all patients with Paget's disease have a relative with the disorder. The cause of Paget's disease is unknown, although a viral etiology has been proposed. Regions of the skeleton commonly affected are the pelvis, long bones, spine, ribs, and cranium.

Clinical Manifestations
In milder forms of Paget's disease, patients may remain free of symptoms, and the disease may be discovered incidentally on x-ray or serum chemistry.
- Initial manifestations are usually an insidious development of skeletal pain (which may progress to severe intractable pain), fatigue, and progressive development of a waddling gait.
- Pathologic fracture is the most common complication and may be the first indication of the disease. Other complications include malignant osteosarcoma, osteoclastoma (giant cell) tumors, or fibrosarcoma.

Diagnostic Studies
- There are markedly elevated serum alkaline phosphatase (ALP) levels in advanced forms of the disease.
- X-rays may reveal that the normal contour of the affected bone is curved and the bone cortex is thickened, especially in weight-bearing bones and the cranium.
- Bone scans using a radiolabeled bisphosphate demonstrate bone lesions.

Nursing and Collaborative Management
Management is usually limited to symptomatic and supportive care and correction of secondary deformities by either surgical intervention or braces. Bone resorption, relief of acute symptoms, and lowering of the serum ALP levels may be significantly influenced by the administration of calcitonin, which inhibits osteoclastic activity. Response to calcitonin therapy is not permanent and often stops when therapy is discontinued.

- Bisphosphonate drugs such as etidronate (Didronel), alendronate (Fosamax), pamidronate (Aredia), risedronate (Actonel), clodronate (Bonefos), tiludronate (Skelid), and ibandronate (Boniva) are also used to retard bone resorption.
- Calcium and vitamin D are often given to decrease hypocalcemia, a common side effect of bisphosphonates.
- Pain is usually managed by nonsteroidal antiinflammatory drugs (NSAIDs).
- Orthopedic surgery for fractures, hip and knee replacements, and knee realignment may be necessary.

A firm mattress should be used to provide back support and to relieve pain. The patient may be required to wear a corset or light brace to relieve back pain and provide support when in the upright position. The patient should be proficient in the correct application of such devices and know how to regularly examine areas of the skin for friction damage.

- Activities such as lifting and twisting should be discouraged. Good body mechanics are essential. Physical therapy may increase muscle strength.
- A properly balanced nutritional program, especially as it pertains to vitamin D, calcium, and protein, is important for bone formation.

Because metabolic bone disorders increase the possibility of pathologic fractures, the nurse must use extreme caution when the patient is turned or moved. It is important to keep the patient as active as possible to retard demineralization resulting from disuse or extended immobilization. A supervised exercise program is an essential part of the treatment program. If the patient's condition permits, ambulation without causing fatigue must be encouraged.

- Prevention measures such as patient education, the use of an assistive device, and environmental changes should be actively pursued to prevent falls and subsequent fractures.

PANCREATIC CANCER

Description

Pancreatic cancer is the fourth leading cause of death from cancer in North America, with the peak incidence occurring between 65 and 80 years. Most pancreatic tumors are adenocarcinomas occurring in the head of the pancreas. As the tumor grows, the common bile duct becomes obstructed and obstructive jaundice develops.

The majority of cancers have metastasized at the time of diagnosis, and the prognosis is poor. Most patients die within 5 to 12 months of the initial diagnosis, and the 5-year survival rate is only about 10%.

Pathophysiology
The cause of pancreatic cancer is unknown. Major risk factors are diabetes mellitus; chronic pancreatitis; family history of pancreatic cancer; a high-fat, high-meat diet; and exposure to chemicals such as benzedine and coke. Pancreatic cancer develops twice as frequently in smokers as in nonsmokers.

Clinical Manifestations
Manifestations include abdominal pain (dull or aching), anorexia, rapid and progressive weight loss, nausea, and jaundice.
- Pain is common and related to the tumor location. Extreme, unrelenting pain is related to the extension of the cancer into the retroperitoneal tissues and nerve plexuses. The pain is frequently located in the upper abdomen or left hypochondrium and radiates to the back. It is commonly related to eating, and it also occurs at night. Weight loss is due to poor digestion and absorption caused by lack of pancreatic digestive enzymes.

Diagnostic Studies
Better diagnostic measures are needed for detection of pancreatic cancer because most of the current methods detect only advanced stages.
- Transabdominal ultrasound and computed tomography (CT) scan are the most commonly used imaging techniques.
- Magnetic resonance imaging (MRI) and MR cholangiopancreatography (MRCP) may be used for diagnosing and staging pancreatic cancer.
- Endoscopic retrograde cholangiography (ERCP) allows for visualization of and collection of secretions and tissues from the pancreatic duct and biliary system.
- Endoscopic ultrasound allows for pancreas imaging and fine needle aspiration of tumor.
- Tumor markers such as CA19-9 are used for establishing the diagnosis and monitoring treatment response.

Collaborative Care
Surgery provides the most effective treatment, but only 15% to 20% of patients have resectable tumors. The classic surgery is a *radical pancreaticoduodenectomy* or *Whipple's procedure*. This

procedure is a resection of the proximal pancreas (proximal pancreatectomy), the adjoining duodenum (duodenectomy), the distal portion of the stomach (partial gastrectomy), and the distal segment of the common bile duct. An anastomosis of the pancreatic duct, common bile duct, and stomach to the jejunum is done.

- Radiation therapy alters survival rates little but is effective for pain relief. External radiation is usually used, but implantation of internal radiation seeds into the tumor has also been used.
- The role of chemotherapy in pancreatic cancer is limited. Chemotherapy usually consists of gemcitabine (Gemzar) either alone or in combination with agents such as capecitabine (Xeloda) or erlotinib (Tarceva). However, response rates are less than 15%, with minor effects on overall survival.

Nursing Management

Because the patient with pancreatic cancer has many of the same problems as the patient with pancreatitis, nursing care includes the same measures (see Pancreatitis, Acute, below).

- The nurse should provide symptomatic and supportive nursing care. Medications and comfort measures to relieve pain should be provided before the patient reaches the peak of pain.
- Psychologic support is essential, especially during times of anxiety or depression.
- Adequate nutrition is an important part of the nursing care plan. Frequent and supplemental feedings may be necessary. Measures to stimulate the appetite as much as possible and to overcome anorexia, nausea, and vomiting should be included.
- A significant component of the nursing care is helping the patient and the family or significant others through the grieving process.

PANCREATITIS, ACUTE

Description

Acute pancreatitis is an acute inflammatory process of the pancreas, with the degree of inflammation varying from mild edema to severe hemorrhagic necrosis. Some patients recover completely;

others have recurring attacks; still others develop chronic pancreatitis. Acute pancreatitis can be life threatening.

- It is most common in middle-aged men and women, and it affects men more than women.

P

Pathophysiology

Many factors can cause injury to the pancreas. The primary etiologic factors are biliary tract disease (more common in women) and alcoholism (more common in men). In the United States the most common cause is gallbladder disease, followed by alcoholism. Less common causes of acute pancreatitis include trauma (postsurgical, abdominal), viral infections (mumps), penetrating duodenal ulcers, cysts, abscesses, cystic fibrosis, certain drugs (corticosteroids, sulfonamides, nonsteroidal antiinflammatory drugs [NSAIDs]), and metabolic disorders, such as hyperparathyroidism and renal failure. In some cases the cause is not known (idiopathic).

- The most common pathogenic mechanism is believed to be autodigestion of the pancreas. The etiologic factors cause injury to pancreatic cells or activation of the pancreatic enzymes in the pancreas rather than in the intestine.

The pathophysiologic involvement of acute pancreatitis ranges from *edematous pancreatitis* (which is mild and self-limiting) to *necrotizing pancreatitis* (which is severe and increases the risk for organ failure and sepsis).

Clinical Manifestations

Abdominal pain is the predominant symptom. The pain is usually located in the left upper quadrant but may be in the mid-epigastrium. It commonly radiates to the back because of the retroperitoneal location of the pancreas.

- The pain has a sudden onset and is described as severe, deep, piercing, and continuous or steady. It is aggravated by eating and frequently has its onset when the patient is recumbent; it is not relieved by vomiting. The pain may be accompanied by flushing, cyanosis, and dyspnea.

Other manifestations include nausea and vomiting, low-grade fever, leukocytosis, hypotension, tachycardia, and jaundice. Abdominal tenderness with muscle guarding is common. Bowel sounds may be decreased or absent. Ileus may occur and causes marked abdominal distention. The lungs are frequently involved, with crackles present.

- Intravascular damage from circulating trypsin may cause areas of cyanosis or greenish to yellow-brown discoloration of the abdominal wall. Other areas of ecchymoses are the

flanks (*Grey Turner's spots* or *sign*, a bluish flank discoloration) and the periumbilical area (*Cullen's sign,* a bluish periumbilical discoloration).
- Shock may occur because of hemorrhage into the pancreas, toxemia from the activated pancreatic enzymes, or hypovolemia as a result of massive fluid shifts into the retroperitoneal space.

Complications

Local complications of acute pancreatitis are pseudocyst and abscess.
- A pancreatic *pseudocyst* is a cavity continuous with or surrounding the outside of the pancreas. Symptoms are abdominal pain, palpable epigastric mass, nausea, vomiting, and anorexia. The serum amylase level frequently remains elevated. These cysts usually resolve spontaneously within a few weeks, but they may perforate, causing peritonitis, or rupture into the stomach or duodenum. They are treated with an internal drainage procedure with an anastomosis between the pancreatic duct and the jejunum.
- A *pancreatic abscess* is a large fluid-containing cavity within the pancreas. It results from extensive necrosis in the pancreas. It may become infected or perforate into adjacent organs. Manifestations include upper abdominal pain, abdominal mass, high fever, and leukocytosis. Pancreatic abscesses require prompt surgical drainage to prevent sepsis.

Systemic complications of acute pancreatitis include pleural effusion, atelectasis, pneumonia, hypotension, and hypocalcemia leading to tetany.

Diagnostic Studies

- Elevations of serum amylase (pancreatic isoamylase), serum lipase, and urinary amylase are primary diagnostic findings.
- Other laboratory abnormalities include hyperglycemia, hyperlipidemia, and hypocalcemia.
- Trypsinogen activation peptide (TAP) is produced by the conversion of trypsinogen to active trypsin, and urinary levels may be useful in detection of early acute pancreatitis.
- An abdominal ultrasound, x-ray, or contrast-enhanced computed tomography (CECT) can be used to identify pancreatic problems, including pseudocysts and abscesses. Other diagnostic tests include endoscopic retrograde cholangiopancreatography (ERCP), endoscopic ultrasound (EUS), magnetic resonance cholangiopancreatography (MRCP), and angiography.

Collaborative Care

Objectives of management for acute pancreatitis include relief of pain, prevention or alleviation of shock, reduction of pancreatic secretions, control of fluid and electrolyte imbalance, prevention or treatment of infections, and removal of the precipitating cause, if possible.

- A primary consideration is the relief and control of pain. Morphine may be used and may be combined with an antispasmodic.
- If shock is present, blood volume replacements and expanders such as dextran or albumin may be given.

It is important to reduce or suppress pancreatic enzymes to decrease stimulation of the pancreas and allow it to rest. The patient is allowed to take nothing by mouth (NPO). Nasogastric (NG) suction may be used to reduce vomiting and gastric distention and to prevent gastric digestive juices from entering the duodenum. Drugs that neutralize or suppress formation of hydrochloric (HCl) acid in the stomach, such as antacids, histamine H_2-receptor antagonists, and proton pump inhibitors, also help suppress pancreatic activity.

- Inflamed and necrotic pancreatic tissue is a good medium source for bacterial growth. Antibiotic therapy should be instituted early if an infection occurs.
- When food is allowed, small, frequent feedings are given. The diet is usually high in carbohydrate content because it is the least stimulating to the exocrine portion of the pancreas.

Surgical intervention may be indicated when the diagnosis is uncertain and in patients who do not respond to conservative therapy. Surgery is necessary for an abscess, acute pseudocyst, and severe peritonitis. Percutaneous drainage of a pseudocyst can be performed, and a drainage tube is left in place. Surgical treatment of associated biliary tract disease such as gallstones may be necessary.

Several different drugs may be used in the treatment of both acute and chronic pancreatitis (see Table 44-21, Lewis and others, *Medical-Surgical Nursing,* edition 7, p. 1121).

Nursing Management
Goals

The patient with acute pancreatitis will have relief of pain, normal fluid and electrolyte balance, minimal to no complications, and no recurrent attacks.

See NCP 44-3 for the patient with acute pancreatitis, Lewis and others, *Medical-Surgical Nursing,* edition 7, pp. 1122 to 1123.

Nursing Diagnoses
- Acute pain
- Deficient fluid volume
- Imbalanced nutrition: less than body requirements
- Ineffective therapeutic regimen management

Nursing Interventions

Health promotion interventions include encouragement of the early diagnosis and treatment of alcohol abuse and biliary tract disease, such as cholelithiasis.

During the acute phase, a major focus of nursing care is the relief of pain. Pain and restlessness can increase the metabolic rate and subsequent stimulation of pancreatic enzymes. Morphine may be used for pain relief, and giving analgesics before the pain becomes too severe makes the medication more effective. Measures such as comfortable positioning, frequent changes in position, and relief of nausea and vomiting assist in reducing the restlessness that usually accompanies the pain.

- Some patients experience reduced pain by assuming positions that flex the trunk and draw the knees up to the abdomen. A side-lying position with the head elevated 45 degrees decreases tension on the abdomen and may help ease the pain.

Nursing measures for the patient who is on NPO status or has an NG tube should be used. Frequent oral and nasal care to relieve the dryness of the mouth and nose is comforting to the patient.

- Observation for fever and other manifestations of infection is important. Respiratory infections are common because the retroperitoneal fluid raises the diaphragm, which causes the patient to take shallow, guarded abdominal breaths. Prevention of respiratory infections includes turning, coughing, deep breathing, and assuming a semi-Fowler's position.

Most patients need follow-up home care. The patient may have lost physical reserve and muscle strength. Physical therapy may be needed. Continued care to prevent infection and detect any complications is important.

▼ **Patient and Family Teaching**

- The patient should be encouraged to eliminate alcohol intake, especially if there have been any previous episodes of pancreatitis. Attacks of pancreatitis become milder or disappear with the discontinuance of alcohol use.
- Beverages with caffeine should not be consumed. Because smoking and stressful situations can overstimulate the pancreas, they should also be avoided.
- Dietary teaching should include the restriction of fats because they stimulate the secretion of cholecystokinin, which then

stimulates the pancreas. Carbohydrates are less stimulating to the pancreas, so they should be encouraged. The patient should be instructed to avoid crash dieting and bingeing because these can precipitate attacks.

- The patient and family should be given instructions regarding the recognition and reporting of symptoms of infection, diabetes mellitus (DM), or steatorrhea (foul-smelling, frothy stools). These changes indicate possible destruction of pancreatic tissue.
- The nurse should make sure the patient fully understands the prescribed regimen. Each aspect must be explained. The importance of taking required medications and following the recommended diet should be stressed.

PANCREATITIS, CHRONIC

Description
Chronic pancreatitis is a continuous, prolonged, inflammatory, and fibrosing process of the pancreas. The pancreas is destroyed as it is replaced with fibrotic tissue. Chronic pancreatitis may follow acute pancreatitis, but it may also occur in the absence of any history of an acute condition. The two major types are chronic obstructive pancreatitis and chronic calcifying pancreatitis.

Pathophysiology
Chronic obstructive pancreatitis is associated with biliary disease. The most common cause is inflammation of the sphincter of Oddi associated with cholelithiasis. Cancers of the ampulla of Vater, duodenum, or pancreas are additional causes.

   Chronic calcifying pancreatitis is associated with inflammation and sclerosis that mainly occurs in the head of the pancreas and around the pancreatic duct. It is also called alcohol-induced pancreatitis and is the most common form. The ducts are obstructed with protein precipitates that block the pancreatic duct and eventually calcify. This is followed by fibrosis and glandular atrophy. Pseudocysts and abscesses commonly develop.

Clinical Manifestations
As with acute pancreatitis, a major manifestation of chronic pancreatitis is abdominal pain. The patient may have episodes of acute pain, but it usually is chronic (recurrent attacks at intervals of months or years). The attacks may become more and more fre-

quent until they are almost constant, or they may diminish as the pancreatic fibrosis develops. The pain is located in the same areas as in acute pancreatitis but is usually described as a heavy, gnawing feeling or sometimes as burning and cramplike. The pain is not relieved with food or antacids.

- Other manifestations include symptoms of pancreatic insufficiency, including malabsorption with weight loss, constipation, mild jaundice with dark urine, steatorrhea, and diabetes mellitus (DM). The steatorrhea may become quite severe with voluminous, foul, fatty stools. Urine and stool may be frothy. Some abdominal tenderness may be found.
- Complications of chronic pancreatitis may include pseudocyst formation, bile duct or duodenal obstruction, pancreatic ascites or pleural effusion, and pancreatic cancer.

Diagnostic Studies
Confirming the diagnosis of chronic pancreatitis can be challenging and is based on the patient's signs and symptoms, lab studies, and imaging.

- Serum amylase and lipase levels may be elevated slightly or not at all.
- Serum bilirubin and alkaline phosphatase levels may be elevated.
- Mild leukocytosis and elevated sedimentation rate may be found.
- Endoscopic retrograde cholangiopancreatography (ERCP) is used to visualize changes in the pancreatic and biliary ductal system.
- Imaging studies such as computed tomography (CT), magnetic resonance imaging (MRI), MR cholangiopancreatography (MRCP), transabdominal ultrasound, and endoscopic ultrasound may be useful.

Nursing and Collaborative Management
When the patient with chronic pancreatitis is experiencing an acute attack, the therapy is identical to that for acute pancreatitis. At other times the focus is on the prevention of further attacks, the relief of pain, and the control of pancreatic exocrine and endocrine insufficiency. It sometimes takes large, frequent doses of analgesics to relieve the pain.

- Diet, pancreatic enzyme replacement (e.g., Viokase, Cotazym), and control of diabetes mellitus (DM) are measures used to control the pancreatic insufficiency. The diet is bland, low in fat, and high in carbohydrates. Alcohol must be totally eliminated.

- Treatment of chronic pancreatitis sometimes requires surgery. When biliary disease is present or if obstruction or pseudocyst develops, surgery may be indicated to divert bile flow or relieve ductal obstruction.

▼ **Patient and Family Teaching**

- The patient should be instructed to take measures to prevent further attacks. Dietary control, along with consistency of other treatment measures such as taking pancreatic enzymes, is essential. Pancreatic extracts are usually given with meals or can be given with a snack. The patient's stools need to be observed for steatorrhea to help determine the effectiveness of the enzymes. The patient and family need instructions regarding observation of stools.
- Alcohol must be avoided, and the patient may need assistance with this problem. If the patient has developed a dependence on alcohol, a referral to other agencies or resources may be necessary.
- If DM has developed, the patient needs instruction regarding testing of blood glucose levels and drugs (see Diabetes Mellitus, p. 164).
- The nurse should teach the patient who is taking antacids to take them as ordered to help control gastric acidity. Antacids should be taken after meals.

PARKINSON'S DISEASE

Description

Parkinson's disease (PD) is a disease of the basal ganglia characterized by slowness in the initiation and execution of movement *(bradykinesia),* increased muscle tonus *(rigidity),* tremor at rest, and impaired postural reflexes. PD is the most common form of *parkinsonism* (a syndrome characterized by similar symptoms).

The prevalence of PD is about 160 per 100,000 people. The diagnosis increases with age, with the peak onset in the sixth decade. To date, more than 10 autosomal dominant and recessive genes have been linked to familial PD.

Pathophysiology

There are many forms of parkinsonism other than PD. Encephalitis lethargica, or type A encephalitis, has been clearly associated with the onset of parkinsonism. Parkinson-like symptoms have also occurred after intoxication with a variety of chemicals, including carbon monoxide, manganese (among copper miners),

and an analog of meperidine (MPTP). Drug-induced parkinsonism can follow reserpine (Serpasil), methyldopa (Aldomet),
lithium, haloperidol (Haldol), and phenothiazine (Thorazine)
therapy. It is also seen following the use of amphetamine and
methamphetamine.

- The pathology of PD involves the degeneration of the dopa-
  mine-producing neurons in the substantia nigra of the mid-
  brain, which in turn disrupts the normal balance between
  dopamine (DA) and acetylcholine (ACh) in the basal
  ganglia.
- Dopamine is a neurotransmitter essential for normal functioning of the extrapyramidal motor system, including
  control of posture, support, and voluntary motion. Symptoms do not occur until 80% of neurons in the substantia
  nigra are lost.

Clinical Manifestations

Onset of PD is gradual and insidious, with a prolonged progression
and course. Classic manifestations include tremor, rigidity, and
bradykinesia, which are often called the triad of PD. In the beginning stages, only a mild tremor, slight limp, or decreased arm
swing may be evident. Later the patient may have a shuffling,
propulsive gait with arms flexed and loss of postural reflexes. In
some patients there may be a slight change in speech patterns.

- *Tremor,* often the first sign, may initially be minimal, so
  that the patient is the only one who notices it. This tremor
  is more prominent at rest and is aggravated by emotional
  stress or increased concentration. The hand tremor is
  described as "pill rolling" because the thumb and forefinger
  appear to move in a rotary fashion as if rolling a pill, coin,
  or other small object. Tremor can involve the diaphragm,
  tongue, lips, and jaw.
- *Rigidity* is increased resistance to passive motion when the
  limbs are moved through their range of motion. Parkinso-
  nian rigidity is typified by a jerky quality, as if there were
  intermittent catches in the movement of a cogwheel, when
  the joint is moved. This is called *cogwheel rigidity.*
- *Bradykinesia* (slow and retarded movement) is particularly
  evident in the loss of automatic movements, which is secondary to the physical and chemical alteration of the basal
  ganglia. In the unaffected person, automatic movements are
  involuntary and occur subconsciously; these include the
  blinking of the eyelids, swinging of the arms while walking,
  swallowing of saliva, self-expression with facial and hand
  movements, and minor movement of postural adjustment.

The patient with PD does not execute these movements. This lack of spontaneous activity accounts for the "old man" image with stooped posture, masked facies ("deadpan" expression), drooling of saliva, and shuffling gait. There is difficulty in initiating movement.

- Nonmotor symptoms include depression, anxiety, apathy, fatigue, pain, impotence, and short-term memory impairment.
- As the disease progresses, complications such as *dyskinesia, akinesia,* dementia, and neuropsychiatric problems occur. Dementia occurs in up to 40% of patients with PD.
- Swallowing may become very difficult *(dysphagia)*, leading to malnutrition or aspiration.
- General debilitation may lead to pneumonia, urinary tract infections, and skin breakdown.
- Orthostatic hypotension may occur and, along with the loss of postural reflexes, may result in falls or other injury.

Diagnostic Studies
Because there is no specific diagnostic test for PD, the diagnosis is based solely on the history and clinical features.

- A definitive diagnosis can be made only when there are at least two of the three characteristic signs of the classic triad: tremor, rigidity, and bradykinesia.
- The ultimate confirmation is a positive response to antiparkinsonian medication.

Collaborative Care
Because there is no cure, management is aimed at relieving symptoms.

Drug Therapy
Drug therapy for PD is aimed at correcting the imbalance of central nervous system (CNS) neurotransmitters. Antiparkinsonian drugs either enhance the release or supply of DA (dopaminergic) or antagonize or block the effects of acetylcholine (ACh) in the striatum. Levodopa with carbidopa (Sinemet) is often the first drug to be used. Levodopa is a precursor of dopamine and can cross the blood-brain barrier. It is converted to dopamine in the basal ganglia.

- Anticholinergic drugs are also used to manage PD. These drugs act by decreasing ACh activity. Antihistamines with anticholinergic properties or a β-adrenergic blocker (e.g., propranolol [Inderal]) are used to manage tremors. The antiviral agent amantadine (Symmetrel) is also an effective antiparkinsonian drug.

- Select monoamine oxidase (MAO) inhibitors (e.g., selegi-
  line [Eldepryl]) may be used in combination with Sinemet,
  and catechol-*O*-methyltransferase (COMT) inhibitors (e.g.,
  entacapone [Comtan], tolcapone [Tasmar]) may be used as
  adjuncts to levodopa.

Table 65 summarizes drugs commonly used in Parkinson's
disease, symptoms they relieve, and their common side effects.

Surgical Therapy

Surgical therapy is usually used to relieve symptoms in patients
with PD who are unresponsive to drug therapy or who have
developed severe motor complications. Procedures fall into three
categories: ablation (destruction), deep brain stimulation (DBS),
and transplantation. Ablation therapy involves stereotactic ablation of areas in the thalamus, globus pallidus, and subthalamic
nucleus. Ablative procedures have been largely replaced by DBS,
which involves placing an electrode in the thalamus, globus pallidus, or subthalamic nucleus that delivers a specific current to
the targeted brain location. Ablative and DBS procedures work
by reducing the increased neuronal activity produced by
DA depletion.

Transplantation of fetal neural tissue into the basal ganglia is
designed to provide DA-producing cells in the brain, but this form
of therapy is still in experimental stages.

Nutritional Therapy

Diet is of major importance because malnutrition and constipation can be serious consequences of inadequate nutrition. Patients
who have dysphagia and bradykinesia need appetizing foods
that are easily chewed and swallowed. The diet should contain
adequate roughage and fruit to avoid constipation. Ample time
should be planned for eating to avoid frustration and encourage
independence.

Nursing Management

Goals

The patient with PD will maximize neurologic function, maintain
independence in activities of daily living for as long as possible,
and optimize psychosocial well-being.

See NCP 59-4 for the patient with PD, Lewis and others,
Medical-Surgical Nursing, edition 7, pp. 1554 to 1555.

Nursing Diagnoses

- Impaired physical mobility
- Impaired verbal communication
- Imbalanced nutrition: less than body requirements
- Deficient diversional activity

Table 65   Drug Therapy: Parkinson's Disease

Drug	Symptoms Relieved	Side Effects and Precautions
Dopaminergic		
levodopa (L-dopa)	Bradykinesia, tremor, rigidity	Nausea, dyskinesia, hypotension, palpitations, dysrhythmias; agitation, hallucinations, confusion (in older patients); avoidance of vitamin pills and diet high in vitamin B_6 (reversal of effect of levodopa); contraindicated in narrow-angle glaucoma
levodopa/carbidopa (Sinemet, Parcopa)	Bradykinesia, tremor, rigidity	Less nausea but greater chance of dyskinesia, confusion, hallucinations; periodic check of BUN, AST, WBCs, Hct; contraindicated in melanoma, narrow-angle glaucoma, combination with reserpine, methyldopa, guanethidine, antipsychotics
bromocriptine mesylate (Parlodel)	Bradykinesia, tremor, rigidity	Orthostatic hypotension, nausea, vomiting, toxic psychosis, limb edema, phlebitis, dizziness, headache, insomnia
pergolide (Permax)	Same as above	Same as above
pramipexole (Mirapex)	Same as above	
ropinirole (Requip)	Same as above	
amantadine (Symmetrel)	Rigidity, akinesia	Nervousness, insomnia, confusion, hallucinations, dry mouth, nausea, edema, orthostatic hypotension

AST, Aspartate aminotransferase; BUN, blood urea nitrogen; Hct, hematocrit; WBCs, white blood cells.

Continued

Table 65 Drug Therapy: Parkinson's Disease—cont'd

Drug	Symptoms Relieved	Side Effects and Precautions
apomorphine (Apokyn)	Hypomobility, including difficulty starting movements, muscle stiffness, slow movements	Causes severe nausea and vomiting; needs to be taken with antiemetic drug; dyskinesia, sleepiness, dizziness, runny nose, chest pain, increased sweating, flushing
Anticholinergic trihexyphenidyl (Artane) benztropine (Cogentin) biperiden (Akineton)	Tremor	Dry mouth, blurred vision, constipation, delirium, anxiety, agitation, hallucinations; avoidance of drugs with similar actions, including over-the-counter drugs containing scopolamine or antihistamines (e.g., Sominex), antispasmodics (e.g., Donnatal, Bellergal), tricyclic antidepressants (e.g. imipramine [Tofranil], amitriptyline [Elavil])
Antihistamine diphenhydramine (Benadryl)	Tremor, rigidity	Sedation, same precautions as for anticholinergic drugs
Monoamine Oxidase Inhibitor selegiline (Eldepryl, Carbex) rasagiline (Azilect)	Bradykinesia, rigidity, tremor	Similar to dopaminergic drugs
Catechol-O-Methyltransferase (COMT) Inhibitors entacapone (Comtan) tolcapone (Tasmar)	By blocking COMT, these drugs slow the breakdown of levodopa, thus prolonging the action of levodopa	Similar to dopaminergic drugs; these drugs are used in combination with levodopa Tolcapone requires additional monitoring for liver function

Nursing Interventions

Promotion of physical exercise and a well-balanced diet are major concerns for nursing care. Exercise can limit the consequences of decreased mobility such as muscle atrophy, contractures, and constipation. Overall muscle tone as well as specific exercises to strengthen the muscles involved with speaking and swallowing should be included.

Because PD is a chronic degenerative disorder with no acute exacerbations, nurses should note that teaching and nursing care are directed toward the maintenance of good health, encouragement of independence, and avoidance of complications such as contractures.

▼ Patient and Family Teaching

- Instructions for patients who tend to "freeze" while walking include these: think consciously about stepping over imaginary lines on the floor, drop rice kernels and step over them, rock from side to side, lift the toes when stepping, take one step backward and two steps forward.
- Getting out of a chair can be facilitated by using an upright chair with arms and placing the back legs on small (2-inch) blocks.
- Rugs and excess furniture should be removed to avoid stumbling.
- Clothing can be simplified by the use of slip-on shoes and Velcro hook-and-loop fasteners or zippers on clothing instead of buttons and hooks.
- An elevated toilet seat can facilitate getting on and off the toilet.
- As the disease progresses, the impact on the psychologic well-being of the patient and family also increases. The nurse can assist the patient and family caregivers through listening, providing education, encouraging social interactions, and referral to the American Parkinson Disease Association (*www.apdaparkinson.org*).

PELVIC INFLAMMATORY DISEASE

Description

Pelvic inflammatory disease (PID) is an infectious condition of the pelvic cavity that may involve the fallopian tubes (salpingitis), ovaries (oophoritis), and pelvic peritoneum (peritonitis). PID remains a major cause of infertility and is often the result of untreated cervicitis.

Pelvic pain may be of a chronic nature. *Chronic pelvic pain* is noncyclical pain greater than 6 months in duration, involving the pelvis, lower back, buttocks and abdomen. Up to one-third of women have chronic pelvic pain after PID. Factors also associated with chronic pelvic pain include interstitial cystitis, lower genital tract inflammation, irritable bowel syndrome, untreated uterine fibroids, endometriosis, and dysmennorhea.

Pathophysiology
The most frequent causative organisms of PID are *Chlamydia trachomatis* and *Neisseria gonorrhoeae.* These organisms, as well as mycoplasma, streptococci, and anaerobes, may gain entrance during sexual intercourse or after pregnancy termination, pelvic surgery, or childbirth.

Clinical Manifestations
The woman with PID usually goes to a health care provider because of lower abdominal pain.
- The pain starts gradually and is constant. The intensity may vary from mild to severe; movements such as walking increase the pain.
- Spotting after intercourse and abnormal vaginal discharge are common.
- Fever and chills may also be present.
- Women with less acute symptoms notice increased cramping pain with menses, irregular bleeding, and some pain with intercourse. Women who have mild symptoms may go untreated either because they did not seek care or the health care provider misdiagnosed their complaints.

Complications
Immediate complications of PID include septic shock and *Fitz-Hugh–Curtis syndrome,* a perihepatitis that can occur when PID spreads through the peritoneum to the liver. The patient has symptoms of right upper quadrant pain, but liver function tests are normal. Pelvic and tubal ovarian abscesses may "leak" or rupture, resulting in pelvic or generalized peritonitis.
- Long-term complications include ectopic pregnancy, infertility, and chronic pelvic pain. PID can cause adhesions and strictures to develop in the fallopian tubes.

Diagnostic Studies
The diagnosis is based on data obtained during the bimanual portion of the pelvic examination. Women with PID have lower abdominal tenderness, bilateral adnexal tenderness, and positive cervical motion tenderness.

- Diagnostic criteria also include fever and abnormal vaginal or cervical discharge.
- Cultures for gonorrhea and chlamydia should be obtained from the endocervix.
- A pregnancy test should be done to rule out an ectopic pregnancy.
- When pain or obesity compromises the pelvic examination and a tubo-ovarian abscess may be present, a vaginal ultrasound is indicated.

Collaborative Care

Treatment of PID is usually on an outpatient basis. The patient is given a combination of antibiotics such as cefoxitin (Mefoxin) and doxycycline (Vibramycin) to provide broad coverage against the causative organisms. Instructions are given to avoid intercourse for 3 weeks and to return to the clinic for reevaluation in 48 to 72 hours even if symptoms are improving. Her partner or partners must be examined and treated.

If outpatient treatment is not successful or if the patient is acutely ill or in severe pain, admission to the hospital is indicated. Maximum doses of parenteral antibiotics are given in the hospital. Some providers believe the addition of corticosteroids to the antibiotic regimen reduces inflammation and improves subsequent fertility. Analgesics to relieve pain and intravenous (IV) fluids to prevent dehydration are also prescribed.

Application of heat to the lower abdomen or sitz baths may be used to improve circulation and decrease pain. Bed rest in semi-Fowler's position promotes drainage of the pelvic cavity by gravity and may prevent the development of abscesses high in the abdomen.

Indications for surgery include the presence of abscesses that fail to resolve with IV antibiotics. The abscesses may be drained by laparotomy or laparoscopy. Childbearing function in young women is preserved whenever possible.

Treatment for chronic pelvic pain should focus on the underlying disorder. If the source of the pain is unknown, treatment is directed at managing the symptoms.

Nursing Management

Prevention, early recognition, and prompt treatment of vaginal and cervical infections can help prevent PID and its serious complications. Nurses can provide information regarding factors that place a woman at increased risk for PID, such as multiple sexual partners.

During hospitalization for PID, the nurse has an important role in implementing drug therapy, monitoring the patient's health status, and providing symptom relief and patient education. Vital signs and the character, amount, color, and odor of the vaginal discharge are recorded. Explanations about the need for limited activity (bed rest in a semi-Fowler's position) and increased fluid intake should increase patient cooperation.

- The patient may have guilt feelings about PID, especially if it was associated with a sexually transmitted disease. She may also be concerned about the complications associated with PID, such as adhesions and strictures of the fallopian tubes, infertility, and the increased incidence of ectopic pregnancy. Discussion with the patient and significant others regarding these feelings and concerns can assist her to cope more effectively with them.

PEPTIC ULCER DISEASE

Description

Peptic ulcer disease is an erosion of the gastrointestinal (GI) mucosa resulting from the digestive action of hydrochloric (HCl) acid and pepsin. Any portion of the GI tract that comes into contact with gastric secretions is susceptible to ulcer development, including the lower esophagus, stomach, duodenum, and at the margin of a gastrojejunal anastomosis site after surgical procedures.

Peptic ulcers can be classified as acute or chronic, depending on the degree of mucosal involvement, and gastric or duodenal, according to the location.

- An *acute ulcer* is associated with superficial erosion and minimal inflammation. It is of short duration and resolves quickly when the cause is identified and removed.
- A *chronic ulcer* is of long duration, eroding through the muscular wall with the formation of fibrous tissue. It is continuously present for many months or intermittently throughout the person's lifetime. A chronic ulcer is at least four times as common as an acute ulcer.
- *Gastric* and *duodenal* ulcers, although defined as peptic ulcers, are distinctly different in etiology, incidence, and clinical manifestations (Table 66). Generally, the treatment of all ulcer types is similar.

Pathophysiology

Peptic ulcers develop only in the presence of an acid environment. The stomach is normally protected from autodigestion and damage

Table 66	Comparison of Gastric and Duodenal Ulcers

Gastric Ulcers	Duodenal Ulcers
Lesion Superficial; smooth margins; round, oval, or cone shaped	Penetrating (associated with deformity of duodenal bulb from healing of recurrent ulcers)
Location of lesion Predominantly antrum, also in body and fundus of stomach	First 1-2 cm of duodenum
Gastric secretion Normal to decreased	Increased
Incidence ■ Greater in women ■ Peak age 50-60 yr ■ More common in persons of lower socioeconomic status and in unskilled laborers ■ Increased with smoking, drugs (aspirin, NSAIDs), and alcohol use ■ Increased with incompetent pyloric sphincter and bile reflux	■ Greater in men but increasing in women, especially postmenopausal ■ Peak age 35-45 yr ■ Associated with psychologic stress ■ Increased with smoking, drugs, and alcohol use ■ Associated with other diseases (e.g., chronic obstructive pulmonary disease, pancreatic disease, hyperparathyroidism, Zollinger-Ellison syndrome, chronic renal failure)
Clinical manifestations ■ Burning or gaseous pressure in high left epigastrium and back and upper abdomen ■ Pain 1-2 hr after meals; if penetrating ulcer, aggravation of discomfort with food ■ Occasional nausea and vomiting, weight loss	■ Burning, cramping, pressure-like pain across mid-epigastrium and upper abdomen; back pain with posterior ulcers ■ Pain 2-4 hr after meals and mid-morning, mid-afternoon, middle of night, periodic and episodic ■ Pain relief with antacids and food; occasional nausea and vomiting

NSAIDs, Nonsteroidal antiinflammatory drugs.

Continued

Table 66	Comparison of Gastric and Duodenal Ulcers—cont'd

Gastric Ulcers	Duodenal Ulcers
Recurrence rate	
High	High
Complications	
Hemorrhage, perforation, outlet obstruction, intractability (higher risk than duodenal ulcers)	Hemorrhage, perforation, obstruction

by the gastric mucosal barrier. Under specific circumstances the mucosal barrier can be impaired and back-diffusion of HCl acid and pepsin can occur (Fig. 12). When the barrier is broken, HCl acid freely enters the mucosa and cellular destruction and inflammation occur. Histamine is released from the damaged mucosa, resulting in vasodilation, increased capillary permeability, and further secretion of acid and pepsin. A variety of agents are known to destroy the mucosal barrier (see Gastritis, p. 238). The critical pathologic process in gastric ulcer formation may not be the amount of acid that is secreted but the amount that is able to penetrate the mucosal barrier.

- Medications such as nonsteroidal antiinflammatory drugs (NSAIDs), aspirin, and reserpine (Serpasil) are known to cause gastric ulcers.
- *Helicobacter pylori* is a dominant factor in the promotion of peptic ulcer formation. This organism promotes gastric mucosal destruction (see Gastritis, p. 238).

Clinical Manifestations

It is common with gastric or duodenal ulcers to have no pain or other symptoms (gastric and duodenal mucosa have few pain sensory fibers). When pain does occur with a duodenal ulcer, it is described as burning or cramplike and is most often located in the mid-epigastrium region beneath the xiphoid process.

Pain associated with gastric ulcer is located high in the epigastrium and occurs spontaneously about 1 to 2 hours after meals. The pain is described as burning or gaseous. The pain can occur when the stomach is empty or when food has been ingested. Some persons do not experience any pain until a serious complication such as hemorrhage or perforation occurs.

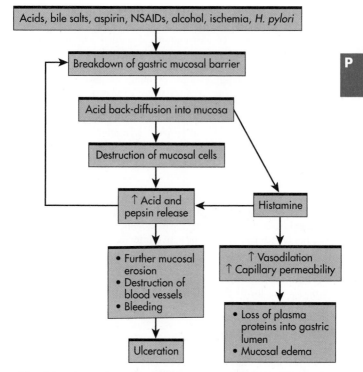

Fig. 12. Disruption of gastric mucosa and pathophysiologic consequences of back-diffusion of acids.

Complications

Major complications of peptic ulcers are hemorrhage, perforation, and gastric outlet obstruction. All are considered emergency situations and are initially treated conservatively; however, surgery may become necessary at any time during treatment.

Hemorrhage is the most common complication. It develops from the erosion of granulation tissue at the base of the ulcer during healing or from the erosion of an ulcer through a major blood vessel. Duodenal ulcers account for a greater percentage of upper GI bleeding than gastric ulcers.

Perforation, the most lethal complication, occurs when the ulcer penetrates the serosal surface with spillage of either gastric or duodenal contents into the peritoneal cavity. Contents may contain air, saliva, food particles, HCl acid, pepsin, bacteria, bile, and pancreatic fluid and enzymes. Bacterial peritonitis may occur within 6 to 12 hours.

- Manifestations of perforation are sudden with a dramatic onset and include severe upper abdominal pain that quickly spreads throughout the abdomen. Respirations become shallow and rapid, and bowel sounds are usually absent.

Gastric outlet obstruction may occur over time as a result of edema, inflammation, and pylorospasm associated with active ulcer formation. The patient with gastric outlet obstruction generally has a long history of ulcer pain. Symptoms include upper abdomen discomfort and swelling, loud peristalsis, visible peristaltic waves, vomiting (often projectile), and constipation.

Diagnostic Studies

- Endoscopy is used to determine the characteristics and nature of the ulcer, obtain a tissue biopsy, obtain specimens to test for *H. pylori,* and assess the degree of ulcer healing after treatment.
- Urea breath test checks for active infection by *H. pylori.*
- Barium x-ray studies can diagnose gastric outlet obstruction.
- Complete blood count (CBC), urinalysis, liver enzyme studies, serum amylase determination, and stool examination may be performed for further diagnostic information.

Collaborative Care

Conservative Therapy

The regimen consists of adequate rest, dietary manifestations, drug therapy, elimination of smoking, and long-term follow-up care. Drugs are a vital part of therapy, and strict adherence to the prescribed regimen of drugs is important because peptic ulcer recurrence is high without treatment.

Drug therapy includes the use of histamine H_2-receptor antagonists (e.g., cimetidine [Tagamet], famotidine [Pepcid]), protein pump inhibitors (e.g., omeprazole [Prilosec]), antisecretory agents (e.g., misoprostol [Cytotec]), cytoprotective agents (e.g., sucralfate [Carafate]), antacids, and anticholinergics. Aspirin and NSAIDs should be discontinued. The patient is given antibiotics to eradicate *H. pylori* infection. See Drug Therapy Tables 42-20 to 42-22, Lewis and others, *Medical-Surgical Nursing,* edition 7, pp. 1019 and 1020.

Healing of a peptic ulcer requires many weeks of therapy. Pain disappears after 3 to 6 days, but ulcer healing is much slower. Complete healing may take 3 to 9 weeks, depending on the ulcer size and the treatment regimen used.

Acute exacerbation of peptic ulcer can usually be treated with the same regimen used for conservative therapy. Blood products may be given for bleeding. The situation is considered more serious, however, because of the chronicity of the ulcer and possible complications of perforation, hemorrhage, and gastric outlet obstruction.

- One method of symptom relief is to keep the stomach empty for 24 to 48 hours by means of a nasogastric (NG) tube and intermittent suctioning, with IV fluid and electrolyte infusions given.
- In perforation, the focus of therapy is to stop the spillage of gastric contents by NG tube or surgery. Blood volume is replaced with lactated Ringer's and albumin solutions, and packed red blood cells (RBCs) may be necesssary. Broad-spectrum antibiotic therapy is started immediately to treat bacterial peritonitis. Pain medication is also given.
- In gastric outlet obstruction the aim of therapy is to decompress the stomach by way of an NG tube.

Nutritional Therapy

Nutritional therapy is individualized, with instructions to eat and drink foods and fluid that do not cause any distressing symptoms. Dietary instructions should include a sample diet with a list of foods that usually cause distress and should therefore be eliminated from the diet. Protein is considered the best neutralizing food, but it also stimulates gastric secretions. Carbohydrates and fats are the least stimulating to HCl acid secretion, but they do not neutralize well. The patient must determine a suitable combination of these essential nutrients without causing undue distress. Small, frequent (six per day) meals may be recommended.

Surgical Therapy

Surgery may be performed after other therapy has been tried and proven unsuccessful. Types of surgery to treat ulcers include partial gastrectomy, vagotomy, or pyloroplasty. Partial gastrectomy with removal of the distal two thirds of the stomach and anastomosis of the gastric stump to the duodenum is called a *gastroduodenostomy* or *Billroth I* operation; removal of the distal two thirds of the stomach with anastomosis of the gastric stump to the jejunum is called a *gastrojejunostomy* or *Billroth II* operation.

Postoperative complications from surgery are dumping syndrome, postprandial hypoglycemia, and bile reflux gastritis.

- *Dumping syndrome* occurs when surgery drastically reduces the reservoir capacity of the stomach and causes loss of control over the amount of gastric chyme entering the small intestine. The large bolus of hypertonic fluid entering the intestine causes a fluid shift into the bowel, creating a decrease in plasma volume along with distention of the bowel lumen and rapid intestinal transit. The patient usually

describes feelings of generalized weakness, sweating, palpitations, and dizziness caused by the decrease in plasma
volume. The patient also complains of abdominal cramps,
borborygmi, and the urge to defecate as a result of fluid being
drawn into the bowel lumen. The onset of symptoms occurs
at the end of a meal or within 15 to 30 minutes of eating,
and symptoms usually last about 1 hour after meals.

- *Postprandial hypoglycemia* is considered a variant of
dumping syndrome, since it is the result of uncontrolled
gastric emptying of a bolus of fluid high in carbohydrates,
resulting in hyperglycemia and the release of excessive
amounts of insulin into the circulation. A secondary
hypoglycemia then occurs with symptoms typical of any
hypoglycemia: sweating, weakness, mental confusion,
palpitations, and tachycardia.

- The major symptom associated with *bile reflux gastritis* is
continual epigastric distress that increases after meals.
Vomiting relieves distress but only temporarily. The administration of cholestyramine (Questran) to bind with the bile
salts, either before or with meals, has met with success.

Because of surgical changes, the stomach's reservoir is diminished and meal size must be reduced accordingly. Dry foods with
a low-carbohydrate content and moderate protein and fat content
are better tolerated initially. Fluids should be taken between meals
but not with the meal, and the patient should plan rest periods of
at least 30 minutes after each meal.

Nursing Management
Goals
The overall goals are that the patient with peptic ulcer disease will
comply with the prescribed therapeutic regimen, experience
a reduction or absence of discomfort, exhibit no signs of GI
complications, have complete healing of the peptic ulcer, and
make appropriate lifestyle changes to prevent recurrence.

See NCP 42-2 for the patient with peptic ulcer disease, Lewis and
others, *Medical-Surgical Nursing,* edition 7, pp. 1023 to 1024.
Nursing Diagnoses/Collaborative Problem
- Acute pain
- Ineffective therapeutic regimen management
- Nausea
- Potential complication: perforation of GI mucosa
Nursing Interventions
During an acute phase with pain and nausea and vomiting, the
patient may be maintained on nothing by mouth (NPO) status,
have an NG tube inserted and connected to intermittent suction,

and have IV fluid replacement. The volume of fluid lost, signs and symptoms of the patient, and laboratory test results determine the type and amount of IV fluids administered. The anxious patient and family must be informed that when the stomach is kept empty of gastric secretions, the ulcer pain diminishes and ulcer healing begins. Vital signs are taken at least hourly, with hematocrit (Hct) and hemoglobin (Hb) levels monitored so that hemorrhage and perforation can be detected early.

If the patient has surgery, postoperative care is similar to postoperative care after abdominal laparotomy (see Abdominal Pain, Acute, p. 3). Additional considerations for a patient with a partial gastrectomy include:

- Gastric aspirate from the NG tube must be carefully observed for color, amount, and odor during the immediate postoperative period.
- It is essential that the NG suction is working and that the tube remains patent so that accumulated gastric secretions do not put a strain on the anastomosis.
- Observe the patient for signs of decreased peristalsis and lower abdominal discomfort that may indicate impending intestinal obstruction.
- Keep the patient comfortable and free of pain by the administration of prescribed medications and by frequent changes in position.
- Observe the dressing for signs of bleeding or odor and drainage indicative of an infection.
- Ambulation is encouraged and is increased daily.
- Because the patient is usually returning to the same home and work environment, there is always the danger of ulcer redevelopment, especially at the site of the anastomosis. Adequate rest, nutrition, and avoidance of known stressors are keys to complete recovery.

▼ Patient and Family Teaching

General instructions for newly diagnosed patients and their family should cover aspects of the disease process itself, nutritional therapy, medication, possible changes in lifestyle, and regular follow-up care (Table 67).

- Stress-reduction techniques should be taught to the patient because relaxation results in decreased acid production and reduction in pain.
- The need for long-term follow-up care must be stressed. Because successful treatment is frequently followed by a recurrence of ulcer disease, the patient should be encouraged to seek immediate intervention if symptoms such as pain and discomfort recur or if blood is noted in stools or vomitus.

| Table 67 | Patient and Family Teaching Guide: Peptic Ulcer Disease |

The following are teaching guidelines for the patient and family:

1. Explain dietary modifications, including avoidance of foods that cause epigastric distress. This may include black pepper, spicy foods, and acidic foods. Small frequent meals are better tolerated than large meals.
2. Explain the rationale for avoiding cigarettes. In addition to promoting ulcer development, smoking will delay ulcer healing.
3. Encourage the need to reduce or eliminate alcohol ingestion.
4. Explain the rationale for avoiding OTC medications unless approved by the patient's care provider. Many preparations contain ingredients, such as aspirin, that should not be taken unless approved by the health care provider. Check with the care provider regarding the use of nonsteroidal antiinflammatory drugs.
5. Explain the rationale for not interchanging brands of antacids and H_2-receptor blockers that can be purchased OTC without checking with the health care provider. This can lead to harmful side effects.
6. Teach the need to take all medications as prescribed. This includes both antisecretory and antibiotic medications. Failure to take medications as prescribed can result in relapse.
7. Explain the importance of reporting any of the following:
   - Increased nausea and/or vomiting
   - Increased epigastric pain
   - Bloody emesis or tarry stools
8. Explain the relationship between symptoms and stress. Stress-reducing activities or relaxation strategies are encouraged.
9. Encourage patient and family to share concerns about lifestyle changes and living with a chronic illness.

OTC, Over-the-counter.

PERICARDITIS, ACUTE

Description

Pericarditis is a condition caused by inflammation of the pericardium that may occur on an acute basis. The pericardium provides lubrication to decrease friction during systolic and diastolic heart movements and assists in preventing excessive dilation of the heart during diastole.

Pathophysiology

Acute pericarditis is most often idiopathic with a variety of suspected viral causes. The coxsackievirus B group is the most commonly identified virus. In addition to idiopathic or viral pericarditis, other causes of this syndrome include uremia, bacterial infection, acute myocardial infarction (MI), tuberculosis, neoplasm, and trauma.

Pericarditis in the patient with an acute MI may be described as two distinct syndromes. *Acute pericarditis* may occur within the initial 48- to 72-hour period after an MI. The second is *Dressler's syndrome (late pericarditis),* which appears 2 to 4 weeks after infarction.

An inflammatory response is the characteristic pathologic finding in acute pericarditis. There is an influx of neutrophils, increased pericardial vascularity, and eventual fibrin deposition on the visceral pericardium.

Clinical Manifestations

Characteristic manifestations found in acute pericarditis include chest pain, dyspnea, and a pericardial friction rub.

- Progressive, frequently severe, pleuritic chest pain is generally worse with deep inspiration and when lying supine. The pain may radiate to the neck, arms, or left shoulder, mimicking angina, but pericardial pain has the distinction of referral to the trapezius muscle. The pain is relieved by sitting up and leaning forward.
- Dyspnea is related to the patient's need to breathe in rapid, shallow breaths to avoid chest pain and may be aggravated by fever and anxiety.
- The hallmark finding is the *pericardial friction rub.* The rub is a scratching, grating, high-pitched sound believed to arise from friction between the roughened pericardial and epicardial surfaces. It is best heard with the stethoscope diaphragm firmly placed at the lower left sternal border of the chest. The pericardial friction rub does not radiate widely or vary in timing from the heartbeat. It can require frequent auscultation to identify because it may be elusive and transient. Timing the pericardial friction rub with the pulse (and not respirations) helps to distinguish it from pleural rub.

Complications

Complications that may result from acute pericarditis are pericardial effusion and cardiac tamponade.

Pericardial effusion is an accumulation of excess fluid in the pericardium. Large effusions may compress adjoining structures.

Pulmonary tissue compression can cause cough, dyspnea, and tachypnea. Phrenic nerve compression can induce hiccups, and compression of the recurrent laryngeal nerve may result in hoarseness. Heart sounds are generally distant and muffled. Blood pressure (BP) is usually maintained by compensatory changes.

Cardiac tamponade develops as the pericardial effusion increases in size, compressing the heart. The patient may report chest pain and is often confused, agitated, and restless. Heart sounds become muffled, pulse pressure is narrowed, and the patient develops tachypnea, tachycardia, and decreased cardiac output. The neck veins are usually markedly distended because of jugular venous pressure elevation, and a significant pulsus paradoxus is present. *Pulsus paradoxus* is a decrease in systolic BP with inspiration that is exaggerated in cardiac tamponade. (See Table 37-8, Lewis and others, *Medical-Surgical Nursing,* edition 7, p. 873 for measurement technique.)

Diagnostic Studies

- Auscultation of the chest to assess for pericardial friction rub.
- Electrocardiogram (ECG) may be normal or exhibit changes over a period of hours to days to weeks.
- Echocardiography is used to determine the presence of pericardial effusion or cardiac tamponade.
- Tissue Doppler imaging and color M-mode of early left-ventricular flow help assess diastolic function.
- Pericardiocentesis and pericardial biopsy may be done to determine the cause of pericarditis.
- Computed tomography (CT) scan and magnetic resonance imaging (MRI) provide for visualization of the pericardium and pericardial space.

Collaborative Care

Management is directed toward identification and treatment of the underlying problem. Antibiotics should be used to treat bacterial pericarditis. Corticosteroids are generally reserved for patients with pericarditis secondary to systemic lupus erythematosus, patients already taking corticosteroids for a rheumatologic or other immune system condition, or patients who do not respond to nonsteroidal antiinflammatory drugs (NSAIDs). When necessary, prednisone is usually given in a tapering dosage schedule. Pain and inflammation are usually treated with high-dose salicylates (300 to 900 mg orally [po] four times per day) or NSAIDs (e.g., ibuprofen).

- Pericardiocentesis is usually performed for acute cardiac tamponade, purulent pericarditis, or a high suspicion of a neoplasm. Hemodynamic support as the patient is prepared for the pericardiocentesis may include the administration of volume expanders and inotropic agents (e.g., dopamine [Intropin]).

P

Nursing Management

Management of the patient's pain and anxiety are primary nursing considerations. Assessment of the amount, quality, and location of the pain is important, particularly in distinguishing the pain of acute MI (or reinfarction) from the pain of pericarditis. Pericarditic pain is usually located in the precordium or left trapezius ridge and has a sharp, pleuritic quality that increases with inspiration. Relief from this pain is often obtained by sitting or leaning forward and is worsened when lying supine (recumbency).

- Pain relief measures include maintaining the patient on bed rest with the head of the bed elevated to 45 degrees and providing a padded overbed table.
- Antiinflammatory medications help to alleviate the patient's pain. Because of the potential for gastrointestinal (GI) problems with the use of high doses of these medications, specific nursing interventions should include administration of these drugs with food or milk and instructions to the patient to avoid alcoholic beverages while taking these medications.
- Monitoring for the signs and symptoms of tamponade and making preparations for possible pericardiocentesis are important nursing responsibilities.
- Anxiety-reducing measures for the patient include providing simple, complete explanations of all procedures performed. These explanations are particularly important for the patient whose diagnosis is being established and for the patient who has already experienced an acute MI and has Dressler's syndrome.

PERIPHERAL ARTERIAL DISEASE (LOWER EXTREMITIES)

Description

Peripheral arterial disease (PAD) of the lower extremities may affect the aortoiliac, femoral, popliteal, or tibial arteries; the peroneal vessels; or any combination of these arteries.

Pathophysiology

The leading cause of PAD is *atherosclerosis,* a gradual thickening of the intima and media of arteries, which leads to progressive narrowing of the vessel lumen. These pathologic changes consist of migration and replication of smooth muscle cells, deposition of connective tissue, lymphocyte and macrophage infiltration, and accumulation of lipids. Significant risk factors for PAD are cigarette smoking, hyperlipidemia, hypertension, and diabetes mellitus, with the highest risk being cigarette smoking.

Clinical Manifestations

Severity of the manifestations depends on the site, extent of obstruction, and extent and amount of collateral circulation.

- The classic symptom is *intermittent claudication,* which is ischemic muscle ache or pain that is precipitated by exercise and relieved by resting.
- Paresthesia, manifested as numbness or tingling in the toes or feet, may result from nerve tissue ischemia. Gradually diminishing perfusion to neurons produces loss of both sensation and deep pain.
- Pallor or blanching of the foot is noted in response to leg elevation. *Reactive hyperemia* (redness) and a bluish or dusky appearance are observed when the limb is allowed to hang in a dependent position *(dependent rubor).* The skin becomes shiny and taut, and there is hair loss on the lower legs. Diminished or absent pedal, popliteal, or femoral pulses may also be noted.
- As the disease process advances and involves multiple arterial segments, continuous pain develops at rest. Rest pain most often occurs in the forefoot or toes and is aggravated by limb elevation.

Complications are nonhealing arterial ulcers and gangrene, which may result in lower extremity amputation. If atherosclerosis has been present for an extended period, collateral circulation may prevent gangrene of the extremity.

Diagnostic Studies

- Doppler ultrasound can determine blood flow.
- Duplex imaging is done.
- Segmental blood pressure (BP) readings of leg show low pressures.
- Angiography or magnetic resonance angiography (MRA) delineates location and extent of disease.

Collaborative Care

The first treatment goal is to aggressively modify cardiovascular risk factors because of the high risk for myocardial infarction (MI), ischemic stroke, and cardiovascular-related death in all patients with PAD. Smoking cessation is essential. Hyperlipidemia can be controlled with lipid-lowering agents such as a statin (e.g., simvastatin [Zocor]), and statin use has been associated with improved walking distance and speed in patient with PAD. Hypertension and diabetes mellitus also need to be properly controlled.

Antiplatelet agents such as aspirin, ticlopidine (Ticlid), and clopidogrel (Plavix) are important for reducing the risks of MI, ischemic stroke, and cardiovascular-related death in patients with PAD.

- Based on the best available evidence, first-line oral anti-platelet therapy for patients with PAD should be aspirin (160 to 325 mg/day) or clopidogrel.
- Early evidence indicates that treatment of PAD patients with angiotensin-converting enzyme (ACE) inhibitors (e.g., ramipril [Altace]) appears to decrease cardiovascular morbidity and mortality as well as increase peripheral blood flow and walking distance.
- Two drugs approved specifically to treat intermittent claudication are pentoxifylline (Trental) and cilostazol (Pletal). Pentoxifylline increases erythrocyte flexibility and reduces blood viscosity, whereas cilostazol is a phosphodiesterase inhibitor that inhibits platelet aggregation and increases vasodilation.

The primary nonpharmacologic treatment for claudication is a formal exercise-training program. It improves oxygen extraction in the legs and skeletal muscle metabolism. Walking is the most effective exercise. The patient should be instructed to walk to the point of discomfort, stop and rest, and then resume walking until the discomfort recurs. Walking should be done for 30 to 40 minutes per day, three to five times per week.

- The patient with PAD should be taught how to alter the dietary intake. Overall caloric intake should be adjusted so that ideal body weight can be achieved and maintained, dietary cholesterol should be less than 200 mg/day, and sodium intake should be no more than 2 g/day.
- Ginkgo biloba is effective in increasing walking distance for patients with intermittent claudication. Patients taking antiplatelet agents, nonsteroidal antiinflammatory agents, or anticoagulants should consult with their health care

provider before using ginkgo biloba because of bleeding risks.

Conservative management goals of the patient with critical limb ischemia resulting from PAD include protecting the extremity from trauma, decreasing vasospasm, preventing and controlling infection, and maximizing arterial perfusion. Careful inspection, cleansing, and lubrication of both feet are advised to prevent cracking of the skin and infection.

Interventional radiologic procedures are indicated when intermittent claudication symptoms become incapacitating, the patient experiences pain at rest, or ulceration or gangrene threatens the viability of the limb.

- *Percutaneous transluminal balloon angioplasty* involves the insertion of a catheter through the femoral artery. The balloon dilates the vessel by cracking the confining atherosclerotic intimal shell while also stretching the underlying media.
- Placement of intravascular stents with balloon angioplasty helps to relieve the problems of restenosis and arterial dissection.

Various surgical approaches can be used to improve arterial blood flow beyond a stenotic or occluded artery. The most common is a peripheral arterial bypass operation with autogenous vein or synthetic graft material to bypass or carry blood around the lesion.

- Other surgical options include *endarterectomy* (opening the artery and removing the obstructing plaque) and *patch graft angioplasty* (opening the artery, removing plaque, and sewing a patch to the opening to widen the lumen).
- Amputation is the least desirable surgical option, but it may be required if gangrene is extensive, infection is present in the bone (osteomyelitis), or all major arteries in the limb are occluded.

Nursing Management
Goals
The patient with PAD will have adequate tissue perfusion, relief of pain, increased exercise tolerance, and intact, healthy skin on extremities.

See NCP 38-1 for the patient with peripheral arterial disease of the lower extremities, Lewis and others, *Medical-Surgical Nursing*, edition 7, pp. 905 to 906.

Nursing Diagnoses
- Ineffective tissue perfusion (peripheral)
- Risk for impaired skin integrity

- Activity intolerance
- Ineffective therapeutic regimen management

Nursing Interventions

After surgical or radiologic intervention, the operative extremity should be checked every 15 minutes initially and then hourly for color, temperature, capillary refill, presence of peripheral pulses distal to the operative site, and extremity movement and sensation. Loss of palpable pulses necessitates immediate intervention.

After transfer from the recovery area, nursing care should focus on continued circulatory assessment and monitoring for the development of potential complications. These include bleeding, hematoma, thrombosis, embolization, and compartment syndrome. A dramatic increase in pain level, loss of palpable pulse or pulses, decreasing ankle-brachial indices, numbness or tingling, or cold extremity temperature may indicate occlusion of the bypass graft and should be reported to the surgeon immediately.

- Knee-flexed positions should be avoided except for exercise. Sitting for long periods is discouraged because leg dependency may cause edema, resulting in discomfort and stress to suture lines and increased risk of deep vein thrombosis. If significant swelling develops, a reclining position is preferred, with the edematous leg elevated above heart level. Walking even short distances is desirable.

▼ **Patient and Family Teaching**

- Emphasize that because atherosclerosis is a systemic disease that is not just localized to the lower extremities, cardiovascular risk management is essential.
- The patient should be strongly encouraged to stop smoking. Instruction regarding diet modification to reduce the intake of animal fat and refined sugars, proper foot care, and avoidance of injury to the extremities is also important.
- Promotion of a progressive exercise program often increases the patient's tolerance for exercise, enhances venous return, and improves the development of collateral circulation.
- Encourage rest when pain occurs so that tissue ischemia and pain are relieved or reduced, and explain rationale to patient to increase cooperation.
- Instruct the patient that footwear should be soft, roomy, and protective. Patients should learn to inspect their legs and feet daily for skin color changes, mottling, alterations in skin texture and subcutaneous fat, and reduction or absence of hair growth. Any ulceration or inflammation must be reported to the health care provider. Skin temperature should be noted with capillary refill of fingers and toes.

PERITONITIS

Description
Peritonitis results from a localized or generalized inflammatory process of the peritoneum. Primary peritonitis occurs when blood-borne organisms enter the peritoneal cavity. Secondary peritonitis is much more common and occurs when abdominal organs perforate or rupture and release their contents (bile, enzymes, bacteria) into the peritoneal cavity. Common causes are listed in Table 68.

Pathophysiology
The introduction of microorganisms or the leakage of gastro-intestinal (GI) contents into the peritoneal cavity results in infection and inflammation. No matter the cause, the resulting inflammatory response leads to massive fluid shifts (peritoneal edema) and adhesions as the body attempts to wall off the infection.

Clinical Manifestations
- Abdominal pain is the most common symptom.
- A universal sign is tenderness over the involved area. Rebound tenderness, muscular rigidity, and spasm are other major signs of peritoneum irritation.
- Abdominal distention or ascites, fever, tachycardia, tachypnea, nausea, vomiting, and altered bowel habits may also be present.

Table 68	Causes of Peritonitis
Primary	**Secondary**
Blood-borne organisms	Appendicitis with rupture
Genital tract organisms	Blunt or penetrating trauma to
Cirrhosis with ascites	abdominal organs
	Diverticulitis with rupture
	Ischemic bowel disorders
	Obstruction in the gastrointestinal tract
	Pancreatitis
	Perforated peptic ulcer
	Peritoneal dialysis
	Postoperative (breakage of anastomosis)

Complications include hypovolemic shock, sepsis, intraabdominal abscess formation, paralytic ileus, and acute respiratory distress syndrome. If treatment is delayed, death may occur.

Diagnostic Studies

- Complete blood count (CBC) will determine hemoconcentration and leukocytosis.
- Peritoneal fluid aspiration and analysis can detect blood, bile, pus, bacteria, fungi, and amylase content.
- Abdominal x-ray may show dilated loops of bowel consistent with paralytic ileus, free air if there is a perforation, or air and fluid levels if an obstruction is present.
- Computed tomography (CT) scan or ultrasound will identify ascites or abscesses.
- Peritoneoscopy may be helpful in patients without ascites.

Collaborative Care

Surgery is usually indicated to locate the cause, drain purulent fluid, and repair the damage. Patients with milder cases of peritonitis or those who are poor surgical risks may be managed nonsurgically. Treatment consists of antibiotics, nasogastric (NG) suction, analgesics, and intravenous (IV) fluid administration. Patients who require surgery need preoperative preparation.

Nursing Management

Goals

The patient with peritonitis will have resolution of inflammation, relief of abdominal pain, freedom from complications (especially hypovolemic shock), and normal nutritional status.

Nursing Diagnoses

- Acute pain
- Risk for deficient fluid volume
- Imbalanced nutrition: less than body requirements
- Anxiety

Nursing Interventions

The patient with peritonitis is extremely ill and needs skilled supportive care. An IV line is inserted to replace fluids lost to the peritoneal cavity and as an access for antibiotic therapy. The patient is monitored for pain and response to analgesic therapy. The patient may be positioned with knees flexed to increase comfort. The nurse should provide rest and a quiet environment. Sedatives may be given to allay anxiety.

- Accurate monitoring of fluid intake and output and electrolyte status is necessary to determine replacement therapy. Vital signs are monitored frequently.

- Antiemetics may be administered to decrease nausea and vomiting and prevent further fluid and electrolyte losses. The patient is on nothing by mouth (NPO) status and may have an NG tube in place to decrease gastric distention.

If the patient has an open-incision surgical procedure, drains are inserted to remove purulent drainage and excessive fluid. Postoperative care of the patient is similar to the care of the patient with an exploratory laparotomy (see Abdominal Pain, Acute, p. 3).

PNEUMONIA

Description

Pneumonia is an acute inflammation of the lung parenchyma caused by a microbial agent. Despite the availability of antimicrobial agents to treat pneumonia, it is still common and, as the seventh leading cause of death in the United States, is associated with significant morbidity and mortality rates. Pneumonia can be caused by bacteria, viruses, *Mycoplasma,* fungi, parasites, and chemicals.

A clinically effective way to classify pneumonia is to classify it as *community-acquired pneumonia* (CAP) or *hospital-acquired pneumonia* (HAP) (Table 69). This classification identifies likely causative organisms and appropriate antibiotics for treatment.

- *CAP* is defined as a lower respiratory tract infection of the lung parenchyma with onset in the community or during the first 2 days of hospitalization. Incidence is highest in the winter months.
- HAP is pneumonia occurring 48 hours or longer after hospital admission and not incubating at the time of hospitalization. HAP is further classified into ventilator-associated pneumonia (VAP) and health care–associated pneumonia (HCAP). HAP is the second most common nosocomial infection, second only to urinary tract infection.

Other causes of of pneumonia include fungi, aspiration, and opportunistic pathogens.

Pathophysiology

Normally the airway distal to the larynx is sterile because of protective defense mechanisms. Pneumonia is more likely to result when defense mechanisms become incompetent or are overwhelmed by infectious agents. Risk factors for pneumonia are varied and include:

| Table 69 | Organisms Associated with Pneumonia |

Community-Acquired	Hospital-Acquired
Streptococcus pneumoniae*	Pseudomonas aeruginosa
Mycoplasma pneumoniae	Enterobacter
Haemophilus influenzae	Escherichia coli
Respiratory viruses	Proteus
Chlamydia pneumoniae	Klebsiella
Legionella pneumophila	Staphylococcus aureus
Oral anaerobes	Streptococcus pneumoniae
Moraxella catarrhalis	Oral anaerobes
Staphylococcus aureus	
Nocardia	
Enteric aerobic gram-negative bacteria (e.g., Klebsiella)	
Fungi	
Mycobacterium tuberculosis	

* Most common cause of community-acquired pneumonia (CAP).

- Altered consciousness, which depresses the cough and epiglottal reflexes
- Tracheal intubation, which interferes with the normal cough reflex and the mucociliary escalator mechanism
- Impaired mucociliary mechanism caused by air pollution, cigarette smoking, viral upper respiratory tract infections, and normal aging changes
- Malnutrition, in which the function of lymphocytes and polymorphonuclear leukocytes is altered
- Certain diseases such as leukemia, alcoholism, and diabetes mellitus, which are associated with an increased frequency of gram-negative bacilli in the oropharynx
- Altered oropharyngeal flora, which can occur secondary to antibiotic therapy given for an infection elsewhere in the body

Organisms that cause pneumonia reach the lungs by aspiration from the nasopharynx or oropharynx, inhalation of microbes present in the air, or hematogenous spread from an infection elsewhere in the body.

There are four characteristic stages of *pneumococcal pneumonia*:

1. *Congestion.* After the pneumococcus organisms reach the alveoli by way of droplets or saliva, there is an outpouring

of fluid into the alveoli. Organisms multiply in the serous fluid, spreading the infection.

2. *Red hepatization.* Massive dilation of capillaries; alveoli are filled with organisms, neutrophils, red blood cells (RBCs), and fibrin. The lung appears red and granular, or liverlike, which is why the process is called hepatization.

3. *Gray hepatization.* Blood flow decreases, and leukocytes and fibrin consolidate in the affected part of the lung.

4. *Resolution.* Complete resolution and healing occur if there are no complications.

The exudate becomes lysed and is processed by the macrophages. Normal lung tissue and the person's gas-exchange ability both return to normal. The pathophysiology of other types of pneumonia is similar.

Clinical Manifestations and Complications

Patients with a typical pneumonia syndrome usually have a sudden onset of fever, chills, cough productive of purulent sputum, and pleuritic chest pain (in some cases). In the older or debilitated patient, confusion or stupor (possibly related to hypoxia) may be the only finding.

- On physical examination signs of pulmonary consolidation, such as dullness to percussion, increased fremitus, bronchial breath sounds, and crackles, may be found.
- The typical pneumonia syndrome is usually caused by *Streptococcus pneumoniae,* the most common pathogen in CAP, but can also be due to other bacterial pathogens, such as *Haemophilus influenzae.*

Pneumonia may also present atypically with a more gradual onset, dry cough, and extrapulmonary manifestations such as headache, myalgias, fatigue, sore throat, nausea, vomiting, and diarrhea. On physical examination crackles are often heard. This presentation is classically produced by *Mycoplasma pneumoniae* but can also be caused by *Legionella pneumophilia* and *Chlamydia pneumoniae.*

Viruses also cause pneumonia that is usually characterized by an atypical presentation with chills, fever, dry nonproductive cough, and extrapulmonary symptoms.

- Primary viral pneumonia can be caused by influenza virus infections.

Most cases of pneumonia generally run an uncomplicated course. Complications can occur and develop more frequently in individuals with underlying chronic diseases and other risk factors.

Complications include pleurisy (inflammation of the pleura), pleural effusion, atelectasis (collapsed, airless alveoli), bacteremia, lung abscess, empyema (accumulation of purulent exudate in pleural cavity), pericarditis, arthritis, meningitis, and endocarditis.

Diagnostic Studies

- History, physical examination, and chest x-ray often provide enough information for making management decisions without further testing.
- Chest x-ray often shows a pattern characteristic of the infecting organism.
- Sputum culture and sensitivity test may be done.
- Gram stain of sputum and blood cultures are used to identify causative organism.
- Arterial blood gases (ABGs) and pulse oximetry usually reveal hypoxemia.
- Complete blood count (CBC) with a white blood count (WBC) count may reveal leukocytosis .

Collaborative Care

Prompt treatment with appropriate antibiotics almost always cures bacterial and *Mycoplasma* pneumonia. Table 28-4 in Lewis and others, *Medical-Surgical Nursing,* edition 7, p. 563, outlines the drug therapies used in the treatment of CAP.

In uncomplicated cases, the patient responds to drug therapy within 48 to 72 hours. Indications of improvement include decreased temperature, improved breathing, and reduced chest pain.

- Supportive measures may be used, including oxygen therapy, analgesics to relieve chest pain, and antipyretics such as aspirin or acetaminophen. During the acute febrile phase, the patient's activity should be restricted and rest should be encouraged and planned.
- Fluid intake of at least 3 L/day should be maintained. Nutritional intake should be provided to meet the increased metabolic needs of the patient. Small, frequent meals are better tolerated by the dyspneic patient.

Currently there is no definitive treatment for viral pneumonia. Two antiviral drugs, amantadine (Symmetrel) and rimantadine (Flumadine), are approved for use within 48 hours of onset of symptoms in the treatment of influenza A virus. The neuraminidase inhibitors, zanamivir (Relenza) and oseltamivir (Tamiflu), are active against both influenza A and B.

- During outbreaks of influenza, the Centers for Disease Control and Prevention (CDC) encourage the use of amantadine or rimantadine for chemoprophylaxis and use of oseltamivir or zanamivir for treatment.

- Vaccination against influenza is the mainstay of prevention and recommended annually for individuals considered to be at risk.
- Pneumococcal vaccine is indicated primarily for the individual considered at increased risk who (1) has chronic illnesses such as lung and heart disease and diabetes mellitus, (2) is recovering from a severe illness, (3) is at least 65 years old, or (4) is in a long-term care facility. In the immunosuppressed individual at increased risk for development of fatal pneumococcal infection, revaccination is recommended after 5 years.

Nursing Management
Goals
The patient with pneumonia will have clear breath sounds, normal breathing patterns, normal chest x-ray, and no complications related to pneumonia.

See NCP 28-1 for the patient with pneumonia, Lewis and others, *Medical-Surgical Nursing,* edition 7, p. 568.

Nursing Diagnoses
- Ineffective breathing pattern
- Ineffective airway clearance
- Acute pain

Nursing Interventions
Interventions focus on preventing the occurrence of pneumonia. If possible, exposure to upper respiratory infections (URIs) should be avoided. If a URI occurs, it should be treated promptly with supportive measures (e.g., rest, fluids). If symptoms persist for more than 7 days, the person should obtain medical care. The individual at increased risk for pneumonia should be encouraged to obtain both influenza and pneumococcal vaccines.

- In the hospital, the nursing role involves identifying the patient at risk and taking measures to prevent the development of pneumonia.
- The patient with altered consciousness should be placed in positions (e.g., side-lying, upright) that will prevent or minimize aspiration. The patient should be turned and repositioned at least every 2 hours to facilitate adequate lung expansion and to discourage the pooling of secretions.
- The patient who has a feeding tube requires attention to prevent aspiration.
- Intubated patients should be placed in a semirecumbent position (30 to 45 degrees) with continuous aspiration of subglottic secretions above the tracheal tube cuff with a

specially designed endotracheal tube to prevent risk of ventilator-associated pneumonia.

- The patient who has difficulty swallowing (e.g., a stroke patient) needs assistance in eating, drinking, and taking medication to prevent aspiration. The gag reflex should be present in the individual who has had local anesthesia to the throat before the administration of fluids or food.
- Overmedication with opioids or sedatives, which can cause a depressed cough reflex and fluid accumulation in the lungs, should be avoided.
- Strict medical asepsis and adherence to infection control guidelines should be practiced to reduce the incidence of nosocomial infections.

The essential components of nursing care for patients with pneumonia include monitoring physical assessment parameters, facilitating laboratory and diagnostic tests, providing treatment, and monitoring the patient's response to treatment. Therapeutic positioning may identify the best positioning for the patient based on lung disease and patient response to positioning. Exercise and early ambulation augment bronchial hygiene and are encouraged as tolerated.

▼ Patient and Family Teaching

- Instruct the patient to prevent the occurrence of pneumonia by practicing good health habits, such as proper diet and hygiene, adequate rest, and regular exercise.
- It is extremely important to emphasize to the patient the need to take all of the prescribed medication and to return for follow-up medical care and evaluation.
- Adequate rest is needed to maintain progress toward recovery and to prevent relapse. The patient needs to be told that it may be weeks before the usual vigor and sense of well-being are felt.
- The patient considered to be at increased risk for pneumonia should be told about available vaccines and should discuss them with the health care provider.
- Deep-breathing exercises should be practiced for 6 to 8 weeks after the patient is discharged from the hospital.

PNEUMOTHORAX

Description

Pneumothorax is a complete or partial collapse of a lung as a result of an accumulation of air in the pleural space. This condition should be suspected after any blunt trauma to the chest wall. A pneumothorax may be closed or open.

Pathophysiology

Closed pneumothorax has no associated external wound; the most common form is spontaneous pneumothorax, which is caused by the rupture of small blebs on the visceral pleural space. The cause of blebs is unknown, but they occur most commonly in underweight male cigarette smokers between 20 and 40 years old. There is a tendency for spontaneous pneumothorax to recur.

- Other causes of closed pneumothorax include injury to the lungs from mechanical ventilation, insertion of a subclavian catheter, perforation of the esophagus, injury to the lungs from broken ribs (see Flail Chest, p. 225), and ruptured blebs or bullae in a patient with chronic obstructive pulmonary disease (COPD).

Open pneumothorax occurs when air enters the pleural space through an opening in the chest wall. Examples include stab or gunshot wounds and surgical thoracotomy. A penetrating chest wound is often referred to as a sucking chest wound.

Tension pneumothorax results when a rapid accumulation of air in the pleural space causes high intrapleural pressures that create tension on the heart and great vessels. It may result from an open or closed pneumothorax. In an open chest wound, a flap may act as a one-way valve; thus air can enter on inspiration but cannot escape. Intrathoracic pressure increases, the lung collapses, and the mediastinum shifts toward the unaffected side, which is subsequently compressed. As intrathoracic pressure increases, cardiac output (CO) is altered because there is decreased venous return and compression of the great vessels.

- Tension pneumothorax is a medical emergency because both the respiratory and circulatory systems are affected. It usually occurs with mechanical ventilation or resuscitative efforts.
- Tension pneumothorax can also occur if chest tubes are clamped or become blocked after insertion for a pneumothorax. Unclamping the tube or relieving the obstruction will remedy the situation.

Hemothorax is an accumulation of blood in the intrapleural space. It is frequently found in association with open pneumothorax and is then called a *hemopneumothorax*. The causes of hemothorax include chest trauma, lung malignancy, complication of anticoagulant therapy, and pulmonary embolus.

Clinical Manifestations

If the pneumothorax is small, only mild tachycardia and dyspnea may be present. If it is a large pneumothorax, shallow, rapid respirations, dyspnea, air hunger, and oxygen desaturation may occur.

- Chest pain and a cough with or without hemoptysis may also be present.
- On auscultation there are no breath sounds over the affected area, and hyperresonance may be heard.
- Chest x-ray shows the presence of pneumothorax.

If a tension pneumothorax develops, severe respiratory distress, tachycardia, and hypotension occur. Mediastinal displacement occurs, and the trachea shifts to the unaffected side.

Collaborative Care

If the amount of air or fluid accumulated in the intrapleural space is minimal, no treatment may be needed because the pneumothorax resolves spontaneously, or the pleural space can be aspirated with a large-bore needle.

- An open pneumothorax should be covered with a vented dressing. (A vented dressing is one secured on three sides with the fourth side left untaped.) This allows air to escape from the vent and decreases the likelihood of tension pneumothorax developing. If the object that caused the open chest wound is still in place, it should not be removed until a physician is present.

The most common treatment for a pneumothorax and hemothorax is to insert a chest tube and connect it to water-seal drainage (see Chest Tubes and Pleural Drainage, p. 718). Repeated spontaneous pneumothoraces may need to be treated surgically by a partial pleurectomy, stapling, or pleurodesis to promote the adherence of pleurae to one another.

POLYCYSTIC KIDNEY DISEASE

Polycystic kidney disease (PKD) is the most common life-threatening genetic disease in the world. It is characterized by large, thin-walled cysts that fill the cortex and the medulla and destroy surrounding tissue by compression. The cysts range in size from several millimeters to several centimeters in diameter, involve both kidneys, and are filled with fluid, including blood or pus.

The *childhood form* of PKD is a rare autosomal recessive disorder that is often rapidly progressive. The *adult form* of PKD is an autosomal dominant disorder that is latent for many years and usually manifests between 30 and 40 years old.

Symptoms appear when the cysts begin to enlarge. Often the first manifestations are hypertension, hematuria (from rupture of cysts), or a feeling of heaviness in the back, side, or abdomen. On physical examination, palpable bilateral enlarged kidneys are often found.

- Sometimes the first manifestations are a urinary tract infection (UTI) and/or urinary calculi.
- Chronic pain is one of the most common problems, and in some people it can be constant and quite severe.
- Other manifestations include hematuria and hypertension.
- Usually the disease progresses to end-stage renal failure.

Diagnosis is based on clinical manifestations, family history, intravenous pyelogram (IVP), ultrasound (best screening measure), or computed tomography (CT) scan.

There is no specific treatment for PKD. A major aim of treatment is to prevent infections of the urinary tract or to treat them with appropriate antibiotics if they occur. Nephrectomy may be necessary if pain, bleeding, or infection becomes a chronic, serious problem. When the patient begins to experience progressive renal failure, interventions are determined by the remaining renal function. Kidney transplant remains the only cure.

Nursing measures are those used for management of end-stage renal disease (see Kidney Disease, Chronic, p. 372). They include diet modification, fluid restriction, medications (e.g., antihypertensives), helping the patient to accept the chronic disease process, assisting the patient and family to deal with financial concerns, and other issues related to the hereditary nature of the disease.

- The patient needs appropriate counseling regarding plans for having children. Genetic counseling should also be provided for the children because each child of a parent with polycystic kidney disease has a 50% chance of having the disease.

POLYCYTHEMIA

Description

Polycythemia is the production and presence of increased number of red blood cells (RBCs). The increase in erythrocytes can be so great that blood circulation is impaired as a result of the increased blood viscosity (hyperviscosity) and volume (hypervolemia).

Pathophysiology

The two types of polycythemia are *primary polycythemia (polycythemia vera)* and *secondary polycythemia* (Fig. 13). Their

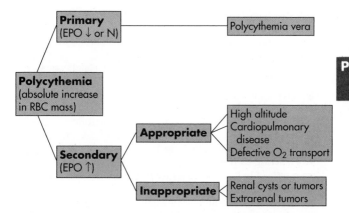

Fig. 13. Differentiating between primary and secondary polycythemia. *EPO,* Erythropoietin; *N,* normal; *O₂,* oxygen; *RBC,* red blood cell.

etiologies and pathogeneses differ, although their complications and clinical manifestations are similar.

Polycythemia vera is considered a myeloproliferative disorder arising from a chromosomal mutation in a single pluripotent stem cell. Therefore not only are RBCs involved, but also granulocytes and platelets, leading to increased production of each of these blood cells. The disease develops insidiously and follows a chronic, vacillating course. The median age at diagnosis is 60 years old. Patients have enhanced blood viscosity and blood volume and congestion of organs and tissues with blood. Splenomegaly and hepatomegaly are common.

- The major cause of morbidity and mortality from polycythemia vera is thrombosis.

Secondary polycythemia can be either *hypoxia driven* or *hypoxia independent.* In hypoxia-driven polycythemia, hypoxia stimulates erythropoietin (EPO) production in the kidney, which in turn stimulates erythrocyte production. The hypoxia may be due to high altitude, pulmonary and cardiovascular disease, defective O_2 transport, or tissue hypoxia. In this situation, secondary polycythemia is a physiologic response in which the body tries to compensate for a problem. In hypoxia-independent polycythemia, EPO is produced by a malignant or benign tumor tissue.

Clinical Manifestations

Initial manifestations from hypertension caused by hypervolemia and hyperviscosity include:

- Complaints of headache, vertigo, dizziness, tinnitus, and visual disturbances

Manifestations caused by blood vessel distention, circulatory stasis, thrombosis, and tissue hypoxia include:

- Angina, heart failure (HF), intermittent claudication, and venous thrombosis

Hemorrhage caused by either vessel rupture from overdistention or inadequate platelet function may result in:

- Petechiae, ecchymoses, epistaxis, or gastrointestinal (GI) bleeding

Other clinical manifestations include:

- Generalized pruritus that may be a striking symptom and is related to histamine release from an increased number of basophils
- Hepatomegaly and splenomegaly that contribute to patient complaints of satiety and fullness
- Pain resulting from peptic ulcer resulting from increased gastric secretions
- Paresthesia and erythromelalgia (painful burning and redness of the hands and feet)
- Plethora (ruddy complexion) may be present
- Hyperuricemia resulting from the increase in RBC destruction that accompanies excessive RBC production; may cause a form of gout

Diagnostic Studies

- Elevated hemoglobin (Hb) and RBC count with microcytosis
- Low to normal EPO level (polycythemia vera); high EPO level (secondary polycythemia)
- Elevated white blood cell (WBC) count with basophilia
- Elevated platelets (thrombocytosis) and platelet dysfunction
- Elevated leukocyte alkaline phosphatase, uric acid, and cobalamin levels
- Elevated histamine levels
- Bone marrow examination showing hypercellularity of RBCs, WBCs, and platelets
- Splenomegaly found in 90% of patients with primary polycythemia

Collaborative Care

Treatment of polycythemia vera is directed toward reducing blood volume and viscosity and bone marrow activity. Phlebotomy is the mainstay of treatment. At the time of diagnosis 300 to 500 ml of blood may be removed every other day until the hematocrit (Hct) level is reduced to normal. The aim of phlebotomy is to reduce and keep the Hct to less than 45% to 48%. An individual managed with repeated phlebotomies eventually becomes iron deficient, although this effect is rarely symptomatic. Iron supplementation should be avoided.

- Hydration therapy is used to reduce the blood's viscosity.
- Myelosuppressive agents such as busulfan (Myleran), hydroxyurea (Hydrea), melphalan (Alkeran), and radioactive phosphorus may be given to inhibit bone marrow activity.
- Paroxetine (Paxil) or low-dose aspirin may be used to alleviate erythromelalgia. Interferon alpha (IFN-α) is used in women of childbearing age or those with intractable pruritus.
- Anagrelide (Agrylin) may be used to reduce the platelet count and inhibit platelet aggregation.
- Allopurinol (Zyloprim) may reduce the number of acute gouty attacks.

Nursing Management

Primary polycythemia vera is not preventable. However, because hypoxia-driven polycythemia is generated by any source of hypoxia, maintaining adequate oxygenation may prevent problems. Therefore controlling chronic pulmonary disease, stopping smoking, and avoiding high altitudes may be important.

When acute exacerbations of polycythemia vera develop, the nurse may either assist with or perform phlebotomies, depending on the institution's policies.

- Fluid intake and output must be evaluated during hydration therapy to avoid fluid overload (which further complicates circulatory congestion) and underhydration (which can cause even greater blood viscosity).
- If myelosuppressive agents are used, the nurse must administer the drugs as ordered, observe the patient, and teach the patient about medication side effects.
- An assessment of the patient's nutritional status in collaboration with the dietitian may be necessary to offset the inadequate food intake that can result from GI symptoms of fullness, pain, and dyspepsia.
- Activity is needed to decrease thrombus formation. The major cause of morbidity and mortality from polycythemia vera is related to thrombosis. Active or passive leg exercises and ambulation when possible should be initiated.
- Because of its chronic nature, polycythemia vera requires ongoing evaluation. Phlebotomy may need to be done every 2 to 3 months. The nurse must evaluate the patient for the development of complications.

PRESSURE ULCER

Description
A pressure ulcer is a localized area of tissue necrosis caused by unrelieved pressure that occludes blood flow to the tissues. The most common site for pressure ulcers is the sacrum, with heels being second. Factors influencing development of pressure ulcers include amount of pressure (intensity), length of time pressure is exerted on the skin (duration), and ability of the patient's tissue to tolerate externally applied pressure. Besides pressure, shearing force (pressure exerted on skin when it adheres to the bed and skin layers slide in the direction of body movement), friction (two surfaces rubbing against each other), and excessive moisture contribute to pressure ulcer formation.

- Factors that put a patient at risk for the development of pressure ulcers include immobility, advanced age, obesity, impaired circulation, incontinence, diabetes mellitus, neurologic disorders, contractures, anemia, and prolonged surgery.

Clinical Manifestations
Pressure ulcers are graded or staged according to their deepest level of tissue damage or "wounding." Table 70 describes the four pressure ulcer stages.

- When eschar is present, accurate staging is not possible until the eschar is removed by debridement. If the pressure ulcer becomes infected, signs of systemic infection, such as leukocytosis and fever, may occur.

Collaborative Care
Care of a patient with a pressure ulcer requires local wound care as well as support measures such as adequate nutrition, pain management, and pressure relief. The current trend is to keep a pressure sore slightly moist, rather than dry, to enhance reepithelialization. Both conservative and surgical strategies are used in the treatment of pressure ulcers, depending on the ulcer's stage and condition.

Nursing Management
Goals
The patient with a pressure ulcer will have no deterioration of the ulcer stage, reduce or eliminate the factors that lead to pressure ulcers, not develop an infection in the pressure ulcer, and have no recurrence.

Table 70	Staging of Pressure Ulcers

Definition/Description
Stage I
  A stage I pressure ulcer is an observable pressure-related
    alteration of intact skin whose indicators, as compared with
    an adjacent or opposite area on the body, may include
    changes in one or more of the following:
      skin temperature (warmth or coolness)
      tissue consistency (firm or boggy feel)
      sensation (pain, itching)
  The ulcer appears as a defined area of persistent redness in
    lightly pigmented skin, whereas in darker skin tones, the ulcer
    may appear with persistent red, blue, or purple hues.
Stage II
  Partial-thickness skin loss involving epidermis, dermis, or both.
    The ulcer is superficial and presents clinically as an abrasion,
    blister, or shallow crater.
Stage III
  Full-thickness skin loss involving damage to or necrosis of
    subcutaneous tissue that may extend down to, but not
    through, underlying fascia. The ulcer presents clinically as a
    deep crater with or without undermining of adjacent tissue.
Stage IV
  Full-thickness skin loss with extensive destruction, tissue necrosis,
    or damage to muscle, bone, or supporting structures (e.g.,
    tendon, joint capsule). Undermining and sinus tracts may also
    be associated with stage IV pressure ulcers.

Source: National Pressure Ulcer Advisory Board. Staging criteria were undergoing final revisions at publication. Check website for National Pressure Ulcer
Advisory Panel Board at *www.npuap.org*.

Nursing Diagnosis
  ■ Impaired skin integrity
Nursing Interventions
Patients should be assessed for pressure ulcer risk initially on
admission and at periodic intervals. Risk assessment should be
done using a validated assessment tool, such as the Braden scale
(see Table 13-12, Lewis and others, *Medical-Surgical Nursing*,
edition 7, p. 208). Prevention remains the best treatment for pressure ulcers.
  ■ Devices such as alternating pressure mattresses, foam mat-
    tresses with adequate stiffness and thickness, wheelchair
    cushions, padded commode seats, foam boots, and lift
    sheets are useful in reducing pressure and shearing force.

However, they are not adequate substitutes for frequent repositioning.

- Once a person has been identified as being at risk for pressure ulcer development, prevention strategies should be implemented. Table 13-15 and NCP 13-1, Lewis and others, *Medical-Surgical Nursing,* edition 7, p. 210, list guidelines for preventing pressure ulcers.

Once a pressure ulcer has developed, the nurse should initiate interventions based on the ulcer's characteristics (e.g., size, stage, location, presence of infection or pain) and the patient's general status. Documentation should be made of the pressure ulcer size.

Local ulcer care may involve debridement, wound cleaning, relief of pressure, and the application of a dressing.

- A pressure ulcer that has necrotic tissue or eschar (except for dry, stable necrotic heels) must have the tissue removed by surgical, mechanical, enzymatic, or autolytic debridement methods. Once the pressure ulcer has been successfully debrided and has a clean granulating base, the goal is to provide an appropriate wound environment that supports moist wound healing and prevents disruption of newly formed granulation tissue.
- Reconstruction of the pressure ulcer site by operative repair, including skin grafting, skin flaps, musculocutaneous flaps, or free flaps, may be necessary.
- Pressure ulcers should be cleaned with noncytotoxic solutions that do not kill or damage cells, such as fibroblasts.
- After the pressure ulcer has been cleansed, it needs to be covered with an appropriate dressing. (Dressings are discussed in Table 13-9, Lewis and others, *Medical-Surgical Nursing,* edition 7, p. 205.)

Maintenance of adequate nutrition is an important nursing responsibility for the patient with a pressure ulcer. Often the patient is debilitated and has a poor appetite secondary to the disease process or other reasons.

- Oral feedings must be adequate in calories, protein, fluids, vitamins, and minerals to meet the patient's nutritional requirements.
- Nasogastric (NG) or gastrostomy feedings can be used to supplement oral feedings. If necessary, parenteral nutrition may be used.

▼ **Patient and Family Teaching**

Because recurrence of pressure ulcers is common, education of both the patient and the care provider in prevention techniques is extremely important (Table 71).

Table 71	Patient and Family Teaching Guide: Pressure Ulcer

1. Identify and explain risk factors and etiology of pressure ulcers to patient and family.
2. Assess all at-risk patients at time of first hospital and/or home visit or whenever the patient's condition changes. Thereafter assess at regular intervals based on care setting (48 hours for acute care or every visit in home care).
3. Teach family care techniques for incontinence. If incontinence occurs, cleanse skin at time of soiling, use topical moisture barriers, and use pads or briefs that are absorbent.
4. Demonstrate correct positioning to decrease risk of skin breakdown. Instruct family to reposition bed-bound patient at least every 2 hours, chair-bound patient every hour. Never position the patient directly on the pressure ulcer.
5. Assess resources (i.e., adequacy of caregiver availability and skill, finances, equipment) of patients requiring pressure ulcer care at home. When selecting ulcer care dressing, consider cost and amount of caregiver time.
6. Teach patient and/or caregiver to use clean dressings over sterile dressings using "no touch" technique when changing dressings. Instruct family on disposal of contaminated dressings.
7. Teach patient and family to inspect skin daily. Assess and document pressure ulcer status at least weekly; may require help from patient and family.
8. Teach patient and family the importance of good nutrition to enhance ulcer healing.
9. Evaluate program effectiveness.

- The care provider needs to know the etiology of pressure ulcers, prevention techniques, early signs, nutritional support, and care techniques for pressure ulcers.
- Because the patient with a pressure ulcer often requires extensive care for other health problems, it is important that the nurse support the care provider.

PROSTATE CANCER

Description
Prostate cancer is the most common form of cancer in men, with one in five men developing prostate cancer at some point in their lives. It is the second leading cause of cancer death in men after

lung cancer. Most cases occur in men older than age 65 years, but many cases occur in younger men, who sometimes have a more aggressive type of cancer. A large increase in incidence of prostate cancer noted between 1988 and 1992 is attributed to the use of prostate-specific antigen (PSA) screening, and the incidence has now leveled off.

Age, ethnicity, and family history are three nonmodifiable risk factors for prostate cancer. Eighty percent of men diagnosed with prostate cancer are older than 65 years.

- African American men have a higher incidence of prostate cancer than any other male group worldwide.
- A history of benign prostatic hyperplasia (BPH) is not a risk factor for prostate cancer.

Pathophysiology

Prostate cancer is an androgen-dependent adenocarcinoma. The tumor usually is slow growing and occurs in the outer portion of the prostate. Tumor spread is by three routes: direct extension, lymphatics, and bloodstream. Spread by direct extension involves the seminal vesicles, urethral mucosa, bladder wall, and external sphincter. Later spread occurs through the lymphatic system to the regional lymph nodes. Venous spread from the prostate involves the pelvic bones, head of the femur, lower lumbar spine, liver, and lungs.

Clinical Manifestations

Prostate cancer is often asymptomatic in the early stages. Eventually the patient may have symptoms similar to those of BPH, including dysuria, hesitancy, dribbling, frequency, urgency, hematuria, nocturia, and retention.

- Pain in the lumbosacral area that radiates down to the hips or legs, when coupled with urinary symptoms, may indicate metastasis. As the cancer spreads to the bones, pain can become severe, especially in the back and legs because of spinal cord compression and bone destruction.

Diagnostic Studies

- In a digital rectal examination (DRE) of the prostate gland, it may feel hard, nodular, and asymmetric.
- Elevated levels of prostate specific antigen (PSA) are indicative of prostatic pathologic conditions, but not necessarily prostate cancer.
- Elevated prostatic acid phosphatase (PAP) levels are specific for prostate cancer.
- Transrectal ultrasonography scan allows visualization of the prostate gland.

- Biopsy of the prostate gland is done when a suspicious lesion is noted.
- Computed tomography (CT) scan, bone scan, or magnetic resonance imaging (MRI) can assess cancer spread.
- Elevated serum alkaline phosphatase may indicate bone metastasis.

Collaborative Care

The management of prostate cancer depends on the stage and grade of the cancer. Prostate cancer is staged on the basis of tumor growth and spread (Whitmore-Jewett stages A to D) and graded on tumor histology. The 5-year survival rate with an initial diagnosis at stage A is 100%.

At all stages, there is more than one possible treatment option. The decision of which treatment course to pursue is a joint decision between the patient and the health care provider. Various treatment options are summarized in Table 55-6, Lewis and others, *Medical-Surgical Nursing,* edition 7, p. 1424.

- A conservative approach to slow-growing tumors is "watchful waiting" that involves follow-up with frequent PSA testing and DREs to monitor the progress of the disease. Significant changes in PSA, DRE, or symptoms warrant a reevaluation of treatment options.
- Surgical therapy for patients with a stage A or B tumor involves a radical prostatectomy as the treatment of choice for long-term survival. With radical prostatectomy, the entire prostate gland, seminal vesicles, and part of the bladder neck (ampulla) are removed. A retroperitoneal lymph node dissection is also usually done. The two most common approaches for radical prostatectomy are retropubic (low abdominal incision) and perineal (incision between the scrotum and anus).
- Surgery is usually not considered an option for stage D cancer, except to relieve obstruction, because metastasis outside the prostate has already occurred.

The two major complications following a radical prostatectomy are erectile dysfunction and urinary incontinence.

- A nerve-sparing technique is sometimes used to prevent erectile dysfunction caused by radical prostatectomy. This surgery is the preferred choice for most men undergoing prostatectomy in the early stage of disease with cancer confined to the prostate gland. The degree of success varies.
- In advanced cases of prostate cancer, surgical removal of the prostate followed by an orchiectomy (removal of the testes) eliminates the source of 90% of circulating andro-

gens. Orchiectomy often provides rapid relief of bone pain and may induce sufficient shrinkage of the prostate to relieve urinary obstruction in the later stages of disease when surgery is not an option.

- Cryosurgery, which destroys cancer cells by freezing, may be used. The treatment takes about 2 hours, with the patient under general or spinal anesthesia.
- Radiation therapy is a common option for prostate cancer, especially for men older than 70 years, patients who are poor surgical risks, or those who wish to avoid surgery. External beam radiation is the most widely used method. Brachytherapy using radioactive seed implants placed in the prostate gland is best suited for patients with stage A or B prostate cancer. Radiation therapy may be offered as the only treatment, or it may be offered in combination with surgery or with hormonal therapy.
- Chemotherapy is generally reserved for late-stage disease and has not been shown to improve survival. The goal of chemotherapy is palliation.

Prostate cancer growth is largely dependent on the presence of androgens. Therefore androgen deprivation is a primary therapeutic approach. Hormone therapy focuses on reducing the levels of circulating androgens to reduce tumor growth.

- Luteinizing hormone–releasing hormone (LHRH) agonists (e.g., leuprolide [Lupron, Eligard, Viadur], goserelin [Zoladex], triptorelin [Trelstar]) produce a chemical castration similar to the effects of an orchiectomy.
- Androgen receptor blockers (e.g., flutamide [Eulexin], nilutamide [Nilandron], bicalutamide [Casodex]) compete with circulating androgens at the receptor sites and can be used in combination with goserelin or leuprolide.
- Estrogen has been used as a form of androgen deprivation therapy but is declining in popularity because of development of more effective hormone therapies.

Nursing Management
Goals
The patient with prostate cancer will be an active participant in the treatment plan, have satisfactory pain control, follow the therapeutic plan, understand the effect of the therapeutic plan on sexual function, and find a satisfactory way to manage the impact on bladder or bowel function.
Nursing Diagnoses
- Decisional conflict
- Acute pain

- Urinary retention
- Impaired urinary elimination
- Constipation or diarrhea
- Sexual dysfunction
- Anxiety

Nursing Interventions

One of the most important roles for nurses in relation to prostate cancer is to encourage patients to have an annual prostate screening (PSA and DRE) starting at the age of 50 years or younger if risk factors are present.

- The nurse needs to provide psychologic support for the patient and the family to help them cope with the cancer diagnosis and decisions regarding treatment choices.
- Preoperative and postoperative phases of therapy are the same as for open prostatectomy (see Benign Prostatic Hyperplasia, p. 67).
- Pain control is the primary nursing intervention for the terminally ill patient.
- In advanced prostate cancer, hospice care is often appropriate and beneficial to the patient and family. (Hospice care is discussed in Chapter 11, Lewis and others, *Medical-Surgical Nursing,* edition 7.)

▼ **Patient and Family Teaching**

If the patient is discharged with an indwelling catheter in place, the nurse must teach appropriate catheter care.

- The patient should be instructed to clean the urethral meatus with soap and water once each day; maintain a high fluid intake; keep the collecting bag lower than the bladder at all times; keep the catheter securely anchored to the inner thigh or abdomen; and report any signs of bladder infection, such as bladder spasms, fever, or hematuria.
- If urinary incontinence is a problem, the patient should be encouraged to practice pelvic floor muscle exercises (Kegel) at every urination and throughout the day. Continuous practice during the 4- to 6-week healing process improves the success rate.

PULMONARY EMBOLISM

Description

Pulmonary embolism (PE) is blockage of pulmonary arteries by a thrombus, fat, or air embolus or tumor tissue. Pulmonary embolism is one of the most common causes of preventable death in hospitalized patients. It is estimated to cause more than 200,000 deaths annually in the United States.

The most common risk factors for PE are immobilization, surgery within the last 3 months, stroke, history of DVT, and malignancy. An increased risk in women is also associated with obesity, cigarette smoking, and hypertension.

Pathophysiology

Most PEs arise from thrombi in the deep leg veins. Other sites of origin include the right side of the heart (especially with atrial fibrillation), upper extremities (rare), and the pelvic veins (especially after surgery or childbirth). Lethal pulmonary emboli originate most commonly in the femoral or iliac veins. *Emboli* are mobile clots that generally do not stop moving until they lodge at a narrowed part of the circulatory system.The lungs are an ideal location for emboli to lodge because of their extensive arterial and capillary network. The lower lobes are most frequently affected because they have a higher blood flow than other lobes. The presence of deep venous thrombosis (DVT) is often unsuspected until a PE occurs.

- Thrombi in the deep veins can dislodge spontaneously. However, a more common mechanism is jarring of the thrombus by mechanical forces, such as sudden standing, and changes in the rate of blood flow, such as those that occur with the Valsalva maneuver.

Clinical Manifestations

The severity of manifestations depends on the size of the emboli and the size and number of blood vessels occluded. The most common manifestations are anxiety and the sudden onset of unexplained dyspnea, tachypnea, and tachycardia. A classic triad of dyspnea, pleuritic chest pain, and hemoptysis occurs in only about 20% of patients.

- Other signs are cough, chest pain, crackles, fever, accentuation of the pulmonic heart sound, and a sudden change in mental status resulting from hypoxemia.

Massive emboli may produce a sudden collapse of the patient with shock, pallor, severe dyspnea, and crushing chest pain. However, some people with massive PE do not have pain. The pulse is rapid and weak, the blood pressure (BP) is low, and an electrocardiogram (ECG) indicates right ventricular strain. When rapid obstruction of 50% or more of the pulmonary vascular bed occurs, acute cor pulmonale may result because the right ventricle can no longer pump blood into the lungs. The mortality rate of those with massive PE and shock is approximately 33%.

Medium-sized emboli often cause pleuritic chest pain accompanied by dyspnea, slight fever, and a productive cough with blood-streaked sputum. A physical examination may indicate tachycardia and a pleural friction rub.

Small emboli frequently go undetected or produce vague, transient symptoms. The exception to this is the patient with underlying cardiopulmonary disease, in whom even small or medium-sized emboli may result in severe cardiopulmonary compromise.

Complications

Pulmonary infarction (death of lung tissue) is most likely when (1) the occlusion is of a large or medium-sized pulmonary vessel (>2 mm in diameter), (2) insufficient collateral blood flows from the bronchial circulation, or (3) preexisting lung disease is present. Infarction results in alveolar necrosis and hemorrhage. Concomitant pleural effusion is frequently found.

Pulmonary hypertension occurs when more than 50% of the cross-sectional area of the normal pulmonary bed is compromised. Pulmonary hypertension also results from hypoxemia. As a single event an embolus does not cause pulmonary hypertension unless it is massive. However, recurrent small to medium-sized emboli may result in chronic pulmonary hypertension. Pulmonary hypertension eventually results in dilation and hypertrophy of the right ventricle. Depending on the degree of pulmonary hypertension and its rate of development, outcomes can vary, with some patients dying within months of the diagnosis and others living for decades (see Pulmonary Hypertension, p. 521).

Diagnostic Studies

- Ventilation-perfusion lung scan is the most frequently used test for PE.
- Plasma D-dimer testing screens for an embolism.
- Spiral (or helical) computed tomography (CT) scan can diagnose embolism.
- Pulmonary angiography is a definitive test for embolism.
- Venous ultrasound can detect DVT as the source of PE.
- Arterial blood gases (ABGs) are abnormal with pulmonary occlusion but are not diagnostic of PE.

Collaborative Care

Objectives of treatment are to (1) prevent further growth or multiplication of thrombi in the lower extremities, (2) prevent embolization from the upper or lower extremities to the pulmonary vascular system, and (3) provide cardiopulmonary support if indicated. Supportive therapy for the patient's cardiopulmonary status varies according to the severity of the pulmonary embolism.

- Administration of oxygen (O_2) by mask or cannula may be adequate for some patients. O_2 is given in a concentration determined by ABG analysis. In some situations, endotracheal intubation and mechanical ventilation may be needed to maintain adequate oxygenation.
- Respiratory measures such as turning, coughing, and deep breathing are important to prevent or treat atelectasis.
- If shock is present, vasopressor agents may be necessary to support systemic circulation. If heart failure is present, digitalis and diuretics are used.

Pain resulting from pleural irritation or reduced coronary blood flow is treated with opioids, usually morphine. Properly managed anticoagulant therapy is effective for many patients. Low-molecular-weight heparin (e.g., enoxaparin [Lovenox], dalteparin [Fragmin]), and warfarin (Coumadin) are the drugs of choice. Heparin should be started immediately and is continued while warfarin is initiated. Warfarin is usually administered for 3 to 6 months. Anticoagulant therapy may not be indicated in the presence of blood dyscrasias, hepatic dysfunction causing an alteration in the clotting mechanism, overt bleeding, a history of hemorrhagic stroke, or neurologic conditions. Fibrinolytic agents, such as tissue plasminogen activator (tPA [Activase]), may be used to dissolve the PE as well as the thrombus source.

If the degree of pulmonary arterial obstruction is severe (usually >50%) and the patient does not respond to conservative therapy, an immediate embolectomy may be indicated. This is a rarely performed procedure that has a 50% mortality rate.

- To prevent further pulmonary embolization, an inferior vena cava (IVC) filter may be surgically placed in the vena cava to prevent migration of large clots from the lower extremities into the pulmonary system. It can be used for patients with absolute contraindications to anticoagulant therapy or for patients at high risk for PE (see Venous Thrombosis, p. 680).

Nursing Management

Nursing measures aimed at prevention of pulmonary embolism parallel those for the prevention of venous thrombosis (see Venous Thrombosis, p. 680).

The prognosis of a patient with pulmonary emboli is good if therapy is promptly instituted. The patient should be kept in bed in a semi-Fowler's position to facilitate breathing. An intravenous (IV) line should be maintained for medications and fluid therapy. O_2 therapy should be administered as ordered. Careful monitoring of vital signs, electrocardiogram (ECG), blood gases, and lung sounds is critical to assess the patient's status.

- The patient is usually anxious because of pain, an inability to breathe, and a fear of death. The nurse carefully explains the situation and provides emotional support and reassurance to help relieve the patient's anxiety. During the acute phase someone should be with the patient as much as possible.

In addition to thromboembolic problems, the patient may have an underlying chronic illness requiring long-term treatment. To provide supportive therapy, the nurse must understand and differentiate between the various problems caused by the underlying disease and those related to thromboembolic disease.

▼ **Patient and Family Teaching**

- Long-term management is similar to that for the patient with venous thrombosis (see p. 684).
- Patient teaching regarding long-term anticoagulant therapy is critical. The anticoagulant therapy continues for at least 3 to 6 months; patients with recurrent emboli are treated indefinitely. Follow-up appointments at a nurse-managed or pharmacist-managed anticoagulation clinic are often used to monitor medication and adjust dosages.
- Discharge planning is aimed at limiting the progression of the condition and preventing complications. The nurse must reinforce the need for the patient to return to the health care facility for regular follow-up examinations.

PULMONARY HYPERTENSION

Description

Pulmonary hypertension can occur as a primary disease *(primary pulmonary hypertension [PPH])* or as a secondary complication of a respiratory, cardiac, autoimmune, or hepatic disorder *(secondary pulmonary hypertension)*. Pulmonary hypertension is elevated pulmonary pressures caused by an increase in pulmonary vascular resistance to blood flow.

Primary Pulmonary Hypertension

PPH is a rare, potentially fatal disease whose exact cause is unknown. It is characterized by mean pulmonary arterial pressure above 25 mm Hg at rest (normal 12 to 16 mm Hg) or above 30 mm Hg with exercise in the absence of a demonstrable cause. PPH

affects more women than men, and it may have a genetic component because the incidence is higher in families. The mean age
is 36 years.

Pathophysiology
PPH has been linked to the use of fenfluramine in the drug
Fen-Phen that was used as an appetite suppressant to treat obesity.
The drug was withdrawn from the market in 1996.
- Normally the pulmonary circulation is characterized by low
  resistance and low pressure. In pulmonary hypertension the
  pulmonary pressures are elevated.
- A key mechanism involved in PPH is a deficient release of
  vasodilator mediators from the pulmonary epithelium with
  a resultant cascade of injury.
- Vasoconstriction, remodeling of the walls of the pulmonary
  vessels, and thrombosis in situ are the three elements that
  combine to increase vascular resistance.

Clinical Manifestations
Classic symptoms are dyspnea on exertion and fatigue. Exertional
chest pain, dizziness, and exertional syncope are other symptoms.
Eventually, as the disease progresses, dyspnea occurs at rest.
Pulmonary hypertension increases the workload of the right ventricle and causes right ventricular hypertrophy (a condition called
cor pulmonale) and eventually heart failure (see Cor Pulmonale,
p. 149).
   PPH is a diagnosis of exclusion, and evaluation includes electrocardiogram (ECG), chest x-ray, echocardiogram, and spiral
computed tomography (CT). Cardiac catheterization is done to
measure pulmonary artery pressures and cardiac output.
- Chest x-ray generally shows enlarged central pulmonary
  arteries and clear lung fields. An enlarged right heart may
  be seen.
- Echocardiogram usually reveals right ventricular
  hypertrophy.

Collaborative Care
Although there is no cure for PPH, treatment can relieve symptoms, increase quality of life, and prolong life.
- Diuretic therapy relieves dyspnea and peripheral edema and
  may be useful in reducing right ventricular volume
  overload.
- Anticoagulation therapy is recommended for patients
  with severe pulmonary hypertension to prevent thrombus
  formation.

- Hypoxia is a potent pulmonary vasoconstrictor, and use of low-flow oxygen provides symptomatic relief.
- Vasodilator therapy is used to reduce right ventricular overload by dilating pulmonary vessels. Some patients with pulmonary hypertension can be effectively managed with calcium channel blocker therapy.

Epoprostenol (Flolan), a prostacyclin that promotes pulmonary vasodilation and reduces pulmonary vascular resistance, has revolutionized PPH management. It is now the treatment of choice for selected patients unresponsive to calcium channel blockers. Its administration requires the placement of an indwelling central line catheter and continuous infusion pump. If the central line is disrupted, stopped, or dislodged for any reason, clinical deterioration can occur within minutes. With careful teaching and training of the patient and family, epoprostenol has been successful in improving the quality of life of patients with PPH.

Other prostacyclin preparations are possible alternatives to epoprostenol:

- Treprostinil (Remodulin) is used as a continuous subcutaneous injection and has been recently approved for continuous intravenous use.
- Bosentan (Tracleer) is a form of prostacyclin and the only oral vasodilator currently approved for the treatment of pulmonary hypertension.

Lung transplantation is recommended for those patients who do not respond to drug therapy and progress to severe right-sided heart failure. Recurrence of the disease has not been reported in individuals who have undergone transplantation.

- A patient education and support site for pulmonary hypertension is located at *www.phassociation.org*.

Secondary Pulmonary Hypertension

Secondary pulmonary hypertension (SPH) occurs when a primary disease causes a chronic increase in pulmonary artery pressures. The disease pathology may result in anatomic or vascular changes causing pulmonary hypertension.

Anatomic changes causing increased vascular resistance include loss of capillaries as a result of alveolar wall damage (e.g., chronic obstructive pulmonary disease [COPD]), stiffening pulmonary vasculature (e.g., pulmonary fibrosis connective tissue disorders), and obstruction of blood flow (chronic emboli).

Vasomotor increases in pulmonary vascular resistance are found in conditions characterized by alveolar hypoxia. Hypoxia causes localized vasoconstriction and shunting of blood away from poorly ventilated alveoli.

- It is possible to have a combination of anatomic restriction
  and vasomotor constriction. This is found in the patient with
  long-standing chronic bronchitis who has chronic hypoxia
  in addition to loss of lung tissue.

Symptoms and diagnosis of SPH are similar to PPH, but some
symptoms of SPH are directly attributable to the underlying diseases of COPD, pulmonary fibrosis, or chronic pulmonary emboli.

- Treatment of SPH consists mainly of treating the underlying
  primary disorder. When irreversible pulmonary vascular
  damage has occurred, therapies used for PPH are initiated.

PYELONEPHRITIS

Description

Pyelonephritis is an acute or chronic inflammation of the renal
parenchyma and the collecting system (including the renal pelvis).
Urosepsis is a systemic infection arising from a urologic source.
Its prompt diagnosis and effective treatment are critical because
it can lead to septic shock, the outcome of unresolved bacteremia
involving a gram-negative organism (see Shock, p. 565).

Pathophysiology

Pyelonephritis usually begins with colonization and infection of
the lower urinary tract by way of the ascending urethral route.
Bacteria normally found in the intestinal tract, such as *Escherichia
coli,* frequently cause pyelonephritis.

A preexisting factor is often present, such as *vesicoureteral
reflux* (retrograde or backward movement of urine from lower to
upper urinary tract) or dysfunction of lower urinary tract function,
such as obstruction from benign prostatic hyperplasia or a urinary
stone. In residents of long-term care facilities, urinary tract
catheterization and the use of indwelling catheters are common
causes of pyelonephritis.

Acute pyelonephritis commonly starts in the renal medulla and
spreads to the adjacent cortex. Recurring episodes of pyelonephritis, especially in the presence of obstructive abnormalities, can
lead to scarred, poorly functioning kidneys and a condition called
chronic pyelonephritis.

Chronic pyelonephritis may also occur in the absence of an
existing infection, recent infection, or history of urinary tract
infections (UTIs). It often progresses to end-stage renal disease
when both kidneys are involved, even if the underlying infection

or problem is successfully eradicated (see Kidney Disease, Chronic, p. 372).

Clinical Manifestations

Acute pyelonephritis manifestations vary from mild fatigue to the sudden onset of chills, fever, vomiting, malaise, flank pain, and costovertebral tenderness on the affected side. Dysuria, urinary urgency, and frequency that are characteristic of bladder infections may also be present.

Acute manifestations generally subside within a few days even without specific therapy, although bacteriuria or pyuria usually persists.

Diagnostic Studies

- Urinalysis for culture, sensitivity, and Gram stain
- Urinalysis also to detect pyuria, bacteriuria, hematuria, and white blood cell (WBC) casts
- Complete blood cell (CBC) count with WBC differential to identify leukocytosis
- Blood culture if bacteremia or urosepsis suspected
- Intravenous pyelogram (IVP) and computed tomography (CT) not recommended in early stages to prevent spread of infection
- Ultrasound to identify anatomic abnormalities, hydrone-phrosis, renal abscesses, or stones

Chronic pyelonephritis is diagnosed by radiologic and histologic testing rather than clinical features. Pathologic analysis reveals loss of functioning nephrons, infiltration of the parenchyma with inflammatory cells, and fibrosis.

Collaborative Care

Patients with severe infections or complicating factors such as nausea and vomiting with dehydration require hospital admission. Parenteral antibiotics are often given initially in the hospital to rapidly establish high serum and urinary drug levels.

The patient with mild symptoms may be treated as an outpatient with antibiotics for 14 to 21 days. Symptoms and signs typically improve or resolve within 48 to 72 hours after starting therapy. Relapses may be treated with a 6-week course of antibiotics. Antibiotic prophylaxis may also be used for recurrent infections.

Nursing Management

Goals

The patient with pyelonephritis will have normal renal function, normal body temperature, no complications, relief of pain, and no recurrence of symptoms.

See NCP 46-1 for the patient with a UTI, Lewis and others, *Medical-Surgical Nursing,* edition 7, p. 1160.

Nursing Diagnoses/Collaborative Problem

- Impaired urinary elimination
- Ineffective therapeutic regimen management
- Potential complication: urosepsis

Nursing Interventions

Because the patient with structural abnormalities of the urinary tract is at increased risk for infection, the need for regular medical care should be stressed.

- Instruct the patient regarding the need to continue medications as prescribed and the need for follow-up urine cultures to ensure proper management and identification of recurrence of infection or relapse.
- In addition to antibiotic therapy, the patient should be encouraged to drink at least eight glasses of fluid every day even after the infection has been treated.
- Rest is often indicated to increase patient comfort.
- The patient with frequent relapses or reinfections may be treated with long-term, low-dose antibiotics. Understanding the rationale for therapy is important to enhance patient compliance.

RAYNAUD'S PHENOMENON

Description

Raynaud's phenomenon is an episodic vasospastic disorder of the small cutaneous arteries, most frequently involving the fingers and toes. The condition occurs primarily in young women; the exact etiology is unknown. It may occur secondary to an exaggerated response to sympathetic nervous system stimulation. Other contributing factors include occupationally related trauma and pressure to fingertips as noted in typists, pianists, and those who use hand-held vibrating equipment. Exposure to heavy metals may also be a contributing etiologic factor. Symptoms are usually precipitated by exposure to cold, emotional upsets, caffeine, and tobacco use.

Clinical Manifestations

- The disorder is characterized by vasospasm-induced color changes (white, red, and blue) of the fingers, toes, ears, and nose. Decreased perfusion as a result of arteriole vasospasm produces pallor (white), followed by cyanosis (bluish purple).

These changes are subsequently followed by rubor or hyperemia.

- The patient usually describes cold and numbness in the vaso-constrictive phase, with throbbing and aching pain, tingling, and swelling in the hyperemic phase. This type of episode usually lasts only minutes, but in severe cases it may persist for several hours.
- Complications from severe cases include punctate (small hole) lesions of the fingertips and superficial gangrenous ulcers in advanced stages.

Nursing and Collaborative Management

There is no simple diagnostic test for Raynaud's phenomenon. If symptoms persist for at least 2 years in the absence of an associated underlying disorder, a diagnosis of primary *Raynaud's disease* is made. In contrast, if symptoms exist in conjunction with a connective tissue or autoimmune disease, the diagnosis of *secondary Raynaud's phenomenon* is made. Because Raynaud's phenomenon can be associated with rheumatic disorders, routine follow-up is advised.

Calcium channel blockers (e.g., nifedipine [Procardia], diltiazem [Cardizem]) are the first-line drug therapy when other therapies are ineffective. Sympathectomy is considered only in advanced cases.

▼ Patient and Family Teaching

Teaching should be directed toward prevention of recurrent episodes.

- Loose, warm clothing should be worn for protection from cold, including gloves when the refrigerator-freezer is used or when cold objects are being handled.
- Temperature extremes should be avoided. Immersing hands in warm water often decreases the spasm.
- Patients should stop using all tobacco products and avoid caffeine and other drugs with vasoconstrictive effects.
- Biofeedback, relaxation training, and stress management are effective for some patients whose symptoms are exacerbated by stress.

REACTIVE ARTHRITIS

Reactive arthritis (*Reiter's syndrome*) is associated with a symptom complex that includes urethritis or cervicitis, conjunctivitis, and mucocutaneous lesions. It occurs more commonly in young men as compared with young women. Although the exact etiology is unknown, reactive arthritis appears to occur after a genitourinary or gastrointestinal tract infection. *Chlamydia trachomatis* is most often implicated in sexually transmitted reactive arthritis. Men and women appear to have equal risk for developing dysenteric reactive arthritis, which typically occurs within days or weeks after infection with *Shigella, Salmonella, Campylobacter,* or *Yersinia.* A genetic predisposition is suggested in that individuals with inherited HLA-B27 are at increased risk of developing reactive arthritis after contact or exposure to certain enteric pathogens.

- Urethritis develops within 1 to 2 weeks after sexual contact or dysentery. Low-grade fever, conjunctivitis, and arthritis may occur over the next several weeks.
- This arthritis tends to be asymmetric, frequently involving large joints of the lower extremities and toes. Lower back pain may occur with severe disease.
- Mucocutaneous lesions commonly occur as small, painless, superficial ulcerations on the tongue, oral mucosa, and glans penis. Soft tissue manifestations commonly affect tendons and ligaments.
- Few laboratory abnormalities occur, although the erythrocyte sedimentation rate (ESR) may be elevated.

Prognosis is favorable, with most patients recovering after 2 to 16 weeks. Because reactive arthritis is often associated with *Chlamydia trachomatis* infection, treatment of patients and their sexual partners with doxycycline (Vibramycin) is widely recommended.

Joints heal completely, and many patients have complete remission with full joint function. Up to 50% may develop chronic or recurring disease, which can result in major disability. Treatment of chronic reactive arthritis is symptomatic.

REFRACTIVE ERRORS

Refractive errors are the most common visual problem. This defect in vision prevents light rays from converging into a single focus on the retina. Defects are due to corneal curvature irregularities, lens-focusing power, or eye length.

Types of refractive errors include the following:

- *Myopia* (nearsightedness), the most common refractive error, is caused by light rays focusing in front of the retina, resulting in an inability to accommodate for objects at a distance.

- *Hyperopia* (farsightedness) is caused by light rays focusing behind the retina and requires the person to use accommodation to focus the light rays on the retina for near and far objects.
- *Presbyopia* is a loss of accommodation resulting from age, with the crystalline lens becoming larger, firmer, and less elastic. This condition generally appears about the age of 45 years and results in an inability to accommodate for near objects.
- *Astigmatism* is caused by an irregular corneal curvature so that incoming light rays are bent unequally and light rays do not come to a single point of focus on the retina.
- *Aphakia* is the absence of the crystalline lens resulting from a congenital defect or cataract extraction surgery.
- The major symptom of refractive errors is blurred vision. Additional complaints may include ocular discomfort, eye strain, or headaches.
- Management of refractive errors is correction, which may include eyeglasses, contact lenses, refractive surgery, or surgical implantation of an artificial lens to improve the focus of light rays on the retina.

RENAL FAILURE, ACUTE

Description

Renal failure is a partial or complete impairment of kidney function. Renal failure is classified as acute or chronic. Acute renal failure (ARF) has a rapid onset. In contrast, chronic kidney disease (CKD) usually develops slowly over months to years.

- ARF is a clinical syndrome characterized by a rapid loss of renal function with progressive *azotemia* (an accumulation of nitrogenous waste products such as blood urea nitrogen [BUN]) and increasing levels of serum creatinine. *Uremia* is the condition in which renal function declines to the point that symptoms develop in multiple body systems.
- ARF is often associated with *oliguria* (<400 ml of urine in 24 hours), although it is possible to have normal or increased urinary output.
- ARF usually develops over hours or days. It most commonly follows severe, prolonged hypotension, hypovolemia, or exposure to a nephrotoxic agent.

Pathophysiology

ARF is categorized according to pathogenesis into prerenal, intrarenal (or intrinsic), and postrenal causes.

- *Prerenal* ARF is due to factors external to the kidneys that reduce renal blood flow and lead to decreased glomerular perfusion and filtration. Prerenal causes are the most common, accounting for 60% to 70% of all cases of ARF. Examples include hypovolemia, decreased cardiac output (CO), decreased peripheral vascular resistance, and vascular obstruction. Prerenal disease can lead to intrarenal disease (acute tubular necrosis) if renal ischemia is prolonged.

- *Intrarenal* causes include conditions that cause direct damage to the renal tissue (parenchyma), resulting in impaired nephron function. Primary renal diseases such as systemic lupus erythematosus and acute pyelonephritis may also cause ARF. Intrarenal ARF is usually due to prolonged ischemia, nephrotoxins (e.g., antibiotics), myoglobin released from necrotic muscle cells, or hemoglobin released from hemolyzed red blood cells (RBCs). Acute tubular necrosis (ATN) is a type of intrarenal ARF resulting from ischemia and nephrotoxins.

- *Postrenal* causes involve a mechanical obstruction of urinary outflow. As the flow of urine is obstructed, urine refluxes into the renal pelvis, impairing kidney function. The most common causes are prostate cancer, benign prostatic hyperplasia (BPH), urinary tract calculi, trauma, and extrarenal tumors. Postrenal ARF is almost always treatable if identified before permanent kidney damage occurs.

Clinical Manifestations

Acute renal failure may progress through four phases: initiating, oliguric, diuretic, and recovery. In some situations the patient does not recover from ARF, and CKD results (see Kidney Disease, Chronic, p. 372).

The *initiating phase* begins at the time of the insult and continues until the signs and symptoms become apparent. It can last hours to days.

The *oliguric phase* reflects a reduction in the glomerular filtration rate (GFR) that causes oliguria. Oliguria resulting from prerenal causes reflects compensatory mechanisms (e.g., activation of renin-angiotensin-aldosterone system, norepinephrine and antidiuretic hormone secretion) and is usually reversible. Oliguria resulting from intrarenal causes reflects injured tubules that cannot respond to compensatory mechanisms. The oliguric phase usually occurs within 1 to 7 days of the causative event and lasts an average of 10 to 14 days. The longer the oliguric phase lasts, the poorer the prognosis for recovery of complete renal function.

- In addition to oliguria, other urinary changes include bloody urine with casts, RBCs, white blood cells (WBCs), a specific gravity fixed at around 1.010, and urine osmolality around 300 mOsm/kg (300 mmol/kg). This is the same specific gravity and osmolality as plasma.
- Fluid retention occurs as urinary output decreases; neck veins become distended with a bounding pulse, and edema and hypertension may develop. Fluid overload can lead to heart failure (HF), pulmonary edema, and pericardial and pleural effusions.
- Metabolic acidosis results when the kidneys cannot synthesize ammonia, which is needed for excretion of hydrogen (H^+). The patient may develop Kussmaul (rapid, deep) respirations to increase the excretion of carbon dioxide (CO_2).
- Serum sodium and potassium levels are altered. Damaged tubules cannot conserve sodium; urinary excretion of sodium may increase, resulting in decreased serum sodium. Serum potassium levels may exceed 6.0 mEq/L (6 mmol/L) because the kidneys cannot excrete potassium. Treatment must be initiated immediately if cardiac dysrhythmias are identified.
- Anemia occurs because renal failure results in impaired erythropoietin production. Platelet abnormalities can lead to bleeding from multiple sources (gastrointestinal [GI] tract, brain). WBCs are also altered, causing immunodeficiency.
- Calcium deficit and phosphate excess occur as the kidneys are unable to activate vitamin D for calcium absorption from the bowel and are unable to excrete phosphate.
- Neurologic changes can occur as nitrogenous waste products accumulate in the brain and other nervous tissue. Symptoms can be as mild as fatigue and difficulty concentrating and can escalate to seizures, stupor, and coma.

The *diuretic phase* begins with a gradual increase in urine output of 1 to 3 L/day but may reach 3 to 5 L/day or more. In this phase the kidneys have recovered their ability to excrete wastes but not to concentrate urine. Uremia may still be severe.

- The diuretic phase may last 1 to 3 weeks, with the patient's acid-base, electrolyte, and waste product values beginning to normalize. Because of large losses of fluid and electrolytes, the patient must be monitored for hypovolemia, hypotension, hyponatremia, and hypokalemia.

The *recovery phase* begins when the GFR increases, allowing the BUN and serum creatinine levels to plateau and then decrease. Although major improvements occur in the first 1 to 2 weeks of this phase, renal function may take up to 12 months to stabilize.

- The outcome of ARF is influenced by the patient's overall health, the severity of renal failure, and the number and type of complications. Some patients do not recover and progress to CKD. Of those who recover, the majority achieve clinically normal kidney function with no complications.

Diagnostic Studies

- History is essential for determining the etiology.
- Serum creatinine and BUN levels are elevated initially.
- Serum electrolytes, especially K^+, are altered.
- Urine osmolality, sodium content, and specific gravity help to differentiate the three different types of ARF. Urinalysis is also done to assess sediment, casts, hematuria, pyuria, and crystals.
- Retrograde pyelogram, renal scan, and ultrasound are done to assess renal blood flow and integrity of the collecting system.
- Computed tomography (CT) scan or magnetic resonance imaging (MRI) can identify masses and vascular abnormalities.

Collaborative Care

Because ARF is potentially reversible, the primary goals of treatment are to eliminate the cause, manage the signs and symptoms, and prevent complications while the kidneys recover. The first step is to determine if there is adequate intravascular volume and CO to ensure adequate perfusion of the kidneys. Diuretic therapy is often administered along with volume expanders to prevent fluid overload. If ARF is already established, forcing fluids and diuretics is not effective and may, in fact, be harmful. Conservative therapy may be all that is necessary until renal function improves.

- Fluid intake must be closely monitored during the oliguric phase.
- Hyperkalemia is one of the most serious complications because it can cause cardiac dysrhythmias. Both insulin and sodium bicarbonate temporarily shift potassium into the cells, but it eventually shifts back out. Calcium gluconate raises the threshold at which dysrhythmias occur. Only sodium polystyrene sulfonate (Kayexalate) and dialysis actually remove potassium from the body.

The general trend in management of ARF is to initiate early and frequent dialysis to minimize symptoms and prevent complications. Continuous renal replacement therapy is technically similar to hemodialysis but provides a more gradual removal of excess

fluid and solutes. It is the preferred treatment in the hemodynamically unstable patient with mild to moderate ARF with fluid
overload.

Nutritional Therapy. The challenge of nutritional management is
to provide adequate calories to prevent catabolism despite the
restrictions required to prevent electrolyte and fluid disorders and
azotemia. Adequate energy should be primarily from carbohydrate and fat sources to prevent ketosis from endogenous fat breakdown and gluconeogenesis from muscle protein breakdown.

- Daily caloric intake should be about 30 to 35 kcal/kg. Protein
  intake is adjusted according to the patient's condition but is
  generally 0.6 g/kg/day to control nitrogenous waste production. Essential amino acid supplements (e.g., Amin-Aid) can
  be given for amino acid and caloric supplementation.
- Potassium (K^+) and sodium (Na^+) are regulated in accordance with plasma levels. Na^+ is restricted as needed to
  prevent edema, hypertension, and heart failure. Potassium
  is also restricted.
- Intralipid (fat emulsions) infusions can also be given as a
  nutritional supplement and provide a good source of non-
  protein calories.

When the GI tract is not functional, parenteral nutrition is necessary for the provision of adequate nutrition (see Parenteral
Nutrition, p. 743).

Nursing Management

Goals
The patient with ARF will completely recover without any loss of
kidney function, be maintained in normal fluid and electrolyte
balance, have decreased anxiety, and comply with and understand
the need for careful follow-up monitoring.

Nursing Diagnoses/Collaborative Problems
- Excess fluid volume
- Risk for infection
- Imbalanced nutrition: less than body requirements
- Disturbed thought processes
- Fatigue
- Anxiety
- Potential complication: dysrhythmias
- Potential complication: metabolic acidosis

Nursing Interventions
Prevention of ARF is essential because of the high mortality rate
and is primarily directed toward (1) identifying and monitoring
high-risk populations, (2) controlling exposure to industrial chemicals and nephrotoxic drugs, and (3) preventing prolonged epi-

sodes of hypotension and hypovolemia. In the hospital the factors that increase the risk for developing ARF are advanced age, massive trauma, extensive burns, cardiac failure, obstetric complications, or the presence of renal insufficiency resulting from hypertension or diabetes mellitus.

- Patients must be monitored carefully for intake and output, as well as for fluid and electrolyte balance. Extrarenal losses of fluid from vomiting, diarrhea, and hemorrhage must be assessed and recorded.
- Prompt replacement of significant fluid losses helps prevent ischemic tubular damage associated with trauma, burns, and extensive surgery. Intake and output records and the patient's weight provide valuable indicators of fluid volume status.
- Aggressive diuretic therapy for the patient with fluid overload resulting from any cause can lead to inadequate renal vascular perfusion.
- Streptococcal infections must be identified and treated. Compliance with the antibiotic regimen is critical to eliminate the source of infection and prevent complications such as acute poststreptococcal glomerulonephritis and rheumatic heart disease.
- The individual who is taking drugs that are potentially nephrotoxic must have renal function monitored. Nephrotoxic medications should be used sparingly in the high-risk patient.
- Patients undergoing diagnostic studies requiring nephrotoxic intravenous contrast media may be pretreated with acetylcysteine (Mucomyst) or sodium bicarbonate to reduce contrast-induced nephropathy.

Acute intervention involves managing the fluid and electrolyte balance during the oliguric and diuretic phases. This includes accurate intake and output records and daily weights.

- The nurse must be knowledgeable about common signs and symptoms of hypervolemia (in the oliguric phase) or hypovolemia (in the diuretic phase), K^+ and Na^+ disturbances, and other electrolyte imbalances that may occur in ARF.
- Because infection is the leading cause of death in ARF, meticulous aseptic technique is critical.
- Respiratory complications, especially pneumonitis, can be prevented. Humidified oxygen (O_2), incentive spirometry; turning, coughing, deep breathing; and ambulation are measures the nurse can use to help the patient maintain adequate respiratory ventilation.
- Skin care and measures to prevent pressure ulcers should be performed because the patient usually develops edema,

as well as a loss of muscle tone. Mouth care is important to prevent stomatitis.

▼ **Patient and Family Teaching**
- Once kidney function has returned, follow-up care and regular evaluation of renal function should be emphasized.
- The patient should be taught the signs and symptoms of recurrent renal disease. Measures to prevent recurrence of ARF must be emphasized.

R

RESPIRATORY FAILURE, ACUTE

Description
The major function of the respiratory system is gas exchange, which involves the transfer of oxygen (O_2) and carbon dioxide (CO_2) between the atmosphere and the blood. Respiratory failure results when one or both of these gas-exchanging functions are inadequate. Respiratory failure is not a disease; it is a condition that occurs as a result of one or more diseases involving the lungs or other body system (Table 72). Respiratory failure can be classified as hypoxemic or hypercapnic.

- *Hypoxemic respiratory failure* is also referred to as oxygenation failure because the primary problem is inadequate O_2 transfer between the alveoli and the pulmonary capillary bed. Although no universal definition exists, hypoxemic respiratory failure is commonly defined as a partial pressure of oxygen in arterial blood (PaO_2) of 60 mm Hg or less when the patient is receiving an inspired O_2 concentration of 60% or greater.
- *Hypercapnic respiratory failure* is also referred to as ventilatory failure because the primary problem is insufficient CO_2 removal. Hypercapnic respiratory failure is commonly defined as a partial pressure of carbon dioxide in arterial blood ($PaCO_2$) above normal (>45 mm Hg) in combination with acidemia (pH < 7.35).

Many patients experience both hypoxemic and hypercapnic respiratory failure.

Pathophysiology
Hypoxemic Respiratory Failure. Common diseases and conditions that cause hypoxemic respiratory failure are listed in Table 72. Four physiologic mechanisms may cause hypoxemia and subsequent hypoxemic respiratory failure: (1) mismatch between ventilation (V) and perfusion (Q) commonly referred to as V/Q

Table 72	Types of Respiratory Failure and Common Causes

Hypoxemic Respiratory Failure*	Hypercapnic Respiratory Failure*
Respiratory System Acute respiratory distress syndrome Pneumonia Toxic inhalation (smoke inhalation) Hepatopulmonary syndrome (low-resistance flow state, V/Q mismatch) Massive pulmonary embolism (e.g., thrombus emboli, fat emboli) Pulmonary artery laceration and hemorrhage **Cardiac System** Anatomic shunt (ventricular septal defect) Cardiogenic pulmonary edema Shock (decreasing blood flow through pulmonary vasculature)	**Respiratory System** Asthma COPD Cystic fibrosis **Central Nervous System** Brainstem infarction Sedative and opioid overdose Spinal cord injury Severe head injury **Chest Wall** Thoracic trauma (e.g., flail chest) Kyphoscoliosis Pain Massive obesity **Neuromuscular System** Myasthenia gravis Critical illness polyneuropathy Acute myopathy Toxic ingestion (e.g., tree tobacco) Amyotrophic lateral sclerosis Phrenic nerve injury Guillain-Barré syndrome Poliomyelitis Muscular dystrophy Multiple sclerosis

COPD, Chronic obstructive pulmonary disease.
* This list is not all inclusive.

mismatch, (2) shunt, (3) diffusion limitation, and (4) hypoventilation. The most common causes are V/Q mismatch and shunt.

- Many diseases and conditions cause *V/Q mismatch.* The most common are those in which increased secretions are present in the airways (e.g., chronic obstructive pulmonary disease [COPD]) or alveoli (e.g., pneumonia) or when bronchospasm is present (e.g., asthma). V/Q mismatch may also result when alveoli collapse (atelectasis) or as a result of pain.

- *Shunt* occurs when blood exits the heart without having participated in gas exchange. A shunt can be viewed as an extreme V/Q mismatch. There are two types of shunt: anatomic and intrapulmonary. O_2 therapy alone may be ineffective in increasing the PaO_2 if hypoxemia is due to shunt because (1) blood passes from the right to the left side of the heart without passing through the lungs (anatomic shunt), or (2) the alveoli are filled with fluid, which prevents gas exchange (intrapulmonary shunt).

- *Diffusion limitation* occurs when a process that thickens or destroys the membrane compromises the gas exchange across the alveolar-capillary membrane. Diffusion limitation may worsen by conditions that affect the pulmonary vascular bed, such as severe emphysema or recurrent pulmonary emboli. Some diseases cause the alveolar-capillary membrane to become thicker (fibrotic), which slows gas transport. These diseases include pulmonary fibrosis, interstitial lung disease, and acute respiratory distress syndrome (ARDS). The classic sign of diffusion limitation is hypoxemia that is present during exercise but not at rest.

- *Alveolar hypoventilation* is a generalized decrease in ventilation that results in an increase in the $PaCO_2$ and a consequent decrease in PaO_2. Alveolar hypoventilation may be the result of restrictive lung disease, central nervous system (CNS) disease, chest wall dysfunction, or neuromuscular disease.

- Frequently, hypoxemic respiratory failure is caused by a combination of V/Q mismatch, shunting, diffusion limitation, and hypoventilation.

Hypercapnic Respiratory Failure. Hypercapnic respiratory failure results from an imbalance between ventilatory supply and ventilatory demand. Normally, ventilatory supply far exceeds ventilatory demand. However, patients with preexisting lung disease such as severe COPD cannot effectively increase lung ventilation in response to exercise or metabolic demands. Hypercapnic respiratory failure is sometimes called ventilatory failure because the primary problem is the inability of the respiratory system to ventilate out sufficient CO_2 to maintain a normal $PaCO_2$.

- Many diseases can cause a limitation in ventilatory supply (see Table 72). They can be grouped into four categories: (1) abnormalities of the airways and alveoli, (2) abnormalities of the CNS, (3) abnormalities of the chest wall, and (4) neuromuscular conditions.

Clinical Manifestations

Respiratory failure may develop suddenly (in minutes or hours) or gradually (taking several days or longer). A sudden decrease in PaO_2 or a rapid rise in $PaCO_2$ implies a serious condition that can rapidly become a life-threatening emergency.

- Manifestations are related to the extent of the change in PaO_2 and $PaCO_2$, the rapidity of change (acute versus chronic), and the ability to compensate to overcome this change. When the patient's compensatory mechanisms fail, respiratory failure occurs. Because manifestations are variable, it is important to monitor arterial blood gas (ABG) values or use pulse oximetry to evaluate the extent of change.

- Mental status changes such as restlessness, confusion, and combative behavior will occur early, frequently before ABG results indicate changes.

- Tachycardia and mild hypertension are also early signs. A severe morning headache may suggest that hypercapnia may have occurred during the night. Rapid shallow breaths suggest that the tidal volume may be inadequate to remove CO_2 from the lungs.

- As the PaO_2 decreases and acidosis increases, the heart may become dysfunctional, resulting in decreased cardiac output and dysrhythmias. Permanent brain damage may occur because of O_2 deprivation. Renal function may be impaired, and sodium (Na^+) retention, edema formation, acute tubular necrosis, and uremia may result.

- The patient may have a rapid, shallow breathing pattern or a respiratory rate that is slower than normal. A change from a rapid to a slower rate in a patient in acute respiratory distress suggests extreme fatigue and the possibility of an impending respiratory arrest.

- Respiratory behaviors such as assumption of tripod position, pursed-lip beathing, and two-word or three-word dyspnea also indicate respiratory distress.

- There may be a change in the inspiratory (I) to expiratory (E) (I/E) ratio. Normally the I/E ratio is 1:2. In patients in respiratory distress, the ratio may increase to 1:3 or 1:4. This change signifies airflow obstruction.

- The nurse may observe *retraction* (inward movement) of the intercostal spaces or the supraclavicular area and the use of accessory muscles during inspiration or expiration. Use of the accessory muscles signifies moderate distress. Paradoxic breathing indicates severe distress.

- Any deterioration in mental status, such as combative behavior, confusion, or a decreased level of consciousness

(LOC), should be reported immediately, because this change may indicate the onset of rapid deterioration and the need for mechanical ventilation.

Diagnostic Studies
- ABG analysis is used to determine $PaCO_2$, PaO_2, and blood pH.
- A catheter may be inserted into a peripheral artery for monitoring blood pressure (BP) and obtaining ABGs.
- Pulse oximetry is used for the monitoring of oxygenation status, but in respiratory failure, ABGs are necessary to obtain oxygenation (PaO_2) and ventilation ($PaCO_2$) status, as well as acid-base information.
- Other studies may include a chest x-ray, complete blood count (CBC), serum electrolytes, urinalysis, pulmonary function tests, and electrocardiogram (ECG).
- Cultures of sputum and blood are obtained as necessary to determine sources of possible infection.
- If pulmonary embolus is suspected, a ventilation-perfusion lung scan or pulmonary angiography may be done.
- In severe respiratory failure, the measurement of cardiac output (CO) and mixed oxygen saturation gases by pulmonary artery catheter may be performed. Pulmonary artery, pulmonary artery wedge, and left atrial pressures are monitored.

Nursing and Collaborative Management
Because many different problems can cause respiratory failure, specific care of the patient varies.

Goals
The patient in acute respiratory failure will have ABG values within the patient's baseline, baseline breath sounds, breathing patterns within the patient's baseline, and an effective cough with the ability to clear secretions.

See NCP 68-1 for the patient with acute respiratory failure, Lewis and others, *Medical-Surgical Nursing,* ed. 7, pp. 1807 to 1809.

Nursing Diagnoses
Nursing diagnoses for the patient with acute respiratory failure include, but are not limited to, those presented under Acute Respiratory Distress Syndrome, p. 13.

Respiratory Therapy
The major goals of care for acute respiratory failure include maintaining adequate oxygenation and ventilation. This goal is accomplished by collaboration among nursing, medical, and respiratory care teams. Interventions include O_2 therapy, mobilization of secretions, and positive pressure ventilation (PPV).

O_2 Therapy. The primary goal of O_2 therapy is to correct hypoxemia (see Oxygen Therapy, p. 734). If hypoxemia is secondary to V/Q mismatch, supplemental O_2 administered at 1 to 3 L/min by nasal cannula or 24% to 32% by simple face mask or Venturi mask should improve the PaO_2 and SpO_2. Hypoxemia secondary to an intrapulmonary shunt is usually not responsive to high O_2 concentrations, and the patient usually requires PPV (see Mechanical Ventilation, p. 726).

- Patients with chronic hypercapnia frequently have CO_2 narcosis and should receive O_2 through a low-flow device, such as a nasal cannula at 1 to 2 L/min or a Venturi mask at 24% to 28%. They should be closely monitored for changes in mental status, respiratory rate, and ABG results until their PaO_2 level has reached their baseline normal value.

Mobilization of Secretions. Retained pulmonary secretions may cause or exacerbate acute respiratory failure by blocking O_2 movement into the alveoli and pulmonary capillary blood. Secretions can be mobilized through effective coughing, adequate hydration and humidification, chest physical therapy, and tracheal suctioning.

Effective Coughing and Positioning. If secretions are obstructing the airway, the patient should be encouraged to cough. The patient with a neuromuscular weakness from disease or exhaustion may not be able to generate sufficient airway pressures to produce an effective cough. *Augmented coughing (quad coughing)* may be helpful. It is performed by placing the palm of the hand or hands on the abdomen below the xiphoid process. As the patient ends a deep inspiration and begins the expiration, the hands should be moved forcefully downward, increasing abdominal pressure and facilitating the cough.

- Positioning the patient by elevating the head of the bed to at least 45 degrees or by using a reclining chair bed may assist to maximize thoracic expansion.
- All patients should be side-lying if there is a possibility that the tongue will obstruct the airway or that aspiration may occur. An oral or nasal artificial airway should be kept at the bedside for use if necessary.

Hydration and Humidification. Thick and viscous secretions are difficult to raise and should be thinned. Adequate fluid intake (2 to 3 L/day) is necessary to keep secretions thin and easy to expel. If the patient is unable to take sufficient fluids orally, intravenous (IV) hydration will be used. Appropriate humidification with humidifiers or aerosol therapy may also be used to liquefy secretions.

Airway Suctioning. If the patient is unable to expectorate secretions, nasopharyngeal, oropharyngeal, or nasotracheal suctioning is indicated. Suctioning through an artificial airway, such as endotracheal or tracheostomy tubes, may also be performed. At all times, suctioning is done cautiously since it may precipitate hypoxia.

Positive Pressure Ventilation. If intensive measures fail to improve ventilation and oxygenation, ventilatory assistance may be initiated. See Mechanical Ventilation, p. 726.

Drug Therapy

Goals of drug therapy for patients in acute respiratory failure include relief of bronchospasm, reduction of airway inflammation and pulmonary congestion, treatment of pulmonary infection, and reduction of severe anxiety and restlessness.

Relief of Bronchospasm. Alveolar ventilation is increased with the relief of bronchospasm. Short-acting bronchodilators, such as metaproterenol (Alupent) and albuterol (Ventolin), are frequently administered to reverse bronchospasm, using either a hand-held nebulizer or a metered-dose inhaler with a spacer. These drugs may be given at 15- to 30-minute intervals until it can be determined that a response is occurring.

Reduction of Airway Inflammation. IV corticosteroids may be used in conjunction with bronchodilating agents when bronchospasms and inflammation are present. Inhaled corticosteroids are not used for acute respiratory failure, because they require 4 to 5 days before optimum effects are seen.

Reduction of Pulmonary Congestion. IV diuretics (e.g., furosemide [Lasix]) and nitroglycerin (e.g., Tridil) are used to decrease the pulmonary congestion caused by heart failure. If atrial fibrillation is also present, calcium channel blockers and β-adrenergic blockers may be used to decrease heart rate and improve cardiac output.

Treatment of Pulmonary Infections. Pulmonary infections can either cause or exacerbate acute respiratory failure. IV antibiotics are frequently administered to inhibit bacterial growth.

Reduction of Severe Anxiety and Restlessness. Anxiety, restlessness, and agitation result from cerebral hypoxia. In addition, fear caused by the inability to breathe and a sense of loss of control may exacerbate anxiety. The anxiety, pain, and agitation in turn increase O_2 consumption and CO_2 production and may worsen the degree of hypoxemia.

- Sedation and analgesia with drug therapy may be used to decrease anxiety, agitation, and pain. Patients receiving any sedative medication must be monitored closely for respiratory and cardiovascular depression. In the critical care setting, sedation and neuromuscular paralysis are commonly used for severely restless, anxious, and agitated patients in acute respiratory failure.

Collaborative Care
The primary therapeutic goal is to treat the underlying cause of the respiratory failure. Other goals include maintaining an adequate cardiac output and hemoglobin concentration.

- Interventions are directed toward reversing the disease process that resulted in the development of acute respiratory failure.
- Decreased cardiac output is treated by administration of IV fluids, medications, or both.
- If hemoglobin concentration is <9 g/dl (<90 g/L), packed red blood cells may be transfused.

Nutritional Therapy
The maintenance of protein and energy stores is especially important because nutritional depletion causes a loss of muscle mass, including the respiratory muscles, and may prolong recovery. During the acute manifestations of respiratory failure, the risk of aspiration typically prevents oral nutritional intake. Enteral or parenteral nutrition may therefore be administered until acute manifestations subside.

RESTLESS LEGS SYNDROME

Description
Restless legs syndrome (RLS) is characterized by unpleasant sensory (paresthesias) and motor abnormalities of one or both legs. Prevalence rates vary from 1% to 15%, although the numbers may be higher, because the condition is underdiagnosed.

- Although the exact cause of RLS is not known, probably more than one half of all cases are transmitted in an autosomal dominant pattern. There are two distinct types of RLS, primary (idiopathic) and secondary.
- *Primary RLS* is the most common, and many patients with this type of RLS report a positive family history.
- *Secondary RLS* can be seen in metabolic abnormalities associated with iron deficiency, renal failure, polyneuropathy associated with diabetes mellitus, rheumatic disorders (e.g., rheumatoid arthritis), or pregnancy.

Pathophysiology
Idiopathic RLS is related to abnormal iron metabolism and functional alterations in central dopaminergic neurotransmitter systems. Although the exact etiology remains to be determined,

theories include (1) an alteration in dopaminergic transmission in the basal ganglia, (2) axonal neuropathy, or (3) a brainstem disinhibition phenomenon resulting in motor and sensory disturbances.

Clinical Manifestations

The severity of RLS sensory symptoms ranges from infrequent minor discomfort (paresthesias including numbness, tingling, "pins and needles") to severe pain. Sensory symptoms often appear first and are manifested as an annoying and uncomfortable (but usually not painful) sensation in the legs.

- The sensation is often compared with the sensation of bugs creeping or crawling on the skin.
- Patients can also experience pain in the upper extremities and trunk that occurs when the patient is sedentary and usually in the evening or at night.
- Pain at night can produce sleep disruptions and is often relieved by physical activity such as walking, stretching, rocking, or kicking.

Motor abnormalities associated with RLS consist of voluntary restlessness and periodic, involuntary movements that usually occur during sleep. Symptoms are aggravated by fatigue. Over time, RLS advances to more frequent and more severe episodes.

Diagnostic Studies

RLS is a clinical diagnosis based in large part on the patient's history or the report of the bed partner related to nighttime activities. Proposed diagnostic criteria include (1) desire to move the limbs, (2) motor restlessness, (3) symptoms that are worse or exclusively present at rest with at least partial and temporary relief by activity, and (4) symptoms that are worse in the evening or night.

- Polysomnography studies during sleep may be performed to distinguish the problem from other clinical conditions (e.g., sleep apnea).

Nursing and Collaborative Management

The goal of collaborative management is to reduce patient discomfort and distress and to improve sleep quality. When RLS is secondary to uremia or iron deficiency, correction of these conditions will decrease symptoms.

- Nonpharmacologic approaches include establishing regular sleep habits, encouraging exercise, avoiding activities that cause symptoms, and eliminating aggravating factors such as alcohol, caffeine, and certain drugs (neuroleptics, lithium, antihistamines, antidepressants).

If nonpharmacologic measures fail to provide symptom relief, drug therapy may be started. The drugs of choice in treating RLS are dopaminergic agents such as carbidopa-levodopa (Sinemet) and dopamine agonists (e.g., pergolide [Permax], bromocriptine [Parlodel], pramipexole [Mirapex]). Ropinirole (Requip), a drug used to treat Parkinson's disease, is used to treat moderate to severe RLS. These agents are effective in managing sensory and motor symptoms.

Other agents that may be used include antiseizure drugs, benzodiazepines, clonidine (Catapres), and propranolol (Inderal). Opioids (e.g., oxycodone) are usually reserved for those patients with severe symptoms who fail to respond to other drug therapies.

RETINAL DETACHMENT

Description
Retinal detachment is a separation of the sensory retina and underlying pigment epithelium with fluid accumulation between the two layers. Risk factors include increasing age, severe myopia, aphakia, diabetic retinopathy, cataract or glaucoma surgery, eye trauma, and family or personal history.

Pathophysiology
The most common cause is a retinal break, which is an interruption in the full thickness of the retinal tissue. Additional causes for detachment include retinal holes with spontaneous atrophic breaks and retinal tears where the vitreous shrinks with aging and pulls on the retina.

Once there is a retinal break, liquid vitreous enters between the sensory and retinal pigment epithelium layers, causing detachment. Untreated retinal detachment leads to blindness in the involved eye.

Clinical Manifestations
Symptoms of a detaching retina include photopsia ("light flashes"), floaters, and a "cobweb" or ring in the vision field. Once the retina is detached, a painless loss of peripheral or central vision is described.

Diagnostic Studies
- Visual acuity measurements
- Direct visualization of the retina using direct and indirect ophthalmoscopy or slit lamp microscopy
- Ultrasound to help identify a detachment

Collaborative Care

Retinal breaks are evaluated to determine if prophylactic laser photocoagulation or cryopexy is necessary to avoid retinal detachment. Some breaks do not progress to detachment, so the patient may be observed and given precise information about the warning signs of impending detachment and instructions to seek immediate evaluation if these signs occur. The ophthalmologist usually refers the patient with a retinal detachment to a retinal specialist.

Treatment of retinal detachment has two objectives: (1) to seal any retinal breaks and (2) to relieve inward traction on the retina. Surgical treatment to seal breaks may include laser photocoagulation and cryopexy. Management of inward retinal traction can involve scleral buckling, pneumatic retinopexy, and vitrectomy.

- Reattachment is successful in 90% of all cases, with visual prognosis dependent on the extent, length, and area of detachment.

Nursing Management

Goals

The patient with a retinal detachment will experience minimal anxiety throughout the event and maintain an acceptable level of comfort postoperatively.

Nursing Diagnoses

- Acute pain
- Anxiety
- Risk for infection

Nursing Interventions

Retinal detachment is a situation with an urgent need for surgery. The patient needs emotional support, especially during the immediate preoperative period.

- The level of activity restriction following retinal detachment surgeries varies greatly. The nurse should verify the prescribed level of activity with each patient's surgeon and help the patient plan for any necessary assistance related to activity restrictions.
- With postoperative pain the nurse should administer prescribed pain medications and teach the patient to take medication as necessary when discharged.
- Discharge planning is important, and the nurse should begin this process as early as possible because the patient may not be hospitalized long.

▼ Patient and Family Teaching

- Instruct the patient with an increased risk of retinal detachment about the signs of detachment and to seek immediate evaluation if any of those signs or symptoms occurs.

- Promote the use of proper protective eyewear to help avoid retinal detachments related to trauma.
- Following eye surgery for retinal detachment, review the signs of retinal detachment with the patient because the risk of detachment in the other eye is increased.

RHEUMATIC FEVER AND HEART DISEASE

Description
Rheumatic fever is an inflammatory disease of the heart. The resulting damage to the heart from rheumatic fever is called *rheumatic heart disease,* a chronic condition characterized by scarring and deformity of the heart valves.

Pathophysiology
Rheumatic fever occurs as a delayed sequela (usually 2 to 3 weeks) after a group A β-hemolytic streptococcal infection of the upper respiratory system, usually a pharyngeal infection. Manifestations of acute rheumatic fever (ARF) appear to be related to an abnormal immunologic response to group A streptococcal cell membrane antigens. ARF affects the heart, joints, central nervous system (CNS), and skin.

About 40% of ARF episodes are marked by carditis, and all layers of the heart (endocardium, myocardium, pericardium) may be involved.

- Rheumatic endocarditis is found primarily in the valves, with swelling and erosion of the valve leaflets. Vegetations form and create a fibrous thickening of the valve leaflets, fusion of commissures and chordae tendineae, and fibrosis of the papillary muscle. Stenosis and regurgitation may occur in valve leaflets. The mitral and aortic valves are most commonly affected.
- Myocardial involvement is characterized by *Aschoff bodies,* which are nodules formed by a reaction to inflammation with accompanying swelling and fragmentation of collagen fibers.
- Rheumatic pericarditis affects both layers of the pericardium, which becomes thickened and covered with a fibrinous exudate.

The lesions of rheumatic fever are systemic, especially involving the connective tissue. The joints (polyarthritis), skin (subcutaneous [SC] nodules), and CNS (chorea) can be involved in rheumatic fever.

A complication that can result from ARF is chronic rheumatic carditis. It results from fibrous tissue growth in valvular structures that may occur months to years after an episode of ARF.

Clinical Manifestations

The presence of two major criteria or one major and two minor criteria indicates a high probability of ARF. Either combination must have evidence of a preceding group A streptococcal infection.

Major Criteria

- *Carditis* is the most important manifestation of ARF and results in three signs: (1) an organic heart murmur or murmurs of mitral or aortic regurgitation, or mitral stenosis; (2) cardiac enlargement and heart failure (HF) occurring secondary to myocarditis; and (3) pericarditis resulting in distant heart sounds, chest pain, a pericardial friction rub, or signs of effusion.
- *Monoarthritis or polyarthritis,* the most common finding in rheumatic fever, involves swelling, heat, redness, tenderness, and limitation of motion. The larger joints are most frequently affected.
- *Chorea (Sydenham's chorea)* is the major CNS manifestation. It is characterized by involuntary movements, especially of the face and limbs, muscle weakness, and disturbances of speech and gait.
- *Erythema marginatum* lesions are a less common feature. The bright pink, nonpruritic, maplike macular lesions occur mainly on the trunk and proximal extremities and may be exacerbated by heat (e.g., a warm bath).
- *Subcutaneous nodules* are firm, small, hard, painless swellings found most commonly over extensor surfaces of the joints, especially knees, wrists, and elbows.

Minor Criteria

Minor clinical manifestations are frequently present and helpful in recognizing the disease. These include fever, polyarthralgia, and laboratory tests that confirm a recent group A streptococcal infection.

Diagnostic Studies

- Antistreptolysin-O (ASO) titer is the most specific test to confirm group A streptococcal infection.
- A throat culture is usually negative at the onset of the disease.
- Erythrocyte sedimentation rate is elevated; C-reactive protein is positive.
- White blood cell (WBC) count is elevated.
- Chest x-ray may show an enlarged heart if HF is present.

- Echocardiogram may show valvular insufficiency and pericardial fluid or thickening.
- Electrocardiogram (ECG) reveals a prolonged PR interval with delayed atrioventricular (AV) conduction.

Collaborative Care

No specific treatment cures rheumatic fever. Treatment consists of drug therapy and supportive measures. Antibiotic therapy does not modify the course of the acute disease or the development of carditis, but it does eliminate residual group A β-hemolytic streptococci remaining in the tonsils and pharynx and prevents the spread of organisms to close contacts. Salicylates, nonsteroidal antiinflammatory drugs (NSAIDs), and corticosteroids are effective in controlling the fever and joint manifestations. Corticosteroids are also used if severe carditis is present.

Nursing Management

Goals

The patient with rheumatic fever will have normal or baseline heart function, resumption of daily activities without joint pain, and verbalization of the ability to manage the disease.

Nursing Diagnoses

- Activity intolerance
- Decreased cardiac output
- Ineffective therapeutic regimen management

Nursing Interventions

Rheumatic fever is one of the few cardiovascular diseases that is preventable. Prevention involves the early detection and immediate treatment of group A β-hemolytic streptococcal pharyngitis. Adequate treatment of streptococcal pharyngitis prevents initial attacks of rheumatic fever. The nurse's role is to educate the community to seek medical attention for symptoms of streptococcal pharyngitis and to emphasize the need for adequate treatment of a streptococcal sore throat.

The primary goals of managing a patient with ARF are to control and eradicate the infecting organism; prevent cardiac complications; and relieve joint pain, fever, and other symptoms.

- The nurse should administer antibiotics as ordered and teach the patient that oral antibiotics require adherence to the full course of therapy.
- Antipyretics, NSAIDs, and corticosteroids should be administered and fluid intake monitored.
- Promotion of optimal rest is essential to reduce the cardiac workload and diminish the metabolic needs of the body. After acute symptoms have subsided, the patient without carditis should ambulate.

- When carditis is present, ambulation is postponed until HF has been controlled with treatment. Full activities should not be resumed until antiinflammatory therapy has been discontinued.
- Painful joints should be positioned for comfort and proper alignment. Heat may be applied and salicylates administered to relieve joint pain.

▼ **Patient and Family Teaching**

- The patient with a previous history of rheumatic fever should be taught about the disease process, possible sequelae, and the need for continued prophylactic antibiotics. Prophylactic antibiotics should continue for life in individuals who develop rheumatic heart disease.
- The patient should be instructed that the dosage of antibiotics used in maintenance prophylaxis is not adequate to prevent infective endocarditis when invasive procedures are performed. Additional prophylaxis is necessary if a patient with known rheumatic heart disease has dental or surgical procedures involving the upper respiratory, gastrointestinal (GI), or genitourinary (GU) tract.
- The patient must be made aware of the high risk of recurrence if a streptococcal infection develops and should be informed about the risk of exposure to individuals with streptococcal infections.
- Ongoing patient education and reinforcement include good nutrition and hygienic practices as well as the importance of adequate rest.
- The patient should be cautioned about the possibility of developing valvular heart disease. The nurse should teach the patient to seek medical attention if symptoms such as excessive fatigue, dizziness, palpitations, or dyspnea on exertion develop.

RHEUMATOID ARTHRITIS

Description

Rheumatoid arthritis (RA) is a chronic, systemic autoimmune disease characterized by inflammation of connective tissue in the diarthrodial (synovial) joints, typically with periods of remission and exacerbation. RA is frequently accompanied by extraarticular manifestations.

RA occurs globally, affecting all ethnic groups. It can occur at any time of life, but the incidence increases with age, peaking between the fourth and sixth decades. Women are affected by RA 3 times more frequently than men. Smoking significantly increases the risk of RA in both men and women who are genetically pre-disposed to the disease.

Pathophysiology

The cause of RA is unknown. No infectious agent has been cul-tured from blood and synovial tissue or fluid with enough repro-ducibility to suggest an infectious cause. An autoimmune etiology is currently the most widely accepted.

1. *Autoimmunity.* The autoimmune theory suggests that changes associated with RA begin when a susceptible host experiences an initial immune response to an antigen. The antigen, which is probably not the same in all patients, trig-gers the formation of an abnormal immunoglobulin G (IgG). RA is characterized by the presence of autoantibodies against this abnormal IgG. The autoantibodies are known as *rheumatoid factor* (RF), and they combine with IgG to form immune complexes that initially deposit on synovial mem-branes or superficial articular cartilage in the joints.

   - Immune complex formation leads to the activation of complement, and an inflammatory response results. Neu-trophils are attracted to the site of inflammation, where they release proteolytic enzymes that damage articular cartilage and cause the synovial lining to thicken.
   - Other components of the inflammatory response include T helper (CD4) cells and proinflammatory cyokines, such as interleukin-1 (IL-1), interleukin-6 (IL-6), and tumor necrosis factor (TNF).
   - Joint changes from chronic inflammation begin when the hypertrophied synovial membrane invades the surround-ing cartilage, ligaments, tendons, and joint capsule. *Pannus* (highly vascular granulation tissue) forms within the joint. It eventually covers and erodes the entire surface of the articular cartilage.

2. *Genetic factors.* Genetic predisposition appears to be impor-tant in the development of RA. The strongest evidence for a familial influence is the increased occurrence of a human leukocyte antigen (HLA) known as HLA-DR4 in white RA patients. Other HLA variants have also been identified in patients from other ethnic groups.

The pathogenesis of RA is more clearly understood than its etiology. If unarrested, the disease progresses through four stages, which are identified in Table 73.

Table 73	Anatomic Stages of Rheumatoid Arthritis

Stage I—Early
No destructive changes on x-ray, possible x-ray evidence of osteoporosis

Stage II—Moderate
X-ray evidence of osteoporosis, with or without slight bone or cartilage destruction, no joint deformities (although possibly limited joint mobility), adjacent muscle atrophy, possible presence of extraarticular soft tissue lesions (e.g., nodules, tenovaginitis)

Stage III—Severe
X-ray evidence of cartilage and bone destruction in addition to osteoporosis; joint deformity, such as subluxation, ulnar deviation, or hyperextension, without fibrous or bony ankylosis; extensive muscle atrophy; possible presence of extraarticular soft tissue lesions (e.g., nodules, tenosynovitis)

Stage IV—Terminal
Fibrous or bony ankylosis, criteria of stage III

From Kirwan JR: Using the Larsen Index to assess radiographic progression in rheumatoid arthritis, *J Rheumatol* 27:264, 2000.

Clinical Manifestations

RA typically develops insidiously. Nonspecific manifestations such as fatigue, anorexia, weight loss, and generalized stiffness may precede the onset of arthritic complaints. The stiffness becomes more localized after weeks to months. Some patients report a history of a precipitating stressful event, such as infection, work stress, physical exertion, childbirth, surgery, or emotional upset.

Articular involvement is manifested by pain, stiffness, limitation of motion, and signs of inflammation (heat, swelling, tenderness). Joint symptoms occur symmetrically and frequently affect the small joints of the hands and feet, as well as the larger peripheral joints, including wrists, elbows, shoulders, knees, hips, ankles, and jaw.

- The patient characteristically has joint stiffness after periods of inactivity. (See Table 62, p. 444, for a comparison of the manifestations of RA and osteoarthritis [OA].)
- As RA progresses, inflammation and fibrosis of the joint capsule and supporting structures may lead to deformity and disability. Atrophy of muscles and destruction of tendons around the joint cause one articular surface to slip past the

other (*subluxation*). Typical hand deformities include "ulnar drift," "swan neck," and boutonniere deformities.

Extraarticular manifestations. RA can affect nearly every system in the body. Extraarticular manifestations of RA are depicted in Fig. 65-5, Lewis and others, *Medical-Surgical Nursing,* edition 7, p. 1705. The three most common manifestations are rheumatoid nodules, Sjögren's syndrome, and Felty's syndrome.

Rheumatoid nodules are present in up to 25% of all patients with RA. They appear subcutaneously as firm, nontender masses and are usually found over the extensor surfaces of joints such as the fingers and elbows. Nodules may also appear on the eye or lungs; these indicate active disease and a poorer prognosis. Nodules develop insidiously and can persist or regress spontaneously. They are usually not removed because of the high probability of recurrence.

Sjögren's syndrome is seen in 10% to 15% of patients with RA. Sjögren's syndrome can occur as a disease by itself or in conjunction with other arthritic disorders, such as RA and systemic lupus erythematosus (SLE). Affected patients have diminished lacrimal and salivary gland secretion, leading to complaints of burning, gritty, itchy eyes. They experience decreased tearing and photosensitivity (see Sjögren Syndrome, p. 583).

Felty syndrome occurs most commonly in patients with severe, nodule-forming RA. It is characterized by inflammatory eye disorders, splenomegaly, lymphadenopathy, pulmonary disease, and blood dyscrasias (anemia, thrombocytopenia, granulocytopenia).

Diagnostic Studies

A diagnosis is often made based on history and physical findings, but some laboratory tests are useful for confirmation and to monitor disease progression.

- Erythrocyte sedimentation rate (ESR) and C-reactive protein are general indicators of active inflammation.
- Positive RF occurs in 80% of patients and rises during active disease.
- Antinuclear antibody (ANA) titers may be noted in some patients.
- Synovial fluid analysis in early disease often shows a straw-colored fluid with many fibrin flecks. The white blood cell (WBC) count of synovial fluid is elevated (up to 25,000/µl).
- Inflammatory changes in the synovium can be confirmed by tissue biopsy.
- X-ray findings (not specifically diagnostic) may reveal bone demineralization and soft tissue swelling during the early months of RA. Later, narrowing of the joint space, destruc-

tion of articular cartilage, erosion, subluxation, and deformity are seen. Malalignment and ankylosis are seen in
advanced disease.

Collaborative Care

Management of RA begins with a comprehensive program of drug
therapy and education. Physical comfort is promoted by nonsteroidal antiinflammatory drugs (NSAIDs) and rest. Education
regarding drug therapy includes correct administration, reporting
of side effects, and frequent medical and laboratory follow-up
visits. Physical therapy maintains joint motion and muscle strength.
Occupational therapy develops upper-extremity function and
encourages joint protection through the use of splints, pacing
techniques, and assistive devices.

Drug Therapy

Drugs remain the cornerstone of RA treatment. Instead of maintaining the patient on high doses of aspirin or NSAIDs until x-
rays show clear evidence of disease, health care providers now
aggressively prescribe disease-modifying antirheumatic drugs
(DMARDs) because irreversible joint changes can occur early in
the disease process. Drugs have the potential to lessen the permanent effects of RA, such as joint erosion and deformity. Choice of
drug is based on disease activity, patient's level of function, and
lifestyle considerations, such as the desire to bear children.

- Methotrexate (Rheumatrex) is usually the first drug of
  choice because it reduces clinical symptoms in days to
  weeks, is inexpensive, and has a lower toxicity compared
  with other drugs.
- Sulfasalazine (Azulfidine) and the antimalarial drug
  hydroxychloroquine (Plaquenil) may be effective DMARDs
  for mild to moderate disease.
- Leflunomide (Arava) is a newer synthetic DMARD that
  blocks immune cell overproduction and has efficacy similar
  to methotrexate and sulfasalazine.
- Combination therapy of two or more drugs, such as a
  DMARD, an NSAID, and a corticosteroid, can slow symptoms and joint damage while improving function.
- Biologic therapy drugs are also used to slow disease progression in patients with moderate to severe disease who
  have not responded to DMARDs or in combination therapy
  with an established DMARD. These agents include
  etanercept (Enbrel), infliximab (Remicade), adalimumab
  (Humira), anakinra (Kineret), and abatacept (Orencia).
- Additional drugs used infrequently for treating RA include
  antibiotics (minocyline [Minocin]), immunosuppressants

(azathioprine [Imuran]), penicillamine (Cuprimine), and gold compounds (auranofin [Ridaura], gold sodium thiomalate [Myochrysine]).

- Corticosteroid therapy can be used to aid in symptom control. Intraarticular injections may temporarily relieve the pain and inflammation associated with disease flare-ups.
- Various NSAIDs and salicylates are included in the drug regimen to treat arthritis pain and inflammation. Aspirin is often used in high dosages of four to six per day (10 to 18 tablets). NSAIDs have antiinflammatory, analgesic, and antipyretic properties. Although many NSAIDs inhibit inflammation, they do not appear to alter the course of RA. A newer generation of NSAIDs, COX-2 inhibitors, is effective in RA as well as in OA. The drug celecoxib (Celebrex) is currently the only available COX-2 inhibitor.

Apheresis

A blood filtration device used in apheresis is infrequently used to remove RF from the patient's blood. Patients are treated once per week for 12 weeks with a decrease in RA signs and symptoms for some patients.

Nursing Management

Goals

The patient with RA will have satisfactory pain relief and minimal loss of functional ability of the affected joints, participate in planning and carrying out the therapeutic regimen, maintain a positive self-image, and perform self-care to the maximum amount possible.

See NCP 65-1 for the patient with rheumatoid arthritis, Lewis and others, *Medical-Surgical Nursing,* edition 7, pp. 1708 to 1710.

Nursing Diagnoses

- Chronic pain
- Impaired physical mobility
- Disturbed body image
- Ineffective therapeutic regimen management
- Self-care deficit (total)

Nursing Interventions

Prevention of RA is not possible at this time. However, community education programs should include information concerning the symptoms of RA to promote early diagnosis and treatment. The primary objectives of acute intervention are reduction of inflammation, management of pain, maintenance of joint function, and prevention or correction of joint deformity.

Nursing interventions begin with a careful physical assessment (joint pain, swelling, range of motion, general health status), psychosocial assessment (family support, sexual satisfaction, emotional stress, financial constraints, vocation and career limitations), and environmental assessment (transportation, home, and work modifications).

- The suppression of inflammation is most effectively achieved through the administration of NSAIDs, DMARDs, and biologic therapies. Education centers around the action and side effects of each drug and the importance of laboratory monitoring. The nurse must make the drug regimen as understandable as possible.

- Nonpharmacologic relief of pain may include the use of therapeutic heat and cold, rest, relaxation techniques, joint protection, biofeedback, transcutaneous electrical nerve stimulation (TENS), and hypnosis.

- Lightweight splints are sometimes used to rest an inflamed joint and prevent deformity from muscle spasms and contractures. These splints should be removed, skin care given, range-of-motion (ROM) exercises performed, and splints reapplied as prescribed.

- Morning care and procedures should be planned around the patient's morning stiffness. Sitting or standing in a warm shower, sitting in a tub with warm towels around the shoulders, or soaking the hands in a basin of warm water may help to relieve joint stiffness and allow the patient to comfortably perform activities of daily living.

- Alternating scheduled rest periods with activity throughout the day helps relieve fatigue and pain. The nurse should assist the patient to modify activities to avoid overexertion.

- Good body alignment while resting can be maintained through the use of a firm mattress or bed board. Positions of extension should be encouraged and positions of flexion avoided. Pillows should never be placed under the knees. A small, flat pillow may be used under the head and shoulders. Splints and casts may be helpful in maintaining proper alignment and promoting rest, especially when joint inflammation is present.

Protecting the joints from stress is important. Nursing interventions include helping the patient identify ways to modify tasks. Sample activities that protect small joints are listed in Table 65-10, Lewis and others, *Medical-Surgical Nursing,* edition 7, p. 1710.

- Patient independence may be increased by occupational therapy training with assistive devices that help simplify tasks, such as built-up utensils, button hooks, and raised toilet seats. A cane or a walker offers support and relief of pain when walking.

- Heat and cold therapy helps to relieve stiffness, pain, and muscle spasm. Application of ice may be beneficial during periods of disease exacerbation, whereas moist heat appears to offer better relief of chronic stiffness.
- The nurse should reinforce participation in an exercise program and ensure that the exercises are being done correctly. Gentle ROM exercises are usually done daily to keep the joints functional.

▼ **Patient and Family Teaching**

Self-management and adherence to an individualized home program are contingent on a thorough understanding of RA, the nature and course of the disease, and the goals of therapy. In addition, the patient's perception of the disease and value system must be considered.

- The nurse can help the patient recognize fears and concerns faced by all people living with a chronic illness. Evaluation of the family support system is important.
- Financial planning may be necessary. Community resources such as a home care nurse, homemaker services, and vocational rehabilitation may be considered. Self-help groups are beneficial for some patients.

SEIZURE DISORDERS

Description

A seizure is the paroxysmal, uncontrolled electrical discharge of neurons in the brain that interrupts normal function. It is frequently a symptom of underlying illness. Seizures may accompany a variety of disorders, or they may occur spontaneously without any apparent cause.

- In the adult, metabolic disturbances that cause seizures include acidosis, electrolyte imbalances, hypoglycemia, hypoxia, alcohol and barbiturate withdrawal, dehydration, and water intoxication.
- Extracranial disorders that can cause seizures include heart, lung, liver, and kidney disease; systemic lupus erythematosus; diabetes mellitus (DM); hypertension; and septicemia.
- Seizures resulting from systemic and metabolic disturbances are not considered epilepsy if the seizures cease when the underlying problem is corrected.

Epilepsy is a condition in which a person has spontaneously recurring seizures caused by a chronic underlying condition. Incidence rates of epilepsy are very high during the first year of life, decline through childhood and adolescence, plateau in middle age, and rise sharply again among the elderly population. The population with the highest rate of new-onset epilepsy is those older than 60 years.

Pathophysiology

The most common causes of seizure during the first 6 months of life are severe birth injury, congenital defects involving the central nervous system (CNS), infections, and inborn errors of metabolism. In individuals between 20 and 30 years old, seizure disorder usually occurs as a result of structural lesions such as trauma, brain tumors, or vascular disease. After the age of 50 years, primary causes of seizure are stroke and metastatic brain tumors. Although many causes of seizure disorders have been identified, three fourths of all cases cannot be attributed to a specific cause and are considered *idiopathic.*

The etiology of recurring seizures (epilepsy) has long been attributed to a group of abnormal neurons (*seizure focus*) that seem to undergo spontaneous firing. This firing spreads by physiologic pathways to involve adjacent or distant areas of the brain. The factor that causes this abnormal firing is not clear. Any stimulus that causes the cell membrane of the neuron to depolarize induces a tendency to spontaneous firing. Often the brain area from which epileptic activity arises is found to have scar tissue (*gliosis*). Scarring is thought to interfere with the normal chemical and structural environment of brain neurons, making them more likely to fire abnormally.

New evidence indicates that *astrocytes,* or cerebral support cells, may play a key role in recurring seizures. Astrocytes release glutamate that triggers synchronous firing of neurons. Drug therapy focused on suppressing astrocyte signaling or decreasing glutamate release might be a mechanism to control seizures.

Clinical Manifestations

The specific clinical manifestations of a seizure are determined by the site of the electrical disturbance. The preferred method of classifying epileptic seizures is the International Classification System (see Table 59-6, Lewis and others, *Medical-Surgical Nursing,* edition 7, p. 1534). The system is based on the clinical and electroencephalographic (EEG) manifestations of seizures.

In this system, seizures are divided into two major classes, *generalized* and *partial.* Depending on the type, a seizure may progress through several phases: (1) *prodromal phase* with signs or activity that precedes a seizure, (2) *aural phase* with a sensory warning, (3) *ictal phase* with full seizure, and (4) *postictal phase,* which is the period of recovery after the seizure.

Generalized Seizures

Generalized seizures are characterized by bilateral synchronous epileptic discharge in the brain. Because the entire brain is affected at the onset of the seizures, there is no warning or aura. In most cases the patient loses consciousness for a few seconds to several minutes.

- *Tonic-clonic* (formerly known as grand mal) seizures are the most common generalized seizures. This type of seizure is characterized by a loss of consciousness and falling to the ground if the patient is upright, followed by stiffening of the body (tonic phase) for 10 to 20 seconds and subsequent jerking of the extremities (clonic phase) for another 30 to 40 seconds. Cyanosis, excessive salivation, tongue or cheek biting, and incontinence may accompany the seizure. In the postictal phase the patient usually has muscle soreness, is very tired, and may sleep for several hours. The patient has no memory of the seizure activity.

- *Typical absence (petit mal)* seizures usually occur only in children and rarely continue beyond adolescence. This type of seizure may cease totally as the child ages, or it may evolve into another type of seizure.The typical clinical manifestation is a brief staring spell that lasts only a few seconds. There may be an extremely brief loss of consciousness. When untreated, the seizures may occur up to 100 times each day. Typical absence seizures are often precipitated by hyperventilation and flashing lights.

- *Atypical absence* seizures are another type of generalized seizure characterized by a staring spell. A brief warning, peculiar behavior during the seizure, and confusion after the seizure are also common.

- Other types of generalized seizures include myoclonic, atonic, tonic, and clonic seizures.

Partial Seizures

Partial (focal) seizures are caused by focal irritations and begin in a specific region of the cortex, as indicated by the EEG and clinical manifestations. Partial seizures may be confined to one side of the brain and remain partial or focal in nature, or they may spread to involve the entire brain, culminating in a generalized tonic-clonic seizure. Any tonic-clonic seizure preceded by an aura or warning is a partial seizure that generalizes secondarily.

- Partial seizures are further divided into simple partial seizures (those with simple motor or sensory phenomena) and complex partial seizures (those with complex symptoms). The terms *focal motor, focal sensory,* and *jacksonian* have been used to describe seizures of the simple partial type.

Complex partial seizures include *temporal lobe seizures,*
temporal lobe absence seizures, and *psychomotor seizures.*

Complications

Status epilepticus is a state of continuous seizure activity or a
condition in which seizures recur in rapid succession without
return to consciousness between seizures. It can occur with any
type of seizure. Status epilepticus is the most serious complication
of epilepsy and is a neurologic emergency.

- During repeated seizures the brain uses more energy than
  can be supplied. Neurons become exhausted and cease to
  function. Permanent brain damage may result.
- Tonic-clonic status epilepticus is the most dangerous
  because it can cause ventilatory insufficiency, hypoxemia,
  cardiac dysrhythmias, and systemic acidosis, all of which
  can be fatal.

Another complication of seizures is severe injury and even
death from trauma experienced during a seizure. Patients who lose
consciousness during a seizure are at greatest risk.

Perhaps the most common complication of seizure disorder is
the effect it has on a patient's lifestyle. Although attitudes have
improved in recent years, epilepsy still carries a social stigma that
can lead to discrimination in employment and educational opportunities. Transportation may also be difficult because of legal
sanctions against driving in most states.

Diagnostic Studies

- Most important in diagnosis are accurate and comprehensive
  descriptions of the seizures and the patient's health history.
- The EEG is useful only if it shows abnormalities. It is not a
  definitive test because some patients who do not have seizure
  disorders have abnormal EEG patterns, whereas many patients
  with seizure disorders have normal EEGs between seizures.
- Complete blood count (CBC), serum chemistries, studies of
  liver and kidney function, and urinalysis can rule out metabolic
  disorders.
- Computed tomography (CT) scan and magnetic resonance
  imaging (MRI) can rule out a structural lesion.
- Cerebral angiography, single photon emission computed tomography (SPECT), magnetic resonance spectroscopy (MRS),
  magnetic resonance angiography (MRA), and positron emission tomography (PET) may be used in selected situations.

Collaborative Care

Most seizures do not require professional emergency medical care
because they are self-limiting and rarely cause body injury.

However, if status epilepticus occurs, if significant body harm occurs, or if the event is a first-time seizure, medical care should be sought immediately. Table 59-8, Lewis and others, *Medical-Surgical Nursing,* edition 7, p. 1537, summarizes the emergency care of the patient with a generalized tonic-clonic seizure.

Drug Therapy

Seizure disorders are treated primarily with antiseizure drugs (see Table 59-9, Lewis and others, *Medical-Surgical Nursing,* edition 7, p. 1538). Medications generally act by stabilizing the nerve cell membranes and preventing the spread of the epileptic discharge.

The primary goal of antiseizure drug therapy is to obtain maximum seizure control with a minimum of toxic side effects. The principle of drug therapy is to begin with a single drug based on patient age and weight with consideration of the type, frequency, and cause of seizure and increase the dosage until the seizures are controlled or toxic side effects occur. If seizure control is not achieved with a single drug, a second drug may be added.

- Newer antiseizure drugs include gabapentin (Neurontin), lamotrigine (Lamictal), topiramate (Topamax), tiagabine (Gabitril), levetiracetam (Keppra), and zonisamide (Zonegran). Some of these drugs are broad spectrum and appear to be effective for multiple seizure types.
- Treatment of status epilepticus requires initiation of a rapid-acting antiseizure medication given intravenously. Drugs most commonly used are lorazepam (Ativan) and diazepam (Valium).
- Antiseizure drugs should not be discontinued abruptly because this can precipitate seizures.
- Alternative therapies, such as vagal nerve stimulation and biofeedback, may also be used.

Surgery may be considered to control intractable seizures, prevent cerebral degeneration from repeated seizures, and improve the quality of life.

Nursing Management
Goals

The patient with seizures will be free from injury during a seizure, have optimal mental and physical functioning while taking antiseizure medication, and have satisfactory psychosocial functioning.

Nursing Diagnoses

- Ineffective breathing pattern
- Risk for injury
- Ineffective coping
- Ineffective therapeutic regimen management

Nursing Interventions

The patient with a seizure disorder should practice good general health habits (e.g., maintaining a proper diet, getting adequate rest, exercising). The patient should be helped to identify events or situations that precipitate the seizures and be given suggestions for avoiding them or handling them better.

The nurse caring for a hospitalized patient or a patient who has had seizures as a result of metabolic factors should focus on observation and treatment of the seizure, education, and psychosocial intervention.

- When a seizure occurs, the nurse should carefully observe and record all aspects of the event because the diagnosis and subsequent treatment depend on the seizure description. The description should include the exact onset of the seizure (which body part was affected first and how); the course and nature of the seizure activity (loss of consciousness, tongue biting, automatisms, stiffening, jerking, total lack of muscle tone); the body parts involved and their sequence of involvement; and the presence of autonomic signs (dilated pupils, excessive salivation, altered breathing, cyanosis, flushing, diaphoresis, or incontinence).

- Assessment of the postictal period should include a detailed description of the level of consciousness (LOC), vital signs, memory loss, muscle soreness, speech disorders (aphasia, dysarthria), weakness or paralysis, sleep period, and the duration of each sign or symptom.

- During the seizure it is important to maintain a patent airway. This may involve supporting and protecting the head, turning the patient to the side, loosening constrictive clothing, or easing the patient to the floor if sitting in a chair. After the seizure the patient may require suctioning and oxygen.

- A seizure can be a frightening experience for the patient and for others who may witness it. The nurse should assess the level of their understanding and provide information about how and why the event occurred.

▼ **Patient and Family Teaching**

The prevention of recurring seizures is the major goal in the treatment of epilepsy. Because seizure disorders cannot be cured, drugs must be taken regularly and continually, often for a lifetime. Table 74 lists patient and family teaching guidelines.

- The nurse should ensure that the patient knows the specifics of the medication regimen and what to do if a dose is missed.

- The patient should be cautioned not to adjust medications without professional guidance because this can increase seizure frequency and even cause status epilepticus.

Table 74	Patient and Family Teaching Guide: Seizure Disorders and Epilepsy

The patient should be taught the following:
1. Drugs must be taken as prescribed. Any and all side effects of medications should be reported to the health care provider. When necessary, blood drawings are done to ensure that therapeutic levels are maintained.
2. Use of nondrug techniques, such as relaxation therapy and biofeedback training, to potentially reduce the number of seizures.
3. Availability of resources in the community.
4. Need to wear a Medic-Alert bracelet, necklace, and identification card.
5. Avoidance of excessive alcohol intake, fatigue, and loss of sleep.
6. Regular meals and snacks in between if feeling shaky, faint, or hungry.

Family members should be taught the following:
1. First aid treatment of tonic-clonic seizure. It is not necessary to call an ambulance or send the patient to the hospital after a single seizure unless the seizure is prolonged, another seizure immediately follows, or extensive injury has occurred.
2. During an acute seizure, it is important to protect the patient from injury. This may involve supporting and protecting the head, turning the patient to the side, loosening constrictive clothing, and easing the patient to the floor, if seated.

- The patient should be encouraged to report any medication side effects and to keep regular appointments with the health care provider.
- The nurse should teach family members and significant others the first-aid treatment of tonic-clonic seizures.
- The nurse should provide psychosocial support for the patient by providing education and helping to identify coping mechanisms.

SEXUALLY TRANSMITTED DISEASES

Sexually transmitted diseases (STDs) are infectious diseases usually transmitted through sexual contact. Historically, they have

| Table 75 | Microorganisms Responsible for Diseases Transmitted by Sexual Activity | |

Organism	Disease
Chlamydia trachomatis	Nongonococcal urethritis (NGU); cervicitis; lymphogranuloma venereum
Cytomegalovirus (CMV)	Multiple diseases
Hepatitis B virus	Hepatitis B
Herpes simplex virus (HSV)	Genital herpes
Human immunodeficiency virus (HIV)	HIV infection, acquired immunodeficiency syndrome (AIDS)
Human papillomavirus	Genital warts
Poxvirus	Molluscum contagiosum
Neisseria gonorrhoeae	Gonorrhea
Treponema pallidum	Syphilis

S

been referred to as *venereal diseases*. Common diseases that are transmitted sexually are listed in Table 75.

- Diseases that are associated with sexual transmission can also be contracted by other routes, such as through blood, blood products, and autoinoculation. See Gonorrhea, p. 251, Syphilis, p. 615, Herpes, Genital, p. 306, Warts, Genital, p. 686, and Chlamydial Infection, p. 112.

An estimated 65 million people in the United States are currently infected with one or more STDs. In the United States all gonorrhea and syphilis and, in most states, chlamydial infection must be reported to the state or local public health authorities. In spite of this requirement there are many unreported cases of these infections.

Many factors contribute to the increased incidence of STDs. Earlier reproductive maturity and increased longevity have resulted in a longer sexual life span. An increase in the total population has resulted in an increase in the number of susceptible hosts.

- Other factors include greater sexual freedom, decreased social control by religious institutions, and an increased emphasis on sexuality in the media.
- Changes in the methods of contraception are also reflected in the incidence of STDs. The preference for oral contraceptives and intrauterine devices (IUDs) that offer no protection against STDs over barrier contraceptives such as condoms increases the risk of transmission of disease.

Nursing Management: Sexually Transmitted Diseases

Goals

The patient with an STD will demonstrate an understanding of the mode of transmission and the risks posed by STDs, complete treatment and return for appropriate follow-up care, notify or assist in notification of sexual contacts about their need for testing and treatment, abstain from intercourse until infection is resolved, and demonstrate knowledge of safe sex practices.

Nursing Diagnoses

- Risk for infection
- Ineffective health maintenance
- Anxiety

Nursing Interventions

The diagnosis of an STD may be met with a variety of emotions, such as shame, guilt, anger, and a desire for vengeance. The nurse should try to help the patient verbalize feelings. A referral for professional counseling to explore ramifications of an STD may be indicated.

All patients should return to the treatment center for a repeat culture from infected sites or for serologic testing at designated times to determine effectiveness of treatment.

- Informing the patient that cures are not always obtained on first treatment can reinforce the need for a follow-up visit.
- The patient should also be advised to inform sexual partners of the need for treatment, regardless of whether they are free of symptoms or experiencing symptoms.

The patient with an STD should have certain hygiene measures emphasized.

- An important measure is frequent hand washing and bathing; this results in destruction of many of the causative organisms of STDs.
- Bathing and cleaning of involved areas can provide local comfort and prevent secondary infection.
- Douching may spread infection and is therefore contraindicated.
- Sexual abstinence is indicated during the communicable phase of the disease. If sexual activity occurs before the patient has completed treatment, the use of condoms may prevent spread of infection and reinfection.

▼ Patient and Family Teaching

- Nurses should be prepared to discuss safe sex practices with all patients, not only those who are perceived to be at risk. These practices include abstinence, monogamy with an uninfected partner, avoidance of certain high-risk sexual practices, and use of condoms and other barriers to limit contact with potentially infectious body fluids or lesions. A patient teaching guide related to the patient with an STD is presented in Table 53-10, Lewis and others, *Medical-Surgical Nursing,* edition 7, p. 1377.

- All sexually active women should be screened for cervical cancer. Women with a history of STDs are at greater risk for cervical cancer than those women without this history.
- The nurse can initiate an interview to establish the patient's risk for contracting an STD. Questions to ask include number of partners, type of birth control used, use of condoms, use of intravenous (IV) drugs, and sexual preference. Patient education can be planned based on responses to these questions.
- An inspection of the sexual partner's genitals before coitus is recommended. The presence of discharge, sores, blisters, or rash should be viewed with concern.
- Men should be told that some protection is provided if they void immediately after intercourse and wash their genitals and adjacent areas with soap and water.
- Women may also benefit from postcoital voiding and washing. Spermicidal jellies and creams have a mild detergent effect that may reduce the risk of contracting STDs.
- Proper use of a latex condom provides a highly effective mechanical barrier to infection. The condom should be undamaged and correctly in place throughout all phases of sexual activity. The use of a spermicide such as nonoxynol-9 (which inactivates most STD organisms) in the vagina and concurrent use of a condom can further reduce risk of disease.
- Sexual contact with persons known or suspected to have human immunodeficiency virus (HIV) infection should be avoided. Sexually active homosexual men may reduce their risk by minimizing the number of sexual contacts. Unprotected anal intercourse should be eliminated, and condoms should be used if sexual contact continues.
- Nurses can actively encourage their communities to provide better education related to STDs for their citizens. Teenagers, who are known to have a high incidence of infection, should be a prime target for such educational programs.

SHOCK

Description

Shock is a syndrome characterized by decreased tissue perfusion and impaired cellular metabolism. Shock is a complex process that often leads to systemic inflammatory response syndrome (SIRS) and multiple organ dysfunction syndrome (MODS) (see p. 617).

■ Although the cause, initial presentation, and management strategies of various types of shock differ, the physiologic responses of the cell to hypoperfusion are similar.

Classification of Shock

Table 76 presents one system that classifies shock as low blood flow (cardiogenic and hypovolemic) shock or maldistribution of blood flow (septic, anaphylactic, and neurogenic) shock.

Low Blood Flow Shock

Cardiogenic shock occurs when either systolic or diastolic dysfunction of the myocardium results in a compromised cardiac output (CO). The heart's inability to pump the blood forward is classified as systolic dysfunction. Systolic dysfunction primarily affects the left ventricle. Figure 67-2 describes the pathophysiology of cardiogenic shock (Lewis and others, *Medical-Surgical Nursing,* edition 7, p. 1774). Causes include myocardial infarction (MI), cardiomyopathies, severe systemic or pulmonary hypertension, blunt cardiac injury, valve rupture, and myocardial depression from metabolic problems.

■ The patient presents with tachycardia, hypotension, and a narrowed pulse pressure. The heart's inability to pump blood forward results in a low CO (<4 L/min) and a low *cardiac index* (<2.1 L/min/m^2).

■ The patient has tachypnea and pulmonary congestion that is evident by the presence of crackles. An increase in the pulmonary artery wedge pressure (PAWP) and pulmonary vascular resistance is also noted.

■ Signs of peripheral hypoperfusion (e.g., cyanosis, pallor, cool and clammy skin, decreased capillary refill time) are apparent.

■ Decreased renal blood flow results in sodium and water retention and decreased urine output. Anxiety and delirium may develop, since cerebral perfusion is impaired.

Studies helpful in diagnosing cardiogenic shock include laboratory studies (e.g., cardiac enzymes, troponin levels), electrocardiogram (ECG), chest x-ray, and echocardiogram.

Hypovolemic shock occurs when there is a loss of intravascular fluid volume. The volume loss may be either an absolute or a relative volume loss (see Table 76).

In hypovolemic shock, the size of the vascular compartment remains unchanged while the volume of blood or plasma decreases. A reduction in intravascular volume results in a decreased venous return to the heart, decreased preload, decreased stroke volume,

| Table 76 | Classification and Precipitating Factors of Shock |

Low Blood Flow	Maldistribution of Blood Flow
Cardiogenic Shock ■ Systolic dysfunction: inability of the heart to pump blood forward (e.g., myocardial infarction, cardiomyopathy) ■ Diastolic dysfunction: inability of the heart to fill during diastole (e.g., cardiac tamponade) ■ Dysrhythmias ■ Structural factors: valvular abnormality (e.g., stenosis or regurgitation), ventricular septal tract, respiratory rupture, tension pneumothorax **Hypovolemic Shock** *Absolute Hypovolemia* ■ External loss of whole blood (e.g., hemorrhage from trauma, surgery, GI bleeding) ■ Loss of other body fluids (e.g., vomiting, diarrhea, excessive diuresis, diabetes insipidus, diabetes mellitus) *Relative Hypovolemia* ■ Pooling of blood or fluids (e.g., bowel obstruction) ■ Fluid shifts (e.g., burn injuries, ascites) ■ Internal bleeding (e.g., fracture of long bones, ruptured spleen, hemothorax, severe pancreatitis) ■ Massive vasodilation (e.g., sepsis)	**Neurogenic Shock** ■ Hemodynamic consequences of injury and/or disease to the spinal cord at or above T5 ■ Spinal anesthesia ■ Vasomotor center depression (e.g., severe pain, drugs, hypoglycemia, injury) **Septic Shock** ■ Infection (e.g., urinary tract, respiratory tract, invasive procedure, indwelling lines and catheters) ■ At-risk patients: older adults, patients with chronic diseases (e.g., diabetes mellitus, chronic kidney disease, heart failure), patients receiving immunosuppressive therapy or who are malnourished or debilitated ■ Gram-negative bacteria most common; also gram-positive bacteria, viruses, fungi, and parasites **Anaphylactic Shock** ■ Contrast media, blood/blood products, drugs, insect bites, anesthetic agents, food/food additives, vaccines, environmental agents, latex

S

GI, Gastrointestinal.

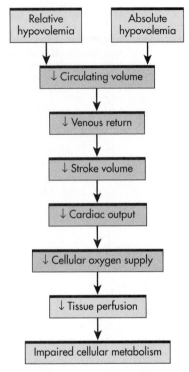

Fig. 14. The pathophysiology of hypovolemic shock.

and decreased CO (Fig. 14). A total blood loss of 15% to 30% results in a sympathetic nervous system (SNS)–mediated response that causes an increase in heart rate, cardiac output, and respiratory rate and depth. If hypovolemia is corrected at this time, tissue dysfunction is generally reversible.

- If volume loss is greater than 30%, blood volume must be replaced aggressively with blood or blood products. A loss of more than 40% of the total blood volume results in irreversible tissue destruction.

Laboratory studies include measurements of serial hemoglobin and hematocrit levels, urine specific gravity, serum electrolytes, and lactic acid.

Maldistribution of Blood Flow Shock

Neurogenic shock is a hemodynamic phenomenon that occurs after a spinal cord injury at the fifth thoracic (T5) vertebra or above. The injury results in a massive vasodilation without compensation, leading to a pooling of blood in the blood vessels, tissue hypoperfusion, and ultimately impaired cellular metabolism. Other causes of neurogenic shock are found in Table 76.

Spinal anesthesia that blocks transmission of impulses from the SNS and depression of the vasomotor center of the medulla by drugs may also cause neurogenic shock.

- Clinical manifestations are hypotension (from massive vasodilation) and bradycardia (from unopposed parasympathetic stimulation).

The patient in neurogenic shock also characteristically presents with hypothalamic dysfunction, which may result in poikilothermy (taking on the temperature of the environment), which combined with massive vasodilation promotes heat loss, often resulting in hypothermia.

The pathophysiology of neurogenic shock is described in Fig. 67-4, Lewis and others, *Medical-Surgical Nursing,* edition 7, p. 1777. Hypoperfusion associated with neurogenic shock also results in impaired tissue perfusion and cellular metabolism.

Anaphylactic shock is an acute and life-threatening hypersensitivity (allergic) reaction to a sensitizing substance, such as a drug, chemical, vaccine, food, or insect venom. It is an immediate reaction that causes massive vasodilation, release of vasoactive mediators, and an increase in capillary permeability.

- As capillary permeability increases, fluid leaks from the vascular space into the interstitial space. Anaphylactic shock can lead to respiratory distress as a result of laryngeal edema or severe bronchospasm, and circulatory failure as a result of massive vasodilation.
- Patients present with a sudden onset of symptoms, including dizziness, chest pain, incontinence, swelling of the lips and tongue, wheezing, and stridor. Skin changes include flushing, pruritus, urticaria, and angioedema.
- A patient can develop a severe allergic reaction, possibly leading to anaphylactic shock after contact, inhalation, ingestion, or injection with an antigen (allergen) to which the person has previously been sensitized (see Table 76).

Septic shock is the presence of sepsis with hypotension despite fluid resuscitation along with the presence of tissue perfusion abnormalities. *Sepsis* is a systemic inflammatory response to an infection. Sepsis progressing to septic shock is the leading cause of death in noncoronary intensive care units (ICUs).

- The primary organisms that cause septic shock are gram-negative and gram-positive bacteria.

- Parasites, fungi, and viruses can also lead to the development of septic shock.

The pathogenesis of septic shock is complex (see Fig. 67-5, Lewis and others, *Medical-Surgical Nursing,* edition 7, p. 1778). When a microorganism enters the body, the normal immune/inflammatory cascade responses are initiated and work together to destroy the antigen. However, in severe sepsis and septic shock the response to an antigen is exaggerated. There is an increase in inflammation and coagulation and a decrease in fibrinolysis. Endotoxins from the microorganism cell wall stimulate the release of cytokines and other proinflammatory mediators. The combined effects of the mediators result in damage to the endothelium, vasodilation, increased capillary permeability, and neutrophil and platelet aggregation and adhesion to the endothelium.

- Clinical manifestations include decreased systemic vascular resistance (SVR), with a compensatory increase in CO, hypotension, tachypnea, and temperature dysregulation (high or low).
- Respiratory failure is common. The patient initially hyperventilates, resulting in respiratory alkalosis. Once the patient can no longer compensate, respiratory acidosis develops.
- Other clinical signs include decreased urine output, alteration in neurologic status, and GI dysfunction, such as GI bleeding and paralytic ileus.

Stages of Shock

The shock continuum begins with the initial stage of shock, followed by the compensatory and progressive stages. If tissue perfusion is not restored, and the progression of the shock is not halted, the patient deteriorates to the refractory (final) stage of shock, from which recovery is unlikely.

The *initial stage of shock* may not be clinically apparent. The patient presents with no outward signs of decreased tissue perfusion. Metabolism changes at the cellular level from aerobic to anaerobic, causing lactic acid buildup. Removal of lactic acid requires oxygen, which is unavailable because of decreased tissue perfusion.

In the *compensatory stage,* the body activates several mechanisms to overcome the increasing consequences of anaerobic metabolism and to maintain homeostasis. Neural, hormonal, and biochemical compensatory mechanisms are involved (see Table 67-6, Lewis and others, *Medical-Surgical Nursing,* edition 7, p. 1781).

- One of the first signs may be a fall in blood pressure (BP). The SNS is activated and stimulates vasoconstriction and the release of epinephrine and norepinephrine; both are potent vasoconstrictors. Blood flow to the most essential organs, the heart and the brain, is maintained; and blood flow to the kidneys, GI tract, and lungs is shunted.
- Decreased blood flow to the kidneys activates the renin-angiotensin-aldosterone system, resulting in vasoconstriction and sodium and water reabsorption.
- Shunting blood from the lungs has an important effect on the patient in shock. Areas of the lungs participating in ventilation are not perfused because of decreased blood flow to the lungs. The patient has a compensatory increase in the rate and depth of respirations.
- The myocardium responds to SNS stimulation and the increase in oxygen demand by increasing heart rate and contractility.

If the perfusion deficit (cause of shock) is corrected at this stage, the patient recovers with few or no residual effects. If the perfusion deficit is not corrected, the patient goes on to the progressive stage of shock.

The *progressive stage* of shock begins as compensatory mechanisms fail. Hallmarks of the stage are decreased cellular perfusion and altered capillary permeability. The patient may have diffuse profound edema (anasarca).

- The combined effects of pulmonary vasoconstriction and bronchoconstriction are impaired gas exchange, decreased compliance, and worsening ventilation-perfusion mismatch. The patient presents with tachypnea, crackles, and an overall increased work of breathing.
- CO begins to fall, with a resultant decrease in BP and peripheral perfusion, including a decrease in coronary artery perfusion. Myocardial dysfunction from decreased perfusion results in dysrhythmias, myocardial ischemia, and potentially myocardial infarction.
- Renal function is markedly impaired. The patient has a decreased urine output and an elevated blood urea nitrogen (BUN) and serum creatinine. Metabolic acidosis occurs from an inability to excrete acids and reabsorb bicarbonate.
- Decreased tissue perfusion predisposes the patient to erosive ulcers and GI bleeding.
- Loss of the functional ability of the liver leads to a failure to metabolize drugs and waste products such as ammonia and lactate. Jaundice results from an accumulation of bilirubin.

- Dysfunction of the hematologic system places the patient at risk for the development of disseminated intravascular coagulation (DIC).

In the final *refractory stage of shock,* decreased perfusion from peripheral vasoconstriction and decreased cardiac output exacerbate anaerobic metabolism (see Fig. 67-8, Lewis and others, *Medical-Surgical Nursing,* edition 7, p. 1784). The loss of intravascular volume worsens hypotension and tachycardia and decreases coronary blood flow. Cerebral blood flow cannot be maintained, and cerebral ischemia results.

- The patient demonstrates profound hypotension and hypoxemia. In this final stage, recovery is unlikely. The organs are in failure, and the body's compensatory mechanisms are overwhelmed.

Diagnostic Studies

- History and physical examination, which provide initial clues for the diagnosis of shock
- Blood studies, which may include complete blood count (CBC), DIC screen, cardiac enzymes, BUN, glucose, electrolytes, arterial blood gases (ABGs), lactate, blood cultures, and liver enzymes
- Urine specific gravity and urine output
- Arterial pressure monitoring, central venous pressure monitoring, and/or pulmonary artery pressure monitoring
- Chest x-ray, which may reveal changes consistent with shock or acute respiratory distress syndrome (ARDS)
- Twelve-lead ECG and cardiac monitor

See Table 67-3, Lewis and others, *Medical-Surgical Nursing,* edition 7, p. 1775 for further information. See Table 67-2 for the hemodynamic effects of shock, *Medical-Surgical Nursing,* p. 1774.

Collaborative Care: General Measures

Critical factors in management are early recognition and treatment. Prompt intervention can alter the shock process and prevent the progressive or refractory stage. Successful management depends on (1) identification of patients at risk for shock; (2) integration of the patient's history, physical examination, and clinical findings to establish a diagnosis; (3) interventions to control or eliminate the cause of the decreased perfusion; (4) protection of target organs from dysfunction; and (5) provision of multisystem supportive care. Emergency care of the patient in shock is presented in Table 77.

General management strategies begin with ensuring that the patient has a patent airway. Once the airway is established, either

Table 77 Emergency Management: Shock

Etiology*	Assessment Findings	Interventions
Surgical ■ Postoperative bleeding ■ Ruptured organ/vessel ■ Gastrointestinal bleeding ■ Aortic dissection ■ Vaginal bleeding ■ Ruptured ectopic pregnancy or ovarian cyst **Medical** ■ Myocardial infarction ■ Dehydration ■ Addisonian crisis ■ Diabetes insipidus ■ Sepsis ■ Diabetes mellitus ■ Pulmonary embolus	■ Restlessness ■ Confusion ■ Anxiety ■ Feeling of impending doom ■ Decreased level of consciousness ■ Weakness ■ Rapid, weak, thready pulses ■ Dysrhythmias ■ Hypotension ■ Narrowed pulse pressure ■ Cool, clammy skin (warm skin in early stage of septic shock and neurogenic shock) ■ Tachypnea, dyspnea, or shallow, irregular respirations ■ Decreased O_2 saturation ■ Extreme thirst	**Initial** ■ Establish and maintain patent airway. ■ Administer high-flow oxygen (100%) by non-rebreather mask or bag-valve-mask. ■ Anticipate need for intubation and mechanical ventilation. ■ Stabilize cervical spine as appropriate. ■ Establish IV access with two large-bore catheters (14-16 gauge), and begin fluid resuscitation with crystalloids (e.g., normal saline solution). ■ Draw blood for lab studies (e.g., blood cultures, lactate, WBCs). ■ Control any external bleeding with direct pressure or pressure dressing.

Continued

IV, Intravenous; WBCs, white blood cells.
* See Table 76 for additional etiologies of shock.

S

Table 77   Emergency Management: Shock—cont'd

Etiology*	Assessment Findings	Interventions
Trauma ■ Ruptured or lacerated vessel or organ (e.g., spleen) ■ Fractures ■ Multisystem or multiorgan injury	■ Nausea and vomiting ■ Chills ■ Pallor ■ Cyanosis ■ Obvious hemorrhage or injury ■ Temperature dysregulation	■ Assess for life-threatening injuries (e.g., cardiac tamponade, liver laceration, tension pneumothorax). ■ Consider vasopressor therapy only after hypovolemia has been corrected. ■ Insert an indwelling urinary catheter and nasogastric tube. ■ Treat dysrhythmias. **Ongoing Monitoring** ■ Level of consciousness ■ Vital signs, including pulse oximetry, peripheral pulses, capillary refill ■ Cardiac rhythm ■ Urine output

with a natural airway or an endotracheal tube, oxygen delivery must be optimized.

- Mechanical ventilation may be necessary to support the delivery of oxygen to maintain an arterial oxygen saturation of 90% or greater (PaO_2 >60 mm Hg) to avoid hypoxemia (see Artificial Airways: Endotracheal Tubes, p. 693, Oxygen Therapy, p. 734, and Mechanical Ventilation, p. 726). The mean arterial pressure and circulating blood volume are optimized with fluid replacement and drug therapy (see Tables 67-8 and 67-9 in Lewis and others, *Medical-Surgical Nursing,* edition 7, pp. 1786 and 1787 to 1788).

In addition to general management of shock, there are specific interventions for different types of shock (Table 78). Drugs used in the treatment of shock are presented in Table 67-9, Lewis and others, *Medical-Surgical Nursing,* edition 7, pp. 1787 to 1788.

Nursing Management
Goals
The patient with shock will have assurance of adequate tissue perfusion, restoration of normal or baseline BP, return/recovery of organ function, and avoidance of complications from prolonged states of hypoperfusion.

See NCP 67-1 for the patient in shock, Lewis and others, *Medical-Surgical Nursing,* edition 7, pp. 1791 to 1792.
Nursing Diagnoses
- Ineffective tissue perfusion: renal, cerebral, cardiopulmonary, gastrointestinal, hepatic, and peripheral
- Fear
Nursing Interventions
To prevent shock, the nurse must first identify persons who are at risk. In general, patients who are older, those with debilitating diseases, and those who are immunocompromised are at increased risk. More specifically, any person who sustains surgical or accidental trauma is at risk of shock resulting from hemorrhage, spinal cord injury, and burn injuries.

Prevention of shock can include interventions such as early stabilization of spinal cord injuries to prevent neurogenic shock, careful monitoring of fluid balance to prevent hypovolemic shock, and monitoring the patient at risk for sepsis for signs of infection. Aseptic technique must be used with all invasive procedures. Frequent hand washing is essential.

The role of the nurse in shock involves (1) monitoring the patient's ongoing physical and emotional status to detect subtle changes in the patient's condition, (2) planning and implementing nursing interventions and therapy, (3) evaluating the patient's

Table 78 Collaborative Care: Specific Strategies for the Treatment of Shock

	Cardiogenic Shock	Hypovolemic Shock	Septic Shock	Neurogenic Shock	Anaphylactic Shock
Oxygenation	■ Provide supplemental O_2 (e.g., nasal cannula, non-rebreather mask) ■ Intubation/mechanical ventilation, if necessary ■ Monitor SvO_2 or $ScvO_2$	■ Provide supplemental O_2 ■ Monitor SvO_2 or $ScvO_2$	■ Provide supplemental O_2 (e.g., nasal cannula, non-rebreather mask) ■ Intubation/mechanical ventilation, if necessary ■ Monitor SvO_2 or $ScvO_2$	■ Maintain patent airway ■ Provide supplemental O_2 ■ Intubation/mechanical ventilation, if necessary	■ Maintain patent airway ■ Optimize oxygenation with supplemental O_2 ■ Intubation/mechanical ventilation, if necessary
Circulation	■ Restore blood flow with thrombolytics, angioplasty with stenting, emergent coronary revascularization	■ Restore fluid volume (e.g., blood/blood products, crystalloids) ■ Rapid fluid replacement using two	■ Aggressive fluid resuscitation ■ End points of fluid resuscitation —CVP 15 mm Hg —PAWP 10-12 mm Hg	■ Cautious administration of fluids	■ Aggressive fluid resuscitation with colloids

- Reduce workload of heart with circulatory assist devices: IABP, VAD

- large-bore (14-16 gauge) peripheral IV lines
- End points of fluid resuscitation
  —CVP 15 mm Hg
  —PAWP 10-12 mm Hg

Drug Therapies
- Nitrates (e.g., nitroglycerin)
- Inotropes (e.g., dobutamine)
- Diuretics (e.g., furosemide)
- β-Adrenergic blockers (contraindicated with ↓ ejection fraction

- Antibiotics as ordered
- Vasopressors (e.g., dopamine)
- Inotropes (e.g., dobutamine)
- Anticoagulation (e.g., low-molecular-weight heparin)

- Vasopressors (e.g., phenylephrine)
- Atropine (for bradycardia)

- Antihistamines (e.g., diphenhydramine)
- Epinephrine subcutaneous, IV, nebulized
- Bronchodilators: nebulized (e.g., albuterol)
- Corticosteroids (if hypotension persists)

Continued

CVP, Central venous pressure; GI, gastrointestinal; IABP, intraaortic balloon pump; IV, intravenous; PAWP, pulmonary artery wedge pressure; VAD, ventricular assist device.

S

Table 78	Collaborative Care: Specific Strategies for the Treatment of Shock—cont'd			
Cardiogenic Shock	Hypovolemic Shock	Septic Shock	Neurogenic Shock	Anaphylactic Shock
Supportive Therapies				
■ Correct dysrhythmias	■ Correct the cause (e.g., stop bleeding, GI losses) ■ Use warmed fluids	■ Obtain cultures (e.g., blood, wound) before beginning antibiotics ■ Monitor temperature ■ Control blood glucose ■ Stress ulcer prophylaxis (e.g., H_2-receptor blockers)	■ Minimize spinal cord trauma with stabilization ■ Monitor temperature	■ Identify and remove offending cause ■ Prevention by avoidance of known allergens ■ Premedication with history of prior sensitivity (e.g., contrast media)

response to therapy, (4) providing emotional support to the patient and family, and (5) collaborating with other members of the health team to coordinate care.

- Ongoing assessment of the patient's clinical status is essential because trends in clinical findings are more meaningful than any single piece of clinical information.

The effects of anxiety and fear in the face of a critical, life-threatening situation on the patient and family are often overlooked or underestimated. Anxiety, fear, and pain may aggravate respiratory distress and increase the release of catecholamines. The nurse should assess and monitor the patient's anxiety and pain, using medication as necessary to decrease the effects of emotions on oxygen demand. Communication with the patient and family can also decrease anxiety and fear. Communication with the patient and family should include:

- Talking to the patient, even if the patient is intubated or appears comatose.
- Simple explanations of procedures for the patient before they are carried out, as well as information regarding the current plan of care and rationale.
- Simple and honest answers if the patient asks questions about his or her progress and prognosis.
- Avoiding conversations about the patient where the patient can overhear them. Hearing is often the last sense to go, and even if the patient cannot respond, he or she may still be able to hear.
- Comfort and support for the patient's family and significant others by keeping them informed of the patient's condition.
- Rehabilitation necessitates the prevention or early treatment of complications and the correction of the precipitating cause of shock. The nurse should continue to assess the patient for indications of complications throughout the recovery period. These complications include chronic kidney disease after acute tubular necrosis or the development of fibrotic lung disease as a result of ARDS.

SICKLE CELL DISEASE

Description

Sickle cell disease (SCD) is a group of inherited, autosomal recessive disorders characterized by the presence of an abnormal form of hemoglobin (Hb) in the erythrocyte. This abnormal hemoglobin,

hemoglobin S (Hb S), causes the erythrocyte to stiffen and elongate, taking on a sickle shape in response to low oxygen (O_2) levels.

SCD is usually identified during infancy or early childhood. It is an incurable disease that is often fatal by middle age from renal and pulmonary failure. The disease affects more than 50,000 people in the United States and is predominant in African Americans, occurring in an estimated prevalence of 1 in about 400 live births. It can also affect persons of Mediterranean, Caribbean, South and Central American, Arabian, or East Indian ancestry.

Pathophysiology

Types of SCD include sickle cell anemia, sickle cell thalassemia, sickle cell Hb C disease, and sickle cell trait. *Sickle cell anemia* is the most severe of the SCD syndromes. It occurs when a person is homozygous for hemoglobin S (Hb SS); the person has inherited Hb S from both parents.

Sickle cell trait occurs when a person is heterozygous for hemoglobin S (Hb AS); the person has inherited hemoglobin S from one parent and normal hemoglobin (hemoglobin A) from the other parent. Sickle cell trait is typically a very mild to asymptomatic condition.

The major pathophysiologic event of SCD is the sickling of erythrocytes. Sickling episodes are most commonly triggered by low O_2 tension in the blood. Hypoxia or deoxygenation of the erythrocytes can be caused by viral or bacterial infection (most common factor), high altitude, emotional stress, surgery, and blood loss. Other triggering events include dehydration, increased hydrogen ion concentration (acidosis), or low body temperature. A sickling episode can also occur without an obvious cause.

- Sickled erythrocytes become rigid and take on an elongated, crescent shape. Sickled cells are unable to easily pass through capillaries or other small vessels and can cause vascular occlusion, leading to acute or chronic tissue injury. The resulting hemostasis promotes a self-perpetuating cycle of local hypoxia, deoxygenation of more erythrocytes, and more sickling.
- Circulating sickled cells are hemolyzed by the spleen, leading to anemia. Initially the sickling of cells is reversible with reoxygenation, but eventually the condition becomes irreversible because of cell membrane damage from recurrent sickling.

Sickle cell crisis is a severe, painful, acute exacerbation of erythrocyte sickling causing a vaso-occlusive crisis. As blood flow is impaired by sickled cells, vasospasm occurs, further restricting blood flow. Tissue ischemia, infarction, and necrosis eventually occur from lack of oxygen. Shock is a possible life-threatening consequence because of severe oxygen depletion of the tissues and a reduction of the circulating fluid volume. Sickle cell crisis can begin suddenly and persist for days to weeks.

- The frequency, extent, and severity of sickling episodes are highly variable and unpredictable, but they largely depend on the percentage of Hb S present. Individuals with sickle cell anemia have the most severe form because erythrocytes contain a high percentage of Hb S.

Clinical Manifestations

The effects of SCD vary greatly from person to person. Many people with sickle cell anemia are in reasonably good health most of the time. The typical patient is anemic but asymptomatic except during sickling episodes.

- Manifestations of chronic anemia include pallor of mucous membranes, fatigue, and decreased exercise tolerance. The skin may have a grayish cast. Because of hemolysis, jaundice is common and patients are prone to gallstones (cholelithiasis).
- The primary symptom associated with sickling is pain. During sickle cell crisis the pain is quite severe as a result of tissue ischemia. The back, chest, extremities, and abdomen are most commonly affected. About one half of episodes are accompanied by fever, swelling, tenderness, tachypnea, hypertension, and nausea and vomiting.

Complications

With repeated episodes of sickling there is gradual involvement of all body systems, especially the spleen, lungs, kidneys, and brain.

- The spleen becomes small and dysfunctional because of repeated infarction and scarring, resulting in a high incidence of infection, especially pneumonia.
- *Acute chest syndrome* describes pulmonary complications that include pneumonia, tissue infarction, and fat embolism, resulting in pulmonary hypertension and cor pulmonale.
- The kidneys may be injured from the lack of oxygen, resulting in renal failure.
- Stroke can result from thrombosis and infarction of cerebral blood vessels.
- The heart may become ischemic and enlarged, leading to heart failure.
- Retinal vessel obstruction may result in hemorrhage, scarring, retinal detachment, and blindness.

- Bone changes may include osteoporosis and osteosclerosis after infarction. Chronic leg ulcers can result from hypoxia.

Diagnostic Studies
- Peripheral blood smear may reveal sickled cells.
- Electrophoresis of hemoglobin identifies the presence of abnormal hemoglobin.
- Findings of hemolysis (jaundice, elevated serum bilirubin levels) and abnormal laboratory test results (see Table 8, p. 31) may be present.
- X-ray, magnetic resonance imaging (MRI), and Doppler studies may be indicated to diagnose end-organ damage.

Nursing and Collaborative Management
Care is directed toward alleviating the symptoms from complications of the disease and minimizing end-organ damage. There is no specific treatment for the disease. Patients with SCD should be taught to avoid high altitudes, maintain adequate fluid intake, and treat infections promptly.

- Pneumovax, *Haemophilus influenzae,* influenza, and hepatitis immunizations should be administered to protect against infection.
- Chronic leg ulcers may be treated with bed rest, antibiotics, warm saline soaks, mechanical or enzyme debridement, and grafting if necessary.
- Sickle cell crises may require hospitalization. O_2 may be administered to treat hypoxia and control sickling. Rest is instituted to reduce metabolic requirements, and fluids and electrolytes are administered to reduce blood viscosity and maintain renal function.
- Transfusion therapy is indicated when an aplastic crisis occurs. These patients, like those with thalassemia major, may require chelation therapy to reduce transfusion-produced iron overload.
- Large doses of continuous (not prn) opioid analgesics are the mainstay of pain management during the acute phase. After discharge patients often continue taking oral opioid analgesics.
- Infection is a frequent complication and needs to be treated. Patients with acute chest syndrome are treated with broad-spectrum antibiotics, O_2 therapy, and fluid therapy.
- Although many antisickling agents have been tried, hydroxyurea (Droxia) is the only one shown to be clinically

beneficial. This drug increases the production of hemoglobin F (fetal hemoglobin), resulting in a proportional decrease in sickled cells.

- Hematopoietic stem cell transplantation (HSCT) is the only available treatment that can cure some patients with SCD. Recent advances in gene therapy technology provide some promise for the future treatment of SCD.

▼ **Patient and Family Teaching**

Patient teaching is important in the long-term care of patients. The patient and family must understand the basis of the disease and the reasons for supportive care.

- The patient must be taught ways to avoid crises. These include taking steps to reduce the chance of developing hypoxia, such as avoiding high altitudes and seeking medical attention quickly to counteract problems including upper respiratory tract infections.
- Teaching about pain control is also needed because the pain during a crisis may be severe and often requires considerable analgesia.

SJÖGREN SYNDROME

Sjögren syndrome is a relatively common autoimmune disease that targets moisture-producing glands, leading to the common symptoms of xerostomia (dry mouth) and keratoconjunctivitis sicca (dry eyes). The nose, throat, airways, and skin can also become dry. The disease can affect other glands as well, including those in the stomach, pancreas, and intestines. The disease is usually diagnosed in women after age 40 years.

In *primary Sjögren syndrome,* symptoms can be traced to problems with the lacrimal and salivary glands. The patient with primary disease is likely to have antibodies against the cytoplasmic antigens SS-A and SS-B, as well as antinuclear antibody (ANA). The patient with *secondary Sjögren syndrome* typically has had another autoimmune disease (e.g., rheumatoid arthritis, systemic lupus erythematosus) before Sjögren's syndrome develops.

- Sjögren syndrome appears to be caused by genetic and environmental factors. The trigger may be a viral or bacterial infection that adversely stimulates the immune system, causing lymphocytes to attack and damage the lacrimal and salivary glands.

Decreased tearing leads to a "gritty" sensation in the eyes, burning, blurred vision, and photosensitivity. Dry mouth produces buccal membrane fissures, altered sense of taste, dysphagia, and increased frequency of mouth infections or dental caries.

- Dry skin and rashes, joint and muscle pain, and thyroid problems may also be present.
- Autoimmune thyroid disorders are common, including Graves' disease or Hashimoto's thyroiditis.
- The disease may become more generalized and involve the lymph nodes, bone marrow, and visceral organs (pseudo-lymphoma). The risk of developing lymphoma is high in Sjögren syndrome.

Ophthalmologic examination (Schirmer's test), salivary flow rates, and lower lip biopsy of minor salivary glands confirm the diagnosis.

Treatment is symptomatic, including instillation of artificial tears as often as necessary to maintain adequate hydration and lubrication, surgical occlusion of the puncta lacrimalia, and increased fluids with meals.

- Dental hygiene is important. Pilocarpine (Salagen) and cevimeline (Evoxac) can be used to treat symptoms of dry mouth.
- Increased humidity at home may reduce respiratory infections. Vaginal lubrication with a water-soluble product such as KY jelly may increase comfort during intercourse.

SPINAL CORD INJURY

Description

The population at highest risk for spinal cord injury (SCI) is young adult men between the ages of 16 and 30 years. The causes of SCI frequently include motor vehicle accidents, falls, violence, and sports injuries. The resulting SCI can be due to cord compression by bone displacement, interruption of blood supply to the cord, or traction resulting from pulling on the cord.

SCIs are classified by the mechanism of injury, level of injury, and completeness or degree of injury. The major mechanisms of injury are flexion, hyperextension, flexion-rotation, extension-rotation, and compression. The level of injury may be cervical, thoracic, or lumbar. Cervical and lumbar injuries are the most common because these levels are associated with the greatest flexibility and movement.

The degree of spinal cord involvement may be either complete or incomplete (partial).

- *Complete cord involvement* results in total loss of sensory and motor function below the level of the lesion (injury). If the cervical cord is involved, paralysis of all four extremities occurs, resulting in *tetraplegia* (paralysis of both arms and legs). If the thoracic or lumbar cord is damaged, the result is *paraplegia* (paralysis and loss of sensation in the legs).
- *Incomplete cord involvement* (partial transection) results in a mixed loss of voluntary motor activity and sensation and leaves some tracts intact. The degree of sensory and motor loss varies depending on the level of the lesion and reflects the specific nerve tracts damaged and those spared. A variety of specific syndromes of incomplete cord involvement have been identified.

Pathophysiology

Penetrating trauma, such as gunshot and stab wounds, can result in tearing and transection of the spinal cord. Complete cord damage in severe trauma is related to autodestruction of the cord.

Shortly after the injury, petechial hemorrhages are noted in the central gray matter of the cord. Within 4 hours there may be infarction in the gray matter. The resulting hypoxia reduces oxygen tension below the level that meets metabolic needs of the spinal cord. Lactate metabolites and an increase in vasoactive substances, including norepinephrine, serotonin, and dopamine, are noted. At high levels, these vasoactive substances cause vasospasms and hypoxia, leading to subsequent necrosis. By 24 hours permanent damage has occurred because of the development of edema. Lack of space for edema results in compression of the cord and extension of edema above and below the injury, increasing the ischemic damage.

The extent of the neurologic damage caused by an SCI results from *primary injury* damage (actual physical disruption of axons) and *secondary injury* damage (ischemia, hypoxia, microhemorrhage, edema). Because secondary injury processes occur over time, the extent of injury and prognosis for recovery are most accurately determined at 72 hours or more after injury.

Spinal and Neurogenic Shock. About 50% of people with acute SCI experience a temporary neurologic syndrome known as *spinal shock* that is characterized by decreased reflexes, loss of sensation, and flaccid paralysis below the level of the injury. This syndrome lasts days to months and may mask postinjury neurologic function. Active rehabilitation may begin in the presence of spinal shock.

Neurogenic shock is due to the loss of vasomotor tone caused by injury and is characterized by hypotension, bradycardia, and warm, dry extremities. Loss of sympathetic innervation causes peripheral vasodilation, venous pooling, and decreased cardiac output. These effects are generally associated with a cervical or high thoracic injury.

Clinical Manifestations

Manifestations of SCI are related to the level and degree of injury. The patient with an incomplete lesion may demonstrate a mixture of symptoms. The higher the injury, the more serious the effects because of the proximity of the cervical cord to the medulla and brainstem. Movement and rehabilitation potential related to specific locations of the SCI are described in Table 61-3, Lewis and others, *Medical-Surgical Nursing,* edition 7, p. 1594. In general, sensory function closely parallels motor function at all levels.

Complications

Immediate postinjury problems include maintaining a patent airway, adequate ventilation, and adequate circulating blood volume and preventing extension of cord damage (secondary injury).

Respiratory System. Cervical injury or fracture above the level of C4 presents with a total loss of respiratory muscle function. Mechanical ventilation is required to keep the patient alive. Injury below the level of C4 can result in diaphragmatic breathing with respiratory insufficiency, hypoventilation, and decreased vital capacity and tidal volume.

Cardiovascular System. Any cord injury above the level of T6 markedly decreases the influence of the sympathetic nervous system. Bradycardia occurs as a result of the unopposed effect of the parasympathetic nervous system on the heart, and peripheral vasodilation results in hypotension. Cardiac monitoring is necessary.

Urinary System. Urinary retention is common in acute spinal cord injuries and spinal shock. While the patient is in spinal shock, the bladder is atonic and becomes overdistended. An indwelling catheter is inserted to drain the bladder. In the postacute phase the bladder may become hyperirritable, with a loss of inhibition from the brain resulting in reflex emptying.

Gastrointestinal System. If the cord injury has occurred above the level of T5, the primary problems are related to hypomotility. Decreased GI activity contributes to the development of a paralytic ileus and gastric distention. A nasogastric (NG) tube for intermittent suctioning may relieve the gastric distention. Histamine H_2-receptor blockers and proton pump inhibitors are frequently used to prevent the development of stress ulcers.

Loss of voluntary neurologic control over the bowel results in a *neurogenic* bowel. With an injury level of T12 or below, the bowel is areflexic and sphincter tone is decreased, resulting in constipation. As reflexes return, the bowel becomes reflexic, sphincter tone is enhanced, and reflex emptying occurs. Bowel programs can be used to manage both types of neurogenic bowel.

Integumentary System. A major consequence of lack of movement is the potential for skin breakdown over bony prominences in areas of decreased sensation. Pressure ulcers can occur quickly and lead to major infection or sepsis. A certain degree of muscle atrophy occurs during the flaccid paralysis state, whereas contractures tend to occur during the spastic state.

Peripheral Vascular Problems. Deep vein thrombosis (DVT) is a common problem accompanying SCI in the first 3 months. Pulmonary embolism is one of the leading causes of death in patients with SCI. Techniques for assessment of DVT include Doppler examination, impedance plethysmography, and measuring of leg and thigh girth.

Autonomic dysreflexia is a massive uncompensated cardiovascular reaction mediated by the sympathetic nervous system. It occurs in response to visceral stimulation after spinal shock is resolved in patients with spinal cord lesions at T6 or higher.

- The condition is a life-threatening situation that requires immediate resolution. If resolution does not occur, this condition can lead to status epilepticus, stroke, and even death.
- The most common precipitating cause is a distended bladder or rectum, although any sensory stimulation may cause autonomic dysreflexia.
- Manifestations include hypertension (up to 300 mm Hg systolic), blurred vision, throbbing headache, marked diaphoresis above the level of the lesion, bradycardia (30 to 40 beats per minute), piloerection (erection of body hair), nasal congestion, and nausea. It is important that blood pressure (BP) be measured when a patient with an SCI complains of a headache.
- Management includes elevation of the head of the bed 45 degrees or sitting the patient upright, notifying the physician, and assessing the cause of the reaction. Interventions to relieve the cause should be implemented immediately (e.g., relieving bladder or bowel distention, removal of all skin stimuli). If symptoms persist after the source has been

relieved, an α-adrenergic blocker (e.g., phentolamine [Regitine]) or an arterial vasodilator (e.g., nifedipine [Procardia]) is administered.

- The patient and family must be taught the causes and symptoms of autonomic dysreflexia (see Table 61-7, Lewis and others, *Medical-Surgical Nursing,* edition 7, p. 1604). They must understand the life-threatening nature of this dysfunction and must know how to relieve the cause.

Diagnostic Studies

After the patient is immobilized, diagnostic studies can be done.

- Complete spine x-rays are performed to assess for vertebral fracture.
- X-rays of C1 through T1 are used to visualize and document presence of vertebral injury.
- Computed tomography (CT) may be used to assess stability of injury, location and degree of bony injury, soft and neural tissue changes, and degree of spinal canal compromise.
- Magnetic resonance imaging (MRI) is used in unexplained neurologic deficit or worsening of neurologic status.
- Patients with cervical injuries who demonstrate altered mental status may need vertebral angiography to rule out vertebral artery damage.

Collaborative Care

After stabilization at the accident scene, the person is transferred to a medical facility. For injury at the cervical level, all body systems must be maintained until the full extent of the damage can be evaluated. A thorough assessment is done to specifically evaluate the degree of deficit and to establish the level and degree of injury. The patient may go directly to surgery after initial immobilization and assessment or to the intensive care unit (ICU) for monitoring and management.

Nonoperative Stablization

Nonoperative treatments are focused on stabilization of the injured spinal segment and decompression, either through traction or realignment, to prevent secondary spinal cord damage caused by repeated contusion or compression.

Surgical Therapy

When cord compression is certain or the neurologic disorder progresses, benefits may be seen following immediate surgery. Surgery stabilizes the spinal column. There is some evidence to suggest that early cord decompression results in reduced secondary injury to the spinal cord and thus better outcomes. Other criteria for early surgery include (1) evidence of cord compression, (2) progressive neurologic deficit, (3) compound fracture of the vertebrae, (4) bony fragments (may dislodge and penetrate the cord), and (5) penetrating wounds of the spinal cord or surrounding structures.

- More common surgical procedures include decompression laminectomy by anterior cervical and thoracic approaches with fusion, posterior laminectomy with the use of acrylic wire mesh and fusion, and the insertion of stabilizing rods (e.g., Harrington rods for the correction and stabilization of thoracic deformities).

Drug Therapy

Vasopressor agents such as dopamine (Intropin) are used in the acute phase to maintain the mean arterial pressure at a level greater than 80 to 90 mm Hg so that perfusion to the spinal cord is improved.

In the past, methylprednisolone (MP) was considered a standard of care for acute SCI treatment to promote greater recovery of neurologic function. Further studies of MP have identified deleterious effects of the drug, including higher risk of complications, higher acute care costs, and longer hospital stays. Today MP is a treatment option that may be used when the physician determines that the potential benefits outweigh the risks. If it is used, it must be given intravenously (IV) within 8 hours of injury for any benefit. It is thought to improve blood flow and reduce edema in the spinal cord.

- Drug therapy is used to treat specific autonomic dysfunctions such as GI hypoactivity, bradycardia, orthostatic hypotension, inadequate emptying of the bladder, and autonomic dysreflexia.

Nursing Management

Goals

The patient with an SCI will maintain an optimal level of neurologic functioning; have minimal or no complications of immobility; learn new skills, gain new knowledge, and acquire new behaviors to be able to care for self or successfully direct others to do so; and return to home and the community at an optimal level of functioning.

See NCP 61-1 for the patient with an SCI, Lewis and others, *Medical-Surgical Nursing*, edition 7, pp. 1598 to 1600.

Nursing Diagnoses

- Impaired gas exchange
- Decreased cardiac output
- Impaired skin integrity

- Constipation
- Impaired urinary elimination
- Impaired physical mobility
- Risk for autonomic dysreflexia
- Ineffective coping
- Interrupted family processes

Nursing Interventions

High cervical injury resulting from flexion-rotation is the most complex SCI and is discussed in this section. Interventions for this type of injury can be modified for patients with less severe problems.

Immobilization. Proper immobilization of the neck involves maintenance of a neutral position. The body should always be correctly aligned, and turning should be performed so that the patient is moved as a unit (e.g., logrolling) to prevent movement of the spine. For cervical injuries, skeletal traction is used less frequently with the development of better surgical stabilization. When skeletal traction is used, realignment or reduction of the injury is usually provided by Crutchfield, Vinke, Gardner-Wells, or other types of skull tongs.

- Infection at the sites of tong insertion is a potential problem. Preventive care includes cleansing the sites twice each day with normal saline solution and applying an antibiotic ointment that acts as a mechanical barrier to the bacteria.
- If skull tongs become displaced, the head should be held in a neutral position and stabilized when the physician reinserts the tongs.
- Meticulous skin care is critical because decreased sensation and circulation make the patient particularly susceptible to skin breakdown.
- Special beds are often used to provide frequent turning to prevent pressure sores and cardiopulmonary complications.
- After cervical fusion or other stabilization surgery, a hard cervical collar or sternal-occipital-mandibular immobilizer brace may provide cervical immobilization with more mobility. A halo apparatus can also be used for cervical immobilization while allowing ambulation.

Respiratory Dysfunction. If the patient is exhausted from labored breathing or arterial blood gases (ABGs) deteriorate (indicating inadequate oxygenation), endotracheal intubation or tracheostomy and mechanical ventilation should be initiated. (See Artificial Airways: Endotracheal Tubes, p. 693, Tracheostomy, p. 746, and Mechanical Ventilation, p. 726.) Respiratory arrest is a possibility that requires careful monitoring and prompt action should it occur. Pneumonia and atelectasis are potential problems because of reduced vital capacity and the loss of intercostal and abdominal muscle function.

- The nurse should regularly assess breath sounds, ABGs, tidal volume, vital capacity, skin color, breathing patterns (especially the use of accessory muscles), subjective comments about the ability to breathe, and the amount and color of sputum.
- In addition to monitoring, the nurse can intervene in maintaining ventilation by the administration of oxygen (O_2) until ABGs stabilize, chest physiotherapy and assisted coughing, incentive spirometry, and tracheal suctioning.

Cardiovascular Instability. If bradycardia is symptomatic, an anticholinergic medication such as atropine is administered. A temporary pacemaker may be inserted in some instances (see Pacemakers, p. 740). Hypotension is managed with a vasopressor agent, such as dopamine, and fluid replacement.

- Compression gradient stockings and pneumatic compression devices can be used to prevent thromboemboli and to promote venous return.
- The nurse should perform range-of-motion (ROM) exercises and heel-cord stretching regularly. The thighs and calves of the legs should be assessed every shift for the signs of DVT.
- The nurse should also monitor the patient for indications of hypovolemic shock secondary to hemorrhage.

Fluid and Nutritional Maintenance. During the first 48 to 72 hours after the injury, the GI tract may stop functioning (paralytic ileus) and an NG tube must be inserted.

- Once bowel sounds are present or flatus is passed, oral food and fluids can gradually be introduced. Because of severe catabolism, a high-protein, high-calorie diet is necessary for energy and tissue repair.
- In patients with high cervical cord injuries, swallowing must be evaluated before starting oral feedings. If the patient is unable to resume eating, enteral tube feedings or parenteral nutrition (PN) may be started to provide nutritional support.

Bowel and Bladder Management. An indwelling catheter is usually inserted as soon as possible after injury. Its patency must be ensured by irrigation and frequent inspection. Strict aseptic technique for catheter care is essential to avoid introducing infection.

Urinary tract infections (UTIs) are a common problem. The best method for preventing UTIs is regular and complete bladder drainage. Cranberry juice may also help prevent UTIs.

Constipation is generally a problem during spinal shock because no voluntary or involuntary (reflex) evacuation of the bowels occurs. A bowel program should be started during acute care. This consists of a rectal stimulant (suppository or mini-enema) inserted daily at a regular time of day followed by gentle digital stimulation or manual evacuation.

Temperature Control. In spinal cord injuries the interruption of the sympathetic nervous system prevents peripheral temperature sensations from reaching the hypothalamus, resulting in the adjustment of body temperature to the room temperature (poikilothermism). In addition, there is no vasoconstriction, piloerection, or heat loss through perspiration below the level of injury. As a result, temperature control is largely external to the patient. The nurse should monitor the environment and the patient's body temperature closely to maintain appropriate temperatures.

Sensory Deprivation. The nurse must compensate for the patient's absent sensations to prevent sensory deprivation. This is done by stimulating the patient above the level of injury. Conversation, music, strong aromas, and interesting flavors should be a part of nursing care. Prism glasses are provided so that the patient can read and watch television. Every effort should be made to prevent the patient from withdrawing from the environment.

Reflexes. Once spinal shock is resolved, reflexes often return with hyperactive and exaggerated responses. Penile erections can occur from a variety of stimuli, causing embarrassment and discomfort. Spasms ranging from mild twitches to convulsive movements below the level of the lesion may also occur. Reflex activity may be interpreted by the patient or family as a return of function, and the nurse must tactfully explain the reason for the activity. Spasms may be controlled with antispasmodic medications, such as baclofen (Lioresal), dantrolene (Dantrium), or tizanidine (Zanaflex).

Rehabilitation. Physiologic and psychologic rehabilitation is complex and involved. Many of the problems identified in the acute period become chronic and continue throughout life. Rehabilitation focuses on refined retraining of physiologic processes and extensive patient and family teaching about how to manage the physiologic and life changes resulting from injury.

SPINAL CORD TUMORS

Description

Tumors that affect the spinal cord account for 0.5% to 1% of all neoplasms. These tumors are classified as primary (arising from some component of cord, dura, nerves, or vessels) or secondary (from primary growths in the breast, prostate, lung, kidney, and other sites).

- Spinal cord tumors are further classified as *extradural tumors* (outside the spinal cord), *intradural-extramedullary tumors* (within the dura but outside the actual spinal cord), and *intradural-intramedullary tumors* (within the spinal cord itself) (see Fig. 61-14 and Table 61-15, Lewis and others, *Medical-Surgical Nursing,* edition 7, pp. 1609 and 1610).

Because many of these tumors are slow growing, their symptoms stem from the mechanical effects of slow compression and irritation of nerve roots, displacement of the cord, or gradual obstruction of the vascular supply. Slowness of growth does not cause autodestruction as in traumatic lesions. Therefore complete functional restoration is possible when the tumor is removed, with the exception of intradural-intramedullary tumors.

Clinical Manifestations

The most common early symptom of a spinal cord tumor outside the cord is pain in the back with a radiation of pain simulating intercostal neuralgia, angina, or herpes zoster. The location of the pain depends on the level of compression. The pain worsens with activity, coughing, straining, and lying down.

- Sensory disruption is later manifested by coldness, numbness, and tingling in an extremity or in several extremities, slowly progressing upward until it reaches the level of the lesion.
- Impaired sensation of pain, temperature, and light touch precedes a deficit in vibration and position sense that may progress to complete anesthesia.
- Motor weakness accompanies sensory disturbances and consists of slowly increasing clumsiness, weakness, and spasticity. The sensory and motor disturbances are ipsilateral to the lesion.
- Bladder disturbances are marked by urgency with difficulty in starting the flow and progressing to retention with overflow incontinence.

Manifestations of intradural spinal tumor develop as progressive damage to the long spinal tracts, producing paralysis, sensory loss, and bladder dysfunction. Pain can be severe as a result of the compression of spinal roots or vertebrae.

Diagnostic Studies

Extradural tumors are seen early on routine spinal x-rays, whereas intradural and intramedullary tumors require magnetic resonance imaging (MRI) or computed tomography (CT) scans for detection. Cerebrospinal fluid (CSF) analysis may reveal tumor cells.

Nursing and Collaborative Management

Compression of the spinal cord is an emergency. Relief of the ischemia related to the compression is the goal of therapy. Corticosteroids, usually dexamethasone (Decadron) in large doses, are generally prescribed immediately to relieve tumor-related edema.

Treatment for nearly all spinal cord tumors is surgical removal. The exception is the metastatic tumor that is sensitive to radiation and that has caused only minimal neurologic deficits in the patient. In general, extradural or intradural-extramedullary tumors can be completely removed surgically.

Radiation therapy after surgery is fairly effective. Chemotherapy may be used in conjunction with radiation therapy.

- Depending on the amount of neurologic dysfunction exhibited, the patient may need to be cared for as though recovering from a spinal cord injury.

SPLEEN DISORDERS

The spleen can be affected by many illnesses, most of which can cause some degree of splenomegaly *(enlarged spleen)*. Some of the many causes of splenomegaly include sickle cell disease, infections, cirrhosis, heart failure (HF), and polycythemia vera. The term *hypersplenism* refers to the occurrence of splenomegaly and peripheral cytopenias (anemia, leukopenia, thrombocytopenia).

- The degree of splenic enlargement varies with the disease. For example, massive splenic enlargement occurs with chronic myelogenous leukemia and thalassemia major, whereas mild splenic enlargement occurs with HF and systemic lupus erythematosus. When the spleen enlarges, its normal filtering and sequestering capacity increases. Consequently, there is often a reduction in the number of circulating blood cells.

A slight to moderate enlargement of the spleen is usually asymptomatic and found during a routine examination of the abdomen. Massive splenomegaly can be well tolerated, but patients may complain of abdominal discomfort and early satiety. In addition to physical examination, other techniques to assess spleen size include Tc-sulfur colloid liver-spleen scan, computed tomography (CT) scan, magnetic resonance imaging (MRI), and ultrasound scan.

Occasionally laparoscopy or open laparotomy and splenectomy are indicated in the evaluation or treatment of splenomegaly. Splenectomy can have a dramatic effect in increasing peripheral red blood cell (RBC), white blood cell (WBC), and platelet counts. Another indication for splenectomy is splenic rupture. The spleen may rupture from trauma, inadvertent tearing during other surgical procedures, and diseases such as mononucleosis, malaria, and lymphoid neoplasms.

Nursing responsibilities for patients with spleen disorders vary depending on the nature of the problem.

- Splenomegaly may be painful and require analgesic administration; care in moving, turning, and positioning; and evaluation of lung expansion, because spleen enlargement may impair diaphragmatic excursion.
- If anemia, thrombocytopenia, or leukopenia develops from splenic enlargement, nursing measures must be instituted to support the patient and prevent life-threatening complications.
- After splenectomy the patient must be observed for hemorrhage, which can lead to shock, fever, and abdominal distention.
- Postsplenectomy patients may develop immunologic deficiencies and have a lifelong risk for infection from encapsulated organisms, such as pneumococcus. This risk is reduced by immunization with polyvalent pneumococcal vaccine (Pneumovax).

STOMACH CANCER

Description

Stomach cancer is an adenocarcinoma of the stomach wall. The rate of stomach cancer has been steadily declining in the United States since the 1930s, but it has a high mortality rate because it is typically at an advanced stage when diagnosed. The incidence of stomach cancer increases with age with most individuals diagnosed in their 70s. More than 50% have advanced disease at the time of diagnosis, and the 5-year survival rate is less than 30% in those with advanced disease. If the tumor is confined to the stomach at diagnosis, the 5-year survival rate is 80%.

Pathophysiology

Many factors have been implicated in stomach cancer. A nonspecific mucosal injury as a result of aging, autoimmunity, or repeated exposure to irritants such as bile, antiinflammatory agents, or smoking may have a carcinogenic effect. Stomach cancer has also been associated with diets containing smoked foods, salted fish and meat, and pickled vegetables. *Helicobacter pylori* infection, especially at an early age, is considered a risk factor for stomach cancer. Other predisposing factors are obesity, family history, atrophic gastritis, pernicious anemia, adenomatous and hyperplastic polyps, and achlorhydria. Whole grains and fresh fruits and vegetables are associated with reduced rates of stomach cancer.

Cancer can occur in any portion of the stomach. Tumors located at the cardia and fundi are associated with a poor prognosis. These tumors spread by direct extension and typically infiltrate rapidly to the surrounding tissue and liver.

- The rich lymphatic plexuses in the stomach facilitate distant metastasis.
- Evidence of spread to the peritoneal cavity is manifested by ascites.

Clinical Manifestations

Stomach cancers often spread to adjacent organs before any distressing symptoms such as indigestion or dysphagia occur. Clinical manifestations include signs and symptoms of anemia, peptic ulcer disease (PUD), or indigestion.

- Anemia commonly occurs with chronic blood loss as the lesion erodes the stomach mucosa. The patient appears pale and weak with fatigue, dizziness, weakness, and positive occult stools.
- Pain and discomfort usually associated with PUD also occur in stomach cancer, including indigestion, signs of vague epigastric fullness with early satiety after meals, weight loss, dysphagia, and constipation.

With more advanced disease, when the appetite is poor and weight loss has been considerable, the patient may appear cachectic. A mass can often be detected beneath the abdominal wall and is seen to move with each inspiration. On palpation the mass may be felt in the epigastrium. The presence of ascites is a poor prognostic sign.

Diagnostic Studies

- Endoscopic examination with biopsy of the stomach is the best diagnostic tool.
- Endoscopic ultrasound and computed tomography (CT) scanning are done for staging of the disease.
- Blood studies detect anemia and its severity and also elevations in liver enzymes and serum amylase that indicate liver and pancreatic involvement.

- Stool examination is done for occult or gross bleeding.
- Carcinoembryonic antigen (CEA) and carbohydrate antigen (CA) 19-9 may be used to detect and monitor progression of malignancy.

Collaborative Care

Treatment of choice is surgical removal of the tumor. Surgical resection can result in 75% 5-year survival in patients with lymph node–negative stomach cancer, but only 10% to 30% 5-year survival if lymph nodes are positive. Surgical procedures used are similar to those used for peptic ulcer disease (see Peptic Ulcer Disease, p. 480).

- Preoperative management focuses on the correction of nutritional deficits and transfusions of packed red blood cells (RBCs) to treat anemia. Gastric decompression may be necessary if gastric outlet obstruction is present, and special preparation of the bowel is needed if the tumor has involved the colon.

Chemotherapy and radiation may be used if a surgical cure is not feasible (see Chemotherapy, p. 712). The combination of chemotherapy and radiation is also now being used for patients who are at high risk for disease recurrence after surgery. The combination of radiation and chemotherapy involving fluorouracil (5-FU) and leucovorin after surgical resection has been shown to prolong life in some patients with stomach cancer.

Nursing Management

Goals
The patient with stomach cancer will experience minimal discomfort, achieve optimal nutritional status, and maintain a degree of spiritual and psychologic well-being appropriate to the disease stage.

Nursing Diagnoses
- Imbalanced nutrition: less than body requirements
- Activity intolerance
- Anxiety
- Acute pain
- Grieving

Nursing Interventions
The nursing role in the early detection of stomach cancer is focused primarily on the identification of patients at risk (e.g., those with pernicious anemia or achlorhydria or those who smoke).

When diagnostic tests confirm the presence of malignancy, the nurse must give emotional and physical support, provide information, clarify test results, and maintain a positive attitude with respect to the patient's immediate recovery and long-term survival.

The preoperative teaching plan is similar to that for PUD surgery (see Peptic Ulcer Disease, p. 480).

Postoperative care is also similar to that following surgery for PUD. Close observation for signs of fluids leaking at the site of anastomosis, as evidenced by an elevation in temperature and increasing dyspnea, is important. If a total gastrectomy is done, dumping syndrome may occur (see p. 485 under Peptic Ulcer Disease).

- Postoperative wound healing may be impaired because of inadequate dietary intake. This necessitates intravenous (IV) or oral replacement of C, D, K, and B-complex vitamins and intramuscular (IM) administration of cobalamin.

Because most radiation therapy and chemotherapy are completed on an outpatient basis, the nurse should assess the patient's knowledge of radiation, skin care, need for good nutrition and fluid intake during therapy, and appropriate use of antiemetic drugs.

▼ **Patient and Family Teaching**

Before discharge, instruction should be given for the relief of pain, including comfort measures and the use of analgesics; additional considerations include the following:

- Wound care, if needed, must be taught to the primary caregiver in the home situation.
- Dressings, special equipment, or special services may be required for the patient's continued care at home.
- A list of community agencies that are available for assistance should be provided.

STROKE

Description

Stroke occurs when there is ischemia to a part of the brain or hemorrhage into the brain that results in brain cell death. Functions, such as movement, sensation, or emotions, that were controlled by the affected brain area are lost or impaired. The severity of the loss of function varies according to the location and extent of the brain area involved.

- Stroke is the third most common cause of death and is a leading cause of serious, long-term disability in the United States and Canada. Strokes are considered a major public health problem in the United States in terms of mortality and morbidity, since an estimated 700,000 persons experience strokes annually.

- About 25% of people who have an initial stroke die within 1 year. This percentage is higher among people age 65 years and older.
- Of those who survive, 50% to 70% will be functionally independent and 15% to 30% will live with permanent disability.

Risk factors associated with stroke can be divided into non-modifiable and modifiable.

- Nonmodifiable risk factors include age, race, and heredity. African Americans experience a higher incidence of stroke, which is associated with an increased incidence of hypertension, obesity, and diabetes mellitus (DM). African American men from the South are almost four times more likely to die from a stroke than Southern white men. Persons with a family history of stroke or transient ischemic attacks (TIAs) are also at higher risk for stroke.
- Modifiable risk factors are hypertension, cardiovascular disease, DM, obesity, sickle cell disease, and certain lifestyle habits, such as cigarette smoking, a diet high in fat, and heavy alcohol consumption. Hypertension is the single most important modifiable risk factor, and its treatment can reduce the risk of stroke by up to 42%.

Transient Ischemic Attack

A TIA is a temporary focal loss of neurologic function caused by ischemia. It lasts less than 24 hours and often lasts less than 15 minutes. Most TIAs resolve within 3 hours. TIAs may be due to microemboli that temporarily block the blood flow and are a warning sign of progressive cerebrovascular disease.

TIA signs and symptoms depend on the blood vessel involved and the brain area that is ischemic.

- If the carotid system is involved, patients may have a temporary loss of vision in one eye, transient hemiparesis, numbness or loss of sensation, or a sudden inability to speak.
- Signs of a TIA involving the vertebrobasilar system may include tinnitus, vertigo, darkened or blurred vision, ptosis, dysphagia, ataxia, and unilateral or bilateral numbness or weakness.

Evaluation must be done to confirm that signs and symptoms of a TIA are not related to other brain lesions, such as a developing subdural hematoma or an increasing tumor mass.

- Computed tomography (CT) of the brain without contrast is the most important initial diagnostic study. Cardiac monitoring and tests may reveal an underlying cardiac condition that is responsible for clot formation.

- Medications that prevent platelet aggregation, such as aspirin, ticlopidine (Ticlid), clopidogrel (Plavix), dipyridamole (Persantine), combined dipyridamole and aspirin (Aggrenox), and anticoagulant medications (e.g., oral warfarin [Coumadin]), may be prescribed for long-term therapy after a TIA.

Types of Strokes

Strokes are classified as ischemic or hemorrhagic based on their underlying pathophysiology (Table 79 and Fig. 15).

- *Ischemic strokes* result from a decreased blood flow to the brain secondary to partial or complete occlusion of an artery. They occur much more frequently than hemorrhagic strokes. The most common types of ischemic stroke are thrombotic and embolic.
- *Hemorrhagic strokes* result from bleeding into the brain tissue itself (intracerebral or intraparenchymal hemorrhage)

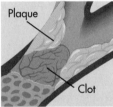

Thrombotic stroke. Cerebral thrombosis is a narrowing of the artery by fatty deposits called *plaque*. Plaque can cause a clot to form, which blocks the passage of blood through the artery.

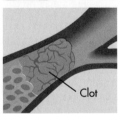

Embolic stroke. An embolus is a blood clot or other debris circulating in the blood. When it reaches an artery in the brain that is too narrow to pass through, it lodges there and blocks the flow of blood.

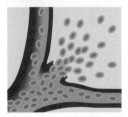

Hemorrhagic stroke. A burst blood vessel may allow blood to seep into and damage brain tissues until clotting shuts off the leak.

Fig. 15. Three types of stroke.

Table 79 Types of Stroke

Type	Gender/Age	Warning	Time of Onset	Course/Prognosis
Ischemic (80%)				
Thrombotic	Men more than women, oldest median age	TIA (30%-50% of cases)	During or after sleep	Stepwise progression, signs and symptoms develop slowly, usually some improvement, recurrence in 20%-25% of survivors
Embolic	Men more than women	TIA (uncommon)	Lack of relationship to activity, sudden onset	Single event, signs and symptoms develop quickly, usually some improvement recurrence common without aggressive treatment of underlying disease
Hemorrhagic (15%)				
Intracerebral	Slightly higher in women	Headache (25% of cases)	Activity (often)	Progression over 24 hr; poor prognosis, fatality more likely with presence of coma
Subarachnoid	Slightly higher in women, youngest median age	Headache (common)	Activity (often), sudden onset Most commonly related to head trauma	Single sudden event usually, fatality more likely with presence of coma

TIA, Transient ischemic attack.

S

or into the subarachnoid space or ventricles (subarachnoid hemorrhage). They account for 15% of all strokes.

Pathophysiology

Thrombotic Stroke. Thrombosis results from the formation of a blood clot that causes narrowing of the lumen of a blood vessel with eventual occlusion and infarction. It is the most common cause of stroke.

- Two thirds of thrombotic strokes are associated with hypertension or DM; both of these conditions accelerate the atherosclerotic process.

Thrombotic strokes may be preceded by a TIA. The extent of the stroke depends on rapidity of onset, size of lesion, and presence of collateral circulation.

- Most patients do not have a decreased level of consciousness in the first 24 hours unless it is due to a brainstem stroke or other conditions, such as seizures, increased intracranial pressure, or hemorrhage.
- Ischemic stroke symptoms may progress in the first 72 hours as infarction and cerebral edema increase.

Embolic Stroke. Cerebral embolism is the occlusion of a cerebral artery by an embolus, resulting in necrosis and edema of the area supplied by the involved blood vessel. Embolism is the second most common cause of stroke.

The majority of emboli originate in the heart. The emboli travel to the cerebral circulation and lodge where a vessel narrows. Emboli are associated with heart conditions such as atrial fibrillation, myocardial infarction (MI), and inflammatory and valvular heart conditions.

- Onset of an embolic stroke is usually sudden and may or may not be related to activity. The patient usually remains conscious, although a headache may develop.
- Recurrence is common unless the underlying cause is aggressively treated.

Hemorrhagic Stroke. **Intracerebral hemorrhage** is bleeding within the brain caused by a rupture of a vessel. Hypertension is the most important cause of intracerebral hemorrhage. Other causes include vascular malformations, coagulation disorders, anticoagulant drugs, trauma, and ruptured aneurysms.

- Hemorrhage commonly occurs during periods of activity. There is most often a sudden onset of symptoms, and progression occurs over minutes to hours as a result of ongoing bleeding.
- Symptoms include neurologic deficits, headache, nausea, vomiting, decreased level of consciousness, and hyperten-

sion. Extent of the symptoms varies depending on amount and duration of bleeding.

- Prognosis of patients with intracerebral hemorrhage is poor, with 40% to 80% of patients dying within 30 days and 50% of the deaths occurring within the first 48 hours. Only about 20% of patients with a hemorrhagic stroke are functionally independent at 6 months.

Subarachnoid hemorrhage occurs when there is intracranial bleeding into the cerebrospinal fluid–filled space between the arachnoid and pia mater membranes on the surface of the brain. Subarachnoid hemorrhage is commonly caused by rupture of a cerebral aneurysm (congenital or acquired weakness and ballooning of vessels). Other causes of subarachnoid hemorrhage include arteriovenous malformations (AVMs), trauma, and illicit drug (cocaine) abuse.

- Characteristic presentation of a ruptured aneurysm is the sudden onset of a severe headache different from a previous headache and typically the "worst headache of one's life." Loss of consciousness may or may not occur, and the patient's level of consciousness may range from alert to comatose, depending on the severity of the bleeding.
- Other symptoms include focal neurologic deficits (including cranial nerve deficits), nausea, vomiting, seizures, and stiff neck.
- Despite improvements in surgical techniques and management, many patients with subarachnoid hemorrhage die or are left with significant disability.

Clinical Manifestations

Manifestations seen with specific cerebral artery involvement are listed in Table 58-2, Lewis and others, *Medical-Surgical Nursing,* edition 7, p. 1507. Figure 16 illustrates manifestations of right-sided and left-sided stroke.

Neuromotor Function. Motor deficits are the most obvious effect of stroke and are caused by destruction of motor neurons in the pyramidal pathway. Because the pyramidal pathway crosses at the level of the medulla, a lesion on one side of the brain affects motor function on the opposite side of the brain (contralateral). This destruction can result in loss of skilled voluntary movements (*akinesia*), impairment of integration of movements, and alterations in muscle tone and reflex activity.

- Hyporeflexia that initially occurs with stroke progresses to hyperreflexia for most patients.

Communication. The left hemisphere is dominant for language skills in all right-handed persons and in most left-handed persons.

- Language disorders involve the expression and comprehension of written or spoken words. The patient may experience *aphasia* (total loss of comprehension and use of language) when a stroke damages the dominant hemisphere of the brain.
- When the stroke involves Wernicke's area of the brain, the patient experiences *receptive aphasia*; neither the sounds of

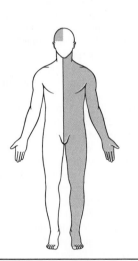 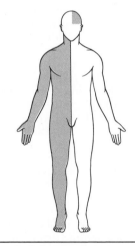

Right brain damage
(Stroke on right side of brain)
- Paralyzed left side: hemiplegia
- Left-sided neglect
- Spatial-perceptual deficits
- Tends to deny or minimize problems
- Rapid performance, short attention span
- Impulsive, safety problems
- Impaired judgment
- Impaired time concepts

Left brain damage
(Stroke on left side of brain)
- Paralyzed right side: hemiplegia
- Impaired speech/language aphasias
- Impaired right/left discrimination
- Slow performance, cautious
- Impaired speech/language
- Aware of deficits: depression, anxiety
- Impaired comprehension related to language, math

Fig. 16. **Manifestations of right-sided and left-sided stroke.**

speech nor its meaning can be understood, and comprehension of both written and spoken language is impaired.

- The stroke causing *expressive aphasia* affects Broca's area, the motor area for speech. This patient has difficulty in speaking and writing.
- Most stroke patients also experience *dysarthria,* a disturbance in the muscular control of speech.

Affect. Patients with a stroke may have difficulty expressing their emotions; emotional responses may be exaggerated or unpredictable. Additional manifestations include impairment of memory and judgment, deficits in spatial-perceptual orientation, and transient problems with bowel and bladder function.

Diagnostic Studies

When symptoms of a stroke occur, diagnostic studies are done to confirm that it is a stroke (and not another brain lesion, such as a subdural hematoma) and to identify the likely cause of the stroke. Tests also guide decisions about therapeutic or surgical treatment to prevent secondary stroke.

- CT scan, the primary diagnostic test, can indicate lesion size and location and differentiate between ischemic and hemorrhagic stroke.
- CT angiography (CTA) provides visualization of vasculature. CTA allows detection of intracranial or extracranial occlusive disease. Serial CT scans may be used to assess effectiveness of treatment and to evaluate recovery.
- Magnetic resonance imaging (MRI) is used to determine extent of brain injury.
- Magnetic resonance angiography (MRA) is a noninvasive method of assessing vascular occlusive disease in the head or neck similar to CTA.
- Other tests used to diagnose stroke and assess extent of tissue damage include positron emission tomography (PET), magnetic resonance spectroscopy (MRS), xenon CT, single photon emission computed tomography (SPECT), and cerebral angiography.
- Angiography can identify cervical and cerebrovascular occlusion, atherosclerotic plaques, and malformation of vessels.
- Intraarterial digital subtraction angiography (DSA) involves injection of a contrast agent to visualize vessels in the neck and the circle of Willis.
- Transcranial Doppler (TCD) ultrasonography has been effective in detecting microemboli and vasospasm in the major cerebral arteries.

- Tests used much less in the diagnosis of stroke are skull x-rays, brain scan, lumbar puncture, and electroencephalogram (EEG).
- If the suspected cause of the stroke includes emboli from the heart, diagnostic cardiac tests should be done.

Collaborative Care
Prevention
The goals of stroke prevention include management of modifiable risk factors to prevent a primary or secondary stroke.

- Patients with known risk factors require close management. In patients who have had a TIA because of atherosclerosis, antiplatelet drugs are usually the chosen treatment to prevent further stroke. Aspirin at a dose of 81 to 325 mg/day is the most frequently used antiplatelet agent. Other drugs include ticlopidine (Ticlid), clopidogrel (Plavix), dipyridamole (Persantine), and combined dipyridamole and aspirin (Aggrenox). Oral anticoagulation using warfarin is the treatment of choice for individuals with atrial fibrillation who have had a TIA.
- Surgical therapy for the patient with TIAs from carotid disease includes carotid endarterectomy, transluminal angioplasty, stenting, and extracranial-intracranial (EC-IC) bypass.

Acute Care
The goals of acute care are preservation of life, prevention of further brain damage, and reduction of disability. Treatment differs according to the type of stroke and as the patient progresses from the acute to the rehabilitation phase.

- The first goal is to maintain a patent airway, which may be compromised as a result of decreased consciousness. Oxygen administration, an artificial airway, intubation, and mechanical ventilation may be indicated.
- The patient is monitored closely for signs of increasing neurologic deficit. Table 58-5, Lewis and others, *Medical-Surgical Nursing,* edition 7, p. 1511 outlines emergency management of the patient with a stroke.
- Patients with ischemia caused by vasospasm following subarachnoid hemorrhage may be treated with hypervolemic hemodilution using crystalloids once the aneurysm has been successfully clipped or coiled (coils placed in aneurysm sac).
- Fluid and electrolyte balance must be controlled carefully. Although the goal is to maintain perfusion to the brain, overhydration may compromise perfusion by increasing

cerebral edema. Adequate fluid intake during acute care by means of oral or intravenous (IV) administration or tube feedings should be 1500 to 2000 ml/day. Urine output is monitored.

- Management of increased intracranial pressure (ICP) focuses on improving venous drainage, including elevation of the head of the bed as ordered, maintaining head and neck in alignment, and avoiding hip flexion.
- Other measures include pain management, avoidance of hypervolemia, and management of constipation. Diuretic medications, such as mannitol (Osmitrol) and furosemide (Lasix), may be used to decrease cerebral edema.

Surgical therapy for stroke may include immediate evacuation of aneurysm-induced hematomas or cerebellar hematomas above 3 cm in size. Treatment of an aneurysm involves clipping, wrapping, or coiling the aneurysm to prevent rebleeding. Figs. 58-8 and 58-9, Lewis and others, *Medical-Surgical Nursing,* edition 7, pp. 1512 and 1513 illustrate surgical approaches.

Drug Therapy

Thrombolytic Therapy. Recombinant tissue plasminogen activator (tPA) is used to reestablish blood flow and prevent cell death for patients with ischemic strokes. This drug must be administered within 3 hours of the onset of clinical signs. Patients are screened carefully before tPA can be given, including a CT or MRI scan to rule out hemorrhagic stroke, blood tests for coagulation disorders, and screening for recent history of GI bleeding, head trauma, or major surgery.

- The major side effect of tPA is cerebral hemorrhage. During infusion the patient's vital signs are monitored to assess for improvement or deterioration related to intracerebral hemorrhage.
- Control of blood pressure (BP) is critical during treatment and for 24 hours after treatment.

Platelet Inhibition/Anticoagulant Therapy. Aspirin is used within 48 hours of an ischemic stroke unless contraindicated because of a history of peptic ulcer disease. Other platelet inhibitors and anticoagulants may also be used to prevent further clot formation. Platelet inhibitors include aspirin, ticlopidine (Ticlid), clopidogrel (Plavix), and dipyridamole (Persantine). Common anticoagulants include heparin and warfarin (Coumadin).

Other Drug Therapies. Anticoagulants and platelet inhibitors are contraindicated in patients with hemorrhagic strokes. The calcium channel blocker nimodipine (Nimotop) is given to patients with subarachnoid hemorrhage to decrease effects of vasospasm and minimize cerebral damage. Because hyperthermia before or during a stroke has been shown to result in negative outcomes, it may be treated with aspirin or acetaminophen (Tylenol). Cooling blankets may also be used cautiously to lower core temperatures. Antiseizure medication such as phenytoin (Dilantin) may be administered if seizures occur.

Nutritional Therapy

Nutritional needs of the patient require prompt attention because the stress of illness contributes to a catabolic state that can interfere with recovery.

- Initially the patient may receive IV fluids. Before the first oral feeding, the gag reflex should be assessed by gently stimulating the back of the throat with a tongue blade. If the gag reflex is absent, feedings should be deferred and exercises to stimulate swallowing should be started. After assessment of swallowing, chewing, gag reflex, and pocketing, oral feedings can be started. The patient should remain in a high Fowler's position, preferably in a chair with the head flexed forward for the feeding and for 30 minutes after feeding.

During the acute phase, patients with severe impairment may require enteral or parenteral nutrition support. After the acute phase, the dietitian can assist in determining the appropriate daily caloric intake for the patient. If the patient is unable to take in an adequate oral diet, enteral feedings by way of a percutaneous gastrostomy (PEG) may be used.

Rehabilitation Care

After the stroke has stabilized for 12 to 24 hours, care shifts from preserving life to lessening disability and attaining optimal function. Depending on the patient's status, the patient's rehabilitation potential, and the available resources, the patient may be transferred to a rehabilitation facility or unit. Other options for rehabilitation include outpatient therapy or home care–based rehabilitation.

Nursing Management
Goals

The patient who has experienced a stroke will maintain a stable or improved level of consciousness, attain maximum physical functioning, maintain stable body functions (e.g., bladder control), maximize communication abilities, attain maximum self-care abilities and skills, maintain adequate nutrition, avoid complications of stroke, and maintain effective personal and family coping.

See NCP 58-1 for the patient with a stroke, Lewis and others, *Medical-Surgical Nursing,* edition 7, pp. 1516 to 1518.

Nursing Diagnoses
- Ineffective tissue perfusion (cerebral)
- Impaired physical mobility
- Self-care deficits
- Impaired swallowing
- Impaired urinary elimination
- Ineffective airway clearance
- Unilateral neglect
- Situational low self-esteem

Nursing Interventions

Respiratory System. During the acute phase of a stroke the nursing priority is management of respiratory function.

- An oropharyngeal airway may be used in comatose patients to hold the tongue in place, prevent airway obstruction, and make suctioning accessible. Interventions include frequent assessment of airway patency and function, suctioning, patient mobility, positioning of the patient to prevent aspiration, and encouragement of deep breathing.

Neurologic System. The patient's neurologic status must be monitored closely to detect changes suggesting extension of the stroke, increased ICP, and vasospasm.

- Neurologic assessment includes the Glasgow Coma Scale (a standardized assessment of level of consciousness), mental status, pupillary responses, and extremity movement and strength. (The Glasgow Coma Scale is shown on p. 783.)
- A decreasing level of consciousness may indicate increasing ICP. Vital signs are closely monitored and documented.

Cardiovascular System. Nursing goals for the cardiovascular system are aimed at maintaining homeostasis.

- Fluid balance requires adequate hydration to promote cerebral perfusion but prevention of fluid overload that can increase cerebral edema and ICP. Intake and output must be closely monitored, and IV therapy is carefully regulated.
- After a stroke the patient is at risk for thrombophlebitis and deep vein thrombosis in the weak or paralyzed lower extremity. The most effective prevention is to keep the patient moving. Active range-of-motion (ROM) exercises should be taught if the patient has voluntary movement in the affected extremity. For the patient with hemiplegia, passive ROM exercises should be done several times each day.
- Other measures used to prevent thrombophlebitis include positioning to minimize the effects of dependent edema and the use of elastic compression gradient stockings.

Musculoskeletal System. The goal for the musculoskeletal system is to maintain optimal function, which is accomplished by prevention of joint contractures and muscle atrophy.

- In the acute phase, ROM exercises and positioning are important interventions. Passive ROM exercise is begun on the first day of hospitalization. Muscle atrophy secondary to lack of innervation and to inactivity can develop within 1 month after stroke.
- The paralyzed or weak side needs special attention when the patient is positioned. Each joint should be positioned higher than the joint proximal to it. Specific deformities on the affected side of the patient with stroke are shoulder adduction; flexion contractures of the hand, wrist, and elbow; external rotation of the hip; and plantar flexion of the foot.

Integumentary System. The patient's skin is particularly susceptible to breakdown because of the loss of sensation, diminished circulation, and immobility.

- The ideal position change schedule for the patient is side-back-side with a maximum duration of 2 hours for any position. Time spent lying on the paralyzed or weak side should be limited to 30 minutes at a time.

Gastrointestinal System. The most common bowel problem is constipation. Absence of a bowel movement daily or every other day requires checking the patient for fecal impaction.

- Depending on the patient's fluid balance status and swallowing ability, fluid intake should include 1800 to 2000 ml/day and fiber intake up to 25 g/day. Physical activity also promotes bowel function.

Urinary System. In the acute stage of stroke, the primary urinary problem is poor bladder control, resulting in incontinence.

- Efforts should be made to promote normal bladder function and avoid the use of an indwelling catheter.
- Long-term use of an indwelling catheter is associated with urinary tract infections and delayed bladder retraining. An intermittent catheterization program may be used for patients with urinary retention.

Communication. During the acute stage the nurse's role in meeting the psychologic needs of the patient is primarily supportive.

- An alert patient is usually anxious because of a lack of understanding of what has happened and the inability to communicate. If the patient cannot understand words, gestures may be used to support verbal cues. It may help to speak slowly and to calmly use relatively simple words.

Sensory-Perceptual Alterations. Homonymous hemianopsia (blindness in the same half of each visual field) is a common problem after a stroke.

- Initially, the nurse helps the patient to compensate by arranging the environment within the patient's perceptual field, such as arranging the food tray so that all food is on the right side or the left side to accommodate for field of vision.
- Later, the patient is instructed to consciously attend to the neglected side. The weak or paralyzed extremities are carefully noted for adequacy of dressing, for hygiene, and for trauma.
- Visual problems may include diplopia, loss of the corneal reflex, and ptosis, particularly if the stroke is in the vertebrobasilar distribution. Diplopia is often treated with the use of an eye patch. If the corneal reflex is absent, the patient is at risk for a corneal abrasion and should be observed closely and protected against eye injuries.

Coping. A stroke is usually a sudden, extremely stressful event for the patient, close family members, and significant others.

- Reactions vary considerably but may involve fear, apprehension, denial of severity of the stroke, depression, anger, and sorrow.
- During the acute phase of caring for the patient and family, nursing interventions designed to facilitate coping involve providing information and emotional support.
- Explanations to the patient about what has happened and about diagnostic and therapeutic procedures should be clear and understandable. It will be particularly challenging to keep the aphasic patient adequately informed.
- Because family members usually have not had time to prepare for the illness, they may need assistance in arranging care for family members or pets and in arranging transportation and finances.

Home Care and Rehabilitation. The patient is usually discharged from the acute care setting to home, an intermediate or long-term care facility, or a rehabilitation facility. Nurses have an excellent opportunity to prepare the patient and family for hospital discharge through education, demonstration and return demonstration, practice, and evaluation of self-care skills before discharge. Total care is considered in discharge planning in relation to medications, nutrition, mobility, exercises, hygiene, and toileting.

- Follow-up care is carefully planned to permit continuing nursing, physical, occupational, and speech therapy, as well as medical care.

The goals of rehabilitation are to prevent deformity and to maintain and improve function.

- These goals are mutually set by the patient, family, nurse, and other members of the rehabilitation team. The goals typically include (1) learning techniques to self-monitor and maintain physical wellness; (2) demonstrating self-care skills; (3) exhibiting problem-solving skills with self-care; (4) avoiding complications associated with stroke; (5) establishing and maintaining a useful communication system; (6) maintaining nutritional and hydration status; (7) listing community resources for equipment, supplies, and support; and (8) establishing flexible role behaviors to promote family cohesiveness.

Rehabilitation and long-term management of the stroke patient are further described in Chapter 58 of Lewis and others, *Medical-Surgical Nursing,* edition 7.

▼ **Patient and Family Teaching**

- The care provider needs instruction and practice in necessary areas of home care while the patient is hospitalized. This allows for support and encouragement, as well as opportunities for feedback. Adjustments in the home environment, such as the removal of a door to accommodate a wheelchair, can be made before discharge.
- Specific areas for instruction related to home care include exercise and ambulation techniques; dietary requirements; recognition of signs indicating the possibility of another stroke (e.g., headache, vertigo, numbness, visual disturbances); understanding of emotional lability and the possibility of depression; medication routine; and time, place, and frequency of follow-up activities, such as occupational therapy and physical therapy.
- To assist the caregiver to stay healthy after the patient is discharged, it is important to plan for respite or time away from caregiving activities on a regular basis.

SYNDROME OF INAPPROPRIATE ANTIDIURETIC HORMONE

Description

The syndrome of inappropriate antidiuretic hormone (SIADH) occurs when excessive antidiuretic hormone (ADH) is released despite normal or low plasma osmolality. It occurs more commonly in older adults.

Pathophysiology

The abnormal production or sustained secretion of ADH leads to fluid retention, serum hypoosmolality, dilutional hyponatremia, hypochloremia, concentrated urine in the presence of normal or increased vascular volume, and normal renal function.

SIADH has various causes, including malignancy, especially small cell lung cancer, and central nervous system disorders such as head injury. Some of the drugs that cause SIADH include general anesthetics, antineoplastic agents, thiazide diuretics, opioids, and tricyclic antidepressants.

Clinical Manifestations

The excess ADH increases renal tubular permeability and reabsorption of water into the circulation. Consequently, extracellular fluid volume expands, plasma osmolality declines, glomerular filtration rate (GFR) rises, and sodium (Na^+) levels decline.

- The patient experiences low urinary output and weight gain without edema.
- The hyponatremia causes muscle cramps and weakness.
- Initially, thirst, dyspnea on exertion, fatigue, and dulled sensorium may be evident.
- As plasma osmolality and serum Na^+ levels continue to decline, cerebral edema may occur, leading to lethargy, anorexia, confusion, headache, seizures, and coma.
- Other effects of hyponatremia include muscle cramps and weakness.

Diagnostic Studies

- Simultaneous measurements of urine and serum osmolality can diagnose SIADH. Serum osmolality level much lower than urine osmolality level indicates inappropriate excretion of concentrated urine in the presence of very dilute serum.

Collaborative Care

Treatment is directed at the underlying cause to restore normal fluid volume and osmolality. Medications that stimulate the release of ADH should be avoided or discontinued. In mild cases, the only treatment may be restriction of fluids to 800 to 1000 ml/day. In cases of severe hyponatremia, intravenous hypertonic saline solution (3% to 5%) may be administered. A diuretic such as furosemide (Lasix) may be used to promote diuresis but only if the serum

sodium is at least 125 mEq/L (125 mmol/L) because it may cause
further sodium loss. Because furosemide increases potassium,
calcium, and magnesium losses, supplements may be needed.
In severe hyponatremia, a fluid restriction of 500 ml/day is
indicated.

- SIADH tends to be self-limiting when caused by head
  trauma or drugs but chronic in nature when associated with
  tumors or metabolic diseases.
- In chronic symptomatic SIADH, demeclocycline (Declo-
  mycin) and lithium may be used. These agents block the
  effect ADH has on renal collecting tubules, thereby allowing a more dilute urine and retention of sodium.

Nursing Management

Patients who are at risk and those who have confirmed SIADH
should undergo an appropriate nursing assessment (see Table
50-2, Lewis and others, *Medical-Surgical Nursing,* edition 7,
p. 1296). The nurse should be alert for low urinary output with a
high specific gravity, sudden weight gain without edema, or a
decrease in serum Na^+. If a patient has SIADH, nursing measures
include:

- Restrict total fluid intake to no more than 1000 ml/day.
- Position head of the bed flat or with no more than 10 degrees
  of elevation to enhance venous return to the heart and
  increase left atrial filling pressure, reducing ADH release.
- Position side rails up because of potential alterations in
  mental status and seizures.
- If patient is bedridden, turn and reposition the patient every
  2 hours and perform range-of-motion (ROM) exercises
  several times each day.
- Assist with ambulation, and provide frequent oral hygiene.

When SIADH is chronic, patients must learn to self-manage
their treatment regimens.

- Fluids are restricted to 800 to 1000 ml/day. Ice chips or
  sugarless candies or chewing gum can help decrease thirst.
  The patient may be treated with a diuretic to remove excess
  fluid volume.
- The diet should be supplemented with Na^+ and K^+, especially if diuretics are prescribed. Solutions of these electrolytes must be well diluted to prevent gastrointestinal (GI)
  irritation or damage.
- Patients should be taught the symptoms of fluid and electrolyte imbalances, especially those involving Na^+ and K^+,
  so that they are able to monitor their own response to
  treatment.

SYPHILIS

Description
Syphilis is a sexually transmitted disease (STD) in which many organs and tissues can become infected by *Treponema pallidum,* a spirochete.

Pathophysiology
The organism *T. pallidum* is thought to enter the body through very small breaks in the skin or mucous membranes. Its entry is facilitated by the minor abrasions that often occur during intercourse. It is extremely fragile and is easily destroyed by drying, heating, or washing.

- Not all people who are exposed to syphilis acquire the disease; about one third become infected after intercourse with an infected person.
- In addition to sexual contact, syphilis may be spread through contact with infectious lesions and through the sharing of needles among intravenous (IV) drug users.
- Congenital syphilis is transmitted from an infected mother to the fetus in utero after the tenth week of pregnancy.
- The incubation period for syphilis ranges from 10 to 90 days.

There is an association between syphilis and human immunodeficiency virus (HIV) infection. Persons at increased risk for acquiring syphilis are also at increased risk for acquiring HIV. Often, both infections are present in the same person. Therefore the evaluation of all patients with syphilis should include serologic testing for HIV with the patient's consent.

Clinical Manifestations
Syphilis presents with a variety of signs and symptoms that can mimic a number of other diseases. Consequently, it is more difficult to recognize syphilis than other STDs. If it is not treated, specific clinical stages are characteristic of the disease progression.

- In the *primary stage, chancres* (painless indurated lesions found on the penis, vulva, and lips and in the mouth, vagina, and rectum) are seen at the site of bacterial invasion. The chancre lasts 3 to 6 weeks, eventually healing on its own. During this time the draining of the microorganisms into the lymph nodes causes regional lymphadenopathy. Genital ulcers may also be present. Without treatment the infection progresses to the secondary stage.

- In the *secondary stage,* syphilis is systemic. During this stage blood-borne bacteria spread to all major organ systems. Manifestations characteristic of the secondary stage include flu-like symptoms and generalized adenopathy. Cutaneous eruptions include a bilateral, symmetric rash usually involving the palms and soles; mucous patches in the mouth, tongue, or cervix; and condylomata (moist papules) in the anal and genital area.
- *Hidden* or *latent* syphilis follows the secondary stage and is a period during which the immune system is able to suppress the infection. There are no signs or symptoms of syphilis during this time.
- The *third stage* (also called *late or tertiary*) of syphilis is the most severe. Because antibiotics can cure syphilis, manifestations of late syphilis are rare. When late syphilis does occur, however, it is responsible for significant morbidity and mortality. *Gummas* (destructive skin, bone, and soft tissue lesions associated with late syphilis) are probably caused by a severe hypersensitivity reaction to the microorganism. Within the cardiovascular system late syphilis may cause aneurysms, heart valve insufficiency, and heart failure. Within the central nervous system the presence of *T. pallidum* in cerebrospinal fluid (CSF) may cause manifestations of neurosyphilis.

Complications
Complications occur in late syphilis. The gummas of late syphilis may produce irreparable damage to bone, liver, or skin but seldom result in death.
- In cardiovascular syphilis, the resulting aneurysm may press on structures such as the intercostal nerves, resulting in pain. Scarring of the aortic valve results in aortic valve insufficiency and eventual heart failure.
- Neurosyphilis (general paresis) is responsible for degeneration of the brain with mental deterioration. Problems related to sensory nerve involvement are a result of tabes dorsalis (progressive locomotor ataxia). There may be sudden attacks of pain anywhere in the body; loss of vision and position sense in the feet and legs can also occur. Walking may become even more difficult as joint stability is lost.

Diagnostic Studies
- Darkfield microscopy confirms diagnosis with the presence of spirochetes from tissue scrapings.
- To screen for syphilis, Venereal Disease Research Laboratory (VDRL) and rapid plasma reagin (RPR) testing can detect

nonspecific antitreponemal antibodies, usually positive 10 to 14 days after chancre appearance.

- To confirm a diagnosis of syphilis, the fluorescent treponemal antibody absorption (FTA-ABS) test and the *T. pallidum* particle agglutination (TP-PA) test can detect specific antitreponemal antibodies.

Collaborative Care

Management is aimed at the eradication of all syphilitic organisms. However, treatment cannot reverse damage that is already present in the late stage of the disease.

- Penicillin G benzathine (Bicillin) or aqueous penicillin G procaine remains the treatment of choice for all stages of syphilis. To date, no evidence suggests a decrease in the effectiveness of penicillin against *T. pallidum*. Table 53-5, Lewis and others, *Medical-Surgical Nursing,* edition 7, p. 1371 describes drug therapy for the various stages of syphilis and is in accordance with U.S. Public Health Service recommendations. All stages of syphilis should be treated.
- Penicillin is effective in preventing the transmission of syphilis from mother to fetus and for treating fetal infection. During pregnancy, treatment should consist of the recommended penicillin regimen appropriate for the stage of syphilis.
- All patients with neurosyphilis must be carefully monitored with periodic serologic testing, clinical evaluation at 6-month intervals, and repeat CSF examinations for at least 3 years.

Nursing Management: Syphilis

See Nursing Management: Sexually Transmitted Diseases, p. 564.

Systemic Inflammatory Response Syndrome (SIRS) and Multiple Organ Dysfunction Syndrome (MODS)

Description

- *Systemic inflammatory response syndrome (SIRS)* is a systemic inflammatory response to a variety of insults, including infection (referred to as sepsis), ischemia, infarct, and injury. Normally the inflammatory response to an insult is

contained within a confined area. However, SIRS is characterized by inflammation in organs remote from the initial
insult. Diagnostic criteria for SIRS include a documented
or suspected infection and some of the following:

- General variables such as fever or hypothermia, tachycardia, tachypnea, altered mental status, positive fluid balance and hyperglycemia in the absence of diabetes mellitus;
- Inflammatory variables including leukocytosis or leukopenia, normal white blood cell (WBC) count with >10% immature forms, and elevated C-reactive protein;
- Hemodynamic variables including arterial hypotension, mixed venous oxygen saturation greater than 70%, and a cardiac index greater than 3.5 L/min/m^2;
- Organ dysfunction variables including arterial hypoxemia, acute oliguria, coagulation abnormalities, ileus, and hyperbilirubinemia; and
- Tissue perfusion variables such as hyperlactatemia and decreased capillary refill or mottling.

Specific values of variables are identified in Table 67-5, Lewis and
others, *Medical-Surgical Nursing,* edition 7, p. 1779.

Multiple organ dysfunction syndrome (MODS) is failure of two
or more organ systems in an acutely ill patient such that homeostasis cannot be maintained without intervention. MODS results
from SIRS, but the transition from SIRS to MODS does not occur
in a clear-cut manner.

- Prognosis for the patient with MODS is poor, with estimated mortality rates at 90% to 95% when three or more organ systems fail.

Pathophysiology and Clinical Manifestations

When the inflammatory response is not controlled, consequences occur. These include activation of inflammatory cells and
release of mediators, direct damage to the endothelium, and
hypermetabolism.

- Vasodilation becomes excessive and leads to decreased systemic vascular resistance (SVR) and hypotension.
- An increase in vascular permeability allows mediators and protein to leak out of the endothelium and into the interstitial space.
- WBCs phagocytize the foreign debris, and the coagulation cascade is activated. Failure of this cascade manifests as disseminated intravascular coagulation (DIC).
- DIC results in simultaneous microvascular clotting and bleeding because of the depletion of clotting factors and platelets in addition to excessive fibrinolysis.

- Organ perfusion may be compromised because of hypotension, decreased perfusion, microemboli, and redistributed or shunted blood flow.

Electrolyte imbalances, which are common, relate to hormonal and metabolic changes and fluid shifts. These changes exacerbate mental status changes, neuromuscular dysfunction, and dysrhythmias.

- Release of antidiuretic hormone and aldosterone results in sodium and water retention; aldosterone increases urinary potassium loss, and catecholamines cause potassium to move into the cells, resulting in hypokalemia.
- Metabolic acidosis results from impaired tissue perfusion, hypoxia, a shift to anaerobic metabolism, and progressive renal dysfunction.
- Hypocalcemia, hypomagnesemia, and hypophosphatemia are common.

The respiratory system is often the first system to show signs of dysfunction in SIRS and MODS. Inflammatory mediators have a direct effect on the pulmonary vasculature. An increase in capillary permeability results in alveolar edema and destruction with decreased surfactant production. The alveoli collapse, and the end result is acute respiratory distress syndrome (ARDS, see p. 13).

Cardiovascular changes include myocardial depression and massive vasodilation in response to increasing tissue demands. To compensate for hypotension, heart rate and stroke volume increase, but increased capillary permeability diminishes venous return and thus preload. Eventually, either perfusion of vital organs becomes insufficient or the cells are unable to use oxygen and their function is further compromised.

Neurologic dysfunction commonly manifests as mental status changes, and mental status changes can be an early sign of MODS. Confusion, agitation, disorientation, lethargy, or coma may occur. Mental changes may be due to hypoxemia, the direct effect of inflammatory mediators, or impaired perfusion.

Acute renal failure (ARF) is frequently seen in SIRS and MODS. ARF can be caused not only by hypoperfusion but also by the effects of the mediators. An additional risk for ARF in this patient is the use of nephrotoxic antibiotics to treat gram-negative bacteremia.

In the early stages of SIRS and MODS, blood is shunted away from the gastrointestinal (GI) mucosa, making it highly vulnerable to injury. Decreased perfusion leads to a breakdown of the mucosal barrier, thereby increasing the risk for ulceration and GI bleeding.

- Breakdown of the mucosal barrier of the gut also results in the potential for bacterial translocation from the GI tract into the circulation.
- GI motility is also decreased in critical illness, causing abdominal distention and paralytic ileus.

Metabolic changes are pronounced in SIRS and MODS. Both syndromes trigger a hypermetabolic response. The net result is a catabolic state, and lean body mass (muscle) is lost.

- The hypermetabolism may last for days and results in liver dysfunction.
- The liver is unable to synthesize albumin that is necessary to maintain plama oncotic pressure, adding to the loss of intravascular fluid to the interstitial space.
- The liver also cannot convert the lactate accumulating as a result of anaerobic metablism to glucose, resulting in both an increase in metabolic acidosis and hypoglycemia.

The defining and clinical manifestations of SIRS and MODS are delineated in Tables 67-5 and 67-11, Lewis and others, *Medical-Surgical Nursing,* edition 7, pp. 1796 to 1797 and 1779.

Nursing and Collaborative Management: SIRS and MODS

The most important goal in the management of SIRS and MODS is to prevent the progression of SIRS to MODS. A critical component of the nursing role is vigilant assessment and ongoing monitoring to detect early signs of deterioration or organ dysfunction.

Collaborative care of patients with MODS focuses on prevention and treatment of infection, maintenance of tissue oxygenation, nutritional and metabolic support, and appropriate support for individual failing organs (see Table 67-11, Lewis and others, *Medical-Surgical Nursing,* edition 7, pp. 1796 to 1797).

- Prevention and treatment of infection are essential to decrease the risk for nosocomial infections. Strict asepsis with the use of invasive devices and procedures is critical. Once an infection is suspected, interventions to control the source must be instituted, and if an organism is identified, appropriate antibiotic therapy should be initiated.
- Hypoxemia frequently occurs in patients with SIRS or MODS. Interventions to decrease oxygen demand and increase oxygen delivery are essential. Sedation, mechanical ventilation, analgesia, paralysis, and rest may decrease oxygen demand and should be considered.
- Hypermetabolism in SIRS or MODS can result in profound weight loss, cachexia, and further organ failure. Nutritional support is vital to preserve organ function. Providing early

and adequate nutrition decreases morbidity and mortality. The use of the enteral route is preferred and may limit translocation of gut bacteria.

Support of any failing organ is a primary goal of therapy. For example, the patient with ARDS requires aggressive oxygen therapy and mechanical ventilation. DIC should be treated appropriately (e.g., blood products). Renal failure may require dialysis or continuous renal replacement therapy.

SYSTEMIC LUPUS ERYTHEMATOSUS

S

Description

Systemic lupus erythematosus (SLE) is a multisystem inflammatory disease of autoimmune origin. It typically affects the skin; joints; serous membranes (pleura, pericardium); and renal, hematologic, and neurologic systems. SLE is characterized by variability within and among persons, and its chronic unpredictable course is marked by alternating periods of exacerbations and remissions. Women are 10 times more likely to develop SLE than men, and it is observed more often in African Americans, Asian Americans, and Native Americans than in whites.

Pathophysiology

The etiology of SLE is unknown, but it is thought to result from interactions among genetic, hormonal, environmental, and immunologic factors. Multiple susceptibility genes from the HLA complex show associations with SLE, including HLA-DR3.

- The role of hormones in the etiology of SLE is reflected in the possible onset or exacerbation of disease symptoms after the onset of menarche, with the use of oral contraceptives, and during and after pregnancy.
- Environmental factors believed to contribute to the occurrence of SLE include sun exposure, burns, and exposure to infectious agents or certain drugs, such as procainamide (Pronestyl), hydralazine (Apresoline), and some antiseizure drugs.

SLE is characterized by the production of a large variety of autoantibodies against nucleic acids (e.g., single- and double-stranded deoxyribonucleic acid [DNA]), erythrocytes, coagulation proteins, lymphocytes, platelets, and many other self-proteins. Most characteristically the autoimmune reactions are directed against constituents of the cell nucleus (antinuclear antibodies [ANA]), particularly DNA. Circulating immune complexes containing antibody against DNA are deposited in the basement membranes of capillaries in the kidneys, heart, skin, brain, and joints. The overaggressive antibody response is also related to B- and T-cell hyperactivity. Specific manifestations of SLE depend on which cell types or organs are involved.

Clinical Manifestations and Complications

No characteristic pattern occurs in the progressive organ involvement. General complaints, including fever, weight loss, arthralgia, and excessive fatigue, may precede an exacerbation of disease activity.

Dermatologic Manifestations. Cutaneous vascular lesions can appear in any location but are most likely to develop in sun-exposed areas. Severe skin reactions can occur in persons who are photosensitive. The classic butterfly rash over the cheeks and bridge of the nose occurs in 50% of patients with SLE.

- Ulcers of the oral or nasopharyngeal membranes can occur. Transient diffuse or patchy hair loss (alopecia) is common. The scalp becomes dry, scaly, and atrophied.

Musculoskeletal Problems. Polyarthralgia with morning stiffness is often the patient's first complaint and may precede the onset of multisystem disease by many years. Arthritis occurs in 90% of all patients with SLE. Diffuse swelling is accompanied by joint and muscle pain.

- Lupus-related arthritis is generally nonerosive, but it may cause deformities such as swan neck, ulnar deviation, and subluxation with hyperlaxity of the joints.

Cardiopulmonary Problems. Tachypnea and cough in patients with SLE are suggestive of restrictive lung disease. Cardiac involvement may include dysrhythmias resulting from fibrosis of the sinoatrial (SA) and atrioventricular (AV) nodes. This occurrence is an ominous sign of advanced disease.

- Clinical factors such as hypertension and hypercholesterolemia require aggressive therapy and careful monitoring. Coronary artery disease is more likely to develop if corticosteroids are being used or renal disease is present.

Renal Problems. Lupus nephritis (LN) occurs in about 40% to 85% of patients with SLE. Manifestations of LN vary from mild proteinuria to rapid, progressive glomerulonephritis. Drug therapy typically includes corticosteroids, cytotoxic agents (cyclophosphamide [Cytoxan]), and immunosuppressive agents (azathioprine [Imuran], cyclosporine [Sandimmune]).

Nervous System Problems. Centralized or focal seizures are the most common neurologic manifestation. They are generally controlled by corticosteroids or antiseizure drug therapy.

- Cognitive dysfunction may result from the deposition of immune complexes within the brain tissue. It is characterized by disordered thought processes, disorientation, memory deficits, and psychiatric symptoms, such as severe depression and psychosis. Occasionally a stroke or aseptic meningitis may be attributable to SLE. Headaches are common and can become severe during a flare (exacerbation).

Hematologic Problems. The formation of antibodies against blood cells such as erythrocytes, leukocytes, thrombocytes, and coagulation factors is a common feature. Anemia, mild leukopenia, and thrombocytopenia are often present. Some patients show a tendency to bleed, whereas others show a tendency toward blood clots.

Infection. Patients appear to have increased susceptibility to infections, possibly related to defects in their ability to phagocytize invading bacteria, deficiencies in the production of antibodies, and the immunosuppressive effect of many antiinflammatory drugs. Infection is a major cause of death, and pneumonia is the most common infection.

Diagnostic Studies

The diagnosis is based on the history, physical examination, and laboratory findings.

- SLE is characterized by the presence of ANA, which establishes the existence of an autoimmune disease. Other antibodies include anti-DNA, antineuronal, anticoagulant, anti–white blood cell (WBC), anti–red blood cell (RBC), antiplatelet, antiphospholipid, and antibasement membrane. The antibody tests that are the most specific for SLE include the anti–double-stranded DNA and the anti-Smith (Sm).
- Lupus erythematosus (LE) cell prep test is nonspecific for SLE and may also be positive in other rheumatic diseases.
- Erythrocyte sedimentation rate (ESR) and C-reactive protein (CRP) levels are not diagnostic of SLE but may be used to monitor disease activity.

Collaborative Care

A challenge in SLE treatment is to manage the active phase of the disease while preventing complications of treatments that cause long-term tissue damage.

Drug Therapy

Nonsteroidal antiinflammatory drugs (NSAIDs) continue to be an important intervention, especially for patients with mild polyarthralgia or polyarthritis. Antimalarial agents such as hydroxychloroquine (Plaquenil) are also often used to treat fatigue and moderate skin and joint problems, as well as prevent flares.

Corticosteroid exposure should be limited, but tapering doses of intravenous (IV) methylprednisolone may be useful in controlling severe exacerbations of polyarthritis. Steroid-sparing drugs such as methotrexate can serve as an alternate treatment. Immunosuppressive drugs such as azathioprine (Imuran) and cyclophosphamide (Cytoxan) may be prescribed to reduce the need for long-term corticosteroid therapy or to treat severe organ-system disease, such as lupus nephritis.

Nursing Management

Goals

The patient with SLE will have satisfactory pain relief, comply with the therapeutic regimen to achieve maximum symptom management, demonstrate awareness of and avoid activities that induce disease exacerbation, and maintain optimal role function and a positive self-image.

See NCP 65-2 for the patient with systemic lupus erythematosus, Lewis and others, *Medical-Surgical Nursing,* edition 7, pp. 1721 to 1722.

Nursing Diagnoses

- Fatigue
- Acute pain
- Impaired skin integrity
- Deficient knowledge

Nursing Interventions

Prevention of SLE is not possible at this time. The education of health professionals and the community should promote a clear understanding of the disease and earlier diagnosis and treatment.

During an exacerbation, patients may become abruptly and dramatically ill. Nursing interventions include accurately recording the severity of symptoms and documenting response to therapy. Fever pattern, joint inflammation, limitation of motion, location and degree of discomfort, and fatigability should be specifically assessed.

- The patient's weight and fluid intake and output should be monitored because of the fluid retention effect of corticosteroids and the possibility of renal failure. Careful collection of 24-hour urine for protein and creatinine clearance may be ordered.
- The nurse should observe for signs of bleeding that result · from drug therapy, such as pallor, skin bruising, petechiae, or tarry stools.
- Careful assessment of neurologic status includes observation for visual disturbances, headaches, personality changes,

and forgetfulness. Psychosis may indicate central nervous system disease or may be the effect of corticosteroid therapy. Irritation of the nerves of the extremities (peripheral neuropathy) may produce numbness, tingling, and weakness of the hands and feet.

- The nurse must explain the nature of the disease, modes of therapy, and all diagnostic procedures. Emotional support for the patient and family is essential.

▼ **Patient and Family Teaching**

The patient with SLE confronts many psychosocial issues. Overwhelming fatigue and pain are the factors that most frequently interfere with quality of life. Education and counseling should focus on issues such as personal relationships, family planning, occupational responsibilities, and recreational activities. The patient must understand that even perfect adherence to the treatment plan is not a guarantee against exacerbation because the disease course is unpredictable. Patient and family education is outlined in Table 80.

The nurse should advise the patient and family that SLE has a good prognosis for the majority of persons. Many couples require pregnancy and sexual counseling. Pacing techniques and relaxation therapy can help keep the patient actively involved.

Table 80	**Patient and Family Teaching Guide: Systemic Lupus Erythematosus**

Teaching related to the disease and appropriate management should include:
1. Disease process
2. Names of medications, actions, side effects, dosage, administration
3. Pain management strategies
4. Energy-conservation and pacing techniques
5. Therapeutic exercise, use of heat therapy (for arthralgia)
6. Avoidance of physical and emotional stress
7. Avoidance of exposure to individuals with infection
8. Avoidance of drying soaps, powders, household chemicals
9. Use of sunscreen protection (at least SPF 15) and protective clothing, with minimal sun exposure from 11 AM to 3 PM
10. Regular medical and laboratory follow-up
11. Marital and pregnancy counseling as needed
12. Community resources and health care agencies

SPF, Sun protection factor.

SYSTEMIC SCLEROSIS (SCLERODERMA)

Description

Systemic sclerosis (SS), or *scleroderma,* is a disorder of the connective tissue characterized by fibrotic, degenerative, and occasionally inflammatory changes in the skin, blood vessels, synovium, skeletal muscle, and internal organs. Two types of SS exist; one is the more common *limited cutaneous disease* (80%), and the second is *diffuse cutaneous disease.*

SS affects women four times more frequently than men. Although symptoms may begin at any time, the usual age at onset is between 30 and 50 years.

Pathophysiology

The exact cause of SS remains unclear. Collagen is overproduced and disrupts the normal functioning of organs such as the lungs, kidney, heart, and gastrointestinal (GI) tract. Disruption of the cell is followed by platelet aggregation and fibrosis. Immunologic dysfunction and vascular abnormalities are believed to play a role in the development of widespread systemic disease. Other etiologic factors include environmental occupational exposure to coal, plastics, and silica dust.

Clinical Manifestations

The manifestations may range from a diffuse cutaneous thickening with rapidly progressive and widespread organ involvement to a more benign variant of limited cutaneous SS. Clinical manifestations can be described by the acronym *CREST*: **C**alcinosis (painful calcium deposits in skin), **R**aynaud's phenomenon, **E**sophageal dysfunction (difficulty swallowing), **S**clerodactyly (tightening of the skin on the fingers), and **T**elangiectasia (red spots on the hands, face, and lips).

Raynaud's phenomenon (paroxysmal vasospasm of the digits) occurs in most patients with SS and is the most common initial complaint in initial disease. Raynaud's phenomenon may precede the onset of systemic disease by months, years, or even decades (see Raynaud's Phenomenon, p. 526).

Symmetric painless swelling or thickening of the skin of the fingers and hands may progress to diffuse scleroderma of the trunk. In limited disease, skin thickening is generally limited to the fingers and face. In more diffuse disease the skin loses elasticity and becomes taut and shiny, producing the typical expressionless facies with tightly pursed lips.

Esophageal fibrosis causes dysphagia and frequent reflux of gastric acid. GI effects include constipation resulting from colonic hypomotility and diarrhea resulting from malabsorption from bacterial overgrowth.

Lung involvement includes pleural thickening, pulmonary fibrosis, pulmonary artery hypertension, and pulmonary function abnormalities.

Primary heart disease consists of pericarditis, pericardial effusion, and cardiac dysrhythmias. Myocardial fibrosis resulting in heart failure occurs most frequently in persons with diffuse SS.

Renal disease is a major cause of death. Malignant hypertension associated with rapidly progressive and irreversible renal insufficiency is often present.

Diagnostic Studies

- Erythrocyte sedimentation rate (ESR) may be mildly elevated with mild hemolytic anemia.
- Anticentromere antibody is seen in many patients with CREST syndrome, and scleroderma antibody SCL-70 is found in systemic SS.
- If renal involvement is present, urinalysis may show proteinuria, microscopic hematuria, and casts.
- X-ray evidence of subcutaneous calcification, distal esophageal hypomotility, and/or bilateral pulmonary fibrosis is diagnostic of SS.
- Pulmonary function studies reveal decreased vital capacity and lung compliance.

Collaborative Care

Management of SS offers no specific treatment with long-term effects. Care is directed toward attempts to prevent or treat the secondary complications of involved organs.

Physical therapy helps maintain joint mobility and preserve muscle strength. Occupational therapy assists the patient in maintaining functional abilities. Gastroesophageal reflux may be treated by antacids and periodic dilation of the esophagus.

Drug Therapy

No specific drugs or combinations of drugs have been proven effective. Vasoactive agents are often prescribed in early disease to manage Raynaud's phenomenon. Calcium channel blockers (nifedipine [Adalat, Procardia], diltiazem [Cardizem]) are a common treatment choice. Other vasoactive drugs include reserpine (Serpasil), iloprost (Ventavis), and losartan (Cozaar).

Corticosteroids are generally reserved for patients with significant joint or muscle involvement or severe skin disease with ulcerations. D-Penicillamine (Cuprimine) increases the solubility of dermal collagen and may cause thinning of the skin, but its possible toxic side effects limit its use.

Topical agents may provide some relief from joint pain. Capsaicin cream may be useful not only as a local analgesic but also as a vasodilator. Other therapies are prescribed to address specific systemic problems, such as tetracycline for diarrhea resulting from bacterial overgrowth, and histamine H_2-receptor blockers (e.g., cimetidine [Tagamet]) and proton pump inhibitors (e.g., omeprazole [Prilosec]) for esophageal symptoms. An antihypertensive agent (e.g., captopril [Capoten], propranolol [Inderal], methyldopa [Aldomet]) may be used to treat hypertension with renal involvement, and a chemotherapeutic agent (e.g., cyclophosphamide [Cytoxan]) may be used for lung disease.

Nursing Management

Because prevention is not possible, nursing interventions often begin during hospitalization for diagnostic purposes. Emotional stress and cold ambient temperatures may aggravate Raynaud's phenomenon. Patients with SS should not have finger stick blood testing done because of compromised circulation and poor healing of the fingers. The nurse may help the patient to resolve feelings of helplessness by providing information about the illness and encouraging active participation in planning care.

- Hands and feet should be protected from cold exposure and possible burns or cuts that might heal slowly. Smoking should be avoided because of its vasoconstricting effect. Lotions may help to alleviate skin dryness and cracking but must be rubbed in for an unusually long time because of skin thickness.
- Dysphagia may be reduced by eating small, frequent meals, chewing carefully and slowly, and drinking fluids. Heartburn may be minimized by using antacids 45 to 60 minutes after each meal and by sitting upright for at least 2 hours after eating.
- Job modifications are often necessary because stair climbing, typing, writing, and cold exposure may pose particular problems.
- Some people need to wear gloves to protect fingertip ulcers and to provide extra warmth. Sensitive areas on the fingertips resulting from ulcers may require padded utensils or special assistive devices to reduce discomfort.
- Daily oral hygiene must be emphasized, or neglect may lead to increased tooth and gingival problems.

- Biofeedback training and relaxation techniques may be used to reduce tension and improve sleeping habits.

The patient must actively carry out therapeutic exercises at home. The nurse should reinforce the use of moist heat applications, the use of assistive devices, and the organization of activities to preserve strength and reduce disability. Sexual dysfunction resulting from body changes, pain, muscular weakness, limited mobility, decreased self-esteem, and decreased vaginal secretions may require sensitive counseling by the nurse.

TESTICULAR CANCER

T

Description

Testicular cancer is relatively rare, but it is the most common type of cancer in young men between 15 and 34 years of age. Testicular tumors are more common in men who have had undescended testicles (cryptorchidism) or a family history of testicular cancer or anomalies.

- Other predisposing factors include orchitis, human immunodeficiency virus (HIV) infection, maternal exposure to diethylstilbestrol (DES), and testicular cancer in the contralateral testis.
- Most testicular cancers develop from embryonic germ cells and include seminomas and nonseminomas.

Clinical Manifestations

Testicular cancer may have a slow or rapid onset depending on the tumor.

- The patient may notice a lump in his scrotum, as well as scrotal swelling and a feeling of heaviness. The scrotal mass is usually nontender and very firm.
- Some patients also complain of a dull ache in the lower abdomen, perianal area, or scrotum.
- Manifestations associated with metastasis include back pain, cough, dyspnea, hemoptysis, dysphagia, alterations in vision or mental status, and seizures.

Diagnostic Studies

Palpation of the scrotal contents is the first step in diagnosing testicular cancer. Ultrasound of the testes and blood serum levels of α-fetoprotein (AFP), lactate dehydrogenase (LDH), and human chorionic gonadotropin (hCG) are done if testicular cancer is suspected. Chest x-ray and computed tomography (CT) scan of the abdomen and pelvis are done to detect metastasis.

Nursing and Collaborative Management

As with many forms of cancer, the patient's survival is closely associated with early tumor recognition. The scrotum is easily examined, and beginning tumors are usually palpable. Every male should be taught and encouraged to perform a monthly testicular self-examination for the purpose of detecting testicular tumors or other scrotal abnormalities such as varicoceles. (See Table 55-9 and Fig. 55-9 for scrotum self-examination guidelines, Lewis and others, *Medical-Surgical Nursing,* edition 7, p. 1433).

- The male may indicate some reluctance to examine his own genitals, but with encouragement he can learn this simple procedure. He should be encouraged to do self-examinations frequently until he is comfortable with the procedure. The scrotum should be examined once each month.

Collaborative management generally involves an orchiectomy or a radical orchiectomy (surgical removal of the affected testis, spermatic cord, and regional lymph nodes). Retroperitoneal lymph node dissection and removal are also done to manage the disease in early stages.

- Postorchiectomy treatment involves surveillance, radiation therapy, or chemotherapy, depending on the stage of the cancer. Chemotherapy protocols use a combination therapy referred to as BEP: **b**leomycin (Blenoxane), **e**toposide (VePesid), and cisplatin (**P**latinol) and one referred to as VIP: **V**ePesid, **I**fex (ifosfamide), and **P**latinol. The prognosis for patients with testicular cancer has improved, and 95% of all patients obtain complete remission if the disease is detected in the early stages.
- All patients with testicular cancer, regardless of pathology or stage, require meticulous follow-up monitoring and regular physical examinations, chest x-ray, CT scan, and assessment of hCG and AFP (if appropriate). The goal is to detect relapse when tumor burden is minimal.
- The man with testicular cancer should have the opportunity to discuss fertility and sperm banking before any treatment.
- The nurse should be sensitive to any psychosocial problems this type of cancer can have on a man's feelings of maleness or self-worth. Treatment has the potential to interfere with both erections and fertility.

TETANUS

Description
Tetanus (lockjaw) is an extremely severe polyradiculitis and poly-neuritis affecting spinal and cranial nerves. It results from the effects of a potent neurotoxin released by the anaerobic bacillus *Clostridium tetani*. The toxin interferes with the function of the reflex arc by blocking inhibitory transmitters at the presynaptic sites in the spinal cord and brainstem. The spores of the bacillus are present in soil, garden mold, and manure. Worldwide, the number of cases per year is estimated to be 1 million. In the United States the number of individuals under the age of 40 years with tetanus is increasing, most likely related to intravenous (IV) drug use. Mortality rates vary according to age, with infants and persons older than 50 years most seriously affected.

Pathophysiology
C. tetani enters the body through a traumatic or suppurative wound, which provides an appropriate low-oxygen environment for the organisms to mature and produce toxin. Other possible sources include dental infection, chronic otitis media, injections of heroin, human and animal bites, frostbite, open fractures, and gunshot wounds.

- Incubation period is usually 7 days but can range from 3 to 21 days, with symptoms frequently appearing after the original wound is healed. In general, the longer the incubation period, the milder the illness and the better the prognosis.

Clinical Manifestations
Manifestations of generalized tetanus include a feeling of stiffness in the jaw *(trismus)* or neck, a slight fever, and other symptoms of general infection. Generalized tonic spasms occur because of the lack of reciprocal innervation.

- As the disease progresses, the neck muscles, back, abdomen, and extremities become progressively rigid. In severe forms, continuous tonic convulsions may occur with *opisthotonos* (extreme arching of the back and retraction of the head). Laryngeal and respiratory spasms cause apnea and anoxia.
- Additional effects are manifested by overstimulation of the sympathetic nervous system; these include profuse diaphoresis, labile hypertension, episodic tachycardia, hyperther-

mia, and dysrhythmias. The slightest noise, jarring motion, or bright light can set off a seizure. These seizures are agonizingly painful.
- Death is usually attributable to asphyxia or heart failure, the result of constantly recurring spasms.
- Residual injury, such as vertebral fracture, muscular contraction, and brain damage secondary to hypoxia, may remain.

Diagnostic Studies
- Serum electrolytes, complete blood count (CBC), albumin, clotting factors, glucose, and arterial blood gases (ABGs) are monitored.
- Electrocardiogram (ECG) monitors cardiac function.

Collaborative Care
Management includes administration of tetanus and diphtheria toxoid booster (Td) and tetanus immune globulin (TIG) in different sites before the onset of symptoms to neutralize circulating toxins. A much larger dose of TIG is given to patients with manifestations of clinical tetanus.
- Because of laryngospasm, a tracheostomy (see Tracheostomy, p. 746) is usually performed early and the patient is maintained on mechanical ventilation.
- Control of spasms is essential and is managed by deep sedation, usually with diazepam (Valium), barbiturates, and, in severe cases, neuromuscular blocking agents such as vecuronium that act to paralyze skeletal muscles.
- If any wound is identified, it should be debrided; any abscesses should be drained. A 10- to 14-day course of penicillin, tetracycline, or doxycycline is recommended to inhibit further growth of the organism.
- Opioid analgesics such as morphine or fentanyl are indicated for pain management.

Nutrition is maintained through parenteral or nasogastric feeding. Those who recover have a long convalescence that includes extensive physical therapy.

Nursing Management
Health teaching is aimed at ensuring tetanus prophylaxis, which is the most important factor influencing the incidence of this disease.
- The patient should be taught that immediate, thorough cleansing of all wounds with soap and water is important in prevention.

- If an open wound occurs and the patient has not been immunized within 5 years, the health care provider should be contacted so that a tetanus booster can be given.

Acute intervention is aimed at supportive care based on the treatment of the clinical manifestations. The patient should be placed in a quiet, darkened room insulated against noise. Judicious sedation should be given.

- Nursing care should be administered with the utmost caution to avoid triggering spasms. For example, the nurse should avoid unnecessary touching, use firm touching when necessary, avoid the use of linens to cover the patient, and maintain a slightly higher than normal ambient temperature.
- Nursing care related to tracheostomy and mechanical ventilation is given as appropriate.
- An indwelling bladder catheter may be used to prevent bladder distention and urinary reflux in the presence of spasms in the muscles of the pelvic floor.
- The patient needs emotional support during the acute phase because the fear of death is real. The family also needs support and education.

THALASSEMIA

Description

Thalassemia is a disease of decreased erythrocyte (red blood cell [RBC]) production resulting from an inadequate production of normal hemoglobin (Hb). Hemolysis also occurs in thalassemia.

- In contrast to iron deficiency anemia, in which heme synthesis is the problem, thalassemia involves a problem with the globin protein. Therefore the basic defect of thalassemia is abnormal Hb synthesis.

Pathophysiology

Thalassemias are a group of autosomal recessive genetic disorders commonly found in members of ethnic groups whose origins are near the Mediterranean Sea or equatorial regions of Asia and Africa. An individual with thalassemia may have a heterozygous or homozygous form of the disease.

- A person who is heterozygous has one thalassemic gene and one normal gene. He or she is said to have *thalassemia minor* or *thalassemic trait,* which is a mild form of the disease.

■ A homozygous person has two thalassemic genes, causing a severe condition known as *thalassemia major*.

Clinical Manifestations

■ The patient with thalassemia minor is frequently asymptomatic, with mild to moderate anemia with microcytosis (small cells) and hypochromia (pale cells).

■ The patient who has thalassemia major is pale and displays other general symptoms of anemia (see Anemia, p. 28). In addition, the person has marked splenomegaly, hepatomegaly, and jaundice from RBC hemolysis. Chronic bone marrow hyperplasia leads to expansion of the marrow space. This may cause thickening of the cranium and maxillary cavity.

■ Thalassemia major is a life-threatening disease in which growth, both physical and mental, is often retarded.

Collaborative Care

The laboratory findings in thalassemia major are summarized in Table 8, p. 31.

■ Thalassemia minor requires no treatment because the body adapts to the reduction of normal Hb.

■ Symptoms of thalassemia major are managed with blood transfusions, intravenous (IV) deferoxamine (Desferal [a chelating agent that binds to iron]), and chelation therapy to reduce the iron overloading that occurs with chronic transfusion therapy. Drug and nutritional therapies are not effective in treating thalassemia. Transfusions are administered to keep the Hb level at about 10 g/dl (100 g/L). This level is low enough to foster the patient's own erythropoiesis without enlarging the spleen.

■ Because RBCs are sequestered in the enlarged spleen, thalassemia may be treated by splenectomy. Even with therapy, however, the person with thalassemia major experiences growth failure; hemochromatosis; and hepatic, pulmonary, and cardiac failure that is often fatal.

THROMBOANGIITIS OBLITERANS (BUERGER'S DISEASE)

Thromboangiitis obliterans (Buerger's disease) is a somewhat rare nonatherosclerotic, segmental, recurrent inflammatory vaso-occlusive disorder that most often affects the medium-sized arteries, veins, and nerves of the upper and lower extremities. The disorder occurs predominantly in younger men under the age of 40 years, but it also occurs in women.

- The underlying cause is not known. There is a very strong relationship to tobacco use.
- In Buerger's disease, an inflammatory process damages the arterial wall. Lymphocytes and giant cells infiltrate the vessel wall, accompanied by fibroblast proliferation. Ultimately, thrombosis and fibrosis occur inside the vessel, causing tissue ischemia.
- The symptom complex of Buerger's disease is often confused with that of peripheral arterial disease and other inflammatory or autoimmune diseases.
- Patients may have intermittent claudication of the feet, hands, or arms. As the disease progresses, pain while at rest and ischemic ulcerations develop.
- Signs and symptoms also can include color and temperature vchanges in the affected limb or limbs, paresthesia, thrombophlebitis, and cold sensitivity.

There are no laboratory or diagnostic tests specific to Buerger's disease. Diagnosis is based on age of onset, history of tobacco usage, clinical symptoms, involvement of distal vessels, presence of ischemic ulcerations, and exclusion of disorders including diabetes mellitus, autoimmune disease, thrombophilia, and a proximal source of emboli.

Treatment includes a complete cessation of tobacco usage and exposure to smoke. Although the amputation rate is significantly lower in patients who stop using tobacco, risk of death is similar in those who continue to use tobacco and those who quit. Other therapies have limited success and include antiplatelet agents, calcium channel blockers, α-adrenergic blockers, and anticoagulants.

THROMBOCYTOPENIC PURPURA

Description

Immune thrombocytopenic purpura (ITP), the most common acquired thrombocytopenia, is a syndrome of abnormal destruction of circulating platelets. It was originally termed idiopathic thrombocytopenic purpura because its cause was unknown; however, it is now known that ITP is an autoimmune disease.

- In ITP, platelets are coated with antibodies. Although these platelets function normally, when they reach the spleen the antibody-coated platelets are recognized as foreign and destroyed by macrophages. Platelets normally survive 8 to 10 days, but in ITP, survival is only 1 to 3 days.
- Chronic ITP occurs most commonly in women between 20 and 40 years old. Chronic ITP has a gradual onset, and transient remissions occur.

Thrombotic thrombocytopenia purpura (TTP) is an uncommon syndrome characterized by hemolytic anemia, thrombocytopenia, neurologic abnormalities, fever (in the absence of infection), and renal abnormalities.

- TTP is almost always associated with hemolytic-uremic syndrome (HUS), a rare autoimmune disorder of primarily children that is associated with infection by one *Escherichia coli* serotype and one *Shigella dysenteriae* serotype.
- The disease is associated with enhanced agglutination of platelets, which form microthrombi that deposit in arterioles and capillaries.
- TTP is seen primarily in adults between the ages of 20 and 50 years old, with a slight female predominance.
- The syndrome is occasionally precipitated by the use of estrogen or by pregnancy.
- TTP is a medical emergency because bleeding and clotting occur simultaneously.

Clinical Manifestations

Many patients with thrombocytopenia are asymptomatic.

- Thrombocytopenia is most commonly manifested by the appearance of small, flat, pinpoint, red or reddish brown microhemorrhages known as *petechiae*. When the platelet count is low, red blood cells (RBCs) may leak out of the blood vessels and into the skin to cause petechiae.
- When petechiae are numerous, the resulting reddish skin bruise is known as *purpura*.
- Larger purplish lesions caused by hemorrhage are called *ecchymoses*. Ecchymoses may be flat or raised; on occasion pain and tenderness are present.
- Prolonged bleeding after routine procedures, such as venipuncture or intramuscular (IM) injection, may indicate thrombocytopenia. Because bleeding may be internal, the nurse must be aware of manifestations that reflect this type of blood loss, including weakness, fainting, dizziness, tachycardia, abdominal pain, and hypotension.

The major complication of thrombocytopenia is hemorrhage, which may be insidious or acute and internal or external. It may occur in any area of the body, including the joints, retina, and brain. Cerebral hemorrhage may be fatal in persons with ITP. Insidious hemorrhage may first be detected by discovering the anemia that accompanies blood loss.

Diagnostic Studies

- Platelet count is decreased below 150,000/µl (150 × 10^9/L); spontaneous life-threatening hemorrhages (e.g., intracranial bleeding) may occur with counts below 20,000/µl (20 × 10^9/L).
- Bleeding time is prolonged.
- Specific assays for antigens help differentiate ITP from other types of thrombocytopenia.
- Bone marrow analysis may show normal or increased megakaryocytes (precursors of platelets); it is done to rule out leukemia, aplastic anemia, and other myeloproliferative disorders.
- Flow cytometry may detect antiplatelet antibodies.
- Hematocrit (Hct) and hemoglobin (Hb) levels are assessed for anemia.

Collaborative Care

Immune Thrombocytopenic Purpura. Multiple therapies are used to manage the patient with ITP.

- Corticosteroids (e.g., prednisone) are used to suppress the phagocytic response of splenic macrophages. This alters the spleen's recognition of platelets and increases platelet life span. In addition, corticosteroids depress antibody formation and reduce capillary fragility and bleeding time.
- Splenectomy is indicated if the patient does not respond to prednisone initially or requires unacceptably high doses to maintain an adequate platelet count. Approximately 80% of patients benefit from splenectomy, which results in a complete or partial remission.
- Treatment may also include high doses of intravenous immunoglobulin (IVIG) in the patient who is unresponsive to corticosteroids or splenectomy. The immunoglobulin works by competing with the antiplatelet antibodies for macrophage receptors. IVIG raises the platelet count, but the beneficial effects are temporary.
- Danazol, an androgen, is often used with glucocorticosteroids in some patients.

- Immunosuppressive agents used in refractory cases includes rituximab (Rituxan), cyclophosphamide (Cytoxan), azathioprine (Imuran), and mycophenolate mofetil (CellCept). High-dose cyclophosamide and combination chemotherapy are third-line therapy.
- Platelet transfusions are not indicated until the count is below 10,000/μl (10×10^9/L) unless the patient is actively bleeding or a procedure is planned. Platelets should not be administered prophylactically because of the possibility of antibody formation.
- Aspirin and aspirin-containing compounds should be avoided.

Thrombotic Thrombocytopenic Purpura. Corticosteroids are used initially. Plasma exchange or plasmapheresis may be needed to aggressively reverse the process. Treatment should be continued daily until the patient is in complete remission. Splenectomy, corticosteroids, dextran 70/75 (an antiplatelet agent), and vincristine (Oncovin) or vinblastine (Velban) have also been used with success.

Nursing Management
Goals
The patient with thrombocytopenia will have no gross or occult bleeding, maintain vascular integrity, and manage home care to prevent any complications related to an increased risk for bleeding.

See NCP 31-2 for the patient with thrombocytopenia, Lewis and others, *Medical-Surgical Nursing,* edition 7, p. 706.

Nursing Diagnoses/Collaborative Problems
- Impaired oral mucous membrane
- Risk for injury
- Ineffective therapeutic regimen management

Nursing Interventions
It is important for the nurse to discourage excessive use of over-the-counter (OTC) medications known to be possible causes of acquired thrombocytopenia. Many medications contain aspirin as an ingredient. Aspirin reduces platelet adhesiveness, thus potentially contributing to bleeding.

The nurse should encourage persons to have a complete medical evaluation if manifestations of bleeding tendencies (e.g., prolonged epistaxis, petechiae) develop. In addition, the nurse must be observant for early signs of thrombocytopenia in patients receiving cancer chemotherapy drugs.

The goal during acute episodes of thrombocytopenia is to prevent or control hemorrhage. In the patient with thrombocytopenia, bleeding is usually from superficial sites; deep bleeding (into the muscles, joints, and abdomen) usually occurs only when clotting factors are diminished. It is important to emphasize that a seemingly minor nosebleed may indicate potential hemorrhage and the physician should be notified.

- In a woman with thrombocytopenia, menstrual blood loss may exceed the usual amount and duration. Counting sanitary napkins or tampons used during menses is an important intervention to detect excess blood loss.
- Proper administration of platelet transfusions is an important nursing responsibility. Platelet concentrates, derived from fresh whole blood, can effectively increase the platelet level.
- All patients with ITP should be monitored for a response to therapy.

▼ **Patient and Family Teaching**
- Discuss complications and signs that should be reported, trauma prevention, the need for a high fluid intake, medication management, and the need for periods of rest and exercise so the patient will be knowledgeable and able to manage his or her own care or direct others in providing care.
- Provide opportunities for the patient to verbalize concerns to decrease his or her anxiety.
- Educate the patient to avoid Valsalva maneuver (e.g., straining at stool), to avoid aspirin or aspirin-containing products, and to cough, sneeze, and blow the nose gently.

TRIGEMINAL NEURALGIA

Description
Trigeminal neuralgia (tic douloureux) is a relatively uncommon cranial nerve disorder. It is seen twice as often in women as in men. The majority of cases are in persons older than 40 years. Although this condition is considered benign, the severity of the pain and the disruption of lifestyle can result in almost total physical and psychologic dysfunction or even suicide.

Pathophysiology
The trigeminal nerve is the fifth cranial nerve (CN V) and has both motor and sensory branches. The sensory branches, primarily the maxillary and mandibular branches, are involved in trigeminal neuralgia.

- Although no specific cause has been identified, one theory is that compression of blood vessels, especially the superior cerebellar artery, occurs and results in chronic irritation of the trigeminal nerve at the root entry zone. Other factors that may result in trigeminal neuralgia include herpesvirus infection, infection of the teeth and jaw, and a brainstem infarct.

- The effectiveness of antiseizure drug therapy may be related to the ability of these drugs to stabilize the neuronal membrane.

Clinical Manifestations

The classic feature of trigeminal neuralgia is an abrupt onset of paroxysms of excruciating pain described as burning or knifelike, or a lightning-like shock in the lips, upper or lower gums, cheek, forehead, or side of the nose.

- Intense pain, twitching, grimacing, and frequent blinking and tearing of the eye occur during the acute attack (giving rise to the term *tic*).
- The attacks are usually brief, lasting seconds to 2 or 3 minutes, and are generally unilateral.
- Recurrences are unpredictable; they may occur several times each day or weeks or months apart.
- After the refractory (pain-free) period, a phenomenon known as *clustering* can occur; it is characterized by a cycle of pain and refractoriness that continues for hours.

The painful episodes are usually initiated by a triggering mechanism of light cutaneous stimulation at specific points (trigger zones) along the distribution of the nerve branches.

- Precipitating stimuli include chewing, teeth brushing, a hot or cold blast of air on the face, washing the face, yawning, or even talking. Touch and tickle seem to predominate as causative triggers rather than pain or changes in temperature.
- As a result, the patient may not eat properly, neglect hygienic practices, wear a cloth over the face, and withdraw from interaction with other individuals. The patient may sleep excessively as a means of coping with the pain.

Diagnostic Studies

- Magnetic resonance imaging (MRI), computed tomography (CT) scan, and lumbar puncture to rule out other problems with similar manifestations
- Complete neurologic assessment with audiologic evaluation
- Electromyography, cerebrospinal fluid analysis, and arteriography and posterior myelography to rule out other pathologic conditions

Collaborative Care

Drug Therapy

The majority of patients obtain adequate relief through antiseizure drugs such as carbamazepine (Tegretol), phenytoin (Dilantin), and valproate (Depakene). Carbamazepine is considered first-line therapy for trigeminal neuralgia. Newer antiseizure drugs that may be used include oxcarbazepine (Trileptal), gabapentin (Neurontin), lamotrigine (Lamictal), and topiramate (Topamax). Antiseizure drugs may prevent an acute attack or promote remission of symptoms, but they may not provide permanent pain relief.

- Nerve blocking with local anesthetics is another treatment possibility. Local nerve blocking results in complete anesthesia of the area supplied by the injected branches. Relief of pain is temporary, lasting 6 to 18 months.
- Biofeedback is another strategy for pain management. In addition to controlling the pain, the patient may experience a strong sense of personal control by mastering the technique and altering certain body functions.

Surgical Therapy

If a conservative approach including drug therapy is not effective, surgical therapy is available.

- *Glycerol rhizotomy* is a percutaneous procedure that consists of an injection of glycerol through the foramen ovale into the trigeminal cistern. It is a more benign procedure with less sensory loss and fewer sensory aberrations than radiofrequency rhizotomy and with comparable or better pain relief.
- *Percutaneous radiofrequency rhizotomy* (electrocoagulation) consists of placing a needle into the trigeminal rootlets that are adjacent to the pons and destroying the area by means of a radiofrequency current. This can result in facial numbness (although some degree of sensation may be retained) or trigeminal motor weakness. This procedure is easily performed with minimal risk to the patient.
- *Microvascular decompression* of the trigeminal nerve is accomplished by displacing and repositioning blood vessels that appear to be compressing the nerve at the root-entry zone where it exits the pons. This procedure relieves pain without residual sensory loss but is potentially dangerous, as is any surgery near the brainstem. This procedure has a long-term success rate equal to or superior to percutaneous procedures without the higher rate of permanent neurologic outcomes, such as numbness.
- Other procedures include gamma knife radiosurgery, retrogasserian rhizotomy, and suboccipital craniotomy.

Nursing Management

Goals

The patient with trigeminal neuralgia will be free of pain, maintain adequate nutritional and oral hygiene status, have minimal to no anxiety, and return to normal or previous socialization and occupational activities.

Nursing Diagnoses

- Acute pain
- Imbalanced nutrition: less than body requirements
- Anxiety
- Impaired oral mucous membrane
- Social isolation

Nursing Interventions

Pain relief is primarily obtained by the administration of the recommended drug therapy. The nurse monitors the patient's response to therapy and notes any side effects. Strong opioids such as morphine should be used cautiously because of the potential for addiction over time. Alternative pain relief measures, such as biofeedback, should be explored for the patient who is not a surgical candidate and whose pain is not controlled by other therapeutic measures.

Environmental management is essential during an acute period to lessen triggering stimuli. The room should be kept at an even, moderate temperature and free of drafts. A private room is preferred during an acute period.

- The nurse must use care to avoid touching the patient's face or jarring the bed. Many patients prefer to carry out their own care, fearing that someone else will inadvertently injure them.

The nurse should instruct the patient about the importance of nutrition, hygiene, and oral care, conveying understanding if previous neglect is apparent.

- The nurse should provide lukewarm water and soft cloths or cotton saturated with solutions not requiring rinsing for cleansing the face. A small, very soft-bristled toothbrush or a warm mouthwash assists in promoting oral care.
- Hygiene activities are best carried out when analgesia is at its peak.

The patient will probably not engage in extensive conversation during the acute period. Alternative communication methods such as paper and pencil should be provided.

Food should be high in protein and calories and easy to chew. It should be served lukewarm and offered frequently. When oral intake is markedly reduced and the patient's nutritional status is compromised, a nasogastric (NG) tube is inserted on the unaffected side for NG feedings.

For the patient who has had surgery, the patient's postoperative pain should be compared with the preoperative level. The corneal reflex, extraocular muscles, hearing, sensation, and facial nerve function are evaluated frequently. General postoperative nursing care after a craniotomy is appropriate if intracranial surgery is performed.

- After a percutaneous radiofrequency procedure, an ice pack is applied to the jaw on the operative side for 3 to 5 hours. To avoid injuring the mouth, the patient should not chew on the operative side until sensation has returned.

▼ **Patient and Family Teaching**

Regular follow-up care should be planned. The patient needs instruction regarding the dosage and side effects of medications. The patient should be encouraged to keep environmental stimuli to a moderate level and to use stress reduction methods.

Long-term management after surgical intervention depends on the residual effects of the procedure used.

- If anesthesia is present or the corneal reflex is altered, the patient should be taught to (1) chew on the unaffected side, (2) avoid hot foods or beverages that can burn the mucous membranes, (3) check the oral cavity after meals to remove food particles, (4) practice meticulous oral hygiene and continue with semiannual dental visits, (5) protect the face against extremes of temperature, (6) use an electric razor, and (7) wear a protective eye shield.
- The patient may have developed protective practices to prevent pain and may need counseling or psychiatric assistance in the readjustment period, especially in reestablishing personal relationships.

TUBERCULOSIS

Description

Tuberculosis (TB) is an infectious disease caused by *Mycobacterium tuberculosis*. It usually involves the lungs, but it can also occur in the kidneys, larynx, bones, lymph nodes, meninges, and adrenal glands. TB can disseminate throughout the body.

TB is the world's second most common cause of death from infectious disease, after human immunodeficiency virus/acquired immunodeficiency syndrome (HIV/AIDS). An estimated one third of the world's population is infected with the *M. tuberculosis* bacterium, with 8 to 9 million new cases each year and approximately 2 million deaths anually. Although TB rates in the United

States have declined, 14,000 new cases per year are being reported. Rates have increased in certain states and populations (e.g., foreign-born persons and ethnic minorities).

- Major factors contributing to the resurgence of TB are high rates of infection among persons with HIV infection and the emergence of multidrug-resistant strains of *M. tuberculosis*. Once a strain of *M. tuberculosis* develops resistance to isoniazid and rifampin, it is defined as multidrug-resistant tuberculosis (MDR-TB). MDR-TB developed because patients had poor compliance with drug therapy, leading to treatment failure, were lost to follow-up treatment, or were placed on drug regimens to which their infections were no longer susceptible.

Pathophysiology

M. tuberculosis, a gram-positive, acid-fast bacillus, is usually spread by way of airborne droplet nuclei, which are produced when the infected individual coughs, sneezes, speaks, or sings.The very small droplet nuclei, 1 to 5 μm in size, are able to remain airborne for minutes to hours.

- Brief exposure to a few tubercle bacilli rarely causes infection.
- TB is not highly infectious, and transmission usually requires close, frequent, or prolonged exposure. The disease cannot be spread by hands, books, glasses, or dishes.
- Once inhaled, these nuclei lodge in alveoli in the small distal airways of the lung.
- The *M. tuberculosis* replicates slowly and spreads by way of the lymphatic system.
- The organisms find favorable environments for growth primarily in the upper lobes of the lungs, kidneys, epiphyses of the bone, cerebral cortex, and adrenal glands.

When the cellular immune system is stimulated by the microorganism, a characteristic tissue *granuloma* is formed from alveolar macrophages that contains the bacteria and prevents further replication.

- At this point the person has *TB infection* and will have a positive tuberculin skin test.
- TB infection occurs when the bacteria are inhaled but there is an effective immune response with formation of a granuloma, and the bacteria become inactive. This person cannot spread the infection to other people.
- TB infection in a person who does not have active disease is not considered a case of TB and is often referred to as *latent TB infection* (LTBI).

- The majority of people mount effective immune responses to encapsulate these organisms for the rest of their life, preventing primary infection from progressing to disease.

If the initial immune response is not adequate, control of the organisms is not maintained and active primary disease results.

- *Tuberculosis disease* is defined as active bacteria that multiply and cause TB disease. People who are immunosuppressed for any reason or have diabetes mellitus are at higher risk for developing active disease.
- Dormant but viable *M. tuberculosis* organisms persist for years. Reactivation TB of latent infection can occur if the host's defense mechanisms become impaired.

Classification of TB according to the American Thoracic Society is presented in Table 81.

Table 81	Classification of Tuberculosis (TB)

Class 0
No TB exposure, not infected (no history of exposure, negative tuberculin skin test)

Class 1
TB exposure, no evidence of infection (history of exposure, negative tuberculin skin test)

Class 2
TB infection without disease (significant reaction to tuberculin skin test, negative bacteriologic studies, no x-ray findings compatible with TB, no clinical evidence of TB)

Class 3
TB infection with clinically active disease (positive bacteriologic studies or both a significant reaction to tuberculin skin test and clinical or x-ray evidence of current disease)

Class 4
No current disease (history of previous episode of TB or abnormal, stable x-ray findings in a person with a significant reaction to tuberculin skin test; negative bacteriologic studies if done; no clinical or x-ray evidence of current disease)

Class 5
TB suspect (diagnosis pending); person should not be in this classification for more than 3 months

From American Thoracic Society, 2000.

Clinical Manifestations

In the early stages the patient is usually free of symptoms.

- Active TB disease may initially present with fatigue, malaise, anorexia, unexplained weight loss, low-grade fevers, and night sweats.

A characteristic pulmonary manifestation is a cough that becomes frequent and produces white frothy sputum. Dyspnea is unusual. Hemoptysis is not a common finding and is usually associated with more advanced cases.

- Sometimes TB has more acute, sudden manifestations; the patient has a high fever, chills, generalized flu-like symptoms, pleuritic pain, and a productive cough.
- The HIV-infected patient with TB often has atypical physical examinations and chest x-ray findings. Classic signs such as fever, cough, and weight loss may be attributed to *Pneumocystis jiroveci* or other HIV-associated opportunistic diseases. Clinical manifestations of respiratory problems in patients with HIV must be carefully investigated to determine the cause.

Complications

Miliary or *hematogenous TB* occurs if a necrotic lesion erodes through a blood vessel, releasing large numbers of organisms into the bloodstream that spread to all body organs.

- The patient may be either acutely ill with fever, dyspnea, and cyanosis or chronically ill with systemic manifestations of weight loss, fever, and gastrointestinal (GI) disturbance.
- Hepatomegaly, splenomegaly, and generalized lymphadenopathy may also be present.

Pleural effusion and *empyema* may occur and are caused by bacteria in the pleural space triggering an inflammatory reaction and plural exudate of protein-rich fluid or pus.

Acute pneumonia may result when large amounts of tubercle bacilli are discharged from granulomas into the lungs or lymph nodes.

- Manifestations are similar to those of bacterial pneumonia, including chills, fever, productive cough, pleuritic pain, and leukocytosis.

Diagnostic Studies

- Tuberculin skin test (TST): positive reaction indicates TB infection (latent or active). See Chapter 26, Lewis and others, *Medical-Surgical Nursing,* edition 7 for guidelines in performing and interpreting TSTs.

- Chest x-ray: diagnosis cannot be based solely on x-ray because other diseases may mimic TB.
- Bacteriologic studies: stained sputum smears for acid-fast bacilli (AFB test) can identify tubercle bacilli; cultures to grow tubercle bacilli to confirm diagnosis.
- QuantiFERON-TB (QFT), a newer, rapid diagnostic test using blood, is an option in detecting TB and may be used in place of TST in health care settings.

Collaborative Care

Most patients with TB are treated on an outpatient basis and continue to work and maintain their lifestyles with few changes. Hospitalization may be used for diagnostic evaluation and for severely ill or debilitated patients.

Drug Therapy

The mainstay of TB treatment is drug therapy. Drug therapy is used to treat an individual with clinical disease, as well as to prevent disease in an infected person. In view of the growing prevalence of multidrug-resistant TB, the patient with active TB should be managed aggressively. Treatment of previously untreated TB usually consists of a combination of at least four drugs to increase therapeutic effectiveness and decrease the development of *M. tuberculosis*–resistant strains. Four different regimen options have been identified by the Centers for Disease Control and Prevention (CDC) (see Table 28-10, Lewis and others, *Medical-Surgical Nursing*, edition 7, p. 574).

- First-line drugs include isoniazid (INH), rifampin (Rifadin), pyrazinamide (PZA), ethambutol (Myambutol), rifabutin (Mycobutin), and rifapentine (Priftin). Combinations of isoniazid and rifampin and of isoniazid, rifampin, and pyrazinamide are available to simplify therapy.
- Second-line drugs are used primarily for the treatment of resistant strains or if the patient develops toxicity to the primary drugs. Newer second-line drugs include the quinolones (e.g., levofloxacin [Levaquin], moxifloxacin [Avelox], gatifloxacin [Tequin]).
- The preferred drug administration strategy for all patients with TB to ensure adherence is directly observed therapy (DOT). This involves providing the antituberculosis drugs directly to the patient and watching as he or she swallows the medications.
- Noncompliance is a major factor in the emergence of multidrug resistance and treatment failures. Many individuals do not adhere to the treatment program in spite of understanding that noncompliance can lead to reactivation of TB

and multidrug-resistant TB. Drug therapy is usually continued for 6 to 9 months.

- The recommended length of 6 to 9 months of drug therapy also contributes to noncompliance.

Drug regimens should be adapted to the resistance pattern evident from sputum culture. In follow-up care for patients receiving long-term therapy, it is important to monitor drug effectiveness and the development of toxic side effects.

- Sputum specimens are usually initially obtained weekly and then monthly to assess effectiveness of medication.

Isoniazid is usually used in the treatment of latent TB infection to prevent the infection from developing into active disease.

Immunization with bacille Calmette-Guérin (BCG) vaccine to prevent tuberculosis is currently used in many parts of the world. However, efficacy of the vaccine is not clear, and development of an effective TB vaccine is an urgent worldwide public health priority.

Nursing Management
Goals
The patient with tuberculosis will comply with the therapeutic regimen, have no recurrence of disease, have normal pulmonary function, and take appropriate measures to prevent the spread of the disease.
Nursing Diagnoses
- Ineffective breathing pattern
- Imbalanced nutrition: less than body requirements
- Noncompliance
- Ineffective health maintenance
- Activity intolerance
Nursing Interventions
The ultimate goal related to TB in the United States is eradication.

- Selective screening programs in known high-risk groups are of value in detecting persons with TB.
- Chest x-rays to assess for the presence of TB in persons with a positive tuberculin skin test should be encouraged.
- Contacts of the individual who has TB should be identified and assessed for the possibility of infection and the need for prophylactic drug treatment.
- When an individual has respiratory symptoms such as cough, dyspnea, or productive sputum, especially if accompanied by night sweats and unexplained weight loss, the nurse should assess for the presence of TB.

If hospitalization is needed for patients suspected of having TB, special measures should be taken.

- Airborne isolation is indicated until the patient has been taking adequate drug therapy for at least 2 weeks, has shown a clinical response to therapy, and has three negative AFB smears.
- High-efficiency particulate air (HEPA) masks molded to fit tightly around the nose and mouth are worn whenever entering the patient's room.

Follow-up care may be indicated during the subsequent 12 months after the medication regimen is completed; this includes bacteriologic studies and chest x-rays.

▼ **Patient and Family Teaching**

- In the hospital the patient should be taught to cover the nose and mouth with paper tissue every time he or she coughs, sneezes, or produces sputum. The patient wears a standard isolation mask to prevent coughing tubercular organisms into the environment.
- The nurse should teach the patient so that the need for dedication to the prescribed medication regimen is fully understood by the patient and family. The patient should be reassured that TB can be cured if the regimen is followed.
- Because approximately 5% of individuals experience relapses, the patient should be taught to recognize symptoms that indicate the recurrence of TB. If these symptoms occur, immediate medical attention should be sought.
- The patient also needs to be instructed about factors that could reactivate TB, such as immunosuppression and malignancy.

ULCERATIVE COLITIS

Ulcerative colitis is an autoimmune disorder that, along with with Crohn's disease, is referrred to as *inflammatory bowel disease* (IBD). See Inflammatory Bowel Disease, p. 352 for a description of the disorder.

URETHRITIS

Urethritis is an inflammation of the urethra. Causes of urethritis include a bacterial or viral infection, trichomonal and monilial infection (especially in women), chlamydia, and gonorrhea (especially in men).

In men, purulent discharge usually indicates a gonococcal urethritis; a clear discharge typically signifies a nongonococcal urethritis.

- Urethritis also produces bothersome lower urinary tract symptoms, including dysuria and frequent urination, similar to those seen with cystitis.

In women, urethritis is difficult to diagnose. It frequently produces bothersome lower urinary tract symptoms as described above, but urethral discharge may not be present.

- Cultures on split urine collections or any urethral discharge may confirm a diagnosis of urethral infection.

Treatment is based on identifying and treating the cause and providing symptomatic relief.

- Sulfamethoxazole with trimethoprim (Bactrim, Septra) and nitrofurantoin (Furadantin) are examples of medications used for bacterial infections. Metronidazole (Flagyl) and clotrimazole (Mycelex) may be used for trichomonal infection. Medications such as nystatin (Mycostatin) or fluconazole (Diflucan) may be prescribed for monilial infections. In chlamydial infections, doxycycline (Vibramycin) may be used.
- Women with negative urine cultures and no pyuria do not usually respond to antibiotics. Warm sitz baths may temporarily relieve the symptoms.

Patients should be instructed to avoid the use of vaginal deodorant sprays, properly cleanse the perineal area after bowel movements and urination, and avoid intercourse until symptoms subside.

URINARY INCONTINENCE AND RETENTION

Description

Urinary incontinence (UI), the uncontrolled leakage of urine, affects an estimated 17 million people in the United States. Although its prevalence is higher among older women and men, it is not a natural consequence of aging. An estimated 80% of incontinence can be cured or significantly improved.

Urinary retention is the inability to empty the bladder despite micturition or the accumulation of urine in the bladder because of an inability to urinate. In certain cases, it is associated with urinary leakage or postvoid dribbling called overflow UI.

Pathophysiology

UI can result from anything that interferes with bladder or urethral sphincter control.

- Causes can include confusion or depression, infection, atropic vaginitis, urinary retention, restricted mobility, fecal impaction, and a wide variety of drugs.
- UI disorders include stress, urge, overflow, and reflex incontinence. (For a complete description of UI, see Table 46-18, Lewis and others, *Medical-Surgical Nursing,* edition 7, p. 1181.)
- Patients may have more than one type of incontinence.

Urinary retention is caused by two different dysfunctions of the urinary system: bladder outlet obstruction and deficient detrusor contraction strength.

- Obstruction leads to urinary retention when the blockage is severe enough that the bladder can no longer evacuate its contents despite a detrusor contraction. A common cause of obstruction in men is an enlarged prostate.
- Common causes of deficient detrusor contraction strength are neurologic diseases affecting the sacral segments 2, 3, and 4; long-standing diabetes mellitus; overdistention; long-term alcoholism; and drugs (e.g., anticholinergic drugs).

Diagnostic Studies

- Focused history, physical assessment, and a voiding record obtain information about the onset of UI, factors that provoke urinary leakage, and associated conditions.
- Pelvic examination assesses for organ prolapse and evaluates pelvic floor muscle strength.
- Urinalysis identifies possible factors contributing to transient incontinence or urinary retention (e.g., urinary infection, diabetes mellitus).
- Postvoid residual (PVR) urine must be measured in the patient undergoing evaluation for urinary incontinence and retention.
- Urodynamic testing is indicated in selected cases of urinary incontinence and retention.
- Imaging studies of upper urinary tract (e.g., ultrasound, intravenous pyelogram [IVP]) are obtained when retention or incontinence is associated with urinary tract infections or when there is evidence of upper urinary tract involvement.

Collaborative Care: Urinary Incontinence

Transient, reversible factors are corrected initially, followed by management of the type of UI. In general, less invasive treatments

652 Urinary Incontinence and Retention

are attempted before more invasive methods (e.g., surgery) are used.

Several behavioral therapies may be used to improve urinary continence.

- Pelvic floor muscle training (Kegel exercises) may help some patients manage stress, urge, or mixed UI.
- Biofeedback is used to assist the patient to identify, isolate, contract, and relax the pelvic muscles.

Drug Therapy

Drug therapy varies according to the type of incontinence.

- Drugs have a very limited role in the management of stress incontinence. α-Adrenergic agonists can be used to increase urethral resistance at the level of the sphincter mechanism. Unfortunately, they exert a limited beneficial effect and are associated with adverse effects, including exacerbation of hypertension and tachycardia.
- Drugs play a more central role in the management of urge or reflex incontinence. Anticholinergic drugs and newer, more specific muscarinic receptor antagonists relax the bladder muscle and inhibit overactive detrusor contractions. These preparations include immediate- and extended-release tolterodine (Detrol, Detrol LA); immediate, extended, and transdermal oxybutynin (Ditropan, Ditropan XL, Oxytrol TDS); twice daily trospium chloride (Sanctura); extended-release solifenacine (VESIcare); and darifenacin (Enablex). Common side effects of anticholingergic drugs include dry mouth, constipation, and dyspepsia.

Surgical Therapy

Surgical techniques also vary according to the type of incontinence.

- Surgical correction of stress UI may reposition the urethra and/or create a backboard of support or otherwise stabilize the urethra and bladder neck to be more receptive to changes in intrabdominal pressure.
- Another technique for stress UI augments the urethral resistance of the intrinsic sphincter unit with a sling or periurethral injectables.
- Placement of a suburethral sling, using autologous fascia, cadaveric fascia, or a synthetic material, is also used to correct stress UI in women.
- An artificial urethral sphincter can be used in men with intrinsic sphincter deficiency and severe stress UI.
- Alternatively, one of several bulking agents can be injected underneath the mucosa of the urethra to correct stress UI in women or men.

Nursing Management: Urinary Incontinence

The nurse must recognize both the physical and the emotional problems associated with incontinence. The patient's dignity, privacy, and feelings of self-worth must be maintained or enhanced.

- This often includes a two-step approach involving containment devices to manage existing urinary leakage and a definitive plan of management designed to reduce or resolve the factors leading to incontinence.
- Consumption of an adequate volume of fluids and reduction or elimination of bladder irritants (particularly caffeine and alcohol) from the diet should be emphasized.
- The patient is advised to maintain a regular, flexible schedule of urination (usually every 2 to 3 hours while awake).
- Patients are strongly advised to quit smoking, since this habit increases the risk of stress UI.
- Aggressive management of constipation, beginning with ensuring adequate fluid intake, increasing dietary fiber, light exercise, and judicious use of stool softeners, is recommended.
- Behavioral treatments include bladder retraining and pelvic floor muscle training. (A patient teaching guide for pelvic floor muscle exercise is found in Table 46-20, Lewis and others, *Medical-Surgical Nursing,* edition 7, p. 1184.)
- The nurse should assess strategies the patient uses to contain UI and share information on products specifically designed to contain urine.
- Prompted toileting is indicated for patients with altered cognitive function and functional incontinence. In this case, caregivers are taught to remind the patient to toilet on a regular basis (usually every 2 to 3 hours); the patient is assisted to the toilet and given praise for successful toileting.
- In inpatient or long-term care facilities, nursing management of UI includes maximizing toilet access. This may take the form of offering the urinal or bedpan or assisting the patient to the bathroom every 2 to 3 hours or at scheduled times.The nurse ensures that toilets are accessible to patients and that there is adequate privacy to allow effective urine elimination.

Collaborative Care: Urinary Retention

Behavioral therapies also may be used in the management of urinary retention. Scheduled toileting and double voiding may be effective in chronic urinary retention with moderate postvoid residual volumes.

- Double voiding is an attempt to maximize bladder evacuation by having the patient urinate, sit on the toilet for 3 to 4 mintues, and urinate again before exiting the bathroom.
- If catheterization is required for acute or chronic urinary retention, intermittent catheterization is preferred. It allows the patient to remain free of an indwelling catheter with its associated risk of urinary tract infection (UTI) and urethral irritation.

Drug Therapy

Several drugs may be administered to promote bladder evacuation. For patients with prostatic hyperplasia, bladder neck dyssynergia, or detrusor sphincter dyssynergia, an α-adrenergic antagonist may be prescribed. These drugs relax the smooth muscle of the bladder neck, prostatic urethra, and possibly dual-innervated rhabdosphincter, diminishing urethral resistance.

Surgical Therapy

Surgical interventions are useful when managing urinary retention caused by obstruction. Transurethral or open surgical techniques are used to treat benign or malignant prostatic enlargement, bladder neck contracture, urethral strictures, or dyssynergia of the bladder neck in selected patients.

- Pelvic reconstruction using an abdominal or transvaginal approach can be used to correct bladder outlet obstruction in women with severe pelvic organ prolapse.

Unfortunately, surgery plays little role in the management of urinary retention caused by deficient detrusor contraction strength.

Nursing Management: Urinary Retention

Acute urinary retention is a medical emergency that requires prompt recognition and bladder drainage. The nurse should insert a catheter (as prescribed) unless otherwise directed.

- The patient with acute urinary retention should be taught strategies to minimize risk, including avoiding intake of large volumes of fluid over a brief period.
- A patient unable to urinate is advised to drink a cup of coffee or brewed caffeinated tea to maximize urinary urgency and to sit in a tub of warm water or take a warm shower and attempt to urinate while in the tub or shower.
- If this does not lead to successful urination, the patient is advised to seek immediate care.
- Patients with chronic urinary retention may be managed by behavioral methods, an indwelling or intermittent catheterization, surgery, or medications.

- Scheduled toileting and double voiding are the primary behavioral interventions used for chronic retention.

URINARY TRACT CALCULI

Description
Each year an estimated 500,000 people in the United States have *nephrolithiasis* (kidney stone disease). Except for struvite stones, associated with urinary tract infection (UTI), stone disorders are more common in men than in women. The majority of patients are between 20 and 55 years old.

- The incidence is also higher in persons with a family history of stone formation. Recurrence of stones can occur in up to 50% of patients.
- The term *calculus* refers to the stone, and *lithiasis* refers to stone formation.

Pathophysiology
Many factors are involved in the incidence and type of stone formation, including metabolic, dietary, genetic, climatic, lifestyle, and occupational influences. Many theories have been proposed to explain the formation of stones in the urinary tract.

- Crystals, when in a supersaturated concentration, can precipitate and unite to form a stone. Keeping urine dilute and free flowing reduces the risk of recurrent stone formation in many individuals.
- Urinary pH, solute load, and inhibitors in the urine affect the formation of stones. The higher the pH, the less soluble are calcium and phosphate. The lower the pH, the less soluble are uric acid and cystine.

Other important factors in the development of stones include obstruction with urinary stasis and urinary infection with urea-splitting bacteria (e.g., *Proteus, Klebsiella, Pseudomonas,* and some species of staphylococci). These bacteria cause the urine to become alkaline and contribute to the formation of struvite (calcium–magnesium–ammonium phosphate) stones.

- Infected stones, when entrapped in the kidney, may assume a staghorn configuration as they enlarge. Infected stones are frequent with an external urinary diversion, long-term indwelling catheter, neurogenic bladder, or urinary retention.
- There are five major categories of stones: calcium phosphate, calcium oxalate, uric acid, cystine, and struvite.

Stone composition may be mixed, although calcium stones are the most common.

Clinical Manifestations

Urinary stones cause manifestations when they obstruct the urinary flow; symptoms include hematuria, abdominal or flank pain, and renal colic.

- The type of pain is determined by the location of the stone. If the stone is nonobstructing, pain may be absent. If it produces obstruction in a calyx or at the ureteropelvic junction (UPJ), the patient may experience dull costovertebral flank pain or even colic. Pain resulting from the passage of a calculus down the ureter is intense and colicky. The patient may be in mild shock with cool, moist skin. As a stone nears the ureterovesical junction (UVJ), pain will be felt in the lateral flank and sometimes down into the testicles, labia, or groin.
- Other manifestations include the presence of urinary infection accompanied by fever, vomiting, nausea, and chills.

Diagnostic Studies

- Serum calcium, phosphorous, sodium, potassium, bicarbonate, uric acid, and creatinine levels and blood urea nitrogen (BUN) assess renal function and stone etiology.
- Urine pH checks for struvite stones and renal tubular necrosis (tendency to alkaline pH) and uric acid stones (tendency to acidic pH).
- X-ray of the abdomen and renal ultrasound will identify larger, radiopaque stones.
- Ultrasonography can be used to identify radiopaque or radiolucent calculi in the renal pelvis, calyx, or proximal ureter.
- Computed tomography (CT) scan differentiates a nonopaque stone from a tumor.
- Intravenous pyelogram (IVP) or retrograde pyelogram localizes the degree and site of obstruction or confirms the presence of nonradiopaque stones (uric acid, cystine).

Collaborative Care

Evaluation and management of the patient with renal lithiasis consist of two concurrent approaches.

The first approach is directed toward management of the acute attack. This involves treating the symptoms of pain, infection, or obstruction. Opioids are typically required at frequent intervals for relief of renal colic pain. Many stones pass spontaneously. However, stones larger than 4 mm in size are unlikely to pass through the ureter.

The second approach is directed toward evaluation of the cause of the stone formation and the prevention of further stone development. Information to be obtained from the patient includes family history of stone formation, geographic residence, nutritional assessment (including intake of vitamins A and D), activity pattern (active or sedentary), history of periods of prolonged illness with immobilization or dehydration, and any history of disease or surgery involving the gastrointestinal (GI) or genitourinary (GU) tract.

Adequate hydration, dietary sodium restrictions, dietary changes, and medications minimize urinary stone formation.

- Various medications are prescribed that prevent stone formation by altering urine pH, preventing excessive urinary excretion of a substance, or correcting a primary disease (e.g., hyperparathyroidism).

Treatment of struvite stones requires control of infection. Acetohydroxamic acid (Lithostat), an inhibitor of the chemical action caused by persistent bacteria, can retard struvite stone formation. If infection cannot be controlled, the stone may have to be removed surgically.

Indications for open surgical, endourologic, or lithotripsy stone removal include:

- Stones too large for spontaneous passage, associated with bacteriuria or symptomatic infection, or causing impaired renal function, persistent pain, nausea, or ileus
- An inability of the patient to be treated medically
- A patient with one kidney

Endourologic procedures include the use of endoscopes to access stones in the urinary tract. *Cystoscopy* can remove small stones in the bladder. For large stones, a *cystolitholapaxy* is performed using a lithotrite to crush stones. A *cystoscopic lithotripsy* uses an ultrasonic lithotrite to pulverize stones. Complications with these cystoscopic procedures include hemorrhage, retained stone fragments, and infection. Flexible *ureteroscopes* can be used to remove stones from the renal pelvis and upper urinary tract with the use of ultrasonic, laser, or electrohydraulic lithotripsy. The same types of lithotripsy can be used during a percutaneous nephrolithotomy by way of a nephroscope inserted through the skin into the kidney pelvis.

Lithotripsy is a procedure for eliminating calculi from the urinary tract with the use of hydraulic, or high-energy, shock waves or a pulsed laser. Specific lithotripsy techniques include percutaneous ultrasonic lithotripsy, electrohydraulic lithotripsy, laser lithotripsy, and extracorporeal shock wave lithotripsy. Extracorporeal shock wave lithotripsy and laser lithotripsy are the most common.

- In *laser lithotripsy* probes are used to fragment lower ureteral and large bladder stones.
- In *extracorporeal shock wave lithotripsy,* a noninvasive
  procedure, the patient is anesthetized (spinal or general)
  and placed in a water bath. Fluoroscopy or ultrasound is
  used to focus the lithotriptor on the affected kidney, and a
  high-voltage spark generator produces high-energy acoustic
  shock waves that shatter the stone without damaging the
  surrounding tissues. The stone is broken down into fine
  sand, which is excreted into the patient's urine within a few
  days of the procedure.

Hematuria is common after lithotripsy procedures. A self-
retaining ureteral stent is often placed after the procedure to
promote passage of this sand and to prevent obstruction caused by
a buildup of sand in the ureter. The stent is removed 1 to 2 weeks
after lithotripsy. A primary advantage of these techniques compared with open surgery is the decrease in the length of hospitalization and the patient's earlier return to normal activities.

A small group of select patients may need open surgical procedures, such as very obese patients or those with complex abnormalities in the calyces or at the UPJ. The type of open surgery
needed depends on the location of the stone.

- A *nephrolithotomy* is an incision into the kidney to remove
  a stone. A *pyelolithotomy* is an incision into the renal pelvis
  to remove a stone. If the stone is located in the ureter, a
  ureterolithotomy is performed. A *cystostomy* may be indicated for bladder calculi. For open surgery on the kidney or
  ureter, a flank incision directly below the diaphragm and
  across the side is usually the preferred surgical approach.

Nutritional Therapy

When an obstructing stone is present, the patient is advised to
drink adequate fluids only to avoid dehydration. Forcing fluids to
assist in flushing a stone through the urinary tract is avoided
because this strategy has not proved effective in "passing" the
stone by way of the urine. In addition, forcing fluids may exacerbate the colic associated with an episode.

A high fluid intake (at least 3000 ml/day) is recommended after
an episode of urolithiasis to produce a urine output of at least
2 L/day and prevent stone formation.

- High urine output prevents supersaturation of minerals (i.e.,
  dilutes the concentration) and flushes them out before they
  have a chance to form a stone.
- Increasing fluid intake is especially important for those who
  live in a dry climate, perform physical exercise, have a

family history of stone formation, or work in an occupation that requires outdoor work that can lead to dehydration.

Dietary intervention may be important in the management of urolithiasis.

- A high level of calcium in the diet, which was previously thought to contribute to kidney stones, may actually lower the risk by reducing the urinary excretion of oxalate, a common factor in many stones.
- Initial nutritional therapy should include limiting oxalate-rich foods, thereby reducing oxalate excretion. Foods high in calcium, oxalate, and purines are presented in Table 46-13, Lewis and others, *Medical-Surgical Nursing,* edition 7, p. 1171.

Nursing Management
Goals
The patient with urinary tract calculi will have relief of pain, no urinary tract obstruction, and an understanding of measures to prevent further recurrence of stones.

See NCP 46-2 for the patient with acute renal lithiasis, Lewis and others, *Medical-Surgical Nursing,* edition 7, pp. 1173 to 1174.

Nursing Diagnoses
- Acute pain
- Impaired urinary elimination
- Ineffective therapeutic regimen management

Nursing Interventions
Preventive measures related to the person who is on bed rest or is relatively immobile for a prolonged time include maintaining an adequate fluid intake, turning the patient every 2 hours, and helping the patient to sit or stand if possible to maximize urinary flow.

Pain management and patient comfort are primary nursing responsibilities when managing a person with an obstructing stone and renal colic.

- All urine voided by the patient should be strained through gauze or a special urine strainer in an effort to detect the stone.
- Ambulation may be encouraged to promote movement of the stone from the upper to lower urinary tract. The patient should not walk unattended when experiencing acute colic, particularly if opioid analgesics are being used.

▼ Patient and Family Teaching
Stone formation can be prevented, and the recurrence rate can be greatly reduced. After the acute phase, it is important for the nurse to teach the patient ways to prevent its recurrence.

- Prevention of stone recurrence always includes adequate fluid intake to produce a urine output of approximately 2 L/day.
- Dietary restriction of oxalate is important for patients who have calcium oxalate stones. Diets that restrict purines may be helpful to patients at risk of developing uric acidstones.
- Follow-up care includes monitoring the patient's compliance with fluid and dietary recommendations.
- Teach the patient the dosage, scheduling, and potential side effects of medications used to reduce the risk of stone formation.
- Selected patients may be taught to self-monitor urinary pH, or they may be asked to measure urinary output.

URINARY TRACT INFECTIONS

Description

Urinary tract infections (UTIs) are the second most common bacterial disease and the most common bacterial infection in women. *Escherichia coli (E. coli)* is the most common pathogen causing a UTI.

- Bacterial counts in the urine of 10^5 colony-forming units per milliliter (CFU/ml) or higher typically indicate a UTI. However, bacterial counts as low as 10^2 to 10^3 CFU/ml in a person with symptoms are also indicative of UTI.
- Fungal and parasitic UTIs are uncommon and are seen most frequently in the patient who is immunosuppressed, has diabetes mellitus (DM), or has taken multiple courses of antibiotics.

Classification

UTIs may be broadly classified as upper and lower UTIs according to their location within the urinary system. Infection of the upper urinary tract (involving the renal parenchyma, pelvis, and ureters) typically causes fever, chills, and flank pain, whereas a UTI confined to the lower urinary tract does not usually have systemic manifestations.

Specific terms are used to further delineate UTI location. For example, *pyelonephritis* implies infection of the renal parenchyma and collecting system, *cystitis* indicates inflammation of the bladder wall, and *urethritis* is inflammation of the urethra. *Urosepsis* is a UTI that has spread into the systemic circulation and is a life-threatening condition requiring emergency treatment.

Classifying a UTI as uncomplicated or complicated is also useful.

- *Uncomplicated infections* are those that occur in an otherwise normal urinary tract.
- *Complicated infections* include the coexisting presence of obstruction, stones, or catheters; the existence of DM or neurologic diseases; or a recurrent infection. The individual with a complicated infection is at an increased risk of kidney damage.
- A *recurrent UTI* is reinfection caused by a second pathogen in a person who experienced a previous infection that was successfully eradicated. If a recurrent UTI occurs because the original infection is not adequately eradicated, it is classified as unresolved bacteriuria or bacterial persistence.

Pathophysiology

The urinary tract above the urethra is normally sterile, and organisms that cause UTIs are usually introduced by way of the ascending route from the urethra. Other less common routes are through the bloodstream or lymphatic system. Most infections are due to gram-negative aerobic bacilli normally found in the gastrointestinal (GI) tract.

- A common factor contributing to ascending infection is urologic instrumentation (e.g., catheterization, cystoscopy). Instrumentation allows bacteria that are normally present at the opening of the urethra to enter the urethra or bladder.
- Sexual intercourse promotes "milking" of bacteria from the vagina and perineum and may cause minor urethral trauma that predisposes women to UTIs.
- Rarely do UTIs result from a hematogenous route, where blood-borne bacteria secondarily invade the kidneys, ureters, or bladder from elsewhere in the body.

An important source of UTIs is hospital-acquired or *nosocomial* infection. The cause is often *E. coli* and, less frequently, *Pseudomonas* organisms. Catheter-acquired UTIs are the most common nosocomial infections and are caused by development of bacterial biofilms that are found on the inner surface of the catheter. Table 82 lists predisposing factors for UTIs.

Clinical Manifestations

Lower urinary tract symptoms are seen in UTIs of both the upper and lower urinary tracts.

- Symptoms include dysuria, frequent urination (more often than every 2 hours), urgency, and suprapubic discomfort or pressure.

- The urine may contain grossly visible blood (hematuria) or sediment, giving it a cloudy appearance.
- Flank pain, chills, and the presence of a fever indicate an infection involving the upper urinary tract (pyelonephritis).

Older adults tend to experience nonlocalized abdominal discomfort rather than dysuria and suprapubic pain. Patients over 80 years old may experience a slight decline in temperature.

Table 82	Predisposing Factors to Urinary Tract Infections

Factors Increasing Urinary Stasis
- Intrinsic obstruction (stone, tumor of urinary tract, urethral stricture, BPH)
- Extrinsic obstruction (tumor, fibrosis compressing urinary tract)
- Urinary retention (including neurogenic bladder and low bladder wall compliance)
- Renal impairment

Foreign Bodies
- Urinary tract calculi
- Catheters (indwelling and intermittent, external condom catheter, ureteral stent, nephrostomy tube)
- Urinary tract instrumentation (cystoscopy, urodynamics)

Anatomic Factors
- Congenital defects leading to obstruction or urinary stasis
- Fistula (abnormal opening) exposing urinary stream to skin, vagina, or fecal stream
- Shorter female urethra and colonization from normal vaginal flora
- Obesity

Factors Compromising Immune Response
- Aging
- Human immunodeficiency virus
- Diabetes mellitus

Functional Disorders
- Constipation
- Voiding dysfunction with detrusor sphincter dyssynergia

Other Factors
- Pregnancy
- Hypoestrogenic state
- Multiple sex partners (women)
- Use of spermicidal agents or contraceptive diaphragm (women)
- Poor personal hygiene

BPH, Benign prostatic hyperplasia.

Multiple factors may produce lower urinary tract symptoms similar to a UTI. For example, patients with bladder tumors or those receiving intravesical chemotherapy or pelvic radiation usually experience urinary frequency, urgency, and dysuria. Interstitial cystitis also produces urinary symptoms that are sometimes confused with a UTI (see Interstitial Cystitis/Painful Bladder Syndrome, p. 359).

Diagnostic Studies

- Dipstick urinalysis is obtained initially to identify presence of nitrites (indicating bacteriuria), white blood cells (WBCs), and leukocyte esterase (an enzyme present in WBCs indicating pyuria).
- After confirmation of bacteriuria and pyuria, a urine culture with sensitivity may be obtained.
- An intravenous pyelogram (IVP) or computed tomography (CT) scan may be obtained when obstruction of the urinary system is suspected.
- Renal ultrasound is the preferred urinary tract imaging technique because it is noninvasive, easy to perform, and relatively inexpensive.

Collaborative Care

Drug Therapy

Once a UTI has been diagnosed, appropriate antimicrobial therapy is initiated. Uncomplicated cystitis can be treated by a short-term course of antibiotics, typically for 1 to 3 days. In contrast, complicated UTIs require longer term treatment, lasting 7 to 14 days or even longer.

- Trimethoprim-sulfamethoxazole (TMP-SMX) or nitrofurantoin (Macrodantin) is often used to empirically treat uncomplicated or initial UTIs.
- Fluoroquinolones (e.g., ciprofloxacin [Cipro], levofloxacin [Levaquin], gatifloxacin [Tequin]) may be used to treat complicated UTIs.
- A number of over-the-counter (OTC) or prescription drugs may be used in combination with antibiotic agents to relieve the discomfort associated with a UTI. Phenazopyridine (Pyridium) provides a soothing effect on the urinary tract mucosa. It also stains the urine a reddish orange that may be mistaken for blood in the urine and that may permanently stain underclothing.
- Combination agents, such as Urised (methenamine, phenylsalicylate, atropine, hyoscyamine), may also be used to relieve symptoms. Patients taking these agents should be advised of their ability to tint the urine blue or green.

Prophylactic or suppressive antibiotics are sometimes administered to patients who experience repeated UTIs. Although suppressive therapy is often effective on a short-term basis, this strategy is limited because of the risk of antibiotic resistance.

Nursing Management
Goals
The patient with a UTI will have relief from bothersome lower urinary tract symptoms, prevention of upper urinary tract involvement, and prevention of recurrence.

See NCP 46-1 for the patient with a UTI, Lewis and others, *Medical-Surgical Nursing,* edition 7, p. 1160.

Nursing Diagnoses/Collaborative Problem
- Impaired urinary elimination
- Ineffective therapeutic regimen management
- Potential complication: urosepsis

Nursing Interventions
Health promotion activities, especially for individuals who are at increased risk for UTI, include teaching preventive measures such as (1) emptying the bladder regularly and completely, (2) evacuating the bowel regularly, (3) wiping the perineal area from front to back after urination and defecation, and (4) drinking an adequate amount of liquid each day.

- Daily intake of cranberry or lingonberry juice or cranberry essence tablets may reduce the risk of certain UTIs. In addition, it is important to teach the patient to seek early treatment if symptoms occur.
- The nurse can play a major role in the prevention of nosocomial infections with avoidance of unnecessary catheterization and early removal of indwelling catheters.

In most cases, acute intervention for a patient with a UTI includes adequate fluid intake. Fluid intake dilutes urine, decreasing bladder irritation, and helps flush out bacteria before they have a chance to colonize in the bladder. Caffeine, alcohol, citrus juices, chocolate, and highly spiced foods or beverages should be avoided because they are potential bladder irritants.

- Application of local heat to the suprapubic area or lower back may relieve the discomfort associated with a UTI. A warm shower or sitting in a tub of warm water filled above the waist can also be effective in providing temporary relief.

▼ Patient and Family Teaching
The patient should be instructed about the prescribed drug therapy including side effects. The nurse should emphasize the importance of taking the full course of antibiotics.

- The patient should be instructed to watch for any changes in the color or consistency of the urine and a decrease in or cessation of symptoms as a sign of therapy effectiveness.
- The patient should be counseled that persistence of bothersome lower urinary tract symptoms beyond the antibiotic treatment course or the onset of flank pain or fever should be reported promptly to the health care provider.
- It is the nurse's responsibility to teach the patient about the need for ongoing home care. This includes taking antimicrobial medication as ordered, maintaining adequate daily fluid intake, regular voiding (approximately every 2 to 4 hours), urinating after intercourse, and temporarily discontinuing the use of a diaphragm (if used).

VAGINAL, CERVICAL, AND VULVAR INFECTIONS

Definition
Infection and inflammation of the vagina, cervix, and vulva tend to occur when the natural defenses of the acid vaginal secretions (maintained by sufficient estrogen levels) and the presence of *Lactobacillus* are disrupted. A woman's resistance may also be decreased as a result of aging, poor nutrition, and the use of drugs (e.g., antibiotics, hormones) that alter the bacterial flora or mucosa.

Pathophysiology
Organisms gain entrance to these areas through contaminated hands, clothing, and douche tips and during intercourse, surgery, and childbirth. Table 83 presents the etiology, clinical manifestations, diagnostic methods, and collaborative care of common infections of the lower genital tract.

- Most lower genital tract infections are related to sexual intercourse. Vulvar infections, such as herpes and genital warts, can be sexually transmitted when no lesions are present (see Herpes, Genital, p. 306, and Warts, Genital, p. 686).
- Oral contraceptives, antibiotics, and corticosteroids may produce changes in the vagina pH and trigger an overgrowth of the organisms present. For example, *Candida albicans* may be present in small numbers in the vagina. An overgrowth of this organism causes vulvovaginitis.

Table 83   Infections of the Lower Genital Tract

Infection/Etiology	Clinical Manifestations and Diagnostic Methods	Drug Therapy
Vulvovaginal candidiasis (VVC) (monilial vaginitis) *Candida albicans*	Commonly found in mouth, GI tract, and vagina; pruritus; thick, white curdy discharge; KOH microscopic examination—pseudohyphae; pH <4.5	Intravaginal agents (cream or suppository): miconazole (Monistat), clotrimazole (Mycelex), butoconazole (Femstat), mycostatin (Nystatin), tioconazole (Vagistat), or terconazole (Terazol) Oral agent: fluconazole (Diflucan)
Trichomoniasis *Trichomonas vaginalis* (protozoa)	Sexually transmitted; pruritus; frothy greenish or gray discharge; hemorrhagic spots on cervix or vaginal walls; saline microscopic examination of vaginal secretions—swimming trichomonads; pH >4.5	metronidazole (Flagyl) orally for patient and partner
Bacterial vaginosis *Gardnerella vaginalis* *Corynebacterium vaginale*	Sexually transmitted; watery discharge with fishy odor; may or may not have other symptoms; saline microscopic examination—epithelial cells; pH >4.5	metronidazole (Flagyl) or clindamycin (Cleocin) orally or intravaginally; examine and treat partner

Cervicitis
Chlamydia trachomatis
Neisseria gonorrhoeae
Staphylococcus aureus

Sexually transmitted; mucopurulent discharge with postcoital spotting from cervical inflammation; culture for chlamydia and gonorrhea

Recommended regimens for chlamydia: azithromycin (Zithromax) or doxycycline; for gonorrhea: cefixime (Suprax), ceftriaxone (Rocephin), ciprofloxacin (Cipro), ofloxacin (Floxin), or levofloxacin (Levaquin) in addition to azithromycin or doxycycline if chlamydia has not been ruled out

Severe recurrent vaginitis
Candida albicans (most often)

May be indication of HIV infection; all women who are unresponsive to first-line treatment should be counseled and offered HIV testing

Drug appropriate to opportunistic organism

GI, Gastrointestinal; *HIV*, human immunodeficiency virus.

Clinical Manifestations

- Abnormal vaginal discharge and reddened vulvar lesions are common.
- In addition to a thick, white, curdy discharge, women with vulvovaginal candidiasis (VVC) often experience intense itching and dysuria.
- The hallmark of bacterial vaginosis is the fishy odor of the discharge.
- Older women may develop gynecologic problems, such as lichen sclerosis, a condition associated with intense itching. The lesions are white initially, although scratching produces changes in the appearance.

Diagnostic Studies

Genital Problems

- History, physical examination, and sexual history need to be obtained.
- Ulcerative lesions need to be cultured for herpes.
- Dark-field microscopy may be used to diagnose syphilis from tissue scrapings of ulcerative lesions.
- Vulvar dystrophies are examined by colposcope, and biopsy specimens are taken for diagnosis.

Vaginal Discharge Problems

- Microscopy and culture of vaginal discharge are done.
- Most common vaginal conditions (bacterial vaginosis, VVC, trichomoniasis) are diagnosed by a wet mount.
- For cervicitis, endocervical cultures are obtained for chlamydia and gonorrhea. If purulent discharge is observed coming from the cervix, endocervical cells may be taken to conduct a Gram stain.

Collaborative Care

Antibiotics taken as directed will cure bacterial infections. Antifungal preparations (in oral or cream preparations) are indicated for VVC. Women with vaginal conditions or cervical infection should abstain from intercourse for at least 1 week. Douching should be avoided, because it disrupts the normal protective mechanisms within the vagina. Sexual partners must be evaluated and treated if the patient is diagnosed with trichomoniasis, chlamydia, gonorrhea, syphilis, or human immunodeficiency virus (HIV).

Drug therapy for vulvar dystrophies is symptomatic because a cure is not available. Treatment involves controlling the itching and hence the scratching. Interrupting the "itch-scratch cycle" prevents further secondary damage to the skin.

Nursing Management

Nurses have the opportunity to educate women about common genital conditions and how women can reduce their risks. Recognizing symptoms that indicate a problem helps women seek care in a timely manner. Matters involving genitals or sexual intercourse are frequently difficult for people to discuss. The nurse's nonjudgmental attitude makes women feel more comfortable and empowers them to ask questions seeking accurate information.

- When a woman is diagnosed with a genital condition, the nurse should ensure that she fully understands the directions for treatment. Taking the full course of medication is especially important to decrease the chance of relapse. Because genitals are such a private area, use of graphs and models is especially helpful for patient teaching.
- When a woman is using a vaginal medication such as an antifungal cream for the first time, showing her the applicator and how to fill it is important. The woman should be taught where and how the applicator should be inserted by using visual aids or models.

VALVULAR HEART DISEASE

Description

Valvular heart disease is defined according to the affected valve or valves (mitral, aortic, tricuspid, pulmonary) and the type of functional alteration *(stenosis* or *regurgitation).*

- The pressure on either side of an open valve is normally equal. However, in a stenotic valve the valve orifice is restricted, impeding the forward flow of blood and creating a pressure gradient difference across an open valve. The degree of stenosis (constriction or narrowing) is reflected in the pressure gradient differences (i.e., the higher the gradient, the greater the stenosis).
- In regurgitation (also called *valvular incompetence* or *insufficiency)* incomplete closure of valve leaflets results in a backward flow of blood.

Valvular disorders occur in children and adolescents primarily from congenital conditions such as tricuspid atresia, pulmonary stenosis, and aortic stenosis. Aortic stenosis and mitral regurgitation are the most common disorders in older adults. New causes of valve disease include disorders related to acquired immunodeficiency syndrome (AIDS) and the use of some antiparkinson drugs (e.g., pergolide [Permax]).

Clinical manifestations of the valve disorders are presented in (Table 84).

Mitral Valve Stenosis

Pathophysiology. The majority of adult cases of mitral stenosis result from rheumatic heart disease. Less common causes include congenital mitral stenosis, rheumatoid arthritis, and systemic lupus erythematosus (SLE).

- Rheumatic endocarditis causes scarring of valve leaflets and chordae tendineae. Contractures develop with adhesions between the commissures (junctional areas) of the two leaflets.
- The stenotic mitral valve assumes a funnel shape because of the thickening and shortening of the structures of the mitral valve. Flow obstruction increases left atrial pressure and volume, resulting in increased pressure in the pulmonary vasculature and eventually the right ventricle.

Clinical Manifestations. Dyspnea, sometimes accompanied by hemoptysis, is the primary symptom of mitral stenosis because of reduced lung compliance. Other clinical manifestations are identified in Table 84.

Mitral Valve Regurgitation

Pathophysiology

- Mitral valve function depends on the integrity of mitral leaflets, chordae tendineae, papillary muscles, left atrium (LA), and left ventricle (LV). Any defect in any of these structures can result in regurgitation. Myocardial infarction with left ventricular failure increases the risk for rupture of the chordae tendineae and acute mitral regurgitation (MR).
- Most cases of MR are caused by myocardial infarction, chronic rheumatic heart disease, mitral valve prolapse, ischemic papillary muscle dysfunction, and infectious endocarditis.
- MR allows blood to flow backward from the LV to the LA because of incomplete valve closure during systole. Both chambers of the left side of the heart work harder to preserve an adequate cardiac output (CO).
- In chronic MR, the volume overload results in atrial enlargement, ventricular dilation, and eventual ventricular hypertrophy.
- In acute MR, abrupt dilation of the LA or LV does not occur. Without dilation to accommodate regurgitant volume, the sudden increase in pressure and volume is transmitted to the pulmonary bed, resulting in pulmonary edema and shock.

Table 84 Clinical Manifestations of Valvular Heart Diseases

Valvular Disorder	Clinical Manifestations
Mitral valve stenosis	Dyspnea on exertion, hemoptysis; fatigue; palpitations; loud, accentuated S_1; low-pitched, rumbling diastolic murmur; atrial fibrillation on ECG
Mitral valve regurgitation	Acute—generally poorly tolerated with fulminating pulmonary edema and shock developing rapidly; new systolic murmur Chronic—weakness, fatigue, exertional dyspnea, palpitations; an S_3 gallop, holosystolic or pansystolic murmur
Mitral valve prolapse	Palpitations, dyspnea, chest pain, activity intolerance, syncope; mid-systolic click, late or holosystolic murmur
Aortic valve stenosis	Angina, syncope, dyspnea on exertion, heart failure, normal or soft S_1, diminished or absent S_2, systolic crescendo-decrescendo murmur; prominent S_4
Aortic valve regurgitation	Acute—abrupt onset of profound dyspnea, orthopnea, PND, chest pain, left ventricular failure and shock Chronic—fatigue, exertional dyspnea, orthopnea, PND, water-hammer pulse; heaving precordial impulse; diminished or absent S_1, S_3, or S_4; soft decrescendo high-pitched diastolic murmur, Austin Flint murmur, systolic ejection click
Tricuspid stenosis and pulmonic stenosis	Tricuspid—peripheral edema, ascites, hepatomegaly; diastolic low-pitched, decrescendo murmur with increased intensity during inspiration Pulmonic—fatigue, loud mid-systolic murmur

ECG, Electrocardiogram; *PND,* paroxysmal nocturnal dyspnea.

Clinical Manifestations. The clinical picture in acute mitral regurgitation is that of pulmonary edema and shock. Patients will have thready, peripheral pulses and cool, clammy extremities. A new systolic murmur may be obscured by low CO.

Patients with chronic mitral regurgitation may remain asymptomatic for many years until the development of some degree of left ventricular failure. Symptoms are identified in Table 84.

Mitral Valve Prolapse

Pathophysiology. Mitral valve prolapse (MVP) is a structural abnormality of the mitral valve leaflets and papillary muscles or chordae that allows the leaflets to prolapse, or buckle, back into the left atrium during systole. It is the most common form of valvular heart disease in the United States.

- Etiology of MVP is unknown but is related to diverse pathogenic mechanisms of the mitral valve apparatus.
- MVP is usually benign, but serious complications can occur, including mitral regurgitation, infective endocarditis, sudden cardiac death, and cerebral ischemia.
- There is an increased familial incidence in some patients resulting from a connective tissue defect affecting only the valve, or as part of Marfan syndrome or other hereditary conditions that influence the structure of collagen in the body.

Clinical Manifestations. MVP encompasses a broad spectrum of severity. Most patients are asymptomatic and remain so for their entire lives. Clinical manifestations may include those identified in Table 84.

- Patients may or may not have chest pain. If episodes of chest pain occur, they tend to occur in clusters, especially during periods of emotional stress. Chest pain may occasionally be accompanied by dyspnea, palpitations, and syncope.

Aortic Valve Stenosis

Pathophysiology. Congenitally abnormal stenotic aortic valves are generally discovered in childhood, adolescence, or young adulthood. In older patients, aortic stenosis is a result of rheumatic fever or senile fibrocalcific degeneration that may have an etiology similar to coronary artery disease.

- In rheumatic valvular disease, the valve leaflets are stiff and retracted, and mitral valve disease accompanies the aortic stenosis. Isolated aortic valve stenosis is almost always non-rheumatic in orgin.
- Aortic stenosis causes obstruction of flow from the left ventricle to the aorta during systole. The effect is left ventricular hypertrophy and increased myocardial oxygen consumption because of the increased myocardial mass.

- As the disease progresses and compensatory mechanisms fail, reduced CO leads to pulmonary hypertension and heart failure.

Clinical Manifestations. Symptoms of aortic stenosis develop when the valve orifice becomes about one third of its normal size and reflect left ventricular failure. Common symptoms are presented in Table 84. Prognosis is poor for a patient whose valve obstruction is not relieved by valve repair or replacement.

Aortic Valve Regurgitation

Pathophysiology. Aortic valve regurgitation may be the result of primary disease of the aortic valve leaflets, the aortic root, or both.

- Acute aortic regurgitation is caused by infective endocarditis, trauma, or aortic dissection and constitutes a life-threatening emergency.
- Chronic aortic regurgitation is generally the result of rheumatic heart disease, a congenital bicuspid aortic valve, syphilis, or chronic arthritic conditions such as ankylosing spondylitis or reactive arthritis.
- The basic physiologic consequence of aortic regurgitation is retrograde blood flow from the ascending aorta into the LV, resulting in volume overload.
- Myocardial contractility eventually declines, and blood volumes increase in the LA and pulmonary vasculature. Ultimately, pulmonary hypertension and right ventricular failure develop.

Clinical Manifestations. Clinical manifestations of acute and chronic aortic valve regurgitation are presented in Table 84.

Tricuspid and Pulmonic Valve Disease

Diseases of the tricuspid and pulmonic valves are uncommon, with stenosis occurring more frequently than regurgitation. Tricuspid stenosis and pulmonic stenosis both result in the backward flow of blood to the right atrium and right ventricle, respectively. Tricuspid stenosis results in right atrial enlargement and elevated systemic venous pressures. Pulmonic stenosis results in right ventricular hypertension and hypertrophy. Table 84 presents clinical manifestations of these valve diseases.

Diagnostic Studies: Valvular Heart Disease

- Chest x-ray reveals heart size, alterations in pulmonary circulation, and valve calcification.
- Electrocardiogram (ECG) shows variations in heart rate (HR), rhythm, and possible ischemia or chamber enlargement.
- Echocardiogram provides information on valve structure and function and on chamber enlargement.

- Cardiac catheterization detects chamber pressure changes and pressure gradients across the valves.

Collaborative Care: Valvular Heart Disease

An important aspect of conservative therapy is the prevention of recurrent rheumatic fever and infective endocarditis. Treatment of valvular heart disease depends on the valve involved and the severity of disease. It focuses on preventing exacerbations of heart failure, acute pulmonary edema, thromboembolism, and recurrent endocarditis. If manifestations of heart failure (HF) develop, vasodilators, positive inotropes, β-adrenergic blockers, diuretics, and a low-sodium diet are recommended.

- Anticoagulant therapy is used to prevent and treat systemic or pulmonary embolization, and it is also used as a prophylactic measure in patients with atrial fibrillation.
- Dysrhythmias, especially atrial dysrhythmias, are common with valvular heart disease and are treated with digitalis, antidysrhythmic drugs, or electrical cardioversion. β-Adrenergic blockers may be used to slow the ventricular rate in patients with atrial fibrillation.

An alternative treatment for some patients with valvular heart disease is the *percutaneous transluminal balloon valvuloplasty* (PTBV) procedure. Balloon valvuloplasty has been used for pulmonic, aortic, and mitral stenosis. The procedure, performed in the cardiac catheterization laboratory, involves threading a balloon-tipped catheter from the femoral artery to the stenotic valve so that the balloon may be inflated in an attempt to separate valve leaflets.

- The PTBV procedure is generally indicated for older adult patients and patients who are poor surgical candidates. PTBV has fewer complications than valve replacement.

Surgical Therapy

The type of surgery used for a particular patient depends on the valves involved, valvular pathologic conditions, the severity of the disease, and the patient's clinical condition.

- Valve repair is typically the surgical procedure of choice. It is often used in mitral or tricuspid valvular heart disease and has a lower operative mortality rate than replacement.
- Mitral *commissurotomy* (valvulotomy) is the procedure of choice for patients with pure mitral stenosis. The open method of commissurotomy (which has largely replaced the older, less precise closed method) requires the use of cardiopulmonary bypass, removal of thrombi from the atrium, excision of the left atrial appendage, commissure incision, and, as indicated, separation of fused chordae, splitting of

underlying papillary muscle, and debriding the valve of calcification.

- Open surgical *valvuloplasty* involves repairing the valve or suturing the torn leaflets, chordae tendineae, and papillary muscles. It is primarily performed to treat mitral regurgitation or tricuspid regurgitation. Valve repair avoids the risks of replacement but may not establish total valve competence.

- Further repair or reconstruction of the valve may be necessary and can be achieved by *annuloplasty,* a procedure also used in cases of mitral or tricuspid regurgitation. Annuloplasty entails reconstruction of valve leaflets and the annulus, with or without the aid of prosthetic rings (e.g., Carpentier ring).

Prosthetic Valves. Valvular replacement may be required for mitral, aortic, tricuspid, and occasionally, pulmonic valvular disease. The surgical treatment of choice for combined aortic stenosis and aortic regurgitation is valvular replacement.

- The two categories of prosthetic valves are *mechanical* and *biologic (tissue) valves.* Mechanical valves are made of combinations of metal alloys, Pyrolite carbon, and Dacron. Biologic valves are constructed from bovine, porcine, and human cardiac tissue. Mechanical prosthetic valves are more durable and last longer than biologic tissue valves but have an increased risk of thromboembolism, which necessitates the use of long-term anticoagulant therapy. Biologic valves offer the patient freedom from anticoagulant therapy as a result of their low thrombogenicity. However, their durability is limited by the tendency for early calcification, tissue degeneration, and stiffening of leaflets.

- Long-term anticoagulation is recommended for all patients with mechanical prostheses and for patients with biologic tissue valves who have atrial fibrillation. Some patients with biologic tissue valves or annuloplasty with prosthetic rings may require anticoagulation during the first few months after surgery.

- The choice of a valvular prosthesis depends on many factors. For example, if a patient cannot take anticoagulant therapy (e.g., women of childbearing age), a biologic valve may be considered. A mechanical valve may be considered for a younger patient because it is more durable and lasts longer. For patients older than 65 years, the importance of durability is less of an issue, but the risks of noncompliance or hemorrhage from anticoagulants may be greater.

Nursing Management

Goals

The patient with valvular heart disease will have normal cardiac function, improved activity tolerance, and an understanding of the disease process and preventive measures.

See NCP 37-2 for the patient with valvular heart disease, Lewis and others, *Medical-Surgical Nursing*, edition 7, pp. 884 to 885.

Nursing Diagnoses

- Activity intolerance
- Excess fluid volume
- Decreased cardiac output
- Deficient knowledge

Nursing Interventions

Diagnosing and treating streptococcal infection and providing prophylactic antibiotics for patients with a history of rheumatic fever are critical to prevent acquired rheumatic valvular disease. Patients at risk for endocarditis and any patient with valvular heart disease must also be treated with prophylactic antibiotics.

- The patient must adhere to the recommended therapies. The individual with a history of rheumatic fever, endocarditis, and congenital heart disease should know the symptoms suggestive of valvular heart disease so that early medical treatment may be obtained.

A patient with progressive valvular heart disease may require hospitalization or outpatient care for the management of HF, endocarditis, embolic disease, or dysrhythmias. HF is the most common reason for ongoing medical care.

The role of the nurse is to implement and evaluate the effectiveness of therapeutic management.

- Activities should be designed after considering the patient's limitations. An appropriate exercise plan can increase cardiac tolerance. However, activities that regularly produce fatigue and dyspnea should be restricted.
- The patient should be assisted in planning activities of daily living (ADLs), with an emphasis on conserving energy, setting priorities, and taking planned rest periods.
- Referral to a vocational counselor may be necessary if the patient has a physically or emotionally demanding job.
- Auscultation of the heart should be performed to monitor the effectiveness of digitalis, β-adrenergic blocking agents, and antidysrhythmic drugs.
- The patient who is receiving anticoagulation therapy after surgery for valve replacement must have the international normalized ratio (INR) checked regularly (usually monthly) to assess the adequacy of therapy.

▼ Patient and Family Teaching

- Explain the nature and cause of the disease process to ensure the patient has an adequate knowledge base on which to make decisions.
- Teach the signs and symptoms of HF, infective endocarditis, or bleeding to ensure early reporting and treatment of complications.
- Explain the need to avoid all invasive surgical or diagnostic procedures that may predispose the patient to bacteremia until prophylactic antibiotics are given. Emphasize the importance of notifying the dentist, urologist, and gynecologist of valvular disease so that prophylactic antibiotic treatment can be initiated before procedures.
- Strongly encourage smoking cessation to decrease all cardiovascular risks.
- Discuss prescribed medications, including dosage, purpose, and side effects, to promote safe and accurate self-medication.
- Instruct patient to wear a Medic-Alert bracelet.
- Emphasize that valve surgery is not a cure and that regular follow-up examinations by the health care provider will be required.

V

VARICOSE VEINS

Description

Varicose veins (varicosities) are dilated, tortuous subcutaneous veins most frequently found in the saphenous system. They may be small and innocuous or large and bulging.

- *Primary* varicose veins (idiopathic) are probably caused by congenital weakness of the veins and are more common in women and patients with a strong family history.
- *Secondary* varicosities typically result from a previous deep vein thrombosis or other identifiable obstruction. Secondary varicose veins may also occur in the esophagus as varices, in the anorectal area as hemorrhoids, and as abnormal arteriovenous connections (AV fistulas and malformations).

Pathophysiology

The etiology of varicose veins is unknown. Risk factors include congenital weakness of the vein structure, use of oral contraceptives or hormone replacement therapy, increasing age, obesity, pregnancy, venous obstruction resulting from thrombosis or extrinsic pressure by tumors, or occupations that require prolonged standing. Superficial veins in the lower extremities become dilated and tortuous, with increased venous pressure.

- As the veins enlarge, valves are stretched and become incompetent, allowing venous blood flow to be reversed. As back pressure increases and the calf muscle pump (muscle movement that squeezes venous blood back toward the heart) fails, further venous distention results.
- Increased venous pressure is transmitted to the capillary bed, and edema develops.

Clinical Manifestations

Discomfort from varicose veins varies dramatically among people and tends to be worsened by superficial thrombophlebitis. The most common symptom is an ache or pain after prolonged standing, which is relieved by walking or by elevating the limb. Some patients feel pressure or a cramp-like sensation. Swelling may accompany the discomfort. Nocturnal leg cramps in the calf may occur.

Superficial thrombophlebitis is the most frequent complication of varicose veins and may occur spontaneously or after trauma, surgical procedures, or pregnancy. Uncommonly, rupture of varicose veins may occur because of weakening of the vessel wall and ulceration of the skin.

Diagnostic Studies

- Duplex ultrasound is the most widely used test to diagnose deep varicose veins since it can detect obstruction and reflux in the venous system with considerable accuracy.

Collaborative Care

Treatment is usually not indicated if varicose veins are only a cosmetic problem. If incompetency of the venous system develops, management involves rest with the affected limb elevated, compression stockings, and walking exercise.

Sclerotherapy involves the injection of a substance that obliterates venous telangiectasis (i.e., spider veins) and small superficial varicose veins. Direct intravenous (IV) injection of a sclerosing agent such as hypertonic saline induces inflammation and results in eventual thrombosis of the vein. This procedure can be performed safely in an office setting and causes minimal discomfort. After injection the leg is wrapped with an elastic bandage for 24 to 72 hours to maintain pressure over the vein. Long-term use of compression stockings is advised to help prevent the development of further varicosities.

Newer, noninvasive options for the treatment of isolated, small venous telangiectasis include laser therapy and high-intensity pulse-light therapy. These methods work by using heat or light to injure the vein endothelium and cause vessel sclerosis.

Surgical intervention is indicated for recurrent thrombophlebitis or when chronic venous insufficiency cannot be controlled with conservative therapy. Traditional surgical intervention involves ligation of the entire vein and dissection and removal of it and its incompetent tributaries. Newer techniques include the use of radiofrequency laser and transilluminated power phlebectomy to obliterate the lumen of the targeted vessel. Surgical treatment for varicose veins typically is done as an outpatient procedure.

Nursing Management

To prevent or manage varicose veins, the patient should be instructed to avoid sitting or standing for long periods, maintain ideal body weight, take precautions against injury to extremities, avoid wearing constrictive clothing, and participate in a daily walking program.

After a patient has vein ligation surgery, encourage deep breathing, which helps promote venous return to the right side of the heart. Patients should be told to check the extremities regularly for color, movement, sensation, temperature, presence of edema, and pedal pulses. Bruising and discoloration are considered normal.

- Postoperatively, the extremities are elevated at a 15-degree angle to prevent edema. Compression stockings are applied, removed every 8 hours for short periods, and reapplied.

Long-term management of varicose veins is directed toward improving circulation, relieving discomfort, improving cosmetic appearance, and avoiding complications such as superficial thrombophlebitis and ulceration. Varicose veins can recur in other veins after surgery.

▼ Patient and Family Teaching

- The patient should be taught proper care of the lower extremities, including cleanliness and the use of individually fitted compression stockings. Instruct the patient to put on the stockings while still lying down, just before rising in the morning.
- The importance of periodic positioning of the legs above the heart should be stressed.
- The overweight patient may need assistance with weight reduction.

- The patient whose occupation requires prolonged periods of standing or sitting should be encouraged to change position as frequently as possible.

VENOUS THROMBOSIS

Description

Venous thrombosis is the formation of a thrombus (clot) in association with inflammation of the vein. Venous thrombosis is classified as either superficial thrombophlebitis or deep vein thrombosis (DVT) (Table 85).

- DVT commonly involves the iliac and femoral veins and is more serious because it can result in embolization of thrombi to the lungs. Pulmonary embolism (PE) is a life-threatening condition and, in the best scenario, results in prolonged hospitalization.

Table 85	Comparison of Superficial Thrombophlebitis and Deep Vein Thrombosis
Superficial Thrombophlebitis	**Deep Vein Thrombosis**
Usual Location	
Superficial veins of arms and legs	Deep veins of arms (axillary, subclavian), legs (femoral), and pelvis (iliac, inferior or superior vena cava)
Clinical Findings	
Tenderness, redness, warmth, pain, inflammation and induration along the course of the superficial vein; vein appears as a palpable cord; edema rarely occurs	Tenderness over involved vein to pressure, induration of overlying muscle, venous distention; edema usually occurs; may have mild to moderate pain; deep reddish color to area because of venous congestion; NOTE: some patients may have no obvious physical changes in the affected extremity
Sequelae	
Embolization rarely occurs	Embolization may occur; chronic venous insufficiency may develop

Pathophysiology

Three important factors *(Virchow's triad)* in the etiology of venous thrombosis are venous stasis, damage of the endothelium (inner lining of the vein), and hypercoagulability of the blood. The patient at risk for venous thrombosis usually has predisposing conditions related to these three disorders.

Venous stasis occurs when the valves are dysfunctional or the muscles of the extremities are inactive.

- Venous stasis occurs more frequently in people who are obese, have chronic heart failure or atrial fibrillation, have been on long trips without regular exercise, undergo a prolonged surgical procedure, or are immobile for long periods (e.g., with spinal cord injuries or fractured hips).

Damage of the endothelium of the vein is caused by trauma or external pressure and occurs any time a venipuncture is performed. Damaged endothelium has decreased fibrinolytic properties, which facilitates thrombus development.

- Endothelial damage occurs when patients are receiving prolonged intravenous (IV) therapy (longer than 72 to 96 hours), especially when receiving irritating substances. Other factors include the use of contaminated IV equipment, a fracture that causes damage to blood vessels, diabetes mellitus (DM), blood pooling, burns, and any unusual physical exertion resulting in muscle strain.

Hypercoagulability of the blood occurs in many hematologic disorders, particularly polycythemia and severe anemias, as well as sepsis and various malignancies.

- Women who smoke, use oral contraceptives or hormone replacement therapy, are older than age 35 years, and have a family history of DVT are at an extremely high risk to develop a thrombotic event.

Thrombus formation results from the adherence of red blood cells (RBCs), white blood cells (WBCs), platelets, and fibrin. A frequent site of thrombus formation is the valve cusps of veins.

- As the thrombus enlarges, blood cells and fibrin collect behind it, producing a larger clot with a "tail" that eventually occludes the lumen of the vein.
- If a thrombus only partially occludes the vein, the thrombus becomes covered by endothelial cells and the thrombotic process stops.
- If the thrombus does not become detached, it undergoes lysis or becomes firmly organized and adherent within 5 to 7 days.
- The organized thrombi may detach and result in emboli. These emboli generally flow through the venous circulation

to the heart and lodge in the pulmonary circulation, becoming PEs.

Clinical Manifestations

- The patient with *superficial thrombophlebitis* may have a palpable, firm, subcutaneous cordlike vein with the surrounding area tender to the touch, reddened, and warm. A mild systemic temperature elevation and leukocytosis may be present. Edema of the extremity may occur. The most common cause of superficial thrombophlebitis in the upper exremities is vein trauma caused by cannulation of a vein or IV therapy. Superficial thrombophlebitis in the lower extremities is related to trauma to varicose veins.

- The patient with DVT may have no symptoms or may have unilateral leg edema, pain, warm skin, erythema, and a temperature above 100.4° F (38° C). If the calf is involved, tenderness may be present on palpation. *Homans' sign,* pain on dorsiflexion of the foot when the leg is raised, is a classic but unreliable sign because it is not specific for DVT. If the inferior vena cava is involved, the lower extremities may be edematous and cyanotic.

Complications

The most serious complications of DVT are PE, chronic venous insufficiency, and phlegmasia cerulea dolens. PE is a life-threatening complication of DVT (see Pulmonary Embolism, p. 517).

- *Chronic venous insufficiency* results from valvular destruction, allowing retrograde flow of venous blood. Persistent edema, increased pigmentation, secondary varicosities, ulceration, and cyanosis of the limb when it is placed in a dependent position may develop in a person with this complication. Signs and symptoms of chronic venous insufficiency often do not develop until several years after DVT.

- *Phlegmasia cerulea dolens* (swollen, blue, painful leg) may develop with severe lower DVT. It causes sudden, massive swelling and intense cyanosis of the extremity. Gangrene occurs as a result of arterial occlusion secondary to venous obstruction.

Diagnostic Studies

- Platelet count, hemoglobin (Hb), hematocrit (Hct), and coagulation tests (bleeding time, prothrombin time [PT], partial thromboplastin time [PTT]) may be altered if underlying blood dyscrasias are present.

- Duplex scanning and venous Doppler evaluation determine location and extent of venous thrombi.
- Venogram (phlebogram) can determine clot location.

Collaborative Care

Management of the patient with superficial thrombophlebitis includes elevation of the affected extremity until the tenderness has subsided.

- Warm, moist heat may be used to relieve pain and treat inflammation.
- Mild oral analgesics such as aspirin or acetaminophen may be used to relieve pain. Aspirin may also be given for its antiplatelet effect. Nonsteroidal antiinflammatory agents, such as ibuprofen (Motrin), have been used to treat the inflammatory process and accompanying pain.
- Anticoagulant therapy is usually not indicated unless the proximal greater saphenous vein or the saphenofemoral junction is involved.

In patients at risk for DVT, various interventions are used to prevent its development.

- Early ambulation and foot and leg exercises for bed-fast patients are the easiest and most cost-effective method to prevent DVT.
- Antiembolism stockings and intermittent compression devices are used to apply pressure to the lower extremities and prevent venous stasis.
- Preventive anticoagulation is used for patients at moderate, high, or very high risk for DVT and PE.

Treatment for DVT involves bed rest, elevation of the extremity, and anticoagulation. Warm compresses may be applied to the affected area.

- Traditionally, strict bed rest with elevation of the affected extremity above the level of the heart has been indicated for patients with DVT until therapeutic levels of anticoagulation are achieved and the edema subsides. However, it has been reported that there were no differences in the development of new PE between patients with DVT or PE receiving anticoagulation therapy who were placed on bed rest versus those who were allowed to walk.
- When the patient is allowed to resume ambulation, elastic compression stockings are recommended. Elastic gradient stockings are recommended for 3 to 6 months to support the vein walls and valves and decrease pain and swelling on ambulation.

- Because hyperhomocystinemia is considered an independent risk factor for DVT, if it is present, patients should be treated with vitamin B_6, cobalamin, and folic acid to reduce homocystine levels. The role of homocystine in arterial endothelial injury and clot promotion is discussed in Coronary Artery Disease, p. 150.
- Anticoagulant therapy is routinely used for DVT. Goals of anticoagulation therapy are to prevent propagation of the clot, development of a new thrombus, and embolization. Agents include vitamin K antagonists (e.g., warfarin [Coumadin]), indirect thrombin inhibitors (e.g., heparin and low-molecular-weight heparins), direct thrombin inhibitors (e.g., hirudin and its derivatives, argatroban [Acova]), and factor Xa inhibitors (e.g., fondaparinux [Arixtra]). Anticoagulation therapy does not dissolve the clot. Lysis of the clot begins spontaneously through the body's intrinsic fibrinolytic system.

Most patients are treated conservatively; a small percentage requires surgical intervention. The primary indication for surgery is to prevent PE. Surgical procedures include venous thrombectomy (rarely performed) and inferior vena cava interruption with devices such as the Greenfield, VenaTech, or TrapEase filters. Venous thrombectomy involves the removal of a DVT clot through an incision in the vein. This procedure is done to prevent PE and chronic venous insufficiency.

Nursing Management
Goals
The patient with venous thrombosis will have relief of pain, decreased edema, no skin ulceration, no complications from anticoagulant therapy, and no evidence of pulmonary emboli.

For the patient with venous thrombosis, see Lewis and others, *Medical-Surgical Nursing*, edition 7, p. 915.

Nursing Diagnoses/Collaborative Problems
- Acute pain
- Ineffective health maintenance
- Risk for impaired skin integrity
- Potential complication: bleeding related to anticoagulant therapy
- Potential complication: pulmonary embolism

Nursing Interventions
Acute care is directed toward the reduction of inflammation and the prevention of emboli formation.

The patient who is receiving anticoagulation therapy should be closely observed for any indications of bleeding, including epistaxis and bleeding gingiva.

- Urine should be assessed daily for gross or microscopic hematuria. A smoky appearance to the urine is sometimes noted if blood is present.
- Particular attention should be paid to the protection of skin areas that may be traumatized. Surgical incisions should be closely observed for bleeding.
- Stools should be tested to determine the presence of occult blood from the gastrointestinal (GI) tract.
- Mental status changes, especially in the older patient, should be assessed as a possible indication of cerebral bleeding.
- PTT, international normalized ratio (INR) for PT, Hb, Hct, and platelet levels should be monitored when the patient is receiving anticoagulant drugs. The nurse should first check the results of clotting studies before administering either heparin or warfarin (Coumadin). The antidote for heparin is protamine sulfate, and vitamin K is used as the antidote for warfarin. These drugs must be immediately available if bleeding occurs. Fresh frozen plasma may be administered to reverse direct thrombin inhibitors or factor Xa inhibitors.

▼ **Patient and Family Teaching**

Discharge teaching should focus on elimination of modifiable risk factors for DVT, the importance of compression stockings and monitoring of laboratory values, medication instructions, and guidelines for follow-up. Modifiable risk factors stress the avoidance of contraceptives for the patient with recurrent thrombophlebitis, the hazards of smoking, the importance of elastic compression stockings, and the need to avoid constrictive girdles or garters.

- Modifiable risk factors include the use of tobacco, use of oral contraceptives or hormone replacement therapy, a sedentary lifestyle, and obesity.
- Exercise programs should be developed with an emphasis on swimming and wading, which are particularly beneficial because of the gentle, even pressure of the water. A balanced program of rest and exercise, along with proper posture and the avoidance of long periods of sitting, improves arterial filling and venous return.
- Dietary considerations for the overweight patient are aimed at limiting caloric intake to achieve and maintain desired weight.
- Review with the patient any medications currently being taken that may interfere with anticoagulant therapy. In addition, the nurse should ask the patient if any herbs are being taken, because they can interfere with anticoagulant therapy.

- Instruct the patient to avoid prolonged standing or sitting in a motionless, leg-dependent position. Frequent knee flexion, ankle rotation, and active walking should be done during long periods of sitting or standing, especially on long trips.
- If the patient is discharged while receiving anticoagulant medication, the patient and family need careful explanations of its dosage, actions, and side effects, as well as the importance of routine blood tests and the need to report symptoms to the health care provider.

WARTS, GENITAL

Description
Genital warts (condylomata acuminata) are caused by many types of the human papillomavirus (HPV). HPV is a highly contagious sexually transmitted disease (STD) seen frequently in young, sexually active adults. Infection with HPV is the most common STD in the United States with an estimated 20 million Americans infected. Most individuals who have HPV do not know they are infected because symptoms are often not present.

- Genital warts are discrete, single, or multiple papillary growths that are white to gray and pink flesh colored.
- They may grow and join together to form large, cauliflower-like masses. Most patients have 1 to 10 lesions.
- In men, the warts may occur on the penis and scrotum, around the anus, or in the urethra.
- In women, the warts may be located on the vulva, vagina, and cervix and in the perianal area.

Most genital warts (papillomavirus [HPV] types 6, 11, 16, and 18) can be prevented by a vaccine (Gardasil) that is given in three doses over a 6-month period with minimal side effects.

A diagnosis is frequently made on the basis of the gross appearance of the lesions. Serologic and cytologic testing can be used to rule out carcinomas or benign neoplasms. The HPV DNA test can determine if women with abnormal Pap test results need further follow-up and can also identify women who are infected with the high-risk HPV strains associated with cervical cancer. HPV cannot be currently confirmed by culture.

The primary goal when treating visible genital warts is the removal of symptomatic warts. Genital warts are difficult to treat and often require multiple office visits with a variety of treatment modalities.

- A common treatment is the use of 80% to 90% trichloro-acetic acid (TCA) applied directly on the wart.
- Podophyllin resin (10% to 25%), a cytotoxic agent, is recommended for small external genital warts.
- Podofilox (Condylox) liquid or gel can be applied by the patient for 3 successive days followed by 4 days of no treatment.
- Imiquimod cream (Aldara), an immune response modifier, can be applied three times per week for up to 16 weeks or until lesions resolve.

If warts do not regress with these therapies, treatments such as cryotherapy with liquid nitrogen, electrocautery, laser therapy, intralesional use of α-interferon, and surgical excision may be indicated.

Because treatment does not destroy the virus, recurrences and reinfection are possible, and careful long-term follow-up care is advised.

Nursing Management: Genital Warts

See Nursing Management: Sexually Transmitted Diseases, p. 564.

W

PART TWO

Treatments and Procedures

Description

Clinical indications for an amputation depend on the underlying disease or trauma. Common indications for amputation include circulatory impairment resulting from a peripheral vascular disorder, traumatic and thermal injuries, malignant tumors, uncontrolled or widespread infection of the extremity (i.e., gas gangrene, osteomyelitis), and congenital disorders. The underlying problem dictates whether the amputation is performed as elective or emergency surgery.

- The goal of amputation surgery is to preserve extremity length and function while removing all infected, pathologic, or ischemic tissue. This improves the possibility of good prosthetic, cosmetic, and functional satisfaction. (See Fig. 63-20 for the levels of amputation of the upper and lower extremities, Lewis and others, *Medical-Surgical Nursing,* edition 7, p. 1659.)

Nursing Management

Most lower limb amputations result from peripheral vascular disease, and most upper limb amputations result from severe trauma. Control of causative illnesses such as peripheral vascular disease, diabetes mellitus (DM), chronic osteomyelitis, and skin ulcers can eliminate or delay the need for amputation.

- Patients with these conditions must be taught to carefully examine the lower extremities daily and report problems, such as change in skin color or temperature, decrease in or absence of sensation, tingling, pain, or the presence of a lesion, to the health care provider.

The nurse must recognize the tremendous psychologic and social implications of an amputation for the patient.

- The disruption in body image caused by an amputation often causes a patient to go through psychologic stages similar to the grieving process. Allowing the patient and the family to go through the grieving process and recognizing it as a normal consequence of the amputation may do much to aid the patient's and family's acceptance of the amputation.

Preoperative Care

Patients should be warned that they might feel as though the amputated limb is still present after surgery. This phenomenon, termed *phantom limb sensation,* occurs in 80% of amputees and may cause patients grave concern unless they are forewarned. If pain was present in the affected limb preoperatively, the patient may experience phantom limb pain postoperatively. The patient may have feelings of coldness and heaviness or cramping, shooting, burning, or crushing pain.

- As recovery and ambulation progress, phantom limb sensation and pain usually subside, although the pain can become chronic.

Postoperative Care

Prevention and detection of complications are important nursing responsibilities during the postoperative period. Careful monitoring of the patient's vital signs and dressing can alert the nurse to hemorrhage in the operative area. Careful attention to sterile technique during dressing changes reduces the potential for wound infection and subsequent interruption of rehabilitation.

- If an immediate postoperative prosthesis has been applied, the nurse must monitor vital signs carefully, since the surgical site is heavily covered and may not be visible.
- A surgical tourniquet must always be available for emergency use. If hemorrhage occurs, the surgeon should be notified immediately and efforts to control the hemorrhage should begin at once.

Not all patients are candidates for prostheses. It is important that the surgeon discuss ambulation possibilities frankly with the patient and family. The seriously ill or debilitated patient may not have the upper body strength or energy required to use a prosthesis. Mobility with a wheelchair may be the most realistic goal for this type of patient.

Flexion contractures may delay the rehabilitation process. The most common and debilitating contracture is hip flexion. Patients should avoid sitting in a chair for more than 1 hour with hips flexed or having pillows under the surgical extremity.

▼ Patient and Family Teaching

As the patient's overall condition improves, the nurse begins instruction in the principles and techniques of transferring from bed to chair and back.

- Active exercise and conditioning are essential in developing ambulation skills. Active range-of-motion exercises of all joints should be started as soon after surgery as the patient's pain level and medical status permit.
- Crutch walking is started as soon as the patient is physically able. If a patient has immediate postsurgical fitting, orders related to weight bearing must be carefully followed to avoid disruption of the skin flap and delay of the healing process.

| Table 86 | Patient and Family Teaching Guide: After an Amputation | A |

1. Inspect the residual limb daily for signs of skin irritation, especially redness and abrasion. Pay particular attention to areas prone to pressure.
2. Discontinue use of the prosthesis if an irritation develops. Have the area checked before resuming use of the prosthesis.
3. Wash residual limb thoroughly each night with warm water and a bacteriostatic soap. Rinse thoroughly, and dry gently. Expose the residual limb to air for 20 minutes.
4. Do not use any substance such as lotions, alcohol, powders, or oil unless prescribed by the health care provider.
5. Wear only a residual limb sock that is in good condition and supplied by the prosthetist.
6. Change residual limb sock daily. Launder in a mild soap, squeeze, and lay flat to dry.
7. Use prescribed pain management techniques.
8. Perform ROM to all joints daily. Perform general strengthening exercises including the upper extremities daily.
9. Do not elevate the residual limb on a pillow.
10. Lie prone with hip extension for 30 minutes three or four times daily.

ROM, Range of motion.

Before discharge, the patient and family need careful instruction related to residual limb care, ambulation, prevention of contractures, recognition of complications, exercise, and follow-up care. Table 86 outlines patient and family teaching after an amputation.

ARTIFICIAL AIRWAYS: ENDOTRACHEAL TUBES

Description

An artificial airway is created by inserting a tube into the trachea, bypassing upper airway and laryngeal structures. A tube is placed into the trachea through the mouth or nose past the larynx (*endotracheal [ET] intubation*). ET intubation is more common in patients in the intensive care unit (ICU). It can be performed quickly without taking the patient to surgery. ET tubes are illustrated in Fig. 17.

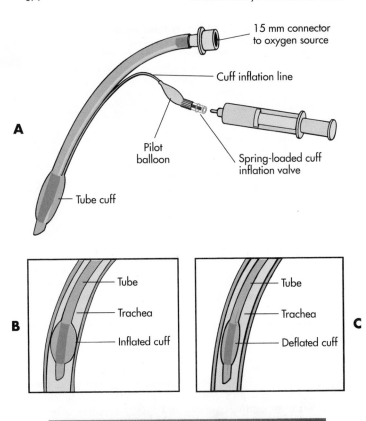

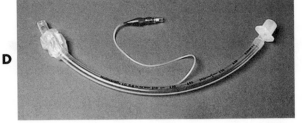

Fig. 17. A, Parts of a cuffed endotracheal tube. **B,** Tube in place with the cuff inflated. **C,** Tube in place with the cuff deflated. **D,** Endotracheal tube.

- Indications for ET intubation include (1) upper airway obstruction, (2) apnea, (3) risk of aspiration, (4) ineffective clearance of secretions, and (5) respiratory distress.

If *oral intubation* is selected, the ET tube is passed through the mouth and vocal cords and into the trachea with the aid of a laryngoscope or bronchoscope.

- Oral ET intubation is the procedure of choice for most emergencies because the airway can be secured rapidly. Compared with the nasal route, a larger-diameter tube can be used for oral intubation. A larger tube provides less airway resistance and easier performance of suctioning and fiberoptic bronchoscopy if needed.
- There are disadvantages of oral ET intubation. It is difficult to place an oral tube if head and neck mobility is limited (e.g., suspected spinal cord injury). Teeth can be chipped or inadvertently dislodged during the procedure. Salivation is increased, and swallowing is difficult. Often a patient will obstruct the ET tube by biting down on it. A bite block or oropharyngeal airway can be used to avoid potential problems. The ET tube and bite block (if used) should be secured (separately) to the face. Mouth care is a challenge.

If *nasal intubation* is selected, insertion is performed by manipulating the tube through the nose, nasopharynx, and vocal cords.

- Nasal ET intubation is sometimes preferred because the tube is more stable than the oral tube and more difficult to dislodge. It can be placed "blindly" without visualizing the larynx; thus it is indicated when head and neck manipulation is risky.
- The nasal tube may be uncomfortable for some because it presses on the septum, whereas others may prefer it because there is no need for a bite block and mouth care is more easily accomplished.
- However, nasal ET tubes are more subject to kinking than oral tubes; the work of breathing is greater because the longer, narrower tube offers more airflow resistance; and suctioning and secretion removal are more difficult. Nasal tubes have been linked with increased incidence of sinus infections, which may be a source of sepsis.
- Before the procedure, the patient and family should be told the reason for ET intubation, the steps that will occur in the procedure, and the patient's role in the procedure (if indicated). It is also important to explain that while intubated, the patient will not be able to speak but that other means of communication will be provided, and

that the patient's hands may be immobilized for safety purposes.

In preparation for ET intubation, all patients need to have a self-inflating *bag-valve-mask* (BVM) (e.g., Ambu bag) available and attached to oxygen, suctioning equipment ready at the bedside, and intravenous access. The procedure for ET intubation is described in Lewis and others, *Medical-Surgical Nursing,* edition 7, p. 1752.

Nursing responsibilities for the patient with an artificial airway include (1) maintaining correct tube placement, (2) maintaining proper cuff inflation, (3) monitoring oxygenation and ventilation, (4) maintaining tube patency, (5) assessing for complications, (6) providing oral care and maintaining skin integrity, and (7) fostering comfort and communication. See NCP 66-1 for the patient on mechanical ventilation, Lewis and others, *Medical-Surgical Nursing,* edition 7, pp. 1754 to 1756.

The nurse monitors tube position by confirming that the exit mark on the tube remains at the point of exit from the body. The nurse observes for the symmetric rise and fall of both sides of the chest and auscultates to confirm bilateral breath sounds.

- An ET tube that is not positioned properly is an emergency. The nurse stays with the patient, maintains the airway, supports ventilation, and secures the appropriate assistance to immediately reposition the tube.
- It may be necessary to ventilate the patient with a BVM device (Ambu bag). If a malpositioned tube is not repositioned, no oxygen will be delivered to the lungs or the entire tidal volume will be delivered to one lung, placing the patient at risk for pneumothorax.

The cuff is an inflatable, pliable sleeve encircling the outer wall of the ET tube. The inflated cuff stabilizes and seals the ET tube within the trachea. It prevents the escape of ventilating gases. However, the cuff can cause tracheal damage.

- To avoid damage, the cuff is inflated with air and the pressure in the cuff is measured and monitored. Normal capillary perfusion is estimated at 30 mm Hg. To ensure adequate tracheal perfusion, cuff pressure should be maintained at 20 to 25 mm Hg.
- The nurse measures and records cuff pressure after intubation and every 8 hours using the minimal occluding volume (MOV) technique.
- The steps in the MOV technique for cuff inflation are as follows: (1) for the mechanically ventilated patient, place a stethoscope over the trachea and inflate the cuff to MOV by

A

adding air until no air leak is heard at peak inspiratory pressure (end of ventilator inspiration); (2) for the spontaneously breathing patient, inflate until no sound is heard after a deep breath or after inhalation with a BVM; (3) use a manometer to verify that cuff pressure is between 20 and 25 mm Hg; and (4) record cuff pressure in the chart.

- If adequate cuff pressure cannot be maintained or larger volumes of air are needed to keep the cuff inflated, the cuff could be leaking or there could be tracheal dilation at the cuff site. In this situation the ET tube should be repositioned or changed and the physician should be notified.

- The nurse should closely monitor the patient with an ET for adequate oxygenation and ventilation by assessing clinical findings, arterial blood gases (ABGs), and other indicators of oxygenation status.

- The patient should be assessed routinely to determine a need for suctioning, but the patient should not be suctioned routinely. Indications for suctioning include visible secretions in the ET tube, sudden onset of respiratory distress with increased respiratory rate and coughing, suspected aspiration of secretions, and auscultation of adventitious breath sounds over the trachea and/or bronchi. See Table 87 for suctioning the patient with an artificial airway.

- The ET tube should be retaped or secured every 24 hours and as needed. If the patient is nasally intubated, the nurse should remove the old tape or ties and clean the skin around the ET tube with saline-soaked gauze or cotton swabs.

- If the patient is orally intubated, the nurse should remove the bite block (if present) and the old tape or ties. The ET tube should be repositioned to the opposite side of the mouth. The nurse replaces the bite block (if appropriate) and reconfirms proper cuff inflation and tube placement.

- If the patient is anxious or uncooperative, it is recommended that two caregivers perform the repositioning procedure to prevent accidental dislodgement. The patient should be monitored for any signs of respiratory distress throughout the procedure.

Oral care, including cleaning of teeth, tongue, and gums, should be performed every 2 to 4 hours and as needed to provide comfort and to prevent injury to the gums and plaque accumulation. If excessive nasal or oral secretions are noted, naso-oropharyngeal suctioning should be performed.

Table 87	Suctioning Procedures for a Patient on a Mechanical Ventilator

General Measures

1. Gather all equipment.
2. Wash hands, and don personal protective equipment.
3. Explain procedure and patient's role in assisting with secretion removal by coughing.
4. Monitor patient's cardiopulmonary status (e.g., vital signs, SpO_2, SvO_2, ECG, level of consciousness) before, during, and after the procedure.
5. Turn on suction, and set vacuum to 100 to 120 mm Hg.
6. Pause ventilator alarms.

Open-Suction Technique

1. Open sterile catheter package using the inside of the package as a sterile field. NOTE: Suction catheter should be no wider than half the diameter of the ET tube (e.g., for a 7-mm ET tube, select a 10-French suction catheter).
2. Fill the sterile solution container with sterile normal saline or water.
3. Don sterile gloves.
4. Pick up sterile suction catheter with dominant hand. Using nondominant hand secure the connecting tube (to suction) to the suction catheter.
5. Check equipment for proper functioning by suctioning a small volume of sterile saline solution from the container (go to step 7).

Closed-Suction Technique

6. Connect the suction tubing to the closed-suction port.
7. Hyperoxygenate the patient for 30 seconds using one of the following methods:
   - Activate the suction hyperoxygenation setting on the ventilator using nondominant hand.
   - Increase FIO_2 to 100%.
   - Disconnect the ventilator tubing from the ET tube, and manually ventilate the patient with 100% O_2 using a BVM device.* Administer five or six breaths over 30 seconds.

Adapted from Chulay M: Suctioning: endotracheal or tracheostomy tube. In Wiegand DL, Carlson KK, editors: *AACN procedure manual for critical care*, ed 5, St Louis, 2005, Mosby.
BVM, Bag-valve-mask; *ECG*, electrocardiogram; *ET*, endotracheal; *FIO₂*, fraction of inspired O_2 concentration, *SpO_2*, functional oxygen saturation; *SvO_2*, venous oxygen saturation.
* Attach a positive end-expiratory pressure (PEEP) valve to the BVM for patients on >5 cm H_2O PEEP.

Table 87	Suctioning Procedures for a Patient on a Mechanical Ventilator—cont'd

8. With suction off, gently and quickly insert the catheter using the dominant hand. When resistance is met, pull back ½ inch.
9. Apply continuous or intermittent suction using the nondominant thumb. Rotate the catheter between the dominant thumb and forefinger, and withdraw the catheter over 10 seconds or less.
10. Hyperoxygenate for 30 seconds as described in step 7.
11. If secretions remain and the patient has tolerated the procedure, two or three suction passes may be performed as described in steps 8 and 9. NOTE: Rinse the suction catheter with sterile saline solution between suctioning passes as needed.
12. Reconnect patient to ventilator (open-suction technique).
13. At the completion of ET tube suctioning, rinse the catheter and connecting tubing with the sterile saline solution.
14. Suction nasal and/or oral pharynx. NOTE: A separate catheter must be used for this step when using the closed-suction technique.
15. Discard the suction catheter, and rinse the connecting tubing with the sterile saline solution (open-suction technique).
16. Reset FIO_2 (if necessary) and ventilator alarms.
17. Reassess patient for signs of effective suctioning.

BIOLOGIC AND TARGETED THERAPY FOR CANCER TREATMENT

Description
Biologic and targeted therapy is used as a type of cancer treatment modality that can be effective alone or in combination with surgery, radiation therapy, and chemotherapy.

- *Biologic therapy,* or *biologic response modifier therapy,* consists of agents that modify the relationship between the host and tumor by altering the biologic response of the host to the tumor cell (Table 88).
- *Targeted therapy* includes drugs that interfere with cancer growth by targeting specific cellular receptors and pathways that are important in tumor growth (see Table 88). Targeted

Table 88 Biologic and Targeted Therapy for Cancer Treatment

Drug	Mechanism of Action	Indications	Side Effects
α-Interferon (Roferon-A, Intron A)	Inhibits DNA and protein synthesis. Suppresses cell proliferation. Increases cytotoxic effects of natural killer (NK) cells	Hairy cell leukemia, chronic myelogenous leukemia, malignant melanoma, renal cell carcinoma, non-Hodgkin's lymphoma, ovarian cancer, multiple myeloma, Kaposi sarcoma, pancreatic carcinoma	Flu-like syndrome (fever, chills, myalgia, headache), cognitive changes, fatigue, nausea, vomiting, anorexia, weight loss
Interleukin-2 (aldesleukin [Proleukin])	Stimulates proliferation of T and B cells. Activates NK cells	Metastatic renal cell cancer, metastatic melanoma	Same as above; capillary leak syndrome resulting in hypotension; bone marrow suppression
levamisole (Ergamisol)	Potentiates monocyte and macrophage function	Duke's stage C colon cancer (given in combination with 5-FU)	Diarrhea, metallic taste, nausea, fever, chills, mouth sores, headache
BCG vaccine (TheraCys)	Induces an immune response which prevents angiogenesis of tumor	In situ bladder cancer	Flu-like syndrome, nausea, vomiting, rash, cough

Tyrosine Kinase Inhibitors		
cetuximab (Erbitux)	Inhibits epidermal growth factor receptor, which is coupled with tyrosine kinase	Colorectal cancer, in combination with radiotherapy for head and neck carcinoma	Rash, dry skin, infusion reactions, interstitial lung disease, fatigue, fever
erlotinib (Tarceva)	Same as above	Non–small cell lung cancer	Rash, diarrhea, interstitial lung disease
gefitinib (Iressa)	Same as above	Non–small cell lung cancer	Same as above
imatinib (Gleevec)	Inhibits Bcr-Abl tyrosine kinase	Chronic myeloid leukemia	Nausea, diarrhea, myalgia, fluid retention
sorafenib (Nexavar)	Inhibits several tyrosine kinases, some of which are involved in angiogenesis	Advanced renal cell carcinoma	Rash, diarrhea, hypertension, redness, pain, swelling, or blisters on hands/feet
Monoclonal Antibody to CD20		
rituximab (Rituxan)	Binds CD20 antigen, causing cytotoxicity	Non-Hodgkin's lymphoma (B cell)	Fever, chills, nausea, headache, angioedema
ibritumomab tiuxetan/ yttrium-90 (Zevalin)	Binds CD20 antigen, causing cytotoxicity and radiation injury	Non-Hodgkin's lymphoma (B cell)	Bone marrow suppression, fatigue, nausea, chills
tositumomab/ tositumomab-^{131}I (Bexxar)	Binds CD20 antigen, causing cytotoxicity and radiation injury	Non-Hodgkin's lymphoma (B cell)	Bone marrow suppression, fever, chills, nausea, headache

Continued

B

Table 88   Biologic and Targeted Therapy for Cancer Treatment—cont'd

Drug	Mechanism of Action	Indications	Side Effects
Angiogenesis Inhibitor bevacizumab (Avastin)	Binds vascular endothelial growth factor, thereby inhibiting angiogenesis	Colorectal cancer	Hypertension, colon bleeding and perforation, impaired wound healing, thromboembolism, diarrhea
Proteasome Inhibitor bortezomib (Velcade)	Inhibits proteasome activity, which function to regulate cell growth	Multiple myeloma	Bone marrow suppression, nausea, vomiting, diarrhea, peripheral neuropathy, fatigue
Monoclonal Antibodies gemtuzumab ozogamicin (Mylotarg)	Binds CD33 antigen (expressed on leukemic cells) to deliver cytotoxic drug into the DNA	Acute myeloid leukemia	Bone marrow suppression, fever, chills, nausea
alemtuzumab (Campath)	Binds CD52 antigen (found on T and B cells, monocytes, NK cells, neutrophils)	Chronic lymphocytic leukemia (B cell)	Bone marrow suppression, chills, fever, vomiting, diarrhea, fatigue
trastuzumab (Herceptin)	Binds human epidermal growth factor receptor 2 (HER-2)	Breast cancer (HER-2 positive)	Cardiotoxicity

therapy anticancer drugs are more selective for specific molecular targets than cytotoxic anticancer drugs and are able to kill cancer cells without damaging normal cells.

Targeted therapies include various tyrosine kinase inhibitors, monoclonal antibodies (MoAb), antiangiogenic agents known as vascular endothelial growth factor (VEGF) receptor inhibitors, and proteasome inhibitors.

- Tyrosine kinase inhibitors block an important enzyme that activates the signaling pathways that regulate cell proliferation and survival.
- Monoclonal antibodies (MoAb) bind to specific target cells and inhibit the internalization of receptor-antibody complexes and signaling pathways. They may also stimulate an immunologic response in the patient.
- Angiogenesis inhibitors work by preventing the mechanisms and pathways necessary for vascularization of tumors.
- Proteasomes are intracellular multienzyme complexes that degrade proteins. Proteasome inhibitors can cause these proteins to accumulate, thus leading to altered cell function.

Indications and side effects of biologic and targeted therapy are included in Table 88.

Nursing Management

The effects of biologic and targeted therapy occur acutely and are dose limited. Critical care nursing may be required for patients who experience capillary leak syndrome and pulmonary edema, but bone marrow depression that occurs with biologic therapy is usually more transient and less severe than that observed with chemotherapy.

- Fatigue associated with biologic therapy can be so severe that it can constitute a dose-limiting toxicity. Because these agents are increasingly combined with cytotoxic therapies, the nurse should monitor the patient for combined and increased therapy-related effects.
- Acetaminophen administered before treatment and every 4 hours after treatment can help relieve the flu-like syndrome associated with biologic agents. Intravenous (IV) meperidine (Demerol) has been used to control the severe chills associated with some biologic agents.

Additional nursing measures include monitoring of vital signs and temperature, planning for periods of rest for the patient, and assisting with activities of daily living (ADLs) and monitoring for adequate oral intake.

CARDIOPULMONARY RESUSCITATION AND BASIC LIFE SUPPORT

Description

Cardiopulmonary resuscitation (CPR) is the process of externally supporting the circulation and respiration of a person who has a cardiac arrest. Resuscitation measures are divided into two components: *basic life support* (BLS) and *advanced cardiac life support* (ACLS). With the invention of the *automatic external defibrillator* (AED), BLS now includes early defibrillation that can be used by trained rescuers.

Basic Life Support

BLS involves the external support of circulation and ventilation for a patient with cardiac or respiratory arrest through CPR. The steps of BLS consist of a series of actions and skills performed by the rescuer or rescuers based on assessment findings.

- The first action performed by the rescuer on finding an adult victim is to assess for responsiveness. If the victim does not respond and the rescuer is alone, the rescuer should activate emergency medical services (EMS), get an AED (if available), return to the victim, and begin CPR. Survival from cardiac arrest is the highest when immediate CPR is provided and defibrillation occurs within 3 to 5 minutes.

- The next step in BLS is to assess the victim's airway to confirm the absence of breathing and to establish a patent airway. The airway is opened by hyperextending the head with the head tilt–chin lift maneuver or, if a cervical spine injury is suspected, a jaw-thrust maneuver.

- If breathing is absent, or the victim is gasping occasionally, ventilation is provided by the rescuer with mouth-to-barrier (recommended) or mouth-to-mouth breathing. Ventilations are given with the victim's nostrils pinched and the rescuer's mouth placed around the victim's mouth to make a tight seal. Face-mask or bag-mask devices can also be used. If airflow is obstructed, the head should be repositioned and ventilation attempted. If the airway obstruction is not relieved, the rescuer should proceed with CPR.

- Health care providers are instructed to assess the pulse in victims who are unresponsive and not breathing. The carotid artery is used to determine the absence of a pulse, and if no pulse is palpated within 10 seconds, chest compression should be administered. *Chest compression* technique consists of serial, rhythmic applications of pressure on the lower half of the sternum with the victim in a supine position on a flat, hard surface.

■ Rescue breathing and chest compression are combined for an effective resuscitation effort of the victim of cardiopulmonary arrest. When the AED or advanced life support team arrives, the victim's rhythm should be assessed. If the victim has a shockable rhythm (e.g., ventricular tachycardia or ventricular fibrillation), one shock should be delivered followed by five cycles of CPR before checking the rhythm. If the rhythm is not a shockable rhythm, CPR should be resumed and the rhythm rechecked every five cycles.

The guidelines for performing BLS with CPR are presented in Tables 89 and 90. Figures 1 through 5 in Appendix A of Lewis and others, *Medical-Surgical Nursing,* edition 7, pp. 1845 to 1849 illustrate CPR techniques.

Table 89	Adult One-Rescuer Cardiopulmonary Resuscitation (CPR)

Assess
1. Determine unresponsiveness:
   ■ Tap or gently shake shoulder.
   ■ Shout "Are you OK?"

Activate Emergency Medical Services (EMS) System*
1. Activate EMS system by calling 911, and get the AED (if available) (outside of hospital).
2. Call a code, and ask for the AED or crash cart (in the hospital).

Airway
1. Position the victim:
   ■ Turn on back (if necessary) using logroll technique.
2. Open the airway using proper technique:
   ■ Head tilt–chin lift maneuver.
   ■ Jaw-thrust maneuver (if cervical spine injury is suspected); if unable to open airway using jaw-thrust maneuver, use head tilt–chin lift maneuver.

From 2005 American Heart Association guidelines for cardiopulmonary resuscitation and emergency cardiovascular care, part 4: adult basic life support, *Circulation* 112:IV-19, 2005.
AED, Automatic external defibrillator; *ACLS,* advanced cardiac life support.
* Rescuers should phone 911 for unresponsive adults before beginning CPR, except in the case of drowning or a likely asphyxiation.

Continued

Table 89	**Adult One-Rescuer Cardiopulmonary Resuscitation (CPR)—cont'd**

Breathing
1. Assess for cessation of breathing:
   LOOK for chest rising and falling.
   LISTEN for air escaping during exhalation.
   FEEL for flow of air.
2. If victim is breathing adequately:
   Continue to protect airway.
   Place victim in recovery position.
3. If victim is unresponsive and gasping or not breathing:
   - Provide two regular breaths each over 1 second.
     Observe chest rise.
     Allow for complete exhalation between breaths.
   - If unable to give two effective breaths:
     Reposition victim to try to open airway
     Look for foreign body, and, if seen, remove.
     Reattempt to ventilate.
   - If ventilation is still unsuccessful, assess circulation.†
   - If adequate spontaneous breathing is restored and signs of circulation are present:
     Maintain open airway.
     Place victim in recovery position.

Circulation
Lay rescuer
1. Begin chest compressions after delivering two initial breaths.
Health care professional
1. Assess for signs of circulation after delivery of the two initial breaths.
2. Feel for carotid pulse (10 seconds).
3. If victim has signs of circulation but is not breathing adequately, continue rescue breathing (1 breath/5 seconds), and recheck circulation every 2 minutes.
4. If there are no signs of circulation, begin chest compressions.

Compressions/Ventilation
1. Compression-ventilation cycle:
   - Compression/ventilation ratio is 30:2.
2. Begin compressions:
   - Get into position for compressions at victim's side (by shoulders).
   - Locate landmark notch (hands in the center of chest, right between the nipples, and two fingers above the xiphoid–sternal notch).
   - Position hands, arms, and shoulders.
   - Elbows are locked, and arms are straight.
   - Rescuer's shoulders are positioned directly over hands.

---

†Lay rescuers are no longer taught a pulse check.

Table 89	Adult One-Rescuer Cardiopulmonary Resuscitation (CPR)—cont'd

Compressions/Ventilation—cont'd
- Begin compressions.
- Compressions should depress victim's sternum approximately 1½ to 2 inches.
- Allow chest to rebound to normal position after each compression.
- Perform compressions hard and fast at the rate of 100/min.
- Maintain correct position at all times.
3. Provide ventilation:
    - Open airway using proper technique.
    - Deliver two slow regular breaths (1 second each) at the end of a cycle of 30 compressions.
    - Return hands to chest.
    - Find proper landmark and hand position.
    - Restart compressions.

Defibrillation
1. If witnessed arrest, use AED as soon as possible.
2. If unwitnessed arrest, deliver five cycles of CPR before using AED.
3. If rhythm is shockable, deliver one shock and then resume CPR for five cycles before rechecking rhythm.
4. If the rhythm is not shockable, resume CPR and recheck rhythm every five cycles.

Continuation of CPR
1. CPR should be continued between rhythm checks and shocks and until ACLS providers arrive or the victim shows signs of improvement.
2. Do not interrupt CPR except in special circumstances.

Table 90	Adult Two-Rescuer Cardiopulmonary Resuscitation (CPR)

Assess/Activate Emergency Medical Services (EMS)*
One rescuer
1. Determine unresponsiveness:
    - Tap or gently shake shoulder.
    - Shout "Are you OK?"

From 2005 American Heart Association guidelines for cardiopulmonary resuscitation and emergency cardiovascular care, part 4: adult basic life support, *Circulation* 112:IV-19, 2005.
AED, Automatic external defibrillator; *ACLS,* advanced cardiac life support.
* Rescuers should phone 911 for unresponsive adults before beginning CPR, except in the case of drowning or a likely asphyxiation.

Continued

| Table 90 | Adult Two-Rescuer Cardiopulmonary Resuscitation (CPR)—cont'd |

Assess/Activate Emergency Medical Services—cont'd

Other rescuer
1. Activate EMS system by calling 911, and get the AED (if available) (outside of hospital).
2. Call a code, and ask for the AED or crash cart (in hospital).

Airway
1. Position the victim:
   Turn on back (if necessary) using logroll technique.
2. Open the airway using proper technique:
   Head tilt–chin lift maneuver.
   Jaw-thrust maneuver (if cervical spine injury is suspected); if unable to open airway using the jaw-thrust maneuver, use the head tilt–chin lift maneuver.

Breathing
1. Assess for cessation of breathing:
   LOOK for chest rising and falling.
   LISTEN for air escaping during exhalation.
   FEEL for flow of air.
2. If victim is breathing adequately:
   Continue to protect airway.
   Place victim in recovery position.
3. If victim is unresponsive and gasping occasionally or not breathing:
   - Provide two regular breaths each over 1 second.
     Observe chest rise.
     Allow for complete exhalation between breaths.
   - If unable to give two effective breaths:
     Reposition victim to try to open airway.
     Look for foreign body, and, if seen, remove.
     Reattempt to ventilate.
   - If ventilation is still unsuccessful, assess circulation.[†]
   - If adequate spontaneous breathing is restored and signs of circulation are present:
     Maintain open airway.
     Place victim in recovery position.

Circulation

Lay rescuers
1. Begin chest compressions after delivering two initial breaths.

Health care professionals
1. Assess for signs of circulation after delivery of the two initial breaths.
2. Feel for carotid pulse (10 seconds).

[†]Lay rescuers are no longer taught a pulse check.

Table 90	**Adult Two-Rescuer Cardiopulmonary Resuscitation (CPR)—cont'd**

Circulation—cont'd

Health care professionals—cont'd

3. If victim has signs of circulation but is not breathing adequately, continue rescue breathing (1 breath/5-6 seconds) and recheck circulation every 2 minutes.
4. If there are no signs of circulation, say "No pulse" and prepare for chest compressions.

Compressions/Ventilation

1. Compression/ventilation ratio is 30:2.

One rescuer/compressor

1. Get into position for compressions at victim's side (by shoulders).
2. Locate landmark notch (hands in the center of chest, right between the nipples, and two fingers above the xiphoid–sternal notch).
3. Position hands, arms, and shoulders:
   - Elbows are locked, and arms are straight.
   - Rescuer's shoulders positioned directly over hands.
4. Begin compressions:
   - Compressions should depress victim's sternum approximately 1½ to 2 inches.
   - Allow chest to rebound to normal position after each compression.
   - Perform compressions hard and fast at the rate of 100/min.
   - Maintain correct position at all times.

Other rescuer/ventilator

1. Get into position at victim's head.
2. Maintain an open airway.
3. Deliver two slow regular breaths (1 second each) at the end of a cycle of 30 compressions.
4. Ensure that chest is rising with each ventilation.
5. Monitor carotid pulse during compressions to verify effectiveness.

Switching

1. Rescuers should change compressor and ventilator roles every 2 minutes to avoid compressor fatigue.
2. Rescuers should exchange positions simultaneously with minimal delay:
   - Ventilator moves to chest.
   - Compressor moves to head.

Defibrillation

1. If witnessed arrest, use AED as soon as possible.
2. If unwitnessed arrest, deliver five cycles of CPR before using AED.

Continued

Table 90	Adult Two-Rescuer Cardiopulmonary Resuscitation (CPR)—cont'd

Defibrillation—cont'd
3. If rhythm is shockable, deliver one shock and then resume CPR for five cycles before rechecking rhythm.
4. If the rhythm is not shockable, resume CPR and recheck rhythm every five cycles.

Continuation of CPR
1. CPR should be continued between rhythm checks and shocks and until ACLS providers arrive or the victim shows signs of improvement.
2. Do not interrupt CPR except in special circumstances.

CASTS

Description
A cast is a temporary circumferential immobilization device. Casting is a common treatment after closed reduction of a fracture. It allows the patient to perform many normal activities of daily living while providing sufficient immobilization to ensure stability.

Types of Cast Material
Cast materials are natural (plaster of Paris), synthetic acrylic, fiberglass free, latex-free polymer, or a hybrid of materials. When plaster of Paris casts are applied, a gauze bandage embedded with plaster is immersed in water and then wrapped and molded around the affected part. The strength of the cast is determined by the number of layers of plaster bandage and the technique of application. Heat is produced during the drying process, and increased edema may result. After the cast is completely dry, it is strong and firm and can withstand stresses.

- The plaster is hard within 15 minutes, so the patient can move around without problems. However, it is not strong enough for weight bearing until it is dry (after about 24 to 48 hours).

Synthetic casting materials are molded to fit the torso or extremity after being activated by submersion in cool or tepid water. Casts made of synthetic materials are being used more than plaster because they are lightweight, are relatively waterproof, and provide for immediate mobilization.

Cast Care

A fresh plaster cast should never be covered with a blanket because air cannot circulate and heat builds up in the cast.

- During the drying period the cast should be kept dry and clean, and direct pressure should be avoided.
- Once the cast is dry, the edges may need to be petaled with tape to protect and smooth the cast edges to avoid skin irritation and prevent plaster crumbs from falling into the cast.

Regardless of the type of material of which it is made, a cast can interfere with circulation and nerve function from being

Table 91	Patient and Family Teaching Guide: Cast Care

Do Not
- Get plaster cast wet
- Remove any padding
- Insert any object inside cast
- Bear weight on new cast for 48 hr (not all casts are made for weight bearing; check with health care provider when unsure)
- Cover cast with plastic for prolonged periods

Do
- Apply ice directly over fracture site for first 24 hr (avoid getting cast wet by keeping ice in plastic bag and protecting cast with cloth)
- Check with health care provider before getting fiberglass cast wet
- Dry cast thoroughly after exposure to water
  Blot dry with towel
  Use hair dryer on low setting until cast is thoroughly dry
- Elevate extremity above level of heart for first 48 hr
- Move joints above and below cast regularly
- Report signs of possible problems to health care provider
  - Increasing pain
  - Swelling associated with pain and discoloration of toes or fingers
  - Pain during movement
  - Burning or tingling under cast
  - Sores or foul odor under the cast
- Keep appointment to have fracture and cast checked

applied too tightly or because of excessive edema after application. Frequent neurovascular assessments of the immobilized extremity are critical as are assessments of abdominal and respiratory status with body casts.

- The nurse should instruct the patient to exercise the joints above and below the cast to prevent stiffness and contractures.

Table 91 summarizes patient and family instructions for cast care.

CHEMOTHERAPY

Description

Chemotherapy is a systemic treatment modality for cancer. It is a mainstay of cancer therapy used in the treatment of most solid tumors and hematologic malignancies (e.g., leukemias, lymphomas). The principle of chemotherapy is to interrupt the cycle of cellular replication and proliferation.

- The two major categories of chemotherapeutic drugs are cell cycle nonspecific and cell cycle phase-specific. These agents are often administered in combination with one another to maximize effectiveness by using agents that function by differing mechanisms and throughout the cell cycle.

Classification of Chemotherapeutic Drugs

Chemotherapy drugs are generally classified according to their molecular structure and mechanisms of action (Table 92).

Methods of Administration

The intravenous (IV) route is the most common route for chemotherapy. Major concerns with IV administration result from the irritant or vesicant characteristics of many chemotherapeutic agents.

- Irritants will damage the intima of the vein, causing phlebitis and sclerosis and limiting future peripheral venous access.
- Vesicants may cause severe local tissue breakdown and necrosis if inadvertently infiltrated into the skin.

To avoid these problems, a central vascular access device may be placed in large blood vessels to permit frequent,

Text continued on p. 717

Table 92 Classification of Chemotherapeutic Drugs

Mechanisms of Action	Examples
Alkylating Agents *Cell cycle phase–nonspecific agents* Damage DNA by causing breaks in the double helix; if repair does not occur, cells will die immediately (cytocidal) or when they attempt to divide (cytostatic)	mechlorethamine (Mustargen), cyclophosphamide (Cytoxan, Neosar), chlorambucil (Leukeran), ifosfamide (Ifex), melphalan (Alkeran), busulfan (Myleran), dacarbazine (DTIC-Dome), temozolomide (Temodar), thiotepa (Thioplex)
Nitrosoureas *Cell cycle phase–nonspecific agents* Like alkylating agents, break DNA helix, interfering with DNA replication; cross blood-brain barrier	carmustine (BiCNU, Gliadel), lomustine (CeeNU), streptozocin (Zanosar)
Platinum Drugs *Cell cycle phase–nonspecific agents* Bind to DNA and RNA, miscoding information and/or DNA; replication is inhibited and cells die	oxaliplatin (Eloxatin), cisplatin (Platinol), carboplatin (Paraplatin)

DNA, Deoxyribonucleic acid; RNA, ribonucleic acid.

Continued

Table 92   Classification of Chemotherapeutic Drugs—cont'd

Mechanisms of Action	Examples
Antimetabolites	
Cell cycle phase-specific agents	
Mimic naturally occurring substances, thus interfering with enzyme function or DNA synthesis; primarily act during S phase; purine and pyrimidine are building blocks of nucleic acids needed for DNA and RNA synthesis	
▪ Interfere with purine metabolism	mercaptopurine (Purinethol), thioguanine, fludarabine (Fludara), pentostatin (Nipent), cladribine (Leustatin)
▪ Interfere with pyrimidine metabolism	capecitabine (Xeloda), cytarabine (Ara-C, Cytosar,DepoCyt), fluorouracil (5-FU), floxuridine (FUDR), gemcitabine (Gemzar)
▪ Interfere with folic acid metabolism	methotrexate (Rheumatrex, Trexall), pemetrexed (Alimta)
▪ Interferes with DNA synthesis	hydroxyurea (Hydrea, Droxia)
Antitumor Antibiotics	
Cell cycle phase-nonspecific agents	
Bind directly to DNA, thus inhibiting the synthesis of DNA and interfering with transcription of RNA	doxorubicin (Adriamycin, Rubex, Doxil), bleomycin (Blenoxane), mitomycin (Mutamycin), daunorubicin (Cerubidine, DaunoXome), dactinomycin (Cosmegen), idarubicin (Idamycin), plicamycin (Mithramycin, Mithracin), epirubicin (Ellence), mitoxantrone (Novantrone), valrubicin (Valstar)

Mitotic Inhibitors

Cell cycle phase–specific agents

Taxanes

Antimicrotubule agents that interfere with mitosis; act during the late G_2 phase and mitosis to stabilize microtubules, thus inhibiting cell division

paclitaxel (Taxol), docetaxel (Taxotere), paclitaxel albumin-bound particles (Abraxane)

Vinca alkaloids

Act in M phase to inhibit mitosis

vinblastine (Velban), vincristine (Oncovin), vinorelbine (Navelbine)

Topoisomerase Inhibitors

Cell cycle phase–specific agents

Inhibit the normal enzymes (topoisomerases) that function to make reversible breaks and repairs in DNA, which allow for flexibility of DNA in replication

irinotecan (Camptosar), topotecan (Hycamtin), etoposide (VePesid), teniposide (Vumon)

Corticosteroids

Cell cycle phase–nonspecific agents

Disrupt the cell membrane and inhibit synthesis of protein; decrease circulating lymphocytes; inhibit mitosis; depress immune system; increase feeling of well-being

cortisone (Cortone), hydrocortisone (Cortef), methylprednisolone (Medrol), prednisone, dexamethasone (Decadron)

Continued

DNA, Deoxyribonucleic acid; RNA, ribonucleic acid.

Table 92   Classification of Chemotherapeutic Drugs—cont'd

Mechanisms of Action	Examples
Hormone Therapy	
Cell cycle phase-nonspecific agents	
Antiestrogens	
Selectively attach to estrogen receptors, causing their down-regulation and inhibiting tumor growth; also known as SERMs (selective estrogen receptor modulators)	tamoxifen (Nolvadex), fulvestrant (Faslodex), raloxifene (Evista), toremifene (Fareston)
Estrogens	
Interfere with hormone receptors and proteins	diethylstilbestrol (DES), estramustine (Emcyt), estrogen (Menest), estradiol (Estrace)
Aromatase inhibitors	
Inhibit aromatase, an enzyme that converts adrenal androgen to estrogen	anastrozole (Arimidex), letrozole (Femara), exemestane (Aromasin)
Miscellaneous	
Inhibit protein synthesis; enzyme derived from the yeast *Erwinia* used to deplete the supply of asparagines for leukemic cells that are dependent on an exogenous source of amino acid	L-asparaginase (Elspar), *Erwinia* asparaginase
Causes changes in DNA in leukemia cells and degrades the fusion protein PML-RAR-α	arsenic trioxide (Trisenox)
Suppresses mitosis at interphase, appears to alter preformed DNA, RNA, and protein	procarbazine (Matulane, Natulan)

DNA, Deoxyribonucleic acid; RNA, ribonucleic acid.

continuous, or intermittent administration of chemotherapy, thus avoiding multiple venipunctures. Three major types of vascular access devices used in oncology patients are tunneled catheters, peripherally inserted central catheters (PICCs), and implanted infusion ports.

- Regional chemotherapy delivers the drug directly to the tumor site. Examples of this type of administration include intraarterial, intraperitoneal, intrathecal (intraventricular), and intravesical bladder chemotherapy.

Effects of Chemotherapy

Chemotherapeutic agents cannot selectively distinguish between normal cells and cancer cells. Chemotherapy-induced side effects are caused by (1) the destruction of normal cells that have a rapid rate of cellular proliferation, (2) the response of the body to products of cellular destruction (cellular waste products in the circulation may cause fatigue, anorexia, and taste alterations), and (3) general cytotoxicity and organ-specific drug toxicities.

The adverse effects of these drugs can be classified as acute, delayed, or chronic.

- Acute toxicity includes anaphylactic and hypersensitivity reactions, extravasation or a flare reaction, anticipatory nausea and vomiting, and dysrhythmias.
- Delayed effects are numerous and include delayed nausea and vomiting, mucositis, alopecia, skin rashes, bone marrow depression, altered bowel function, and a variety of neurotoxicities.
- Chronic toxicities involve damage to organs such as the heart, liver, kidneys, and lungs.

An extensive list of side effects and problems caused by chemotherapy and radiation therapy is provided in Table 16-15, Lewis and others, *Medical-Surgical Nursing,* edition 7, pp. 295 to 296.

Nursing Management

One of the most important responsibilities of the nurse is to differentiate between the toxic effects of the drug and progression of the malignant process. The nurse must also differentiate between tolerable side effects and acute toxic effects of chemotherapeutic agents.

- Myelosuppression is one of the most common effects of chemotherapy and can result in life-threatening and distressing effects, including infection, hemorrhage, and overwhelming fatigue. Monitoring the complete blood count is critical in patients receiving chemotherapy, particularly the neutrophil, platelet, and red blood cell (RBC) counts. White blood cell (WBC) growth factors are routinely used to reduce chemotherapy-induced neutropenia, and platelet transfusions are usually administered when platelet counts fall below 20,000/µl (20×10^9/L).

- Fatigue is a nearly universal symptom, affecting 70% to 100% of patients with cancer. The nurse can help patients recognize that fatigue is a common effect of therapy rather than a sign that treatment is not effective or that their cancer is progressing.

- The intestinal mucosa is one of the most sensitive tissues to chemotherapy, resulting in a variety of gastrointestinal (GI) effects—nausea and vomiting, diarrhea, mucositis, and anorexia—all of which can significantly affect the patient's hydration and nutritional status and sense of well-being. The nurse can successfully manage most of the effects with antiemetic regimens, dietary modification, and other non-pharmacologic interventions.

▼ **Patient and Family Teaching**

Patient and family teaching is an important part of the nurse's role related to chemotherapy. To decrease the fear and anxiety often associated with chemotherapy, the patient must be told what to expect during a course of treatment. The patient's attitude toward treatment should be explored so that any misconception or fear can be discussed.

- The patient must be told of the possible side effects of chemotherapy that may be experienced during treatment. Good nursing judgment is essential to determine the amount of information that the patient and family can assimilate. The patient must be reassured that this is a temporary situation and that the patient should be feeling better within a few weeks after chemotherapy is discontinued.

- The patient should also be informed that supportive care (e.g., antiemetic and antidiarrheal agents, hematopoietic growth factors) will be provided as needed.

CHEST TUBES AND PLEURAL DRAINAGE

Description

Chest tubes are inserted into the pleural space to remove air and fluid from the pleural space and to restore normal intrapleural pressure so that the lungs can reexpand.

Chest Tube Insertion

Chest tubes can be inserted in the emergency department (ED), at the patient's bedside, or in the operating room (OR), depending on the situation. In the OR the chest tube is inserted by way of a thoracotomy incision. In the ED or at the bedside the patient is placed in a sitting position or is lying down with the affected side elevated.

- The area is prepared with antiseptic solution, and the site is infiltrated with a local anesthetic agent. After a small incision is made, one or two chest tubes are inserted into the pleural space.
- During insertion, the tubes are kept clamped.
- To remove air, a tube is placed anteriorly through the second intercostal space; to drain fluid and blood, the tube is placed posteriorly through the eighth or ninth intercostal space (Fig. 18).
- Tubes are sutured to the chest wall, and the puncture wound is covered with a dressing. Some clinicians prefer to use an airtight seal with petroleum gauze; however, continued use of petroleum jelly can irritate the skin.
- After the tubes are in place in the pleural space, they are connected to drainage tubing and pleural drainage. Each tube may be connected to a separate drainage system and suction.
- More commonly a Y connector is used to attach both chest tubes to the same drainage system.

Pleural Drainage

Most pleural drainage systems have three basic compartments, each with a separate function.

- The first compartment, or *collection chamber,* receives fluid and air from the chest cavity. The air in the chamber is vented to the second compartment, called the *water-seal chamber,* which acts as a one-way valve. Air enters from the collection chamber by means of a connector that enters underwater in the second compartment. The air bubbles up through the water, and no air can reenter the collection chamber because of the water seal.
- A third compartment, which is used to apply controlled suction to the system, is called the *suction control chamber.*
- Removal of air from the pleural space is facilitated during periods when the patient's intrathoracic pressure is increased, such as during exhalation, coughing, or sneezing. As a result, more air bubbles are noted in the water-seal chamber during these activities.

■ A lack of bubbling during exhalation or coughing may indicate a blockage in the chest tube (e.g., kinking, clotting) or expansion of the lung with no further air in the pleural space.

A variety of commercial, disposable, plastic chest drainage systems are available. One popular system is the Pleur-evac (Fig. 19).

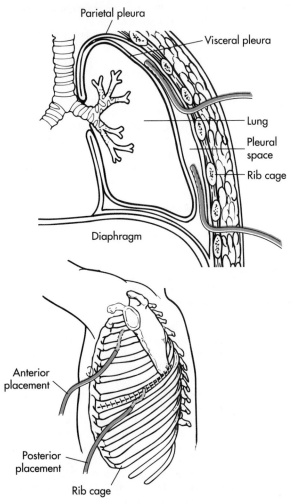

Fig. 18. Placement of chest tubes.

Nursing Management: Chest Drainage

General guidelines for nursing care include the following:

- Keep all tubing as straight as possible and coiled loosely. Do not let the patient lie on the tubing.
- Keep all connections among the chest tubes, drainage tubing, and drainage collector tight, and tape at connections.
- Keep the water-seal chamber and suction control chamber at appropriate water levels by adding sterile water as needed, because water loss by evaporation may occur.
- Mark the time of measurement and the fluid level on the chamber according to prescribed orders. Any change in the quantity or characteristics of drainage should be reported to the physician.
- Observe for air bubbles and fluctuations in the water-seal chamber. If no fluctuations are observed (rising with inspi-

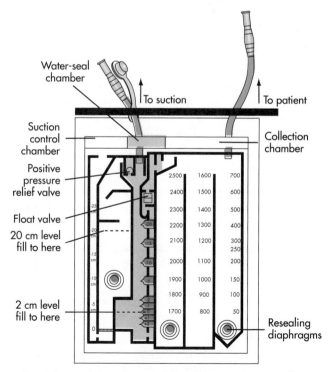

Fig. 19. **Pleur-evac disposable chest suction system.**

ration and falling with expiration in a spontaneously breathing patient; the opposite occurs during positive pressure mechanical ventilation), the drainage system is blocked or the lungs are reexpanded. If bubbling increases, there may be an air leak.

- Bubbling in the water-seal chamber may occur intermittently. When bubbling is continuous and constant, the nurse may determine the source of the air leak by momentarily clamping the tubing at successively distal points away from the patient until the bubbling ceases. Retaping the tubing connections or replacing the drainage apparatus may be necessary to prevent the air leak.
- Monitor the patient's clinical status. Vital signs should be taken frequently, lungs auscultated, and the chest wall observed for any abnormal chest movements.
- Never elevate the drainage system to the level of the patient's chest because this will cause fluid to drain back into the lungs. Drainage systems should not be emptied unless they are in danger of overflowing.
- Encourage the patient to cough and breathe deeply periodically to facilitate lung expansion.
- If the drainage system is overturned and the water seal is disrupted, return it to an upright position and encourage the patient to take a few deep breaths, followed by forced exhalations and cough maneuvers.
- Do not strip or milk chest tubes routinely, because this increases pleural pressures.
- If the drainage system breaks, place the distal end of the chest tubing connection in a sterile water container at a 2-cm level as an emergency water seal.
- Chest tubes are *not clamped routinely*. Clamps with rubber protection are kept at the bedside for special procedures such as changing the chest drainage system and assessment before removal of chest tubes.
- Chest tube malposition is the most common complication. Routine monitoring is done by the nurse to evaluate if the chest drainage is successful by observing for fluctuations in the water-seal chamber, listening for breath sounds over the lung fields, and measuring the amount of fluid drainage.

Chest Tube Removal

Chest tubes are removed when the lungs are reexpanded and fluid drainage has ceased. Suction is usually discontinued and gravity drainage is used for 24 hours before tube removal.

- The tube is removed by cutting the sutures; having the patient take a deep breath, exhale, and bear down (Valsalva maneuver); and then removing the tube.
- The site is covered with an airtight dressing, the pleura will seal itself off, and the wound heals in several days.
- The patient's condition is evaluated with a chest x-ray and close observation of respiratory function.

DIALYSIS

E

Description
Dialysis is a technique in which substances move from the blood through a semipermeable membrane and into a dialysis solution (dialysate). Dialysis is used to correct fluid and electrolyte imbalances and to remove waste products in renal failure. It can also be used to treat drug overdoses.

The two methods of dialysis are *peritoneal dialysis* (PD) and *hemodialysis* (HD).
- In PD the peritoneal membrane acts as the semipermeable membrane.
- In HD an artificial membrane (usually made of cellulose-based or synthetic materials) is used as the semipermeable membrane and is in contact with the patient's blood.
- Generally dialysis is initiated when the glomerular filtration rate (GFR) (or creatinine clearance) of the patient with kidney disease is less than 15 ml/min. This criterion can vary widely in different clinical situations, and the physician determines when to start dialysis based on the patient's clinical status. Certain uremic complications, including encephalopathy, neuropathies, uncontrollable hyperkalemia, pericarditis, and accelerated hypertension, indicate a need for immediate dialysis.

Dialysis is discussed in Lewis and others, *Medical-Surgical Nursing,* edition 7, pp. 1216 to 1224.

EMERGENCY PATIENT: PRIMARY AND SECONDARY SURVEY

Recognition of life-threatening illness or injury is one of the most important aspects of emergency care. Before a diagnosis can be made, recognition of the dangerous clinical signs and symptoms with initiation of interventions to reverse or prevent a crisis is essential.

- A triage system identifies and categorizes patients so the most critical are treated first. *Triage* is a French word meaning "to sort."
- The process is based on the premise that patients with a threat to life, vision, or limb should be treated before other patients.

The emergency nurse must complete an initial assessment to determine the presence of actual or potential threats to life and then rapidly initiate interventions appropriate for the patient's condition. A history is obtained simultaneously with the assessment. A systematic approach to the initial patient assessment decreases the time required to identify potential threats and minimizes the risk of missing a life-threatening condition. Two systematic approaches, a primary and secondary survey, can be used for assessment of any emergency patient.

The **primary survey** focuses on airway, breathing, and circulation and serves to identify life-threatening conditions so that appropriate interventions can be initiated. Life-threatening conditions related to the airway, breathing, and circulation may be identified at any point during the primary survey. When this occurs, interventions are started immediately and before proceeding to the next step of the survey.

After each step of the primary survey is addressed and any lifesaving interventions initiated, the secondary survey begins. The **secondary survey** is a brief, systematic process that is aimed at obtaining a history, identifying *all* injuries, and performing a thorough physical examination.

HEIMLICH MANEUVER

Management of a foreign body airway obstruction depends on whether the person is conscious or unconscious (Table 93). Fig. 20 illustrates the Heimlich maneuver, which is an emergency procedure for dislodging an obstruction from the trachea to prevent asphyxiation. In rare instances when airway obstruction is not relieved by methods in Table 93, additional procedures are necessary. These include transtracheal catheter ventilation and cricothyroidotomy.

Table 93	Management of Foreign Body Airway Obstruction (FBAO)

Conscious Adult Victim
Assessment of victim for airway obstruction
Signs of severe airway obstruction:
- Universal choking sign (victim clutches neck with hands)
- Inability to speak
  Ask the victim "Are you choking?"
- Silent cough
- High-pitched sound or no sound while inhaling
- Increased difficulty breathing
- Cyanosis
  If the victim displays any of the above, severe or complete airway obstruction may be present and the rescuer must take action.

Heimlich maneuver (abdominal thrusts) with standing/sitting victim (Fig. 20, p. 726)

1. Stand behind victim, and wrap arms around waist.
2. Make fist with one hand.
3. Place thumb side of fist against victim's abdomen. Position fist midline, slightly above the umbilicus and well below xiphoid process.
4. Grasp fist with other hand.
5. Press fist into victim's abdomen using quick upward thrusts. Each thrust should be a separate distinct movement. NOTE: If victim is in the late stages of pregnancy or obese, chest thrusts should be used. Position hands (as described) over lower portion of the sternum, and apply quick backward thrusts.
6. Repeat thrusts until object is expelled or victim becomes unresponsive.

Unconscious Adult Victim
Assessment
If rescuer sees victim collapse and knows that FBAO is the cause:
1. Activate the EMS system by calling 911.
2. Be sure victim is supine.
3. Perform tongue-jaw lift; look to see if a foreign body is visible, and, if seen, remove it.
4. Open airway, and attempt to ventilate:
   Give two rescue breaths.
   If breaths are unsuccessful in making victim's chest rise:
      Reposition victim's head.
      Reopen airway.
      Reattempt to ventilate.
5. If efforts to ventilate are still unsuccessful, begin CPR (see Tables 89 and 90, pp. 705 to 710).

From 2005 American Heart Association guidelines for cardiopulmonary resuscitation and emergency cardiovascular care, part 4: adult basic life support, *Circulation* 112:IV-19, 2005.
CPR, Cardiopulmonary resuscitation; *EMS*, Emergency Medical Service.

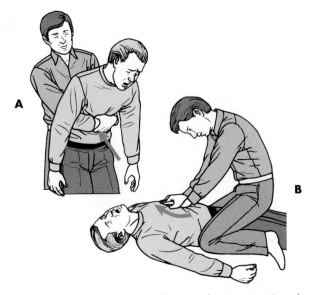

Fig. 20. A, Heimlich maneuver administered to conscious (standing) victim of foreign body airway obstruction. **B,** Heimlich maneuver administered to unconscious (lying) victim of foreign body airway obstruction—astride position.

MECHANICAL VENTILATION

Description

Mechanical ventilation is the process by which room air or oxygen-enriched air is mechanically moved into and out of the lungs. Mechanical ventilation is not curative. It is a means of supporting patients until they recover the ability to breathe independently, as a bridge to long-term mechanical ventilation, or until a decision is made to withdraw ventilatory support. Indications for mechanical ventilation include (1) apnea or an impending inability to breathe, (2) acute respiratory failure, (3) severe hypoxia, and (4) respiratory muscle fatigue.

Types of Mechanical Ventilators

The two major types of mechanical ventilation are negative pressure and positive pressure ventilation.

- *Negative pressure ventilation* involves the use of chambers that encase the chest or body and surround it with intermittent subatmospheric or negative pressure. Intermittent negative pressure around the chest wall causes the chest to be pulled outward. This reduces intrathoracic pressure. Air rushes in through the upper airway, which is outside the sealed chamber. Expiration is passive; the machine cycles off, allowing chest retraction. This type of ventilation is similar to normal ventilation in that decreased intrathoracic pressures produce inspiration. An artificial airway is not required.

- Lightweight, portable negative pressure ventilators are used in the home for patients with neuromuscular diseases, central nervous system disorders, diseases and injuries of the spinal cord, and severe chronic obstructive pulmonary disease (COPD). Negative pressure ventilators are not used extensively for acutely ill patients.

- *Positive pressure ventilation* (PPV) is the primary method used with acutely ill patients. During inspiration the ventilator pushes air into the lungs under positive pressure. Unlike spontaneous ventilation, intrathoracic pressure is raised during lung inflation rather than lowered. Expiration occurs passively as in normal expiration. Positive pressure ventilators are categorized into volume and pressure ventilators.

See the detailed information on mechanical ventilation in Lewis and others, *Medical-Surgical Nursing,* edition 7, pp. 1754 to 1768. Nursing management of the patient receiving mechanical ventilation is presented in NCP 66-1, *Medical-Surgical Nursing,* edition 7, pp. 1754 to 1756.

OSTOMIES

Types of Ostomies

An *ostomy* is a surgical procedure that allows intestinal contents to pass from the bowel through an opening in the skin on the surface of the abdomen. The opening is called a *stoma,* and it is created when the intestine is brought through the abdominal wall and sutured to the skin. An ostomy may be permanent or temporary.

Ostomies are described according to location and type. For example, an ostomy in the ileum is called an *ileostomy,* an ostomy in the sigmoid colon is called a *sigmoid colostomy,* and an ostomy transverse colon is called a *transverse colostomy*. Locations or ostomies are shown in Fig. 21.

The major types of ostomies are end stoma, loop, and double-barrel ostomies.

- An *end stoma* is created by dividing the bowel and bringing the proximal end to the skin and forming a single stoma. The distal portion of the bowel is surgically removed, or the distal segment is sewn closed and left in the abdominal cavity. All of the ostomies in Fig. 21 are end stomas except for the transverse, double-barrel colostomy.

- A *loop stoma* is created by bringing a loop of bowel to the abdominal surface and then opening the anterior part of the bowel to provide fecal diversion. This results in one stoma with a proximal and distal opening and an intact posterior bowel wall that separates the two openings.

- A *double-barrel stoma* is similar to a loop stoma, except that the bowel is divided and both the proximal and distal ends are brought through the abdominal wall as two separate stomas. The proximal stoma is the functioning stoma; the distal, nonfunctioning stoma is referred as the mucous fistula.

Ostomies may be temporary or permanent. Temporary ostomies are used to divert intestinal contents past a diseased or injured part of the bowel until healing occurs. Temporary colostomies are usually located in the transverse colon and are most commonly loop or double-barrel stomas. Cancer involving the rectum requires a permanent ostomy since all bowel distal to the ostomy is removed. A comparison of colostomies and ileostomy is presented in Table 94.

The actual procedures to perform ostomy surgeries are discussed in Lewis and others, *Medical-Surgical Nursing,* edition 7, pp. 1069 to 1079.

Nursing Management

Preoperative Care. Preoperative care that is unique to ostomy surgery includes (1) psychologic preparation for the ostomy; (2) selection of a flat site on the abdomen that allows secure attachment of the collection bag; and (3) selection of a stoma site that will be clearly visible to the patient to facilitate self-care. In the preoperative period it is important to review the information the patient has received from the health care provider. The family and patient usually have many questions concerning the procedures.

- If available, an enterostomal (ET) nurse should visit the patient and select the site where the ostomy should be positioned and mark the abdomen preoperatively. An improp-

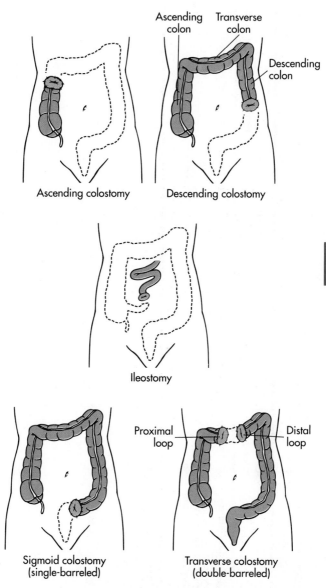

Fig. 21. Types of ostomies.

Table 94   Comparison of Colostomies and Ileostomy

	Ascending Colostomy	Transverse Colostomy	Sigmoid Colostomy	Ileostomy
Stool consistency	Semiliquid	Semiliquid to semiformed	Formed	Liquid to semiliquid
Fluid requirement	Increased	Possibly increased	No change	Increased
Bowel regulation	No	No	Yes (if there is a history of a regular bowel pattern)	No
Pouch and skin barriers	Yes	Yes	Dependent on regulation	Yes
Irrigation	No	No	Possible every 24-48 hr (if patient meets criteria)	No
Indications for surgery	Perforating diverticulitis in lower colon; trauma; inoperable tumors of colon, rectum, or pelvis; rectovaginal fistula	Same as for ascending; birth defect	Cancer of the rectum or rectosigmoidal area; perforating diverticulum; trauma	Ulcerative colitis, Crohn's disease, diseased or injured colon, birth defect, familial polyposis, trauma, cancer

erly placed stoma complicates rehabilitation by increasing the time and expense of the pouch change routine. It can also contribute to skin irritation and poor adaptation.

- If the patient desires a referral and the heath care provider agrees, a trained ostomy visitor from the United Ostomy Association can provide meaningful psychologic support.

Postoperative Care. Postoperative nursing care includes assessment of the stoma and provision of an appropriate pouching system that protects the skin and contains drainage and odor. See NCP 43-3 for the patient with a colostomy or ileostomy, Lewis and others, *Medical-Surgical Nursing,* edition 7, pp. 1073 to 1075.

The stoma should be pink. A dusky-blue stoma indicates ischemia, and a brown-black stoma indicates necrosis. The nurse should assess and document stoma color every 8 hours. There is mild to moderate swelling of the stoma the first 2 to 3 weeks after surgery.

The pouching system consists of a skin barrier and a bag or pouch to collect the feces. The skin barrier is a piece of pectin-based or karaya wafer that has a measurable thickness and hydrocolloid adhesive properties. The skin barrier adheres to the skin and remains in place about 5 to 7 days. The skin should be washed with mild soap, rinsed with warm water, and dried thoroughly before the barrier is applied.

- Pouches come as one- or two-piece systems. The one-piece system has the skin barrier attached, and the two-piece system allows removal of the pouch without removing the skin barrier.
- With an open-ended, transparent, plastic, odor-proof pouch it is easy to protect the skin and to observe and collect the drainage. The pouch must fit snugly to prevent leakage around the stoma. The size of the stoma is determined with a stoma-measuring card. Although the pouch is applied after surgery, the ostomy functions when peristalsis has been adequately restored.
- The volume, color, and consistency of the drainage are recorded. Each time the pouch is changed, the condition of the skin is observed for irritation. A pouch should never be placed directly on irritated skin without the use of a skin barrier.

Colostomy Care

- A colostomy in the ascending and transverse colon has semi-liquid stools. The patient needs to be instructed to use a drainable pouch. A colostomy in the sigmoid or descending colon has semiformed or formed stools and can sometimes be regulated by the irrigation method. The patient may or may not wear a drainage pouch. A nondrainable pouch should have a gas filter.

- For most patients with colostomies, there are few, if any, dietary restrictions. A well-balanced diet and adequate fluid intake are important. For foods and their effects on stomal output, see Table 43-33, Lewis and others, *Medical-Surgical Nursing,* edition 7, p. 1075.

Colostomy irrigations are used to stimulate emptying of the colon in order to achieve a regular bowel pattern. Regularity is only possible when the stoma is in the distal colon or rectum. If control is achieved, there should be little or no spillage between irrigations. The patient who establishes regularity may need to wear only a pad or cover over the stoma. The patient who cannot or chooses not to establish regularity by irrigations must wear a pouch at all times. The procedure for colostomy irrigation is presented in Table 95.

- The procedure should not be rushed; the patient should feel relaxed. The patient or family member must be instructed in the procedure and must be able to demonstrate the ability to irrigate before being independent. This can be done in the outpatient setting.

▼ **Patient and Family Teaching**

- The patient should be able to perform skin care, control odor, care for the stoma, and identify signs and symptoms of complications.
- The patient should know the importance of fluids and food in the diet, have the name and address of the United Ostomy Association, and know when to seek health care.
- Home care and outpatient follow-up care by an ET nurse are highly recommended.
- Patients should be discharged with written pouch change instructions, teaching literature relevant to the type of stoma they have, a list of equipment they use (including names and phone numbers), a list of equipment retailers, outpatient follow-up appointments with the surgeon and ET nurse, and the phone numbers of the surgeon and nurse.

See Table 43-32 for ostomy teaching guidelines, Lewis and others, *Medical-Surgical Nursing,* edition 7, p. 1072.

Ileostomy Care

- Immediately after surgery, intake and output must be accurately monitored. The patient should be observed for signs and symptoms of fluid and electrolyte imbalance, particularly potassium, sodium, and fluid deficits.
- In the first 24 to 48 hours after surgery, the amount of drainage from the stoma may be negligible. Once peristalsis returns, the patient may experience a period of high volume output of 1000

Table 95	Patient and Family Teaching Guide: Colostomy Irrigation

Equipment
Lubricant
Irrigation set (1000- to 2000-ml container, tubing with irrigating
    stoma cone, clamp)
Irrigating sleeve with adhesive or belt
Toilet tissue to clean around the stoma
Disposal sack for soiled dressing

Procedure
1. Place 500 to 1000 ml of lukewarm water (not to exceed
   105° F [40.5° C]) in container. The volume is titrated for the
   individual; use enough irrigant to distend the bowel but not
   enough to cause cramping pain. Most adults use 500-
   1000 ml of water.
2. Ensure comfortable position. Patient may sit in chair in front
   of toilet or on the toilet if the perineal wound is healed.
3. Clear tubing of all air by flushing it with fluid.
4. Hang container on hook or intravenous (IV) pole (18-24
   inches) above stoma (about shoulder height).
5. Apply irrigating sleeve, and place bottom end in toilet bowl.
6. Lubricate cone, insert cone tip gently into the stoma, and
   hold tip securely in place.
7. Allow irrigation solution to flow in steadily for 5-10 min.
8. If cramping occurs, stop the flow of solution for a few
   seconds, leaving the cone in place.
9. Clamp the tubing, and remove irrigating cone when the
   desired amount of irrigant has been delivered or when the
   patient senses colonic distention.
10. Allow 30-45 min for the solution and feces to be expelled.
    Initial evacuation is usually complete in 10-15 min. Close off
    the irrigating sleeve at the bottom to allow ambulation.
11. Clean, rinse, and dry periostomal skin well.
12. Replace the colostomy drainage pouch or desired stoma
    covering.
13. Wash and rinse all equipment, and hang to dry.

to 1800 ml/day. Later on, the average amount can be 500 ml/
day because the proximal small bowel adapts to absorb more
fluid.

▼ **Patient and Family Teaching**
The patient should be instructed to drink at least 2 to 3 L of fluid
daily; more may be necessary when diarrhea occurs and when
perspiration is increased. Diarrhea from an ileostomy produces
acidosis from the loss of bicarbonate. The health care provider

may instruct the patient to take an electrolyte solution at home (e.g., 1 tsp of salt and 1 tsp of baking soda in 1 qt of water). Fluids rich in electrolytes should be encouraged.

- A low-fiber diet is usually ordered initially. Fiber-containing foods are reintroduced gradually. A return to a normal, presurgical diet is the goal.
- The stoma may bleed easily when it is touched because it has a high vascular supply. The patient should be told that minimal oozing of blood is normal.

OXYGEN THERAPY

Description

The goal of oxygen (O_2) therapy is to supply the patient with adequate O_2 to maximize the O_2-carrying ability of the blood. O_2 is usually administered to treat hypoxemia caused by (1) respiratory disorders such as chronic obstructive pulmonary disease (COPD), cor pulmonale, pneumonia, atelectasis, lung cancer, and pulmonary emboli; (2) cardiovascular disorders such as myocardial infarction (MI), dysrhythmias, angina pectoris, and cardiogenic shock; and (3) central nervous system (CNS) disorders such as overdose of opioids, head injury, and disordered sleep (sleep apnea).

Methods of Administration

Various methods of O_2 administration are used (Table 96). The method selected depends on factors such as the fraction of inspired O_2 concentration (FIO_2) and mobility of the patient, humidification required, patient cooperation, comfort, and cost.

- O_2 obtained from cylinders or wall systems is dry. Dry O_2 has an irritating effect on the mucous membranes and dries secretions. Therefore it is important that O_2 be humidified when administered, either by humidification or nebulization.

Complications

O_2 supports combustion and increases the rate of burning. This is why it is important that smoking be prohibited in the area in which O_2 is being used. A "No Smoking" sign should be prominently displayed where oxygen is in use. The patient should also be cautioned against smoking cigarettes with O_2 prongs or a catheter in place.

Text continued on p. 739

Table 96   Methods of Oxygen (O_2) Administration

Advantages	Disadvantages	Nursing Interventions
Low-Flow Delivery Devices *Nasal cannula* Most commonly used device. It is a safe and simple method that is relatively comfortable. It is useful for a patient requiring low O_2 concentrations (e.g., those with chronic CO_2 retention). Patient can eat, talk, or cough while wearing device.	Cannula is difficult to maintain in position and can be easily dislodged. Patient must be alert and cooperative to keep cannula in proper place. High flow rates (>5 L/min) dry nasal membranes and may cause pain in frontal sinuses. Can irritate nares and skin around ears.	Nasal cannula should be stabilized when caring for a restless patient. O_2 concentrations of 24% (1 L/min) to 44% (6 L/min) can be obtained. Amount of O_2 inhaled depends on room air and patient's breathing pattern. Most patients with COPD can tolerate 2 L/min using a cannula. May need to pad cannula where it sits on the ears.

ABGs, Arterial blood gases; *COPD,* chronic obstructive pulmonary disease; *FIO_2,* fraction of inspired O_2 concentration.

Continued

Table 96 Methods of Oxygen (O₂) Administration—cont'd

Advantages	Disadvantages	Nursing Interventions
Simple face mask O_2 can be given quickly for short periods. Useful when transporting patients. O_2 concentrations of 35%-50% can be achieved with flow rates of 6-12 L/min. Mask provides adequate humidification of inspired air.	Lack of patient tolerance results in inadequate therapy. Mask may be uncomfortable because tight seal must be maintained between face and mask. Mask may produce pressure necrosis of the skin. It must be removed to eat or drink.	Wash and dry under mask q2hr. Mask must fit snugly. Nasal cannula may be provided while patient is eating. Watch for pressure necrosis at the top of ears from elastic straps. (Gauze or other padding may be used to alleviate this problem.)
Partial rebreathing mask Mask is lightweight and easy to use. Reservoir bag conserves O_2. Useful for short-term (24-hr) therapy for patients needing higher O_2 concentrations.	Mask cannot be used with a high degree of humidity. Patient may find mask uncomfortable and refuse to wear it.	Method is useful when blood O_2 concentrations must be raised. It is not recommended for patient with COPD. Bag should not be allowed to deflate during inspiration, which is caused by kinking of the reservoir.

Non-rebreathing mask
High concentrations of O_2 can be delivered accurately. O_2 flows into bag and mask during inhalation. Valve prevents expired air from flowing back into bag. Good for short-term (24-hr) therapy for patients needing higher O_2 concentrations.

Mask cannot be used with a high degree of humidity. Patient may find mask uncomfortable and refuse to wear it.

Mask should fit snugly. Flow rate must be sufficient to keep bag from collapsing during inspiration. Make sure valves are open during expiration and closed during inhalation to prevent drastic decrease in FIO_2. Monitor closely because patient may require intubation as the next step.

Transtracheal catheter*
Catheter is less visible. Flow requirement may be reduced approximately 50%-70%, which greatly increases amount of time available from portable source of O_2. Less nasal irritation occurs.

Patient and family must learn entire program of care of tracheostomy and how to replace catheter. Procedure is invasive. Procedure and replacement add costs to O_2 therapy.

Method may not be appropriate for patient with excessive mucous production from mucous plugging because the catheter may frequently become obstructed.

Tracheostomy collar
Collar can deliver high humidity and O_2 by way of a tracheostomy.

Condensed fluid in tubing may drain into tracheostomy. Water traps are usually put in. Secretions collect inside collar and around tracheostomy.

Collar attaches to neck with elastic strap and should be removed and cleaned at least q4hr to prevent aspiration of fluid and infection.

*See Fig. 29-13, Lewis and others, Medical-Surgical Nursing, edition 7, p. 643.

Continued

Table 96 Methods of Oxygen (O_2) Administration—cont'd

Advantages	Disadvantages	Nursing Interventions
Tracheostomy T bar Tight fit allows better O_2 and humidity delivery than tracheostomy collar.	Condensed fluid in tubing may drain into tracheostomy. Water traps are usually put in.	T bar must be removed for suctioning. Mörch swivel may be used to eliminate the need for removal. It should be emptied as necessary.
High-Flow Delivery Device **Venturi mask[†]** Mask can deliver precise, high flow rates of O_2. Lightweight plastic, cone-shaped device is fitted to face. Masks are available for delivery of 24%, 28%, 31%, 35%, 40%, and 50% O_2. Adapters can be applied to increase humidification.	Mask is uncomfortable and must be removed when patient eats. Patient can talk, but voice may be muffled. Other disadvantages are the same as those discussed for the simple face mask.	Entrainment device on mask must be changed to deliver higher concentrations of O_2. Method is especially helpful for administering low, constant O_2 concentration to patients with COPD.

[†]See Fig. 29-11, C, Lewis and others, *Medical-Surgical Nursing*, edition 7, p. 642.

Oxygen toxicity is a complication that can result from prolonged exposure to a high level of O_2. High concentrations of O_2 damage alveolar-capillary membranes, inactivate pulmonary surfactant, cause interstitial and alveolar edema, and decrease compliance. To prevent toxicity the amount of O_2 administered should be just enough to maintain the PaO_2 within a normal or acceptable range for the patient.

Infection can be a major hazard of O_2 administration. Heated nebulizers present the highest risk. Constant use of humidity supports bacterial growth, with the most common infecting organism being *Pseudomonas aeruginosa*. Disposable equipment that operates as a closed system should be used. There should be a hospital policy stating the required frequency of equipment changes based on the type of equipment. Both equipment and respiratory secretions should be Gram stained and cultured frequently.

The administration of high levels of O_2 to patients with COPD has long been considered a potential problem that has recently been questioned. The issue arises from the presence of carbon dioxide (CO_2) narcosis, a condition of elevated CO_2 in the blood. Normally accumulation of CO_2 is the major stimulant of the respiratory center, but in patients with COPD the respiratory center can lose its sensitivity to the high CO_2 levels. For these individuals, there has been concern that hypoxemia becomes the drive to breathe and that administration of oxygen above 2 to 3 L/min can reduce the drive to breathe. This situation is a pervasive myth but is not a serious threat. In fact, not providing adequate O_2 to these patients is much more detrimental, and patients with end-stage COPD require high flow rates and higher concentrations for survival.

Long-Term Oxygen Therapy at Home

Improved prognosis and quality of life have been noted in patients with COPD who receive nocturnal or continuous O_2 to treat hypoxemia. Benefits of long-term continuous O_2 therapy include improved neuropsychologic function, increased exercise tolerance, decreased hematocrit, and reduced pulmonary hypertension. It also improves sleep and may reduce nocturnal dysrhythmias. It should be stresssed with patients that "addiction" to oxygen does not occur and it should be used as prescribed for its positive effects.

- Periodic reevaluations are necessary for the patient who is using long-term supplemental O_2. Generally, the patient should be reevaluated every 30 to 90 days during the first year of therapy and annually after that, as long as the patient remains stable.

Table 97	Patient and Family Teaching Guide: Home Oxygen Use

Mask/Cannula
- Ensure that the straps are not too tight.
- Remove 2 or 3 times/day to wash and dry skin where straps are and stimulate skin.
- Pad any pressure points.
- Observe tops of ears for skin breakdown from pressure points.

Oral and Nasal Mucous Membranes
- Assess oral and nasal mucous membranes 2 or 3 times/day.
- Use water-based gel on lips and nasal mucosa.
- Provide frequent oral hygiene.
- Provide humidification by means of a humidifier or nebulizing device.

Decreasing Risk for Infection
- Remove mask or collar, and cleanse with water 2 or 3 times/day.
- Cleanse skin carefully at this time, and observe for cuts, scratches, and bruises.
- Change disposable equipment frequently.
- Remove secretions that are coughed out.

Decreasing Risk of Fire Injuries
- Post "No Smoking" warning signs in home where they can be seen.
- Do not use electric razors, portable radios, open flames, wool blankets, or mineral oils in the area where oxygen is in use.
- Do not allow smoking in the home.

NOTE: A good resource for patients is *Patient Information Series: Oxygen Therapy* by American Thoracic Society. Available at *www.thoracic.org/ patiented/patedmaterials*.asp

▼ **Patient and Family Teaching**
A home care guide for teaching the patient and family about home O_2 use is given in Table 97.

PACEMAKERS

Description
The artificial cardiac pacemaker is an electronic device used to pace the heart when the normal conduction pathway is damaged or diseased. The basic pacing circuit consists of a power source (battery-

powered pulse generator), one or more conducting leads (pacing leads), and the myocardium. The electrical signal (stimulus) travels from the pacemaker, through the leads, to the wall of the myocardium. The myocardium is "captured" and stimulated to contract.

Types of Pacemakers

Permanent pacemakers are those that are implanted totally within the body, and *temporary pacemakers* are those that have the power source outside the body.

- The permanent pacemaker power source is implanted subcutaneously, usually over the pectoral muscle on the patient's nondominant side. It is attached to pacer leads, which are threaded transvenously to the right atrium and one or both ventricles. Indications for insertion of a permanent pacemaker are listed in Table 98.
- A temporary pacemaker is one that has the power source outside the body. There are three types of temporary pacemakers: transvenous, epicardial, and transcutaneous. Indications for temporary pacing are listed in Table 99.
  - A transvenous pacemaker consists of a lead or leads that are threaded transvenously to the right atrium and/or right ventricle.
  - Epicardial pacing is achieved by attaching an atrial and ventricular pacing lead to the epicardium during heart surgery for use if needed for treatment of dysrhythmias.
  - A transcutaneous pacemaker is used to provide adequate heart rate and rhythm to the patient in an emergency situation and involves the use of external electrode pads.

Table 98	Indications for Permanent Pacemaker Therapy

- Acquired AV block
  - Second-degree AV block
  - Third-degree AV block
- Bundle branch block
- Cardiomyopathy
  - Dilated
  - Hypertrophic
- Heart failure
- Hypersensitive carotid sinus syndrome
- SA node dysfunction
- Tachydysrhythmias

AV, Atrioventricular; SA, sinoatrial.

Table 99	Indications for Temporary Pacing*

- Maintenance of adequate HR and rhythm during special circumstances, such as surgery and postoperative recovery, cardiac catheterization, or coronary angioplasty; during drug therapy that may cause bradycardia; and before implantation of a permanent pacemaker
- As prophylaxis after open heart surgery
- Acute anterior MI with second-degree or third-degree AV block or bundle branch block
- Acute inferior MI with symptomatic bradycardia and AV block
- Electrophysiologic studies to evaluate patient with bradydysrhythmias and tachydysrhythmias

AV, Atrioventricular; HR, heart rate; MI, myocardial infarction.
* This table lists common indications but is not all-inclusive.

Patient Monitoring

Patients with temporary or permanent pacemakers will be monitored by electrocardiogram (ECG) to evaluate the status of the pacemaker. Pacemaker malfunction is primarily manifested by a failure to sense or a failure to capture. *Failure to sense* occurs when the pacemaker fails to recognize spontaneous atrial or ventricular activity and fires inappropriately. Failure to sense may be caused by pacer lead fracture, battery failure, or electrode displacement. *Failure to capture* occurs when the electrical charge to the myocardium is insufficient to produce atrial or ventricular contraction. Failure to capture may be caused by pacer lead fracture, battery failure, electrode displacement, or fibrosis at the electrode tip.

Nursing Management

Nursing interventions after pacemaker insertion include observation of the insertion site for signs of bleeding and infection. Temperature elevation should also be noted. After discharge, pacemaker function is checked on a regular basis to detect problems with sensing or capturing.

- The patient with a newly implanted pacemaker may have many questions about activity restrictions and fears concerning body image after the procedure.
- The goal of pacemaker therapy should be to enhance physiologic functioning and the quality of life. This should be emphasized to the patient, and the nurse should give specific advice on activity restrictions. Patient and family

Table 100	Patient and Family Teaching Guide: Pacemaker

1. Maintain follow-up care with your primary care provider to check the pacemaker site, and begin regular pacemaker function checks.
2. Report any signs of infection at incision site (e.g., redness, swelling, drainage) or fever to your primary care provider immediately.
3. Keep incision dry for 4 days after implantation.
4. Avoid lifting arm on pacemaker side above shoulder until approved by your primary care provider.
5. Avoid direct blows to generator site.
6. Avoid close proximity to high-output electrical generators or to large magnets, such as an MRI scanner. These devices can interfere with the function of the pacemaker.
7. Microwave ovens are safe to use and do not interfere with pacemaker function.
8. Travel without restrictions is allowed. The small metal case of an implanted pacemaker rarely sets off an airport security alarm.
9. Monitor pulse, and inform primary care provider if it drops below predetermined rate.
10. Carry pacemaker information card at all times.
11. A Medic-Alert ID or bracelet should be worn at all times.

P

ID, Identification; *MRI*, magnetic resonance imaging.

teaching for the patient with a pacemaker is outlined in Table 100.

PARENTERAL NUTRITION

Description

Parenteral nutrition (PN) is the administration of nutrients by a route (e.g., bloodstream) other than the gastrointestinal (GI) tract when the GI tract cannot be used for the ingestion, digestion, and absorption of essential nutrients. *Central parenteral nutrition* is the delivery of a nutritionally adequate hypertonic solution consisting of glucose, crystalline amino acids, fat emulsion, minerals, and vitamins using a central venous route.

- The goal of PN is to meet the patient's nutritional needs and to allow for the growth of new body tissue.
- Indications for PN include patients with severe injury, surgery, or burns and those who are malnourished as a

Table 101	Common Indications for Parenteral Nutrition

- Chronic severe diarrhea and vomiting
- Complicated surgery or trauma
- Gastrointestinal obstruction
- Gastrointestinal tract anomalies and fistulas
- Intractable diarrhea
- Severe anorexia nervosa
- Severe malabsorption
- Short bowel syndrome

result of medical treatment or disease processes (Table 101).

Administration of PN

PN may be administered by way of a central line into the superior vena cava (the most common route) or through a single- or double-lumen peripherally inserted central catheter (PICC) usually placed into the basilic or cephalic vein and then advanced into the central circulation.

- *Central PN* is indicated when long-term nutritional support is necessary, such as in cases when the patient has high protein and caloric requirements.
- *Peripheral parenteral nutrition* (PPN) is administered through a large, peripherally inserted catheter or vascular access device that uses a large peripheral vein. PPN is used when (1) nutritional support is needed for only a short time, (2) protein and caloric requirements are not high, (3) the risk of a central catheter is too great, or (4) parenteral support is used to supplement inadequate oral intake.
- Once established for PN, a single-lumen central catheter should not be used for the administration of blood or antibiotics, the drawing of blood samples, or central venous pressure monitoring.

Commercially prepared PN base solutions are available for both central and peripheral use. These base solutions contain dextrose and protein in the form of amino acids. The pharmacy adds the prescribed electrolytes (e.g., sodium, chloride, calcium, magnesium, phosphate), vitamins, and trace elements (e.g., zinc, copper, chromium, manganese) to customize the solution for the patient.

- A three-in-one or total nutrient admixture containing an intravenous (IV) fat emulsion, dextrose, and amino acids is widely used.

- All PN solutions should be prepared by a pharmacist or trained technician using strict aseptic techniques under a laminar flow hood. Nothing should be added to PN solutions after they are prepared by the pharmacy. The danger of drug incompatibilities and contamination is high.
- In general, PN solutions are good for 24 to 36 hours and must be refrigerated until 30 minutes before use.

Nursing Management

Because PN solutions are excellent media for microbial growth, it is essential that proper aseptic techniques be followed.

- Millipore filters should be placed on all parenteral lines: a 0.22-μm filter for parenteral solutions without fat emulsion and a 1.2-μm filter for parenteral solutions with fat emulsion.
- Filters and IV tubing are changed every 24 hours if PN with lipids is being administered and every 72 hours for PN with amino acids and dextrose. The tubing and the filter should be clearly labeled with the date and time they are put into use.

Dressings covering the catheter site are changed according to institutional protocol, from every other day to once per week.

- The insertion site is carefully observed for signs of inflammation and infection. Phlebitis can readily occur in the vein as a result of the hypertonic infusion, and the area can become infected. In immunosuppressed patients and patients receiving chemotherapy, corticosteroids, or antibiotics, signs of inflammation or infection can be subtle, if present at all.
- If an infection is suspected during a dressing change, a culture specimen of the site and drainage should be sent for analysis and the health care provider should be notified immediately.

A metabolic complication of PN is hyperglycemia. Some increase in the blood glucose level is expected during the first few days after PN is started. In general, the dextrose dose of PN should not be increased until the blood glucose concentrations are consistently less than 180 mg/dl.

- Blood glucose levels should be checked at the bedside every 4 to 6 hours with a glucometer. A sliding scale of insulin may be ordered to keep the blood glucose level in the normal range.

An infusion pump must be used during administration of PN so that the infusion rate can be maintained, and an alarm will sound if the tubing becomes obstructed. Even though an infusion pump is being used, the nurse should periodically check the volume infused because pump malfunctions can alter the rate.

Evaluation of the patient's tolerance of PN is an important nursing intervention.

- Vital signs should be monitored every 4 to 8 hours in patients receiving PN. Daily weights give an indication of the patient's hydration status as the therapy progresses. Analysis must be made whether gains or losses in weight are caused by fluid gained from edema, fluid lost through diuresis, or actual increase or decrease in tissue weight.
- Blood levels of glucose, electrolytes, and urea nitrogen, a complete blood count (CBC), and hepatic enzyme studies are monitored three times each week until stable and then weekly as the patient's condition warrants. Monitoring of these important values assists the nurse in assessing the patient's tolerance of PN.

When the catheter is removed, the dressing should be changed daily until the wound heals. Oral nourishment should be encouraged, and a careful record of intake should be maintained.

Additional information related to the nursing management of PN is presented in NCP 40-2 for the patient receiving parenteral nutrition, Lewis and others, *Medical-Surgical Nursing,* edition 7, p. 968.

TRACHEOSTOMY

Description

A *tracheotomy* is a surgical incision into the trachea for the purpose of establishing an airway. A *tracheostomy* is the stoma (opening) that results from a tracheotomy. Previously, a tracheostomy required surgical dissection and was therefore not typically an emergency procedure. A newer procedure, a *percutaneous tracheostomy,* can be performed emergently at the bedside, and has been reported to be a valid alternative to a surgically inserted tracheostomy.

Indications for tracheostomy are to bypass an upper airway obstruction, facilitate the removal of secretions, permit long-term mechanical ventilation, and permit oral intake and speech in the patient requiring long-term mechanical ventilation. When compared with endotracheal tubes, tracheostomies have the following advantages:

- There is less risk of long-term damage to the airway.
- Patient comfort is increased because no tube is present in the mouth.

- The patient can eat with a tracheostomy because the tube enters lower in the airway.
- Because the tube is more secure, patient mobility is increased.

When the patient can adequately exchange air and expectorate secretions, the tracheostomy tube can be removed. The stoma is closed with tape strips and covered with an occlusive dressing. The patient should be instructed to splint the stoma with the fingers when coughing, swallowing, or speaking.

- Epithelial tissue begins to form in 24 to 48 hours, and the opening closes in several days. Surgical intervention to close a tracheostomy is not required.

Nursing Management

Goals

The patient with a tracheostomy will communicate needs, maintain a patent airway, have a normal white blood cell (WBC) count and temperature, have his or her usual appetite with a normal body weight maintained, and have a normal swallowing function.

See NCP 27-1 for the patient with a tracheostomy, Lewis and others, *Medical-Surgical Nursing,* edition 7, pp. 548 to 549.

Nursing Diagnoses

- Ineffective airway clearance
- Impaired verbal communication
- Risk for infection
- Imbalanced nutrition: less than body requirements
- Impaired swallowing
- Ineffective therapeutic regimen management

Nursing Interventions

Before the tracheotomy, the nurse should explain to the patient and family the purpose of the procedure and inform them that the patient will not be able to speak if an inflated cuff is used. A variety of tubes are available to meet patient needs (Fig. 22). Characteristics and nursing management of tracheostomies are described in Table 27-5, Lewis and others, *Medical-Surgical Nursing,* edition 7, p. 544.

Care should be taken not to dislodge the tracheostomy tube during the first few days when the stoma is not mature (healed).

- Retention sutures are often placed in the tracheal cartilage when the tracheotomy is performed. The free ends should be taped to the skin in a place and manner that leaves them accessible if the tube is dislodged.
- Because tube replacement can be difficult, several precautions are required: (1) a replacement tube of equal or smaller

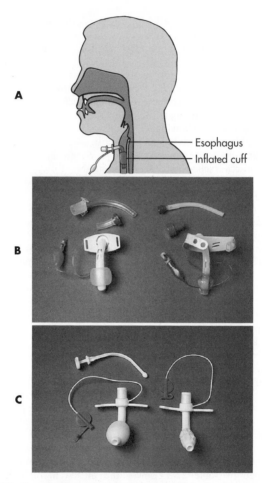

Fig. 22. Types of tracheostomy tubes. **A,** Tracheostomy tube
inserted in airway with inflated cuff. **B,** Shiley and Portex fenestrated
tracheostomy tubes with cuff, inner cannula, decannulation plug, and
pilot balloon. **C,** Bivona (Fome-cuff) tracheostomy tube with foam
cuff and obturator (one cuff is deflated on tracheostomy tube). (See
Table 27-5 and NCP 27-1 in Lewis and others, *Medical-Surgical
Nursing*, edition 7, for related nursing management.)

size is kept at the bedside, readily available for emergency reinsertion, (2) the first tube change is performed by a physician, usually no sooner than 7 days after the tracheotomy, and (3) tracheostomy tapes are not changed for at least 24 hours after the insertion procedure.

- If the tube is accidentally dislodged, the nurse should immediately attempt to replace it. See the discussion of tube replacement techniques on p. 547 of Lewis and others, *Medical-Surgical Nursing,* edition 7.

Care of the patient with a tracheostomy involves suctioning the airway to remove secretions, cleaning around the stoma, changing tracheostomy ties, and inner cannula care if a nondisposable inner cannula is used. See Table 102 for a detailed description of tracheostomy care.

▼ **Patient and Family Teaching**

- Assess ability of the patient and family to provide care at home, and include instructions for tracheostomy tube care, stoma care, suctioning, airway care, and responding to emergencies.
- Make a referral to a home health care nurse to provide ongoing assistance and support.
- Teach patient and family the signs and symptoms to report to health care professionals, such as changes in secretions (color and consistency) and elevated temperature.

Table 102	Tracheostomy Care

1. Explain procedure to patient.
2. Use tracheostomy care kit, or collect necessary sterile equipment (e.g., suction catheter, gloves, water, basin, drape, tracheostomy ties, tube brush or pipe cleaners, 4×4s, hydrogen peroxide [3%], sterile water, and tracheostomy dressing [optional]). NOTE: Clean rather than sterile technique is used at home.
3. Position patient in semi-Fowler's position.
4. Assemble needed materials on bedside table next to patient.
5. Wash hands. Put on goggles and clean gloves.
6. Auscultate chest sounds. If rhonchi or coarse crackles are present, suction the patient if unable to cough up secretions. Remove soiled dressing and clean gloves.
7. Open sterile equipment, pour sterile H_2O and H_2O_2 in basins, and put on sterile gloves.

Continued

Table 102	Tracheostomy Care—cont'd

8. Unlock and remove inner cannula, if present. Many tracheostomy tubes do not have inner cannulas. Care for these tubes includes all steps except for inner cannula care.
9. If disposable inner cannula is used, replace with new cannula. If a nondisposable cannula is used:
   a. Immerse inner cannula in 3% hydrogen peroxide, and clean inside and outside of cannula using tube brush or pipe cleaners.
   b. Drain hydrogen peroxide from cannula. Immerse cannula in sterile water. Remove from sterile water, and shake to dry.
   c. Insert inner cannula into outer cannula with the curved part downward, and lock in place.
10. Remove dried secretions from stoma using 4 × 4 soaked in hydrogen peroxide. Rinse with another 4 × 4 soaked in sterile water. Gently pat area around the stoma dry. Be sure to clean under the tracheostomy face plate, using cotton swabs to reach this area.
11. Maintain position of tracheal retention sutures, if present, by taping above and below the stoma.
12. Change tracheostomy ties. Use a two-person change technique, or secure new ties to flanges before removing the old ones. Tie tracheostomy ties securely with room for one finger between ties and skin. To prevent accidental tube removal, secure the tracheostomy tube by gently applying pressure to flange of the tube during the tie changes. Do not change tracheostomy ties for 24 hr after the tracheotomy procedure.
13. As an alternative, some patients prefer tracheostomy ties made of Velcro, which are easier to adjust.
14. If drainage is excessive, place dressing around tube. A tracheostomy dressing or unlined gauze should be used. Do not cut the gauze because threads may be inhaled or wrap around the tracheostomy tube. Change the dressing frequently. Wet dressings promote infection and stoma irritation.
15. Repeat care three times per day and as needed.

TUBE FEEDING

Tube feeding refers to the administration of a nutritionally balanced liquefied food or formula through a tube inserted into the stomach, duodenum, or jejunum.

Indications for tube feedings as a supplemental form of nutrition include:

- The patient who has a functioning gastrointestinal (GI) tract but cannot take oral nourishment
- Persons with anorexia, orofacial fractures, head and neck cancer, neurologic or psychiatric conditions that prevent oral intake, or extensive burns, or those who are receiving chemotherapy or radiation therapy

Tube feedings are easily administered, safer, more physiologically efficient, and definitely less expensive than parenteral nutrition. Enteral nutrition is used to provide nutrients by way of the GI tract either alone or as a supplement to oral or parenteral nutrition.

Types of commonly used enteral feeding tubes (Fig. 23) include:

- Nastrogastric (NG) tube, which is most commonly used for short-term feeding problems
- Esophagostomy, gastrostomy, or jejunostomy tubes for feeding over an extended time
- Transpyloric (nasointestinal) tube placement used for feeding below the pyloric sphincter

Common delivery options are continuous infusion by pump, intermittent by gravity, intermittent bolus by syringe, and cyclic feedings by infusion pump.

The standard procedure for administration of tube feeding includes (1) having the patient sitting or lying with the head of the bed elevated 30 to 45 degrees; (2) maintaining tube patency by irrigating before and after each feeding; if feedings are continuous, monitoring the built-in alarm on the feeding pump to detect occlusions; and (3) checking proper tube placement and gastric residual volumes before each feeding or every 8 hours with continuous feedings. Feedings should be given at room or body temperature to decrease the likelihood of diarrhea and other GI complaints.

Commercial formulas are preferable to blenderized foods for small-lumen tubes because of the risk of tube clogging, completeness of nutrition, and decreased risk of formula contamination.

Nursing considerations include the following:

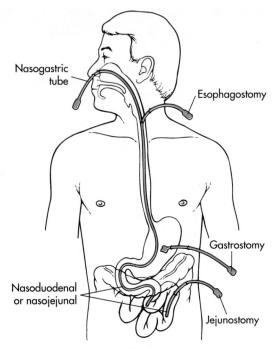

Fig. 23. Common placement locations for enteral feeding tubes.

- Weigh the patient daily or several times per week, and maintain accurate intake and output records.
- Assess for bowel sounds before feeding.
- Check an initial blood glucose level to assess glucose tolerance.
- Discard feedings that have been opened and not refrigerated or feedings that have been infusing longer than 8 hours to minimize bacterial growth.
- Label feedings with the date and time they are initially used.
- If a pump is being used, change the tubing every 24 hours.
- Assess regularly for complications (e.g., aspiration, diarrhea, abdominal distention, hyperglycemia, constipation, fecal impaction).

The types of problems encountered in patients receiving tube feedings and corrective measures are presented in Table

40-17, Lewis and others, *Medical-Surgical Nursing,* edition 7, p. 964.

URINARY CATHETERIZATION

Indications for urinary catheterization are listed in Table 103. Two reasons that *are not* indications for catheterization are (1) the routine acquisition of a urine specimen for laboratory analysis and (2) the convenience of the nursing staff or the patient's family.

- The risks of complications and nosocomial infection are too high to allow catheterization of the patient for convenience.
- Complications of long-term use of indwelling catheters include bladder spasms, periurethral abscess, pain, urinary tract infections (UTIs), urosepsis, urethral trauma/erosion, fistula/stricture formation, and renal stones.

Table 103	Indications for Urinary Catheterization

Indwelling Catheter
1. Relief of urinary retention caused by lower urinary tract obstruction, paralysis, or inability to void
2. Bladder decompression preoperatively and postoperatively for lower abdominal or pelvic surgery
3. Facilitation of surgical repair of urethra and surrounding structures
4. Splinting of ureters or urethra to facilitate healing after surgery or other trauma in area
5. Accurate measurement of urinary output in critically ill patient
6. Measurement of residual urine after urination (referred to as postvoid residual [PVR]) if ultrasound not available
7. Contamination of stage III or IV pressure ulcers with urine that has impeded healing, despite appropriate personal care for incontinence
8. Terminal illness or severe impairment that makes positioning or clothing changes uncomfortable or that is associated with intractable pain

Straight (In and Out) Catheter
1. Study of anatomic structures of urinary system
2. Urodynamic testing
3. Collection of sterile urine sample in selected situations
4. Installation of medications into bladder

U

Catheterization for sterile urine specimens may occasionally be indicated when patients have a history of complicated urinary infections. A catheter should be the last means of providing the patient with a dry environment for the prevention of skin breakdown and protection of dressings or skin lesions.

Scrupulous aseptic technique is mandatory when a urinary catheter is inserted. After insertion, nursing responsibilities include maintaining catheter patency, managing fluid intake, providing for the comfort and safety of the patient, and preventing infection. Concerns of the patient can include embarrassment related to exposure of the body, an altered body image, and fear concerning the care of the catheter that results in increased dependency.

- Catheters vary in construction materials, tip shape, and lumen size. Catheters are sized according to the French scale. Each French unit equals 0.33 mm of diameter. The diameter measured is the internal diameter of the catheter. The size used varies with the size of the individual and the purpose for catheterization.

- The most common route of catheterization is insertion of the catheter through the external meatus into the urethra, past the internal sphincter, and into the bladder.

Suprapubic catheterization is the simplest and oldest method of urinary diversion. The two methods of insertion of a suprapubic catheter into the bladder are (1) through a small incision in the abdominal wall and (2) by the use of a trocar. A suprapubic catheter is placed while the patient is under general anesthesia for another surgical procedure or at the bedside with a local anesthetic. The catheter may be sutured into place.

- The suprapubic catheter is used in temporary situations, such as bladder, prostate, and urethral surgery, and also used long term in selected patients.

- Nursing care includes taping the catheter to prevent dislodgement. The care of the tube and catheter is similar to that of the urethral catheter. A pectin-base skin barrier (e.g., Stomahesive) is effective around the insertion site in protecting the skin from breakdown.

The suprapubic catheter is prone to poor drainage because of mechanical obstruction of the catheter tip by the bladder wall, sediment, and clots. Nursing interventions to ensure the patency of the tube include (1) preventing tube kinking by coiling the excess tubing and maintaining gravity drainage, (2) having the patient turn from side to side, and (3) milking the tube. If these measures are not effective, the catheter is irrigated with sterile technique after a physician's order has been obtained.

- If the patient experiences bladder spasms that are difficult to control, urinary leakage may result. Oxybutynin (Ditropan) or other oral antispasmodics or belladonna and opium (B&O) suppositories may be prescribed to decrease bladder spasms.

An alternative approach to a long-term indwelling catheter is *intermittent catheterization,* also referred to as "straight" or "in and out" catheterization. It is being used with increasing frequency in conditions characterized by neurogenic bladder (e.g., spinal cord injuries, chronic neurologic diseases) or bladder outlet obstruction in men. This type of catheterization may also be used in the oliguric and anuric phases of acute renal failure to reduce the possibility of infection from an indwelling catheter. Intermittent catheterization is also used postoperatively, often after a surgical procedure for female incontinence or following radioactive seed implantation into the prostate.

- The main goal of intermittent catheterization is to prevent urinary retention, stasis, and compromised blood supply to the bladder resulting from prolonged pressure.
- The technique consists of inserting a urethral catheter into the bladder every 3 to 5 hours. Some patients do intermittent catheterization only once or twice each day to measure residual urine and to ensure an empty bladder.
- Patients should be instructed to wash and rinse the catheter and their hands with soap and water before and after catheterization. Lubricant is necessary for men and may make catheterization more comfortable for women.
- The catheter may be inserted by the patient or a care provider. The bladder is emptied, and the catheter is removed.
- Some catheters are single use, but others can be used multiple times.
- When a catheter is reused, it can be dried and placed in a pouch or purse or folded in a paper towel until it is next needed. In general, patients should change the catheter every 7 days.
- In the hospital, sterile technique is used for all urinary catheterizations. For home care, a clean technique that includes good hand washing with soap and water is used.
- The patient is taught to observe for signs of UTI so that treatment can be instituted early. If indicated, some patients are placed on a regimen of prophylactic antibiotics.

PART THREE

Reference Appendix

ABBREVIATIONS

µg*	microgram
µm	micrometer
@	at
ABG	arterial blood gas
ac	before meals
ad lib	freely as desired
ADL	activity of daily living
AIDS	acquired immunodeficiency syndrome
ALS	amyotrophic lateral sclerosis
AM	morning
a.m.a.	against medical advice
AMI	acute myocardial infarction
amp	ampule
ARDS	acute respiratory distress syndrome
BE	barium enema
bid, BID	twice a day
BM, bm	bowel movement
BMR	basal metabolic rate
BP	blood pressure
BPH	benign prostatic hyperplasia
BRP	bathroom privileges
BUN	blood urea nitrogen
c̄	with
c/o	complains of
Ca	calcium, cancer, carcinoma
CAD	coronary artery disease
cap	capsule
cath	catheter, catheterize
CBC	complete blood count
CBR	complete bed rest
CC	chief complaint
cc*	cubic centimeter
CCU	coronary care unit, critical care unit
CDC	Centers for Disease Control and Prevention
CEA	carcinoembryonic antigen
HF	heart failure
CHO	carbohydrate

From Potter PA, Perry AG: *Fundamentals of nursing*, ed 6, St Louis, 2005, Mosby.
Abbreviations in common use can vary widely from place to place. Each institution's list of acceptable abbreviations is the best authority for its records.
*NOTE: See the "prohibited abbreviations" and additional policies concerning the use of abbreviations identified by the Joint Commission on Accreditation for Healthcare Organizations effective January 1, 2004 at the end of this list of abbreviations.

ABBREVIATIONS—cont'd

Cl	chlorine, chloride
cm	centimeter
cm^3	cubic centimeter
CNS	central nervous system
CO	carbon monoxide; cardiac output
CO_2	carbon dioxide
COPD	chronic obstructive pulmonary disease
CPR	cardiopulmonary resuscitation
CSF	cerebrospinal fluid
CT	computed tomography
CVA	cerebrovascular accident, costovertebral angle
CVP	central venous pressure
D&C	dilation and curettage
D5W	5% dextrose in water
db, dB	decibels
dc, D/C*	discontinue
DIC	disseminated intravascular coagulation
diff	differential blood count
DJD	degenerative joint disease
dl	deciliter
DNR	do not resuscitate
DOE	dyspnea on exertion
dx, DX	diagnosis
EBV	Epstein-Barr virus
ECF	extracellular fluid
ECG	electrocardiogram
ED	emergency department
EEG	electroencephalogram
elix	elixir
EMG	electromyogram
ESR	erythrocyte sedimentation rate
ESRD	end-stage renal disease
f℥	fluid ounce
Fe	iron
FEV	forced expiratory volume
FRC	functional residual capacity
FUO	fever of unknown origin
Fx, fx	fracture, fractional urine test
g, gm, Gm	gram (gm and Gm are not preferred)
GI	gastrointestinal
gr	grain
gt, gtt	drop, drops
GTT	glucose tolerance test
GU	genitourinary
GYN, Gyn	gynecologic

Continued

ABBREVIATIONS—cont'd

H_2O	water
hr	hour
H^+	hydrogen ion
h/o	history of
H&P	history and physical examination
HAV	hepatitis A virus
Hb, Hgb	hemoglobin
HBV	hepatitis B virus
Hct, HCT	hematocrit
Hg	mercury
Hb, Hgb	hemoglobin
HIV	human immunodeficiency virus
HLA	human leukocyte antigen
hs*	at bedtime (hour of sleep)
HSV	herpes simplex virus
I&O	intake and output
ICP	intracranial pressure
ICU	intensive care unit
Ig	immunoglobulin
IM	intramuscular
IOP	intraocular pressure
IPPB	intermittent positive pressure breathing
IV	intravenous
IVP	intravenous push, intravenous pyelogram
IVPB	IV piggyback
K	potassium
kg	kilogram
KUB	kidney, ureters, and bladder (x-ray)
KVO	keep vein open
L	liter
L&A	light and accommodation
LBBB	left bundle branch block
LE	lupus erythematosus
LLL	left lower lobe
LLQ	left lower quadrant
LMP	last menstrual period
LP	lumbar puncture
LUL	left upper lobe
LUQ	left upper quadrant
LVH	left ventricular hypertrophy
m	meter
m, min	minim, minute
MAP	mean arterial pressure
mcg	microgram
MCH	mean corpuscular hemoglobin
MCHC	mean corpuscular hemoglobin concentration

ABBREVIATIONS—cont'd

MCV	mean cell volume, mean corpuscular volume
mEq	milliequivalent
mg	milligram
Mg	magnesium
MG	myasthenia gravis
MI	myocardial infarction
MICU	medical intensive care unit
ml	milliliter
mm	millimeter
mm^3	cubic millimeter
mm Hg	millimeters of mercury
MRI	magnetic resonance imaging
MS	multiple sclerosis
N	nitrogen
Na	sodium
NIH	National Institutes of Health
nm	nanometer
NPO	nothing by mouth
NS	normal saline
O_2	oxygen
OD	right eye, optical density, overdose
OOB	out of bed
ORIF	open reduction and internal fixation
OS	left eye
OT	occupational therapy
OTC	over-the-counter
OU	both eyes
oz	ounce
$PaCO_2$	partial pressure of carbon dioxide in arterial blood
PaO_2	partial pressure of oxygen in arterial blood
PAWP	pulmonary artery wedge pressure
pc	after meals
PE	pulmonary embolism, physical examination
PEEP	positive end-expiratory pressure
per	through, by way of
PERRLA	pupils equal, round, and reactive to light and accommodation
PET	positron emission tomography
PG	prostaglandin
pH	hydrogen ion concentration
PID	pelvic inflammatory disease
PM	evening
PMS	premenstrual syndrome
PN	parenteral nutrition

Continued

ABBREVIATIONS—cont'd

PND	paroxysmal nocturnal dyspnea
PO, po	orally
PPD	purified protein derivative
prn	when required, as often as necessary
PT	physical therapy; prothrombin time
PTT	partial thromboplastin time
PVC	premature ventricular contraction
q	every
q2hr	every 2 hours
q3hr	every 3 hours
q4hr	every 4 hours
qhr	every hour
qid, QID	four times a day
R/O	rule out
RA	rheumatoid arthritis
RBBB	right bundle branch block
RDA	recommended daily (dietary) allowance
Rh^+	positive Rh factor
Rh^-	negative Rh factor
RLL	right lower lobe
RLQ	right lower quadrant
ROM	range of motion
ROS	review of systems
RUL	right upper lobe
RUQ	right upper quadrant
$\bar{s}$	without
SICU	surgical intensive care unit
SLE	systemic lupus erythematosus
sol	solution, dissolved
sos	if necessary
sp gr, SG, sg	specific gravity
SQ, subq, SC*	subcutaneous
ss	half
stat, STAT	immediately
STD	sexually transmitted disease
susp	suspension
T&A	tonsillectomy and adenoidectomy
TAH	total abdominal hysterectomy
TB	tuberculosis
TBG	thyroxin-binding globulin
TIA	transient ischemic attack
TIBC	total iron-binding capacity
tid, TID	three times a day
TKO	to keep open
TLC	total lung capacity
TPR	temperature, pulse, and respirations

ABBREVIATIONS—cont'd

tr, tinct	tincture
URI	upper respiratory infection
UTI	urinary tract infection
VC	vital capacity
VD	venereal disease
VDRL	Venereal Disease Research Laboratory (test for syphilis)
VS	vital signs
V_T	tidal volume
WBC	white blood cell
WNL	within normal limits

OFFICIAL "DO NOT USE" ABBREVIATIONS*
**(Identified by the Joint Commission on Accreditation for
Healthcare Organizations effective
January 1, 2004)**

Abbreviation	Preferred Term
U (for unit)	Write "unit"
IU (for international unit)	Write "international unit"
QD and QOD	Write "daily" and "every other day"
Trailing zero (X.0)	Never write zero by itself after a decimal point; always use a zero before a decimal point (0.X mg)

* In addition, each health care organization must identify and apply at least another three "do not use" abbreviations, acronyms, or symbols of its own choosing. Items that should be considered when identifying additional items include:

Abbreviation	Preferred Term
μg (for microgram)	Write "mcg"
HS or hs (for bedtime or half-strength)	Write "at bedtime" or "half-strength"
TIW (for three times per week)	Write "3 times weekly" or "three times weekly"
SC or SQ (for subcutaneous)	Write "Sub-Q," "subQ," or "subcutaneously"
D/C (for discharge)	Write "discharge"
cc (for cubic centimeter)	Write "ml" for milliliters
AS, AD, AU (left, right, or both ears)	Write "left ear," "right ear," or "both ears"

BLOOD GASES
Normal Values

	Arterial (Sea Level)	Venous
pH	7.35-7.45	7.35-7.45
PaO_2*	80-100 mm Hg	40-50 mm Hg
$PaCO_2$	35-45 mm Hg	40-45 mm Hg
HCO_3	22-26 mEq/L	22-26 mEq/L
O_2 saturation	96%-100%	60%-85%
Base excess	± 2.0 mEq/L	± 2.0 mEq/L

* In a patient >60 years old, PaO_2 is equal to 80 mm Hg minus 1 mm Hg for every year over 60. Expected $PaO_2 = FIO_2 \times 5$.

Interpreting Arterial Blood Gases (ABGs)

1. Check pH

   $\uparrow$ = Alkalosis; $\downarrow$ = acidosis

2. Check $PaCO_2$

   $\uparrow$ = CO_2 retention (hypoventilation); respiratory acidosis or compensating for metabolic alkalosis
   $\downarrow$ = CO_2 blown off (hyperventilation); respiratory alkalosis or compensating for metabolic acidosis

3. Check HCO_3

   $\uparrow$ = Nonvolatile acid is lost; HCO_3 gained (metabolic alkalosis or compensating for respiratory acidosis)
   $\downarrow$ = Nonvolatile acid is added; HCO_3 is lost (metabolic acidosis or compensating for respiratory alkalosis)

4. Determine imbalance
5. Determine if compensation exists

Determining the Imbalance in ABGs

If:	Then
If: pH $\uparrow$ and $PaCO_2$ $\downarrow$ or pH $\downarrow$ and $PaCO_2$ $\uparrow$	**Then** respiratory disorder
If: pH $\uparrow$ and HCO_3 $\uparrow$ or pH $\downarrow$ and HCO_3 $\downarrow$	**Then** metabolic disorder
If: $PaCO_2$ $\uparrow$ and HCO_3 $\uparrow$ or $PaCO_2$ $\downarrow$ and HCO_3 $\downarrow$	**Then** compensation is occurring
If: $PaCO_2$ $\uparrow$ and HCO_3 $\downarrow$ or $PaCO_2$ $\downarrow$ and HCO_3 $\uparrow$	**Then** mixed imbalance

BLOOD LABORATORY VALUES

Test	Conventional Units	SI Units
Complete Blood Count		
Red blood cells (RBCs)	$4.5\text{-}6.0 \times 10^6/\mu l$ (males)	$4.5\text{-}6.0 \times 10^{12}/L$
	$4.0\text{-}5.0 \times 10^6/\mu l$ (females)	$4.0\text{-}5.0 \times 10^{12}/L$
White blood cells (WBCs)	$4.0\text{-}11.0 \times 10^3/\mu l$	$4.0\text{-}11.0 \times 10^9/L$
Hemoglobin (Hb)	13.5-18 g/dl (males)	135-180 g/L
	12-16 g/dl (females)	120-160 g/L
Hematocrit (Hct)	40%-51% (males)	0.40-0.51
	38%-44% (females)	0.38-0.44
Chemistry		
Albumin	3.5-5 g/dl	507-725 µmol/L
Alkaline phosphatase	30-120 units/L	0.5-2.0 µkat/L
Alanine aminotransferase (ALT)	5-36 units/L	0.08-0.6 µkat/L
Ammonia	30-70 mcg/dl	17.6-41.1 µmol/L
Amylase	0-130 units/L	0-2.17 µkat/L
Aspartate aminotransferase (AST)	7-40 units/L	0.12-0.67 µkat/L
Bilirubin		
Total	0.2-1.3 mg/dl	3.4-22.0 µmol/L
Direct	0.1-0.3 mg/dl	1.7-5.1 µmol/L
Indirect	0.1-1.0 mg/dl	1.7-17 µmol/L
Blood urea nitrogen (BUN)	10-30 mg/dl	1.8-7.1 mmol/L
BUN:Cr ratio	10:1-15:1	
Calcium	9-11 mg/dl	2.25-2.74 mmol/L
Cholesterol	140-200 mg/dl	3.6-5.2 mmol/L
HDL	(age dependent)	
	>45 mg/dl (males)	>1.2 mmol/L
	>55 mg/dl (females)	>1.4 mmol/L
LDL	<130 mg/dl	<3.4 mmol/L
Chloride	95-105 mEq/L	95-105 mmol/L
CO_2	20-30 mEq/L	20-30 mmol/L
Creatinine	0.5-1.5 mg/dl	44-133 µmol/L
Glucose	70-120 mg/dl	3.89-6.66 mmol/L
Iron	50-150 mcg/dl	9.0-26.9 µmol/L

aPTT, Activated partial thromboplastin time; *FSP,* fibrin split products; *HDL,* high-density lipoprotein; *LDL,* low-density lipoprotein; *PT,* prothrombin time.

BLOOD LABORATORY VALUES—cont'd

Test	Conventional Units	SI Units
Lactic dehydrogenase (LDH)	50-150 units/L	0.83-2.5 μkat/L
Lipase	0-160 units/L	0-2.66 μkat/L
Magnesium	1.5-2.5 mEq/L	0.75-1.25 mmol/L
Osmolality	285-295 mOsm/kg	285-295 mmol/kg
Phosphorus	2.8-4.5 mg/dl	0.90-1.45 mmol/L
Potassium	3.5-5 mEq/L	3.5-5 mmol/L
Protein	6-8 g/dl	60-80 g/L
Sedimentation rate	<15 mm/hr (males) <20 mm/hr (females)	
Sodium	135-145 mEq/L	135-145 mmol/L
T_3	110-230 ng/dl	1.7-3.5 nmol/L
T_4	5-12 mcg/dl	64-154 nmol/L
Triglyceride	40-150 mg/dl	0.45-1.69 mmol/L
Uric acid	2.5-6.5 mg/dl	149-387 μmol/L
Coagulation		
Platelets	$150\text{-}400 \times 10^3/\mu l$	$150\text{-}400 \times 10^9/L$
PT	10-14 sec	Same as conventional unit
aPTT	30-45 sec	Same as conventional unit
FSP	<10 mg/L	Same as conventional unit

BLOOD PRODUCTS*

Description	Special Considerations	Indications for Use
Packed RBCs Packed RBCs are prepared from whole blood by sedimentation or centrifugation. One unit contains 250-350 ml.	Use of RBCs for treatment allows remaining components of blood (e.g., platelets, albumin, plasma) to be used for other purposes. There is less danger of fluid overload. Packed RBCs are preferred RBC source because they are more component specific.	Severe or symptomatic anemia, acute blood loss. In general, one unit of packed RBCs can be expected to increase a patient's hemoglobin level by 1 g/dl or hematocrit by 30%.
Frozen RBCs Frozen RBCs are prepared from RBCs using glycerol for protection and frozen. They can be stored for 10 yr at $-188.6°$ F ($-87°$ C).	They must be used within 24 hr of thawing. Successive washings with saline solution remove majority of WBCs and plasma proteins.	Autotransfusion; stockpiling or rare donors for patients with alloantibodies. Infrequently used because filters remove most WBCs.
Platelets Platelets are prepared from fresh whole blood within 4 hr after collection. One unit contains 30-60 ml of platelet concentrate.	Multiple units of platelets can be obtained from one donor by plateletpheresis. They can be kept at room temperature for 1-5 days. Bag should be agitated periodically. Expected increase is 10,000/µl/unit. Failure to have a rise may be due to fever, sepsis, splenomegaly, or DIC.	Bleeding caused by thrombocytopenia, platelet levels <10,000-20,000/µl (<10-20×10^9/L); may be contraindicated in immune or thrombotic thrombocytopenic purpura and heparin-induced thrombocytopenia except in life-threatening hemorrhage.

Fresh-Frozen Plasma

Liquid portion of whole blood is separated from cells and frozen. One unit contains 200-250 ml.

Plasma is rich in clotting factors but contains no platelets. It may be stored for 1 yr. It must be used within 2 hr after thawing.

Use of plasma in treating hypovolemic shock is being replaced by pure preparations, such as albumin plasma expanders.

Bleeding caused by deficiency in clotting factors (e.g., DIC, hemorrhage, massive transfusion, liver disease, vitamin K deficiency, excess warfarin).

Albumin

Albumin is prepared from plasma. It can be stored for 5 yr. It is available in 5% or 25% solution.

Albumin, 25 g/100 ml, is osmotically equal to 500 ml of plasma. Hyperosmolar solution acts by moving water from extravascular to intravascular space. It is heat treated and does not transmit viruses.

Hypovolemic shock, hypoalbuminemia.

Cryoprecipitates and Commercial Concentrates

Cryoprecipitate is prepared from fresh frozen plasma. It can be stored for 1 yr. Once thawed, must be used.

See Table 31-18 in Lewis and others: Medical-Surgical Nursing, edition 7.

Replacement of clotting factors, especially factor VIII, von Willebrand's disease, and fibrinogen.

DIC, Disseminated intravascular coagulation; RBCs, red blood cells; WBCs, white blood cells.
*Component therapy has replaced the use of whole blood, which accounts for less than 10% of all transfusions. Granulocyte transfusions are not included here because they are rarely used.

BREATH SOUNDS
Normal Sounds

Type	Normal Site	Duration, I/E ratio	Characteristics
Vesicular	Peripheral lung	I > E 3:1	Soft, low-pitched, gentle, rustling sounds; heard over all lung areas except major bronchi; abnormal when heard over the large airways
Bronchovesicular	Sternal border of the major bronchi	I = E 1:1	Medium pitch and intensity; heard anteriorly over the mainstem bronchi on either side of the sternum and posteriorly between the scapulae; abnormal if heard over peripheral lung fields
Bronchial	Trachea and bronchi	I < E 2:3	Louder, higher pitched; resembles air blowing through a hollow pipe; abnormal if heard over peripheral lung

E, Expiration; *I*, inspiration.

BREATH SOUNDS—cont'd
Adventitious Sounds

Characteristics	Possible Clinical Condition
Fine crackles Series of short-duration, discontinuous, high-pitched sounds heard just before the end of inspiration; similar sound to that made by rolling hair between fingers just behind ear	Idiopathic pulmonary fibrosis, interstitial edema (early pulmonary edema), alveolar filling (pneumonia), loss of lung volume (atelectasis), early phase of heart failure
Coarse crackles Series of long-duration, discontinuous, low-pitched sounds caused by air passing through airway intermittently occluded by mucus, unstable bronchial wall, or fold of mucosa; evident on inspiration and, at times, expiration	Heart failure, pulmonary edema, pneumonia with severe congestion, chronic obstructive pulmonary disease (COPD)
Rhonchi Continuous rumbling, snoring, or rattling sounds from obstruction of large airways with secretions; most prominent on expiration	COPD, cystic fibrosis, pneumonia, bronchiectasis
Wheezes Continuous high-pitched squeaking or musical sound caused by rapid vibration of bronchial walls; first evident on expiration but possibly evident on inspiration as obstruction of airway increases	Bronchospasm (caused by asthma), airway obstruction (caused by foreign body, tumor), COPD
Pleural friction rub Creaking or grating sound from roughened, inflamed surfaces of the pleura rubbing together; evident during inspiration, expiration, or both	Pleurisy, pneumonia, pulmonary infarct

CANCER SCREENING GUIDELINES FOR EARLY DETECTION OF CANCER IN ASYMPTOMATIC PEOPLE*

Site	Recommendation
Breast	Women 40 yr and older should have an annual mammogram and an annual clinical breast examination (CBE) by a health care provider. Women aged 20-39 yr should have a CBE by a health care provider every 3 yr. A monthly breast self-examination (BSE) is an option for women starting in their 20s. Women at increased risk should talk to their health care provider about more intensive screening.
Colon and rectum	Beginning at age 50 yr, men and women should follow ONE of the examination schedules below: • Yearly fecal occult blood (FOBT)[†] or fecal immunochemical test (FIT) • Flexible sigmoidoscopy (FSIG) every 5 yr • Yearly FOBT[†] or FIT plus flexible sigmoidoscopy every 5 yr[‡] • Double-contrast barium enema every 5 yr • Colonoscopy every 10 yr
Prostate	Both the prostate-specific antigen (PSA) blood test and digital rectal examination (DRE) should be offered annually, beginning at age 50 yr, to men who have at least a 10-yr life expectancy. Men at high risk (African American men and men with a strong family history of one or more first-degree relatives [father, brothers] diagnosed at an early age) should begin testing at age 45 yr. For both men at average risk and men at high risk, information should be provided to patients about what is known and what is uncertain about the benefits and limitations of early detection and treatment of prostate cancer so that they can make an informed decision about testing.

From *Cancer facts and figures,* Atlanta, 2006, American Cancer Society.
* These recommendations are for people at average risk for cancer. People at increased risk may need to follow a different screening schedule, such as starting at an earlier age or being screened more often.
[†]For FOBT, the take-home multiple sample method should be used.
[‡]The combination of yearly FOBT or FIT plus flexible sigmoidoscopy every 5 yr is preferred over either of these options alone.

**CANCER SCREENING GUIDELINES FOR EARLY DETECTION OF
CANCER IN ASYMPTOMATIC PEOPLE—cont'd**

Site	Recommendation
Uterus	*Cervix:* Screening beginning 3 yr after having vaginal intercourse but no later than 21 yr of age. Conventional Pap test should be performed annually or every 2 yr using liquid-based tests. ■ Beginning at age 30 yr, women who have had three normal Pap test results in a row may get screened every 2-3 yr with either the conventional or liquid- based Pap test. Alternatively, cervical cancer screening with HPV DNA testing and conventional or liquid-based cytology could be performed every 3 yr. ■ Women 70 yr of age or older who have had three or more normal Pap tests in a row and no abnormal Pap test results in the last 10 yr may choose to stop having cervical cancer screening. ■ Women who have had a total hysterectomy may also choose to stop having cervical cancer screening, unless the surgery was done as a treatment for cervical cancer. *Endometrium:* At the time of menopause all women should be informed about the risks and symptoms of endometrial cancer and strongly encouraged to report any unexpected bleeding or spotting to their health care providers. For women with or at high risk for hereditary nonpolyposis colon cancer, annual screening should be offered for endometrial cancer with endometrial biopsy beginning at age 35 yr.
Cancer-related checkup	For individuals undergoing periodic health examinations, a cancer-related checkup should include health counseling and, depending on a person's age and gender, might include examinations for cancers of thyroid, oral cavity, skin, lymph nodes, testes, and ovaries, as well as some nonmalignant diseases.

COMMONLY USED FORMULAS

Parameter	Formula	Normal Range
Anion gap	$Na - (HCO_3 + Cl)$	8-16 mEq/L
Body mass index (BMI)	$\dfrac{\text{Weight in pounds}}{\text{Height in inches}^2} \times 703$	18.5-24.9 kg/m²
Cardiac index (CI)	CO/Body surface area (BSA)	2.2-4.0 L/min/m²
Cardiac output (CO)	$HR \times SV$	4-8 L/min
Cerebral perfusion pressure (CPP)	MAP−ICP	80-100 mm Hg
Ejection fraction (EF)	$\dfrac{SV}{\text{End-diastolic volume}} \times 100$	60% or greater
Heart rate (HR)		60-80 beats/min
Mean arterial pressure (MAP)	$\dfrac{2(DBP) + SBP}{3}$	70-105 mm Hg
Pulmonary vascular resistance (PVR)	$\dfrac{PAMP - PAWP}{CO} \times 80$	<250 dynes/sec/cm⁻⁵

Pulmonary vascular resistance index (PVRI)	$\dfrac{PAMP - PAWP}{CI} \times 80$	160-380 dynes/sec/cm^{-5}/m^2
Stroke volume (SV)	$\dfrac{CO}{HR}$	60-150 ml/beat
Stroke volume index (SVI)	$\dfrac{CI}{HR}$	30-65 ml/beat/m^2
Systemic vascular resistance (SVR)	$\dfrac{MAP - CVP}{CO} \times 80$	800-1200 dyne sec/cm^5
Systemic vascular resistance index (SVRI)	$\dfrac{MAP - CVP}{CI} \times 80$	1970-2390 dyne sec m^2/cm^5

DBP, Diastolic blood pressure; *ICP*, intracranial pressure; *PAMP*, pulmonary artery mean pressure; *PAWP*, pulmonary artery wedge pressure; *SBP*, systolic blood pressure.

COMMONLY USED HERBS*

Name	Examples of Common Uses	Comments
Aloe	Constipation[†] Genital herpes, psoriasis vulgaris[‡]	Use no longer than 7 days for constipation May cause electrolyte imbalances
Bilberry	Cataracts, retinopathy,[§] peripheral vascular disease[§] Varicose veins[§] Diabetes mellitus[§]	May lower blood glucose May lower blood glucose May increase risk of bleeding
Black cohosh	Menopausal symptoms[‡]	Generally safe when used for up to 6 mo in healthy, nonpregnant women
Chamomile	Common cold[§] Gastrointestinal disorders[§] Sleep aid/sedation[§]	Contraindicated with known sensitivity to members of the ragweed family May cause drowsiness May increase risk of bleeding
Echinacea	Treatment of upper respiratory infections[†] Prevention of upper respiratory infections[§] Immune system stimulation[§]	Use with caution in patients with conditions affecting the immune system May lead to liver inflammation Short-term use (10-14 days) recommended
Evening primrose	Eczema, skin irritation[‡]	Contraindicated in individuals with seizure disorders
Feverfew	Migraine headache prevention[†] Rheumatoid arthritis[§]	May increase risk of bleeding Long-term users may experience withdrawal symptoms
Garlic	Hyperlipidemia[‡] Hypertension[§]	Use with caution in patients with bleeding disorders Do not use in large amounts

Ginger	Nausea and vomiting of pregnancy[†] Nausea and vomiting (postoperative or chemotherapy induced)[§] Motion sickness[§]	Use with caution in patients with bleeding disorders Use in pregnancy should not exceed 1 g/day Supervision by health care provider recommended for pregnant women considering use of ginger Generally well tolerated in recommended dosages for up to 6 mo
Ginkgo biloba	Claudication (peripheral vascular disease)[†] Dementia treatment (multi-infarct and Alzheimer's type)[†] Cerebral insufficiency[‡]	May increase risk of bleeding May affect blood glucose
Ginseng (*Panax* species, including Asian and American ginseng)	Improve mental performance[‡] Lower blood glucose in type 2 diabetes mellitus[‡]	Use with caution in diabetic patients Use with caution in patients taking medications, herbs, supplements that affect blood pressure (BP) or heart rhythm
Goldenseal	Heart failure[§] Immunostimulant[§] Infectious diarrhea[§] Upper respiratory tract infection[§]	Generally safe when used for up to 3 mo Should not be used for longer than 2-3 wk Use with caution in patients with cardiovascular disease May increase risk of bleeding
Hawthorn	Heart failure[†] Coronary artery disease[§]	May have additive effect with digoxin or with medications that lower BP

Continued

From Ulbricht CE, Basch EM: *Natural standard herb and supplement reference: evidence-based clinical reviews,* St Louis, 2005, Mosby. Available at www.naturalstandard.com

* Advise patients who are pregnant or lactating to consult a health care practitioner before using any herbs. There is limited scientific evidence for the use of most herbs during pregnancy or lactation.
[†]Strong scientific evidence exists for this use.
[‡]Good scientific evidence exists for this use.
[§]Unclear scientific evidence exists for this use.

COMMONLY USED HERBS—cont'd

Name	Examples of Common Uses	Comments
Kava	Anxiety[†]	Should be used only under the supervision of a health care practitioner
Milk thistle	Hepatitis (chronic)[‡] Cirrhosis[‡]	May cause hepatotoxicity May increase risk of bleeding Generally safe in recommended dosages for up to 4-6 yr Use with caution in diabetic patients
Peppermint	Antispasmodic (gastric spasm)[§] Indigestion[§] Irritable bowel syndrome[§]	Use peppermint oil in small dosages only May interfere with liver's cytochrome P-450 system
St. John's wort	Depressive disorder (mild to moderate)[†] Anxiety[§]	Generally well tolerated for up to 1-3 mo Interacts with many herbs, supplements, medications Advise patients to consult a health care practitioner before using with any herb or medication
Saw palmetto	Benign prostatic hyperplasia (BPH)[†]	Generally well tolerated for up to 3-5 yr May increase risk of bleeding May increase BP
Turmeric	Dyspepsia[§] Osteoarthritis[§]	May cause upset stomach when used in high doses or if taken for a long period of time May increase risk of bleeding
Valerian	Insomnia[†] Anxiety disorder[§]	Generally safe in recommended dosages for up to 4-6 wk Chronic use may result in insomnia

CHARACTERISTICS OF COMMON DYSRHYTHMIAS

Pattern	Rate and Rhythm	P Wave	PR Interval	QRS Complex
NSR	60-100 beats/min and regular	Normal	Normal	Normal
Sinus bradycardia	<60 beats/min and regular	Normal	Normal	Normal
Sinus tachycardia	>100 beats/min and regular	Normal	Normal	Normal
PAC	Usually 60-100 beats/min and irregular	Abnormal shape	Normal	Normal (usually)
PSVT	100-300 beats/min and regular	Abnormal shape, may be hidden	Normal or shortened	Normal (usually)
Atrial flutter	*Atrial:* 250-350 beats/min and regular *Ventricular:* >100 or <100 beats/min and may be regular or irregular	Flutter waves (sawtooth pattern); more flutter waves than QRS complexes;	Not measurable	Normal (usually)
Atrial fibrillation	*Atrial:* 350-600 beats/min and irregular *Ventricular:* >100 or <100 beats/min and irregular	Fibrillatory waves	Not measurable	Normal (usually)
Junctional rhythms	40-140 beats/min and regular	Inverted, may be hidden in QRS	Variable	Normal (usually)

NSR, Normal sinus rhythm; *PAC,* premature atrial contraction; *PSVT,* paroxysmal supraventricular tachycardia; *PVC,* premature ventricular contraction.

Continued

CHARACTERISTICS OF COMMON DYSRHYTHMIAS—cont'd

Pattern	Rate and Rhythm	P Wave	PR Interval	QRS Complex
First-degree heart block	Normal and regular	Normal	>0.20 sec	Normal
Second-degree heart block				
Type I (Mobitz I, Wenckebach)	Atrial: normal and regular Ventricular: slower and irregular	Normal	Progressive lengthening	Normal QRS width, with pattern of one nonconducted (blocked) QRS
Type II (Mobitz II)	Atrial: usually normal and regular Ventricular: slower and regular or irregular	More P waves than QRS complexes (e.g., 2:1, 3:1)	Normal or prolonged	Widened QRS, preceded by two or more P waves, with nonconducted (blocked) QRS
Third-degree heart block	Atrial: regular but may appear irregular because of P waves hidden in QRS complexes Ventricular: 20-40 beats/min and regular	Normal, but no connection with QRS complex	Variable	Normal or widened, no relationship with P waves
PVC	Underlying rhythm can be any rate; regular or irregular rhythm; PVCs occur at variable rates	Not usually present; hidden in the PVC	Not measurable	Wide and distorted
Ventricular tachycardia	100-250 beats/min and regular or irregular	Not usually visible	Not measurable	Wide and distorted
Ventricular fibrillation	Not measurable and irregular	Absent	Not measurable	Not measurable

ELECTROCARDIOGRAM (ECG) MONITORING: WAVEFORM AND NORMAL SINUS RHYTHM

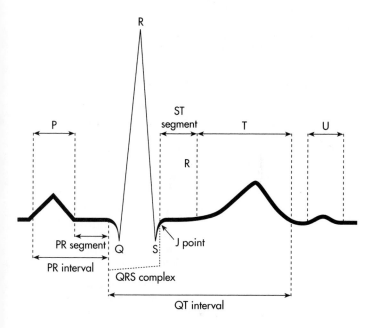

ELECTROCARDIOGRAM (ECG) MONITORING

Wave or Interval	Duration (sec)	Description
P wave	0.06-0.12	Represents time for passage of electrical impulse through the atrium causing atrial depolarization; should be upright
PR interval	0.12-0.20	Represents time required for impulse to travel through the atria, AV node and bundle of His, bundle branches, and Purkinje fibers to a point immediately preceding ventricular contraction
QRS interval	0.04-0.12	Represents depolarization of both ventricles and is measured from beginning of Q wave to end of S wave
ST segment	0.12	Represents the time between ventricular depolarization and repolarization; measured from the S wave of the QRS to the beginning of the T wave; should be flat (isoelectric)
T wave	0.16	Represents the time for ventricular repolarization; should be upright
QT interval	0.34-0.43	Represents total time required for ventricular depolarization and repolarization; measured from beginning of QRS complex to end of T wave

AV, Atrioventricular.

GLASGOW COMA SCALE

Category of Response	Appropriate Stimulus	Response	Score
Eyes open	Approach to bedside Verbal command Pain	Spontaneous response	4
		Opening of eyes to name or command	3
		Lack of opening of eyes to previous stimuli but opening to pain	2
		Lack of opening of eyes to any stimulus	1
		Untestable	U
Best verbal response	Verbal questioning with maximum arousal	Appropriate orientation, conversant, correct identification of self, place, year, and month	5
		Confusion; conversant but disorientation in one or more spheres	4
		Inappropriate or disorganized use of words (e.g., cursing), lack of sustained conversation	3
		Incomprehensible words, sounds (e.g., moaning)	2
		Lack of sound, even with painful stimuli	1
		Untestable	U
Best motor response	Verbal command (e.g., "raise your arm, hold up two fingers") Pain (pressure on proximal nail bed)	Obedience of command	6
		Localization of pain, lack of obedience but presence of attempts to remove offending stimulus	5
		Flexion withdrawal,* flexion of arm in response to pain without abnormal flexion posture	4
		Abnormal flexion, flexing of arm at elbow and pronation, making a fist	3
		Abnormal extension, extension of arm at elbow usually with adduction and internal rotation of arm at shoulder	2
		Lack of response	1
		Untestable	U

* Added to the original scale by many centers.

HEART SOUNDS
Auscultatory Sites

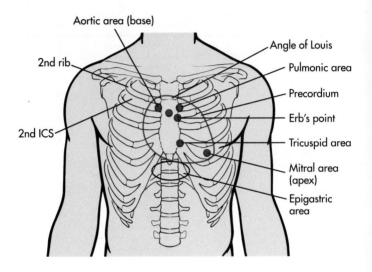

Aortic area (base)

2nd rib

2nd ICS

Angle of Louis

Pulmonic area

Precordium

Erb's point

Tricuspid area

Mitral area (apex)

Epigastric area

CHARACTERISTICS OF HEART SOUNDS

Sound	Auscultation Site	Pitch	Clinical Occurrence
S_1 (M_1 T_1)	Apex	High "lub"	Closing of mitral and tricuspid valves; signals the beginning of systole
S_2 (A_2 P_2)	A_2 at second ICS, RSB; P_2 at second ICS, LSB	High "dub"	Closing of aortic and pulmonic valves; signals the beginning of diastole
S_2 physiologic split	Second ICS, LSB (pulmonic area)	High "dub" sound is split into two sounds	Can be normal and is a split sound that corresponds with the respiratory cycle caused by a normal delay of pulmonic valve during inspiration; can be abnormal if heard during expiration or if it is constant during the respiratory cycle; accentuated during exercise or in individuals with thin chest walls; heard most often in children and young adults
S_3 (ventricular gallop)	Apex	Dull low	Low-intensity vibration of the ventricular wall usually associated with decreased compliance of the ventricles during filling; heard closely after S_2; common in children and young adults and during last trimester of pregnancy
S_4 (atrial gallop)	Apex	Low	Low-frequency vibration caused by atrial filling and contraction against increased resistance in ventricle; precedes S_1 of next cycle; may be normal in infants, children, and athletes; pathologic in patients with heart disease

ICS, Intercostal space; LSB, left sternal border; RSB, right sternal border.

MEDICATION ADMINISTRATION
Equivalent Weights and Measures

Metric	Apothecary	Household
Weight		
1 kg	2.2 pounds	
1000 mg = 1 g	gr xv	
60 or 65 mg	gr i	
30 mg	gr ss (one half)	
0.4 mg	1/150 gr	
1 mcg = 0.0001 mg		
Volume		
1000 ml = 1 L	Approx. 1 quart	Approx. 1 quart
1 L distilled water weighs	1 kg	
500 ml	Approx. 1 pint	16 ounces
240 or 250 ml	℥ viii (8 ounces)	1 cup
30 ml	℥ i (1 fluid ounce)	2 tbs
15 ml	℥ iv (4 fluid drams)	1 tbs
4 to 5 ml	℥ i (1 fluid dram)	1 tsp
1 ml	Minims xv or xvi	

Drug Calculations

Ratio and proportion:
1. To set up a ratio and proportion, put on the right-hand side what you already have or what you already know (e.g., 1000 mg: 1 ml).
2. On the left-hand side put X, or what you want to know (e.g., 750 mg: X).
3. The equation should look like this: 750 mg: X = 1000 mg: 1 ml
4. Multiply the two inside numbers. Multiply the two outside numbers.

$$1000X = 750$$

5. Solve for X:

$$X = \frac{750}{1000} = 0.75 \text{ ml}$$

IV Drip Rate

$$\frac{\text{Total number of milliliters to be infused}}{\text{Total number of minutes infusion is to run}} \times \text{Drop factor} = \frac{\text{Rate}}{(\text{Drops per minute})}$$

Techniques of Administration
Angles of Injection

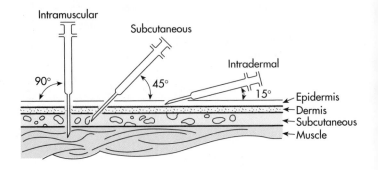

Injection Sites
Subcutaneous

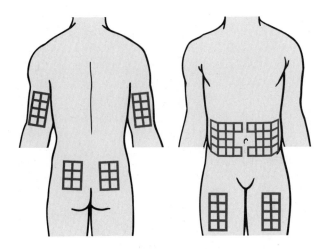

Intramuscular: Deltoid Muscle

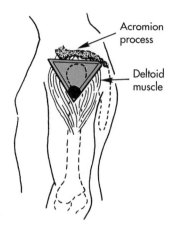

Intramuscular: Dorsogluteal Muscle

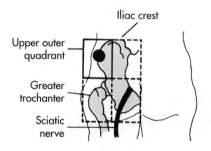

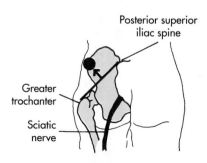

Intramuscular: Vastus Lateralis Muscle

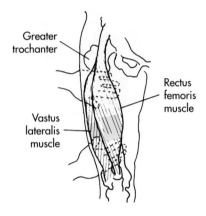

Intramuscular: Ventrogluteal Muscle

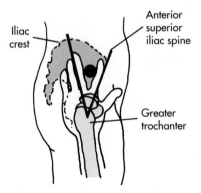

Z-Track Technique

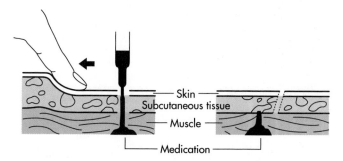

A, In Z-track injection, skin is pulled laterally, then injection is administered. **B,** After needle is withdrawn, skin is released. This technique helps prevent medication from leaking.

Intermittent IV Drug Administration
Peripheral Vein Intermittent Infusion Device
1. Irrigate device with 1 ml of normal saline.
2. Administer prescribed medication.
3. Irrigate device with 1 ml of normal saline after medication administration is completed.
4. If policy, perform a final irrigation with 1 ml of heparin solution (100 units of heparin per milliliter).

Central Vein Intermittent Infusion Device
1. Irrigate device with 2 to 5 ml of normal saline (volume depends on type of infusion catheter and agency policy).
2. Administer prescribed medication.
3. Irrigate device with 2 to 5 ml of normal saline when medication administration is completed.
4. Irrigate device with 2 to 5 ml of heparin solution (100 units of heparin per milliliter).

INTRAVENOUS (IV) SITE COMPLICATIONS

	Infiltration	Phlebitis
Assessment		
Color	Pale	Red
Temperature	Cool to cold	Warm to hot
Swelling	Rounded	Cordlike vein path
Pain	Yes, usually	Yes
Flow	Slowed or stopped	No change or may be slowed
Nursing Actions	Tourniquet proximally (flow continues— infiltration)	Discontinue IV; usually call IV team
	Lower bag (blood in tubing—no infiltration)	Note irritating solution (diazepam [Valium], cephalothin sodium [Keflin], potassium chloride [KCl] running too fast)
	Discontinue IV Call IV team Get order for warm compresses and elevate part	Warm compresses; elevate and immobilize part

PREVENTIVE SERVICES FOR HEALTHY ADULTS
Testing and Immunizations for Asymptomatic Adults*

Service	Who Needs	How Often	Comments
Blood pressure measurement (to detect hypertension)	All adults	Once every 2 yr for those with normal blood pressure	More frequent monitoring for those with readings above 120/80
Cholesterol measurement	All adults	Once every 5 yr; more often if total or LDL ("bad") cholesterol is high, if HDL ("good") is low, and/or if risk factors present	Those at high risk for heart disease need medical advice about lifestyle changes and possibly drug therapy
Diabetes screening (fasting blood glucose test)	Everyone 45 yr and older; earlier for those at high risk	Every 3 yr	African Americans, Hispanics, Asians, Native Americans, obese people, and those with a strong family history need more frequent screening, starting at age 30 yr
Thyroid disease screening	Women 50 yr and older; those with high cholesterol or family history of thyroid disease	On professional advice	Routine screening remains controversial; risk factors should be discussed with health care provider

* Screening tests specific to cancer are found earlier in this appendix in "Cancer Screening Guidelines for Early Detection of Cancer in Asymptomatic People."

Continued

PREVENTIVE SERVICES FOR HEALTHY ADULTS
Testing and Immunizations for Asymptomatic Adults—cont'd

Service	Who Needs	How Often	Comments
Chlamydia screening	Women 25 yr and younger, if sexually active	Annually or more often	Men and women of any age who are at risk for chlamydia, gonorrhea, syphilis, and HIV should be tested
Glaucoma screening	People between 40 and 64 yr of age	Every 2-4 yr	Many eye specialists advise screening all adults every 3-5 yr starting at age 39 yr
	Age 65 yr or older African Americans and those with a family history of glaucoma	More frequently than usual because of increased risk	
		Every 1-2 yr	
Dental checkup	All adults	Every 6 mo or on professional advice	Should include cleaning and examination for oral cancer
Immunizations Tetanus/diphtheria booster	All adults	Every 10 yr; booster recommended with injury if last dose more than 5 yr ago	People older than 50 yr least likely to be adequately immunized

Vaccine	Who should have it	How often	Comments
Influenza vaccine	Everyone 50 yr and older, people with lung or heart disease or cancer, and others at high risk	Annually, in autumn	Even healthy younger adults and health care professionals of all ages can benefit and should consider getting the shot
Pneumococcal vaccine	Those 65 yr and older, and others at high risk for respiratory complications	At least once; a second dose is recommended if more than 5 yr since prior dose and person was younger than 65 yr when initially vaccinated	Effective against most strains of pneumococcal pneumonia; lasts at least 5-10 yr
Measles, mumps, rubella (MMR) vaccine	All adults; especially women of childbearing age	Once	Avoid during pregnancy
Hepatitis B vaccine	All young adults, as well as adults at high risk	On professional advice	All newborns should be vaccinated
Chickenpox vaccine	Anyone who has never had chickenpox	Once; but older than 13 yr; it requires two shots	Not recommended for pregnant women or those with compromised immunity

TEMPERATURE CONVERSION FACTORS

°C	°F	°C	°F	°C	°F
34.0	93.2	37.2	99.0	40.2	104.4
34.2	93.6	37.4	99.3	40.4	104.7
34.4	93.9	37.6	99.7	40.6	105.2
34.6	94.3	37.8	100.0	40.8	105.4
34.8	94.6	38.0	100.4	41.0	105.9
35.0	95.0	38.2	100.8	41.2	106.1
35.2	95.4	38.4	101.1	41.4	106.5
35.4	95.7	38.6	101.5	41.6	106.8
35.6	96.1	38.8	101.8	41.8	107.2
35.8	96.4	39.0	102.2	42.0	107.6
36.0	96.8	39.2	102.6	42.2	108.0
36.2	97.2	39.4	102.9	42.4	108.3
36.4	97.5	39.6	103.3	42.6	108.7
36.6	97.9	39.8	103.6	42.8	109.0
36.8	98.2	40.0	104.0	43.0	109.4
37.0	98.6				

°C = Temperature in Celsius (centigrade) degrees. $(°C \times 9/5) + 32 = °F$.
°F = Temperature in Fahrenheit degrees. $(°F - 32) \times 5/9 = °C$.

TNM CLASSIFICATION SYSTEM

Primary Tumor (T)
T_0 No evidence of primary tumor
T_{is} Carcinoma in situ
T_{1-4} Ascending degrees of increase in tumor size and
            involvement
T_x Tumor cannot be measured or found

Regional Lymph Nodes (N)
N_0 No evidence of disease in lymph nodes
N_{1-4} Ascending degrees of nodal involvement
N_x Regional lymph nodes unable to be assessed clinically

Distant Metastases (M)
M_0 No evidence of distant metastases
M_{1-4} Ascending degrees of metastatic involvement of the host,
            including distant nodes
M_x Cannot be determined

ENGLISH/SPANISH COMMON MEDICAL TERMS

Hints for Pronunciation of Spanish Words
1. *h* is silent.
2. *j* is pronounced as *h*.
3. *ll* is pronounced as a *y* sound.
4. *r* is pronounced with a trilled sound, and *rr* is trilled even more.
5. *v* is pronounced with a *b* sound.
6. A *y* by itself is pronounced with a long *e* sound.
7. Accent marks over the vowel indicate the syllable that is to be stressed.

Introductory

I am _____.	Soy _____.
What is your name?	¿Cómo se llama usted?
I would like to examine you now.	Quisiera examinarlo(a) ahora.

General

How do you feel?	¿Cómo se siente?
Good	Bien
Bad	Mal
Do you feel better today?	¿Se siente mejor hoy?
Where do you work?	¿Dónde trabaja? (Cuál es su profesión o trabajo?) (¿Qué hace usted?)
Are you allergic to anything?	¿Es usted alérgico(a) a algo?
Medications, foods, insect bites?	¿Medicinas, alimentos, picaduras de insectos?
Do you take any medications?	¿Toma usted algunas medicinas?
Do you have any drug allergies?	¿Es usted alérgico(a) a algún médicamento?
Do you have a history of	¿Ha sufrido antes:
Heart disease?	del corazón?
Diabetes?	de diabetes?
Epilepsy?	de epilepsia?
Bronchitis?	de bronquitis?
Emphysema?	de enfisema?
Asthma?	de asma?

Pain

Have you any pain?	¿Tiene dolor?
Where is the pain?	¿Dónde le duele?
Do you have any pain here?	¿Le duele aquí?
How severe is the pain?	¿Qué tan fuerte es el dolor?
Mild, moderate, sharp, or severe?	¿Ligero, moderado, agudo, severo?

Continued

ENGLISH/SPANISH COMMON MEDICAL TERMS—cont'd

Pain—cont'd

What were you doing when the pain started?	¿Qué estaba haciendo cuando le comenzó el dolor?
Have you ever had this pain before?	¿Ha tenido este dolor antes?
Do you have a pain in your side?	¿Tiene usted dolor en el costado?
Is it worse now?	¿Es peor ahora?
Does it still pain you?	¿Le duele todavía?
Did you feel much pain at the time?	¿Sintió mucho dolor entonces?
Show me where.	Muéstreme dónde.
Does it hurt when I press here?	¿Le duele cuando aprieto aquí?

Head

Head	La cabeza
Face	La cara

Eyes

Eye	El ojo

Ears/Nose/Throat

Ears	Los oídos
Eardrum	El tímpano
Laryngitis	La laringitis
Lip	El labio
Mouth	La boca
Nose	La naríz
Tongue	La lengua

Cardiovascular

Heart	El corazón
Heart attack	El ataque del corazón
Heart disease	La enfermedad del corazón
Heart murmur	El soplo del corazón
High blood pressure	Presión alta

Respiratory

Chest	El pecho
Lungs	Los pulmones

ENGLISH/SPANISH COMMON MEDICAL TERMS—cont'd

Gastrointestinal

Abdomen	El abdomen
Intestines/bowels	Los intestinos
Liver	El hígado
Nausea	Náusea
Gastric ulcer	La úlcera gástrica
Stomach	El estómago, la panza, la barriga
Stomachache	El dolor de estómago

Genitourinary

Genitals	Los genitales
Kidney	El riñón
Penis	El pene, el miembro
Urine	La orina

Musculoskeletal

Ankle	El tobillo
Arm	El brazo
Back	La espalda
Bones	Los huesos
Elbow	El codo
Finger	El dedo
Foot	El pie
Fracture	La fractura
Hand	La mano
Hip	La cadera
Knee	La rodilla
Leg	La pierna
Muscles	Los músculos
Rib	La costilla
Shoulder	El hombro
Thigh	El muslo

Neurologic

Brain	El cerebro
Dizziness	El vértigo, el mareo
Epilepsy	La epilepsia
Fainting spell	El desmayo
Unconsciousness (inconsciente, sin sentido)	Pérdida del conocimiento

Endocrine/Reproductive

Uterus	El útero, la matríz
Vagina	La vagina

URINE LABORATORY VALUES

Test	Normal	Abnormal Finding and Significance
Color	Amber yellow	Dark, smoky color suggests hematuria. Yellow-brown to olive green indicates excessive bilirubin. Orange-red or orange-brown is caused by phenazopyridine (Pyridium) or urobilin in excess. Cloudiness of freshly voided urine indicates infection. Colorless urine indicates excessive fluid intake, renal disease, or diabetes insipidus.
Smell	Aromatic	On standing, urine becomes more ammonia-like in smell. In urinary tract infections, urine smells unpleasant.
Protein	0-150 mg/24 hr 0-8 mg/dl	Persistent proteinuria is characteristic of acute and chronic renal disease, especially involving glomeruli: In absence of disease, positive finding may be caused by high-protein diet, strenuous exercise, dehydration, fever, or emotional stress. Vaginal secretions may contaminate urine specimen and give positive finding.
Glucose	None	Glycosuria indicates diabetes mellitus or low renal threshold for glucose reabsorption (if blood glucose level is normal). Small amounts may be found after glucose loading (e.g., glucose tolerance test).
Ketones	None	Altered carbohydrate and fat metabolisms indicate diabetes mellitus and starvation. Findings can also be seen in dehydration, vomiting, and severe diarrhea.
Bilirubin	None	Presence of bilirubinuria is as significant as jaundice in detection of liver disorders. Bilirubin may appear in urine before jaundice becomes visible or may be present in persons with hepatic disorders who do not have recognizable jaundice.

Specific gravity	1.003-1.030	Specific gravity of morning urine specimen reflects maximum concentrating ability of kidney and is 1.025 to 1.030. Low specific gravity indicates dilute urine and possibly excessive diuresis. High specific gravity indicates dehydration. If it becomes fixed at about 1.010, this indicates renal inability to concentrate urine, suggesting that kidney is progressing to end-stage renal disease.
Osmolality	300-1300 mOsm/kg	Measurement is a more accurate method than specific gravity for determining diluting and concentrating ability of kidneys. Deviations from normal indicate tubular dysfunction. Findings indicate if kidney has lost ability to concentrate or dilute urine. (Not part of routine urinalysis.)
pH	4.0-8.0 (average 6.0)	If more than 8.0, finding may be the result of standing of urine or urinary tract infections because bacteria decompose urea to form ammonia. If less than 4.0, may indicate respiratory and metabolic acidosis.
RBCs	0-4/hpf	Bleeding in urinary tract is caused by calculi, cystitis, neoplasm, glomerulonephritis, tuberculosis, kidney biopsy, or trauma.
WBCs	0-5/hpf	Increased number of WBCs in urine (pyuria) indicates urinary tract infection or inflammation.
Casts	None—occasional hyaline	Casts are molds of the renal tubules and may contain protein, WBCs, RBCs, or bacteria. Noncellular casts are hyaline in appearance, and a few may be found in normal urine. Casts indicate renal dysfunction or urinary tract infections.
Culture for organisms	No organisms in bladder, <10⁴ organisms/ml result of normal urethral flora	Bacteria counts >10⁵/ml indicate urinary tract infection. Organisms most commonly found in urinary tract infections are Escherichia coli, enterococci, Klebsiella, Proteus, and streptococci.

hpf, High-powered field; *RBCs,* red blood cells; *WBCs,* white blood cells.

INDEX

A